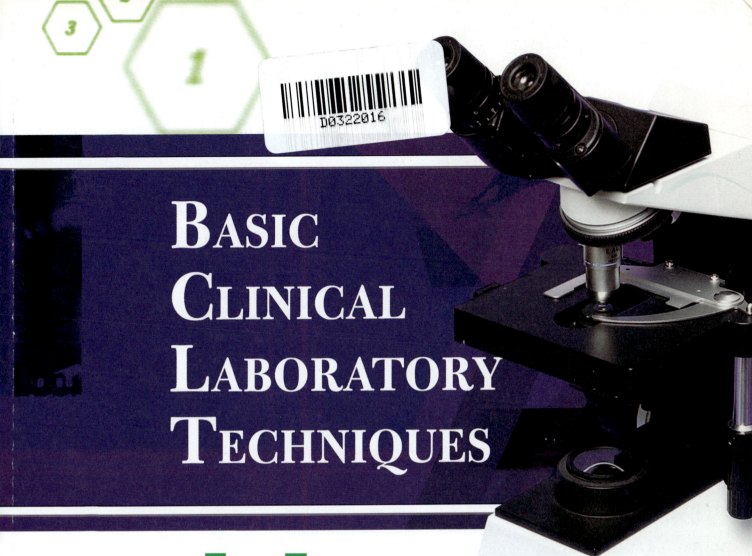

BASIC CLINICAL LABORATORY TECHNIQUES

5TH EDITION

Barbara H. Estridge, BS, MT (ASCP), CLS (NCA)
Anna P. Reynolds, MS, BS, MT (ASCP)

THOMSON

DELMAR LEARNING   Australia   Canada   Mexico   Singapore   Spain   United Kingdom   United States

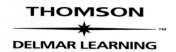

THOMSON

™

DELMAR LEARNING

Basic Clinical Laboratory Techniques, 5th Edition
Barbara H. Estridge, BS, MT (ASCP), CLS (NCA), and Anna P. Reynolds, MS, BS, MT (ASCP)

Vice President, Health Career Business Unit:
William Brottmiller

Director of Learning Solutions:
Matthew Kane

Senior Acquisitions Editor:
Sherry Dickinson

Product Manager:
Natalie Pashoukos

Editorial Assistant:
Angela Doolin

Marketing Director:
Jennifer McAvey

Marketing Manager:
Lynn Henn

Marketing Coordinator:
Andrea Eobstel

Technology Director:
Laurie Davis

Production Director:
Carolyn Miller

Senior Art Director:
Jack Pendleton

Content Project Manager:
Stacey Lamodi

Technology Project Manager:
Carolyn Fox

Library of Congress Cataloging-in-Publication Data
Estridge, Barbara H.
    Basic clinical laboratory techniques / Barbara H. Estridge, Anna P. Reynolds. —
5th ed.
        p. ; cm.
    Rev. ed. of: Basic medical laboratory techniques / Barbara H. Estridge, Anna P. Reynolds, Norma J. Walters. c2000.
Includes bibliographical references and index.
    ISBN 978-1-4180-1279-3
    1. Diagnosis, Laboratory. 2. Medical laboratory technology. I. Reynolds, Anna P. II. Estridge, Barbara H. Basic medical laboratory techniques. III. Title.
    [DNLM: 1. Laboratory Techniques and Procedures. 2. Clinical Laboratory Techniques. QY 25 E825b 2008]
    RB37.W25 2008
616.07'5—dc22   2007016761

NOTICE TO THE READER

Publisher does not warrant or guarantee any of the products described herein or perform any independent analysis in connection with any of the product information contained herein. Publisher does not assume, and expressly disclaims, any obligation to obtain and include information other than that provided to it by the manufacturer.

The reader is expressly warned to consider and adopt all safety precautions that might be indicated by the activities described herein and to avoid all potential hazards. By following the instructions contained herein, the reader willingly assumes all risks in connection with such instructions.

The Publisher makes no representations or warranties of any kind, including but not limited to, the warranties of fitness for particular purpose or merchantability, nor are any such representations implied with respect to the material set forth herein, and the publisher takes no responsibility with respect to such material. The Publisher shall not be liable for any special, consequential, or exemplary damages resulting, in whole or part, from the readers' use of, or reliance upon, this material.

Contents

UNIT 1

Introduction to the Clinical Laboratory   1

UNIT 2

Basic Hematology   159

Unit 3

Basic Hemostasis   309

Unit 4

Basic Immunology and Immunohematology   361

Unit 5

Urinalysis   435

Unit 6

Basic Clinical Chemistry   509

Unit 7

Basic Clinical Microbiology   583

Unit 8

Basic Parasitology   701

Glossary   755

Appendices   767

Index   779

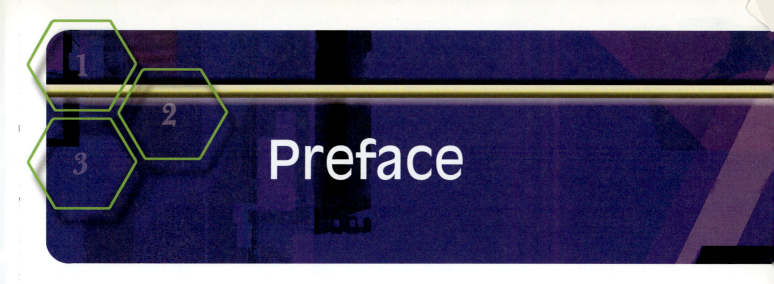

Preface

*Basic Clinical Laboratory Technique*s, 5th edition, is a revision of *Basic Medical Laboratory Techniques,* 4th edition. Over 20 years have passed since the first publication of this text and these years have brought many advances in the field of laboratory medicine. The title of this edition was changed to reflect the evolution of medical technology into the discipline called clinical laboratory science. This text has been revised extensively over the years, but the purpose of the text has remained the same—to provide the foundation of theory, skills, and techniques required for understanding and performing routine laboratory tests. Although this text includes only the most basic procedures, the principles, skills, and techniques presented are core to even the most sophisticated technologies used in the clinical laboratory.

Basic Clinical Laboratory Techniques, 5th edition, is a performance-based text for use in allied health programs at the post-secondary and vocational school levels. It is appropriate for medical laboratory technician and medical assistant programs, as well as for introductory survey courses in medical technology/clinical laboratory science. This text is also useful as a guide for non-laboratory personnel who work at point-of-care (POC) or in physician office laboratories and perform CLIA-waived tests.

TEXT ORGANIZATION

The text provides fundamentals of techniques used throughout the discipline of clinical laboratory science as well as an introduction to current technologies and instrumentation. The text is organized into eight units, encompassing the major departments in the clinical laboratory:

- Introduction to the Clinical Laboratory
- Basic Hematology
- Basic Hemostasis
- Basic Immunology and Immunohematology
- Urinalysis
- Basic Clinical Chemistry
- Basic Clinical Microbiology
- Basic Parasitology

Each unit is a stand-alone unit. Unit 1 should be studied first because it contains basic information used in all other units. Unit 1 includes information about the function of the clinical laboratory; chemical, physical, and biological safety precautions that must be used when working in the laboratory; and other general knowledge that applies to all laboratory departments, including quality assessment policies and procedures, medical terminology, use of the metric system, use of the clinical microscope and general laboratory equipment, and blood collection techniques.

After Unit 1, the remaining units can be studied in any order. Those who choose not to use one or more entire units, might find it useful to have the student study the first lesson of each unit. This would give the student an introduction to that area of clinical laboratory practice, without requiring that they perfect laboratory techniques and skills in that area.

Unit Organization

Instructors who have used previous editions of this text will find that the essential elements present in earlier editions are still here. However, the text has a new look, and lessons have been revised and enhanced with added features. Each unit begins with unit objectives, a brief overview of unit contents, and a list of readings, references, and resources. Each unit is divided into several lessons. Lessons are used rather than chapters, to provide flexibility, while keeping each topic or procedure well-defined within the book.

The first lesson in each unit is an introductory lesson providing general information and principles about the unit topic. Each subsequent lesson covers a particular laboratory procedure, test, or topic within the unit area. With a few exceptions, after the introductory lesson in a unit is studied, the remaining lessons in the unit can be studied in the order of instructor's preference. In general, each lesson contains:

- List of learning objectives to guide the student
- Glossary of new terms with definitions—each term is highlighted when it first occurs in a lesson
- Introductory material, including principle and rationale of the procedure or test

- Safety information and reminders
- Quality assessment information
- Basic theoretical and technical information
- Current topics for extra study
- Case study or critical thinking questions
- Summary
- Review questions
- Suggested student activities, including Web-based activities
- Student Performance Guides: step-by-step guides to performing specific procedures, including worksheets, when appropriate

NEW FEATURES IN THE FIFTH EDITION

The use of full-color throughout this edition gives a new look to the text, enhancing the text and aiding in visual organization and content emphasis. Graphic icons are used to bring attention to safety, critical timing, use of math skills, and other issues in the text and the Student Performance Guides. These icons serve to inform and remind the instructor and student of issues that require special attention in order to avoid injury and to ensure quality results. These icons are:

 Biological hazard—use Standard Precautions

 Chemical hazard—follow chemical safety rules

 Physical hazard—follow safety procedures to protect from hazards such as fire, electrical shock, or cuts from broken glass

 Critical timing—reminder that the procedure requires careful attention to timing

 Quality Assessment—quality assessment policies and techniques must be followed

 Web-based activity

Other new features include:

- Information on current topics
- Case studies or critical thinking questions
- Web activities to augment text information and laboratory practice

It is hoped that these additions to the lessons will pique students' interest and expand their thinking beyond the technical material in the lesson.

CHANGES TO THIS EDITION

In addition to the new look of the text, organizational and content changes have been made. Many new color photographs appear throughout this edition, often replacing line drawings used in the previous edition. All lessons have been updated to reflect current technology and accepted practice at the time of writing. Safety procedures continue to be strongly emphasized, and safety devices and technologies developed to enhance safety are discussed, such as use of plasticware rather than glass tubes and containers, devices designed to prevent needlesticks, and instruments that sample through-the-cap to minimize exposure of personnel to biological specimens. New technologies and instrumentation are discussed, such as immunochromatographic assays and flow cytometry. In particular, look for the following changes:

Unit 1—With the addition of three lessons to Unit 1, the unit can easily be used as a stand-alone introduction to the clinical laboratory. The two lessons on blood collection—Capillary Puncture and Venipuncture—have been moved to Unit 1, since these skills are required for procedures in several other units. By providing this information in the introductory unit, the remaining units can be studied according to the instructor's preference and time constraints. Also moved to Unit 1 is the lesson on reagent preparation and laboratory math, since these principles are also used in all areas of the laboratory.

Unit 2—The hemacytometer has been placed into a lesson by itself to allow the student to understand the dimensions and equations before performing the white blood cell and red blood cell counts. Blood collection techniques have been moved to Unit 1. Information on blood cell morphology is placed into a separate lesson (Lesson 2-8) from the white blood cell differential count (Lesson 2-9), to allow the student more time to concentrate on learning morphology before they perform the differential count. Lesson 2-10, Abnormalities in Peripheral Blood Cell Morphology, is a stand-alone lesson that can be omitted or used, according to the instructor's preference. Students who are interested in hematology might want to explore this introductory information on white blood cell and red blood cell abnormalities on their own.

Unit 4—Unit 4 has a new name, Basic Immunology and Immunohematology. Lesson 4-1, Introduction to Immunology, has been expanded to include the principles of several types of immunological tests. The methodologies incorporated into the latest generation of enzyme immunoassays, called lateral flow assays, immunochromatographic assays, or membrane immunoassays, are explained in Lessons 4-1 and 4-5 (as well as in Lessons 5-6 and 5-7). Test kits using variations of these types of immunoassays are used in all laboratory departments, not just immunology. Lesson 4-2 is new and introduces the reader to the organization and operation of immunohematology, or the blood bank department. The discussions on blood typing include explanation and photographs of gel typing.

Unit 6—Tests for determination of glycated hemoglobin (HbA1c) and triglycerides have been added to the Blood Glucose and Blood Cholesterol lessons, Lessons 6-5 and 6-6, respectively. The lesson on laboratory reagent preparation and laboratory math has been moved to Unit 1.

Unit 7—Unit 7 contains several changes from the previous edition. The lesson that previously included urine culture, colony count, and antibiotic susceptibility has been split into two lessons. Lesson 7-8 includes a discussion of and gives procedures for performing urine culture and colony count. Lesson 7-9, Bacterial Identification and Antibiotic Susceptibility Testing, has been expanded to include more information about identification of bacteria, antibiotic resistance, and susceptibility testing. Two new lessons pertinent to emerging diseases and bioterrorism readiness have been added to this edition. Lesson 7-3, Public Health Threats: I. Emerging Infectious Diseases, includes discussions of agents such as West Nile Virus, SARS, avian influenza virus, Ebola virus, and others. Lesson 7-4, Public Health Threats: II. Biological Agents and Bioterrorism, surveys the types of agents with potential for use as weapons or bioterrorism agents, such as smallpox virus and the anthrax bacterium, and the nation's laboratory readiness program for dealing with these. These lessons are important since certain laboratories will be first responders in the event of an act of bioterrorism.

INSTRUCTOR'S RESOURCES AND SUPPLEMENTS

An Electronic Classroom Manager (ECM) is available for the fifth edition of *Basic Clinical Laboratory Techniques*. It includes:

- Instructor's Manual
- Computerized Test Bank
- PowerPoint Slides
- Student Performance Guides
- Worksheets
- Report Forms

The *Instructor's Manual* contains an objectives list, an overview for each unit, and lesson plans for each lesson. The lesson plans include lesson objectives, glossary terms with definitions, teaching aids and resources, a lesson content outline, student learning activities, case study answers, and lesson review questions and answers. Also included in the *Instructor's Manual* is a resource list of health-care related agencies, societies, and organizations.

The test bank contains over 1,700 questions (and answers) in multiple choice, matching, fill-in-the-blank (completion), and true/false formats. The test bank is in ExamView Pro software, which allows the instructor to mix and match questions to customize a printable test form, as well as to modify questions or add their own questions to the test bank.

A CD containing approximately 350 PowerPoint slides is available, to assist with classroom presentations.

Electronic versions of the Student Performance Guides, Worksheets, and Report Forms from the text are also included on the ECM.

ABOUT THE AUTHORS

Barbara H. Estridge and **Anna P. Reynolds** have over 50 years' combined experience in teaching clinical laboratory courses, biological and biomedical research, and clinical laboratory management. Teaching experience includes instruction in both hospital and university Medical Technology, Medical Laboratory Technician, and Medical Laboratory Assistant Programs, as well university-level basic biological sciences. This includes teaching in the fields of hematology, clinical chemistry, urinalysis, microbiology, mycology, parasitology, immunology, and immunohematology.

ACKNOWLEDGMENTS

We are indebted to the many editors, colleagues, friends, and family members who have provided technical advice, encouragement, and support throughout this project. Since the first edition of this book came to life approximately 25 years ago, this list has continued to grow.

In particular, we would like to thank the following Thomson Delmar Learning editorial and production staff for their guidance and assistance with this edition: Natalie Pashoukos, product manager, Sherry Dickinson, senior acquisitions editor, Marah Bellegarde, managing editor, Angela Doolin, editorial assistant, Jack Pendleton, senior art director, Stacey Lamodi, content project manager, and Darcy Scelsi, product manager.

We also wish to thank those individuals who reviewed the manuscript and offered valuable feedback and suggestions:

Linda A. Dezern, MS, MT (ASCP)
Thomas Nelson Community College
Hampton, VA

Janelle M. Chiasera, Ph.D, MT (ASCP)
The Ohio State University
Columbus, OH

Karen Golemboski, Ph.D, MT (ASCP)
Bellarmine University
Louisville, KY

Donna Larson, Ed.D, MT (ASCP) DLM
Apollo College
Portland, OR

Andrea Rowland, MBA, MT (ASCP)
Southwestern Community College
Sylva, NC

Patricia A. Chappell, MA, MT (ASCP)
Camden County College
Blackwood, NJ

Ernest Dale Hall, MA Ed, MT (ASCP)
Southwestern Community College
Sylva, NC

Phyllis Otto
Ivy Tech State College
Muncie, IN

We would especially like to thank Bob Miglin, Peggy Carroll, Shellie Hassfurter, and the gracious, patient, clinical laboratory staff of Ellis Hospital, Schenectady, New York, for allowing the team of editors, authors, and photographer to use their facilities for many of the photographs in this book. Additionally, we would like to thank the following companies and individuals for providing images, image processing, or access to enhance this edition:

Abbott Laboratories, Abbott Park, IL

Alpha Scientific, Malvern, PA

Bayer Healthcare Diagnostic Division, Norwood, MA

Beckman Coulter, Fullerton, CA

Becton Dickinson and Co., Franklin Lakes, NJ

Bio/Data Corporation, Horsham, PA

bioMérieux, Durham, NC

Biosite, Inc., San Diego, CA

BioTek Instruments, Inc., Winooski, VT

Brevis Corporation, Salt Lake City, UT

Bridgman, R., Hybridoma Facility, Auburn University, AL

Centers for Disease Control and Prevention, Atlanta, GA

Estridge, A., UCLA Medical School, Los Angeles, CA

HemoCue Inc., Lake Forest, CA

Holladay, Jacqueline, Auburn, AL

Hycor Biomedical Inc., Garden Grove, CA

ITC, Edison, NJ

Metrika Inc., Sunnyvale, CA

Mitchell Plastics, Inc., Norton, OH. www.mpicase.com

Nova Biomedical, Waltham, MA

Quidel Corporation, San Diego, CA

Remel, Inc., Lenexa, KS

Roche Diagnostics Corp., Indianapolis, IN

Scientific Device Lab, Des Plaines, IL

Smith's Medical ASD, Inc., Keene, NH

StatSpin, Inc., Norwood, NJ

Sundermann, C. A., Auburn University, AL

Sysmex America, Inc., Mundelein, IL

West, K. M., Medical and Laboratory Technology Program, Auburn University, AL

NOTE TO THE READER

Clinical laboratory science is a rapidly changing field. Instruments and test methods are constantly being improved, modified, updated, and even discontinued. We have performed extensive research to ensure that the information in this work is complete, accurate, and up-to-date. However, because of the possibility of human error and the time lapse between writing and publication, no guarantee can be given that the information contained herein is accurate in every respect by the time this text reaches publication. The authors, publishers, and all other parties involved in this work disclaim all responsibility for errors and/or omissions in this work. Students, instructors, and others who use this work are encouraged to consult other appropriate sources to confirm information. It is especially important to follow established safety guidelines, to always read and follow the operating manuals for the particular instrument being used, and to consult the instructions and package inserts that accompany the reagents and test kits being used. Questions, comments, or suggestions can be made to the authors by contacting the publisher.

Barbara H. Estridge, BS, MT (ASCP), CLS (NCA)
Anna P. Reynolds, MS, BS, MT (ASCP)

Dedication

To our instructors for their guidance, our students for inspiration, our families for their patience, and especially to our husbands, Ron and George, for the unconditional support they have provided through the years

How to Use This Book

OBJECTIVES

Each lesson begins with a list of objectives that highlight the salient points to be learned. Read the objectives before you begin studying the lesson. After completing the lesson, review the objectives to be sure you understand the lesson content.

GLOSSARY

The glossary contains terms that might be new to you and that are critical to understanding the lesson material. Look for the glossary words in bold font the first time they are used and defined in a lesson.

LESSON CONTENT

Introduction.
The introduction gives a brief overview of the lesson and leads into the principle and performance of a procedure.

Principle and Procedure.
Lessons covering a particular test procedure include a description of the procedure principle and a written explanation of how to perform the test. Reference ranges and clinical significance of the tests are also given.

Icons.
Icons are used throughout the text and in the performance guides to remind you of areas that require extra attention to safety, quality assessment, timing, math skills, or procedural details.

Safety Precautions.
Safety Precautions sections call attention to biological, chemical, or physical hazards that might be present when performing a procedure.

Quality Assessment.
Quality Assessment sections remind you of the importance of factors such as proper specimen collection and processing, correct technique, instrument maintenance, and use of controls to the achievement of reliable test results.

Case Studies and Critical Thinking Problems.
Case studies and critical thinking problems present problem-solving situations such as you might encounter in daily laboratory work. These give you a chance to apply your knowledge to a practical real-life situation.

Current Topics.
Current Topics offer interesting and informative material about current topics, such as methicillin-resistant *Staphylococcus* (MRSA) or stem cell research.

Reminders.
Procedural and safety reminders at the end of the lessons reinforce these issues before you begin a laboratory procedure.

Summary.
The summary at the end of each lesson emphasizes the major points in that lesson and helps you recall the information.

REVIEW QUESTIONS

Review questions are provided to test your understanding of the lesson. After you study the unit, if you are unable to answer some of the questions, review the lesson material again.

STUDENT ACTIVITIES AND WEB ACTIVITIES

Student activities help you practice your skills and expand your knowledge using various resources, such as laboratory tours, interviewing laboratory professionals, and comparing test methods. Web activities help you learn about valuable resources available through reliable Web sites that provide a quick way to find useful information.

STUDENT PERFORMANCE GUIDES

Student Performance Guides provide equipment and materials lists and step-by-step instructions for laboratory procedures. Icons alert you to special precautions or considerations that must be observed for personal safety and to achieve quality results. The Guides give you a chance to practice procedures by yourself or with another student until you become confident enough to have your instructor evaluate you as you perform the procedure.

UNIT 1

Introduction to the Clinical Laboratory

UNIT OBJECTIVES

After studying this unit, the student will:

- Discuss the organization and function of the clinical laboratory.
- Discuss the qualifications, job functions, and ethical responsibilities of clinical laboratory personnel.
- Identify and define selected abbreviations and acronyms commonly used in the clinical laboratory.
- Identify and define prefixes, suffixes, and stems in selected medical terms.
- Use the metric system to perform measurements.
- Discuss and implement laboratory safety rules that must be followed to guard against chemical, physical, and biological hazards.
- Discuss the role of quality assessment programs in the clinical laboratory.
- Identify common types of labware and understand their proper uses.
- Discuss and demonstrate use of general laboratory equipment.
- Use the compound brightfield microscope.
- Perform common laboratory calculations and prepare laboratory reagents.
- Perform a capillary puncture.
- Perform a venipuncture.

UNIT OVERVIEW

The clinical laboratory is a place where blood, body fluids, and other biological specimens are tested, analyzed, or evaluated. The observations can be qualitative or quantitative. The tests can be performed manually or using automated analyzers. Precise measurements are made and the results are calculated and interpreted. Because of this, laboratory workers must have the skills necessary to perform a variety of tasks.

Unit 1 is an introduction to the laboratory environment as a workplace and to the profession of medical technology, which is now more commonly called clinical laboratory science. Key concepts and procedures laboratory workers need to know are described.

The organization and function of the clinical laboratory are addressed in Lesson 1-1. Qualifications and job functions of laboratory personnel are reviewed in Lesson 1-2.

As an introduction to the structure of medical terms, Lesson 1-3 gives basic information about medical terminology and abbreviations and acronyms used in the laboratory. As other units are studied, additional vocabulary terms will be introduced and defined.

Because laboratory analyses use metric units, a brief introduction to the metric system is given in Lesson 1-4. Knowledge of the metric system is required for some exercises in Unit 2.

Lessons on laboratory safety (Lessons 1-5 and 1-6) are included in this unit because every worker in the clinical laboratory must be thoroughly aware of potential hazards in the workplace. Workers must understand and follow all safety procedures and practices before any laboratory exercises can be performed.

Methods and procedures for assuring the reliability and accuracy of laboratory analyses are presented in Lesson 1-7, Quality Assessment in the Laboratory. These quality assessment principles are included in this introductory unit because they must be integrated into all aspects of laboratory operations, from employee training and evaluation to specimen collection and processing, specimen analysis, and interpretation and reporting of results.

The care, use, and cleaning of frequently used labware, such as beakers, test tubes, pipets, and flasks, are explained in Lesson 1-8. The use of general laboratory equipment, such as centrifuges, automatic pipets, pH meters, autoclaves, and laboratory balances, is described in Lesson 1-9. The proper care and use of the microscope is included in this unit (Lesson 1-10) because its use is required in the microbiology, hematology, urinalysis, and parasitology units. Basic laboratory calculations and reagent preparation are explained in Lesson 1-11. Lessons 1-12 and 1-13 introduce techniques for collecting capillary and venous blood.

Unit 1 is an introduction to the techniques, rules, and skills needed to perform the exercises in Units 2 through 8. Unit 1 can also be used alone as an introduction to the profession of clinical laboratory science. After Unit 1 has been completed, the remaining units can be studied in order of the instructor's preference depending on available time, laboratory space, and equipment.

READINGS, REFERENCES AND RESOURCES

General—Clinical Laboratory Science

Baker, F. J., et al. (2001). *Baker & Silverton's introduction to medical laboratory technology* (7th ed.). Oxford, UK: Oxford University Press.

Burtis, C. A., et al. (Eds.). (1998). *Tietz textbook of clinical chemistry* (3rd ed.). Philadelphia: W. B. Saunders Company.

Clinical Laboratory Improvement Amendments of 1988. (1992). In *Federal Register* 57(40): 7001–7288.

Henry, J. B. (Ed.). (2006). *Clinical diagnosis & management by laboratory methods* (21st ed.). Philadelphia: W. B. Saunders Company.

Karni, K. (2002). *Opportunities in clinical laboratory science*. Lincolnwood, IL: VGM Career Books, Mc-Graw Hill.

Laposata, M. (1992). *SI unit conversion guide*. Boston: NEJM Books.

Lindh, W. Q., et al. (2002). *Comprehensive medical assisting* (2nd ed.). Clifton Park, NY: Thomson Delmar Learning.

Linné, J. J. & Ringsrud, K. M. (1999). *Clinical laboratory sciences: the basics and routine techniques*. (4th ed.). St. Louis: Mosby.

Simmers, L. (2004). *Diversified health occupations* (6th ed.). Clifton Park, NY: Thomson Delmar Learning.

Westgard, J. O. (2002). *Basic QC practices* (2nd ed.). Washington, DC: AACC Press.

Medical Terminology

Chabner, D. (Ed.). (2005). *The language of medicine* (7th ed.). Philadelphia: W. B. Saunders Company.

Dennerll, J. T., et al. (2002). *Medical terminology made easy* (3rd ed.). Clifton Park, NY: Thomson Delmar Learning.

Dorland, W. A. N. (Ed.). (2003). *Dorland's illustrated medical dictionary* (30th ed.). Philadelphia: W. B. Saunders Company.

Ehrlich, A. & Schroeder, C. L. (2000). *Medical terminology for health professions* (4th ed.). Clifton Park, NY: Thomson Delmar Learning.

Sormunen, C. (2003). *Terminology for allied health professionals* (6th ed.). Clifton Park, NY: Thomson Delmar Learning.

Venes, D., et al. (Eds.). (2005). *Taber's cyclopedic medical dictionary* (20th ed.). Philadelphia: F. A. Davis Company.

Phlebotomy

Hoeltke, L.B. (2006). *The complete textbook of phlebotomy* (3rd ed.). Clifton Park, NY: Thomson Delmar Learning.

Kalanick, K. (2004). *Phlebotomy technician specialist*. Clifton Park, NY: Thomson Delmar Learning.

Turgeon, M. L. (1999). *Clinical hematology theory and procedures* (3rd ed.). Hagerstown, MD: Lippincott Williams & Wilkins.

Safety

American Hospital Association, Division of Quality Resources. (1992). OSHA's final bloodborne pathogens standard: A special briefing.

Centers for Disease Control and Prevention. (1987). Recommendations for prevention of HIV transmission in health-care settings. In *Morbidity mortality weekly report* 36(Suppl. 25):3S–18S.

Centers for Disease Control and Prevention. (2002). Guidelines for hand hygiene in health care settings. In *Morbidity mortality weekly report* 51(No. RR-16):1–45.

Centers for Disease Control and Prevention and National Institutes of Health. (2005). *Biosafety in microbiological and biomedical laboratories* (5th ed.). Washington, D.C.: U.S. Government Printing Office. Available online at www.cdc.gov.

Coastal Training Technologies. Safety training videos, handbooks, and web courses. Available online at www.coastal.com.

Collins, C. H. & Kennedy, D. A. (1999). *Laboratory acquired infections: history, incidence, causes and preventions* (4th ed.). London: Reed Educational and Professional Publishing, Ltd.

Joint Advisory Notice; Department of Labor/Department of Health and Human Services; HBV/HIV. (1982). In *Federal Register* 52(210):41818–41823.

Occupational Safety and Health Administration. Occupational exposure to bloodborne pathogens, final rule, labor. In *Federal Register* 56(235): Rules and regulations. Often referred to as 29 CFR Part 1910.0130.

Occupational Safety and Health Administration. (1987). Hazard communication, labor. In *Federal Register* 52(163): 31852–31886.

Occupational Safety and Health Administration. (1999). How to prevent needlestick injuries: Answers to some important questions (Publication 3161). Washington, D.C.: U.S. Department of Labor.

OSHA Publications. Safety pamphlets. Available online at www.osha.gov.

Safety Alert Network. OSHA-compliant safety training programs. Available online at www.safetyalert.com.

Safety sense: A laboratory guide. (2001). Cold Spring Harbor, NY: Cold Spring Harbor Laboratory Press.

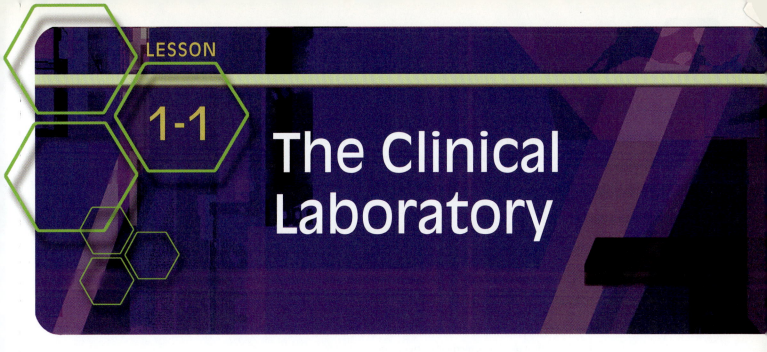

LESSON 1-1

The Clinical Laboratory

LESSON OBJECTIVES

After studying this lesson, the student will:

- Explain the function of a medical or clinical laboratory.
- Discuss the organization of a typical hospital laboratory.
- Describe the functions of the different levels of laboratory personnel.
- List the major departments of a typical clinical laboratory and name a test that would be performed in each department.
- List three examples of nonhospital clinical laboratories.
- Explain how clinical laboratories are regulated.
- Explain the relationship between CMS and CLIA '88.
- Explain how the HIPAA affects the laboratory and laboratory workers.
- Describe the purpose and scope of quality assessment programs in the clinical laboratory.
- Explain the purpose of proficiency testing.
- Explain the purpose of laboratory accreditation.
- Define the glossary terms.

GLOSSARY

accessioning / the process by which specimens are logged in, labeled, and assigned a specimen identification code

accreditation / a voluntary process in which a private, independent agency grants recognition to institutions or programs that meet or exceed established standards of quality

American Association of Blood Banks (AABB) / international association that sets blood bank standards, accredits blood banks, and promotes high standards of performance in the practice of transfusion medicine

bacteriology / the study of bacteria

blood bank / clinical laboratory department where blood components are tested and stored until needed for transfusion; immunohematology department; transfusion services; also the refrigerated unit used for storing blood components

Centers for Disease Control and Prevention (CDC) / central laboratory for the national public health system

Centers for Medicare and Medicaid Services (CMS) / the agency within the Department of Health and Human Services (DHHS) responsible for implementing CLIA '88

5

Clinical and Laboratory Standards Institute (CLSI) / an international, nonprofit organization that establishes standards of best current practice for clinical laboratories; formerly National Committee for Clinical Laboratory Standards (NCCLS)

clinical chemistry / the laboratory section that uses chemical principles to analyze blood and other body fluids

Clinical Laboratory Improvement Amendments of 1988 (CLIA '88) / a federal act that specifies minimum performance standards for clinical laboratories

coagulation / the process of forming a fibrin clot; the laboratory department that performs hemostasis testing

College of American Pathologists (CAP) / agency that offers accreditation to clinical laboratories and certification to clinical laboratory personnel

Commission on Office Laboratory Accreditation (COLA) / agency that offers accreditation to physician office laboratories

Department of Health and Human Services (DHHS) / the governmental agency that oversees public health care matters; commonly called HHS

epidemiology / the study of the factors that cause disease and determine disease frequency and distribution

Food and Drug Administration (FDA) / the division of the Department of Health and Human Services (DHHS) responsible for protecting the public health by assuring the safety and efficacy of foods, drugs, biological products, medical devices, and cosmetics

Health Care Financing Administration (HCFA) / see Centers for Medicare and Medicaid Services (CMS)

hematology / the study of blood and blood-forming tissues

HIPAA / Health Insurance Portability and Accountability Act of 1996

immunohematology / the study of the human blood groups; in the clinical laboratory, often called blood banking or transfusion services

immunology / the branch of medicine encompassing the study of immune processes and immunity

Joint Commission (JC) / an independent agency that accredits hospitals and large health care facilities (formerly known as the Joint Commission on Accreditation of Healthcare Organizations [JCAHO])

Laboratory Response Network (LRN) / a nationwide network of laboratories coordinated by the Centers for Disease Control and Prevention (CDC) with the ability for rapid response to threats to public health

microbiology / the branch of biology dealing with microbes

mycology / the study of fungi

National Committee for Clinical Laboratory Standards (NCCLS) / see Clinical and Laboratory Standards Institute (CLSI)

parasitology / the study of parasites

pathologist / a physician specially trained in the nature and cause of disease

phlebotomist / a health care worker trained in blood collection

physician office laboratory (POL) / small medical laboratory located within a physician office, group practice, or clinic

plasma / the liquid portion of blood in which the blood cells are suspended; the straw-colored liquid remaining after blood cells are removed from anticoagulated blood

point-of-care testing (POCT) / testing outside the traditional laboratory setting; also called bedside testing, off-site testing, or alternate-site testing

proficiency testing (PT) / a program in which a laboratory's accuracy in performing analyses is evaluated at regular intervals and compared to the performance of similar laboratories

Provider-Performed Microscopy Procedure (PPMP) / a certificate category under CLIA '88

quality assessment (QA) / in the laboratory, a program that monitors the total testing process with the aim of providing the highest-quality patient care; a synonym for "quality assurance"

reference laboratory / an independent regional laboratory that offers routine and specialized testing services to hospitals and physicians

serology / the study of antigens and antibodies in serum using immunological methods; laboratory testing based on the immunological properties of serum

serum / the liquid obtained from blood that has been allowed to clot

virology / the study of viruses

INTRODUCTION

Laboratories that perform chemical and microscopic tests on blood, other body fluids, and tissues are called *clinical* or *medical laboratories*. These laboratories play a major role in patient care and are found in a variety of settings, both government and private. A clinical laboratory can be in a large institution, offer sophisticated services, and employ many skilled workers who interact daily with patients and other allied health personnel in the institution. Clinical laboratories can also be small, with only one or two employees.

Today, clinical laboratories, as well as other health care delivery systems, face a variety of challenges. These include coping with rapidly rising costs, maintaining quality personnel, keeping up with advancing technologies, and complying with increased governmental regulations. These issues must be addressed without sacrificing the quality of patient care. This lesson surveys the types of clinical laboratories and describes their organization, function, and regulation.

TYPES OF CLINICAL LABORATORIES

Clinical laboratories can be placed into two groups: hospital laboratories and nonhospital laboratories. Although most people think of hospitals when they think of clinical laboratories, laboratories can also be in clinics, group practices, physician offices, nursing homes, veterinary offices, government agencies, industry, and military installations. Some clinical laboratories, such as regional reference laboratories, are independent of medical facilities.

In 2006, the **Department of Health and Human Services (DHHS), Centers for Medicare and Medicaid Services (CMS)**, formerly known as the **Health Care Financing Administration (HCFA)**, listed more than 196,000 private and commercial laboratories as providing services to humans in the United States. Table 1-1 shows the numbers of U.S. clinical laboratories by type of facility. This number does not include laboratories limited to research or veterinary laboratories.

Hospital Laboratories

Clinical laboratories are found in private hospitals, university teaching hospitals, and government-operated institutions such as military hospitals and veterans' hospitals. The clinical laboratory is one of many hospital departments (Figure 1-1). The level of services available from a hospital laboratory is usually determined by the size of the hospital. A laboratory in a small hospital (less than 100 beds) may perform only very routine test procedures. Complicated or infrequently requested tests may be sent to reference laboratories.

In a clinical laboratory in a medium-size hospital (up to 300 beds), routine tests and many more complicated test procedures are performed. Only the most recently developed tests, infrequently requested tests, or tests with high levels of complexity would need to be sent to reference laboratories.

Clinical laboratories in large hospitals (more than 300 beds) handle large volumes of work and perform complex tests (Figure 1-2).

TABLE 1-1. Numbers and types of clinical laboratories performing tests on humans registered by CMS, June 2006 (From Division of Laboratory Services, CMS, DHHS)

TYPE OF LABORATORY	NUMBER	PERCENT OF TOTAL
Ambulatory surgical center	3809	1.93%
Community clinic	6610	3.34%
Comp. outpatient rehabilitation facility	260	0.13%
Ancillary testing site in health care facility	2749	1.40%
Renal dialysis facility	3978	2.02%
Health fair	508	0.26%
Health maintenance organization	667	0.34%
Home health agency	9654	4.89%
Hospice	1740	0.88%
Hospital	8677	4.41%
Independent	5329	2.71%
Industrial	1702	0.86%
Insurance	45	0.02%
Intermediate care/ mentally retarded	969	0.49%
Mobile laboratory	1120	0.57%
Pharmacy	4085	2.10%
School/student health facility	1873	0.95%
Skilled nursing facility/ nursing facility	14,737	7.47%
Physician office	106,528	54.09%
Other practitioner	2437	1.24%
Tissue bank/repository	35	0.02%
Blood bank	366	0.19%
Rural health clinic	1170	0.59%
Federally qualified health center	389	0.20%
Ambulance	2760	1.40%
Public health laboratory	181	0.09%
Other	14,595	7.41%

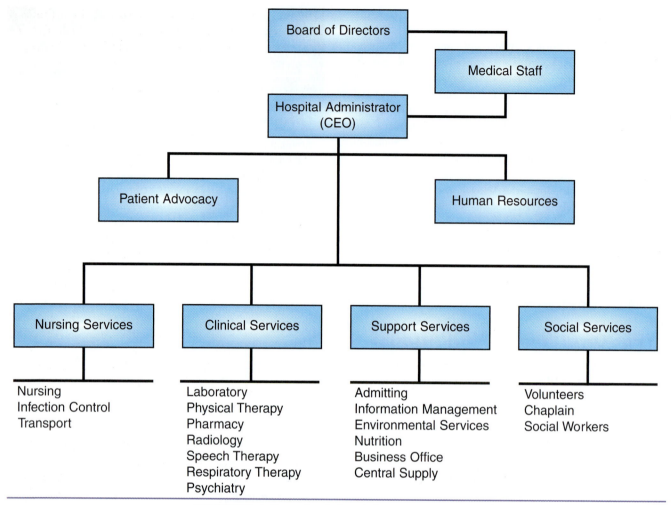

FIGURE 1-1 Example of a hospital organizational chart

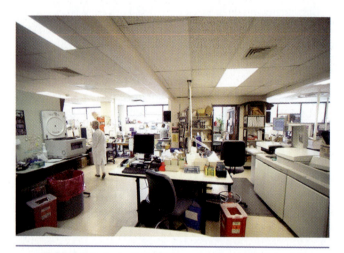

FIGURE 1-2 A clinical laboratory in a large hospital

Nonhospital Clinical Laboratories

Nonhospital clinical laboratories can be publicly (government) or privately operated. They provide a variety of services and employment for many skilled workers. In the United States in 2005, most clinical laboratories were in nonhospital settings (Table 1-1).

Physician Office Laboratories

Physician office laboratories (POLs) are laboratories in a physician's office or small clinic. In 2006, 54% of clinical laboratories listed with the DHHS were classified as POLs. The increased availability of rapid-test kits and small, easy-to-operate analyzers has broadened the scope of testing in the POL. Several common laboratory tests, such as hemoglobin, hematocrit, urine reagent strip, pregnancy, blood glucose, and occult blood, can be performed in the POL by multiskilled personnel such as medical assistants (Table 1-2).

Reference Laboratories

Reference laboratories are usually privately owned, regional laboratories that do high-volume testing and offer a wide variety of tests. Large hospitals use reference laboratories primarily to perform complex or infrequently ordered tests. Small hospitals or physicians' offices use their services for a wide range of tests. Reference laboratories provide courier service to transport specimens from the collection site to the testing laboratory.

Government Laboratories—Federal

The central laboratory for the national public health system is the **Centers for Disease Control and Prevention (CDC)** in Atlanta,

> **TABLE 1-2. Examples of analytes for which there are waived tests under CLIA (as published by FDA, 2005)**
>
> Hemoglobin by copper sulfate
>
> Hemoglobin by single instrument with direct readout
>
> Blood glucose by meters cleared for home use
>
> Glycosylated hemoglobin (HbA1c)
>
> Fecal occult blood
>
> Spun hematocrit
>
> Ovulation tests by color comparison
>
> Urine pregnancy tests by visual color comparison
>
> Urinalysis reagent strip
>
> Microalbumin
>
> Rapid strep test from throat swab
>
> Erythrocyte sedimentation rate
>
> Immunoassay for *Helicobacter pylori*
>
> Prothrombin time
>
> Fructosamine
>
> Cholesterol; high-density lipoprotein (HDL) and low-density lipoprotein (LDL) cholesterol
>
> Infectious mononucleosis antibodies

Georgia. This agency provides consulting services to state public health laboratories as well as to individual physicians. The CDC provides educational materials and safety guidelines for workers in a variety of health care areas as well as for the general public.

Epidemiology is another important function of the CDC. Data are gathered concerning the origin, distribution, and occurrence of various diseases, and outbreaks are investigated to determine the causes. This function of the CDC has gained much public attention because of its role in investigating emerging infectious diseases that have appeared worldwide in recent years.

The CDC also coordinates the **Laboratory Response Network (LRN)**. This laboratory network was established to ensure that state and private laboratories are equipped to respond effectively to threats to public health, such as bioterrorism events or emerging infectious diseases.

Government Laboratories—State

Each U.S. state and territory has a clinical laboratory operated, usually, by the state's department of public health. These state laboratories provide testing and consulting services to hospitals, physicians, and clinics within the state.

Services available from state laboratories vary from state to state. In general, state laboratories perform tests mandated by state regulations, for example, premarital blood tests and phenylketonuria (PKU) testing of newborns. State laboratories also offer tests not routinely available in other laboratories such as culture of fungi, viruses, and mycobacteria (which include the pathogens causing tuberculosis); tests for parasites; confirmatory tests for

reportable infectious diseases such as AIDS; and some environmental testing. Special-case specimens to be sent to the CDC for testing are usually sent via state public health laboratories.

REGULATION OF CLINICAL LABORATORIES

All clinical laboratories, including POLs (but excluding research laboratories), are regulated by both federal and state agencies. The **Clinical Laboratory Improvement Amendments of 1988 (CLIA '88)**, a revision of the Clinical Laboratory Improvement Act of 1967, specifies the minimum performance standards for all clinical laboratories. The objective of CLIA '88 is to ensure quality laboratory testing. Even though CLIA was passed in 1988, the amendments have been continually revised, updated, clarified, and refined since that time.

The Division of Laboratory Services, under the CMS (www.cms.hhs.gov/clia/) has the responsibility for implementing the CLIA '88 Program. Any laboratory performing laboratory tests on humans, except for research laboratories, must obtain a certificate from CMS to be allowed to operate.

Under CLIA '88, laboratories are classified as performing:

- Waived tests
- Tests of moderate and high complexity
- **Provider-Performed Microscopy Procedures (PPMP)**

The classifications are based on the difficulty or complexity of the test procedures and the level of training required to accurately perform the tests. Laboratory personnel standards differ for each of these categories. The more complex the test, the more highly trained the testing personnel must be. Each laboratory must obtain a certificate stating its category. The five certificates are (1) Certificate of Waiver, (2) Certificate for PPMP, (3) Registration Certificate, (4) Certificate of Compliance, and (5) Certificate of Accreditation. Table 1-3 explains conditions under which each certificate would be issued.

Under the CLIA '88 law, laboratories with a certificate of waiver can only perform tests that are determined by the CDC or the **Food and Drug Administration (FDA)** to be so simple that there is little risk of error. These are called *waived tests*, and examples of some analytes for which there are waived tests are listed in Table 1-2. Because of advances in technology, the number and types of waived tests have increased, and the number of laboratories performing waived tests has grown tremendously since CLIA '88 implementation. Laboratories with a PPMP certificate perform microscopy-based tests during the course of a patient visit on specimens that are not easily transportable. Examples of PPMP include urine microscopic examination and wet mounts.

Many POLs perform only waived tests; some others may perform more complex (nonwaived) tests. Most hospital laboratories perform moderate- to high-complexity tests. In 2004, of the more than 180,000 certified laboratories, over 74,000 performed nonwaived tests. This means that, to comply with the law, these facilities must adhere to mandated personnel guidelines, comprehensive recordkeeping, and quality assess-

TABLE 1-3. Types of certificates issued under CLIA '88 and the activity(ies) each certificate permits

CERTIFICATE	ACTIVITY PERMITTED
Certificate of Waiver	Permits a laboratory to perform only CLIA-waived tests
Certificate of Registration	Permits the laboratory to conduct moderate- or high-complexity laboratory testing (or both) until the laboratory is determined by survey to be in compliance with CLIA regulations
Certificate of Compliance	Issued to a laboratory holding a Certificate of Registration after an inspection finds the laboratory to be in compliance with all applicable CLIA regulations
Certificate of Accreditation	Issued to a laboratory that has been accredited by a CMS-approved accrediting organization
PPMP	Issued to a laboratory in which a physician, mid-level practitioner, or dentist performs no tests of complexity other than the microscopy procedures; this certificate also permits the laboratory to perform waived tests

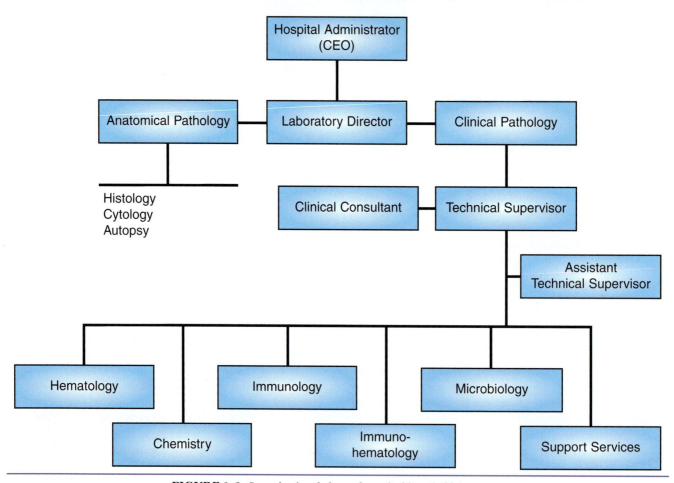

FIGURE 1-3 Organizational chart of a typical hospital laboratory

ment programs; participate in proficiency testing programs; and be subject to government inspections. Laboratories performing moderate- to high-complexity tests must have a certificate of registration, compliance, or accreditation.

States can enact state-specific regulations regarding the operation of laboratories. However, state standards must be at least as stringent as federal regulations and must not violate or counteract federal regulations.

ORGANIZATION OF THE HOSPITAL LABORATORY

The organization schemes of most hospital laboratories follow a general outline (Figure 1-3) that can vary slightly depending on the size of the laboratory. In recent years, some laboratories have changed department and personnel titles to reflect the terminology used in the CLIA '88 rules. Table 1-4 lists personnel titles as

TABLE 1-4. Job titles of clinical laboratory personnel as listed in CLIA '88 Final Rule and commonly used equivalent titles	
CLIA '88 JOB TITLE	**EQUIVALENT JOB TITLE**
Laboratory director	Laboratory director (usually a pathologist)
Technical supervisor	Laboratory manager, chief technologist
Clinical consultant	Consultant
Technical consultant or general supervisor	Department head, section head, section supervisor, technical specialist
Testing personnel	Medical technologist, clinical laboratory scientist, medical laboratory technician, clinical laboratory technician, laboratory assistant

stated in CLIA '88 and gives the commonly used equivalent titles. The personnel qualifications for each category are specified in the Clinical Laboratory Improvement Amendments of 1988, Final Rule, *Federal Register*, Vol. 7, No. 40, February 28, 1992.

Clinical Laboratory Personnel

Laboratory Director

The director of the hospital laboratory has customarily been a **pathologist**, a physician specially trained in the nature and cause of disease. Hospital pathologists usually oversee two branches of pathology, anatomical pathology and clinical pathology. The anatomical pathology department includes cytology, histology, and autopsy services. The clinical laboratory department can also be called clinical pathology or clinical laboratory services.

Under CLIA '88, persons other than pathologists can qualify to be clinical laboratory directors. The type of CMS certificate held by the laboratory determines the qualifications a director must have. In general, the laboratory director must be licensed by the state in which the laboratory operates; hold the degree of doctor of medicine, doctor of osteopathy, or an earned doctorate in a related clinical field; hold certification from an appropriate body; and have supervisory and clinical laboratory experience. The laboratory director has ultimate responsibility for all laboratory operations.

Small hospitals may not have a full-time pathologist on staff or on-site. Depending on the qualifications of the laboratory director, laboratories in these hospitals can be required to contract with certified individuals to serve as *clinical consultants* and/or *technical consultants*. These consultants assist the laboratory director in matters of test appropriateness and interpretation or in technical matters relating to test methods.

Technical Supervisor/Laboratory Manager

Directly under the laboratory director's authority is the technical supervisor or laboratory manager (Figure 1-3). This is someone educated in the clinical laboratory sciences who has additional business or management training or experience.

The technical supervisor (laboratory manager) is responsible for the day-to-day operation of the laboratory. The technical supervisor is also responsible for setting personnel standards, establishing training and evaluation procedures, establishing appropriate quality assessment programs, observing and documenting employee performance and competence, and making sure that all regulatory mandates are followed. The supervisor is responsible for making available to all personnel an up-to-date procedure manual containing instructions for every procedure performed in the laboratory. The **Clinical and Laboratory Standards Institute** (**CLSI**) develops standards of current best practice for clinical laboratory procedures. Laboratory procedure manuals must follow CLSI standards. (CLSI was formerly known as the **National Committee for Clinical Laboratory Standards**, or **NCCLS**).

General Supervisor/Department Head

Each department has a general supervisor or department head responsible for the quality of work performed in the department, training employees, and evaluating employee performance. General supervisors report to the technical supervisor.

Testing Personnel

Testing personnel perform the laboratory analyses (Figure 1-4). These include medical technologists/clinical laboratory scientists and medical laboratory technicians/clinical laboratory technicians. Nonlaboratory personnel such as medical assistants and nursing staff often perform tests in POLs or other settings outside the laboratory proper. Clinical laboratory personnel qualifications are discussed in Lesson 1-2, The Clinical Laboratory Professional.

Departments of the Clinical Laboratory

The number of departments in clinical laboratories varies. Clinical chemistry, hematology, microbiology, blood bank, and support services (phlebotomy and specimen processing) usu-

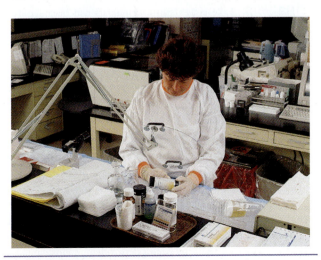

FIGURE 1-4 Testing personnel in a clinical laboratory

ally operate as departments or sections, each with its own department head or general supervisor. The subdivisions within each department differ from one laboratory to another. Large laboratories often have separate departments for urinalysis, coagulation, immunology, and parasitology (Figure 1-3).

Hematology

Most **hematology** tests involve studying the cellular components of blood. Hematology procedures can be qualitative or quantitative. The *quantitative* procedures include counts of the various blood components, such as the number of leukocytes (white blood cells), erythrocytes (red blood cells), or platelets. These counts can be performed manually but are usually performed on a cell counter or hematology analyzer.

In *qualitative* procedures, blood components are observed for qualities such as cell size, shape, and maturity. Using a microscope, a laboratory worker can view a blood smear to determine the types of leukocytes present; estimate the size, shape, and hemoglobin content of erythrocytes; or estimate the number of platelets. Any abnormalities are noted during microscopic examination of the blood smear, including immature leukocytes or erythrocytes.

Hematocrit and hemoglobin are tests commonly performed to help diagnose anemia. Many analyzers are capable of performing several hematological procedures simultaneously.

In large laboratories, complicated tests such as special stains to classify leukemic cells might be performed in a hematology section called *special hematology*. Some tests in special hematology are manual tests.

Coagulation.
Coagulation tests are used to diagnose and monitor patients who have defects in their blood-clotting mechanism or are being treated with anti-clotting drugs. Coagulation tests may be performed in the hematology department or, in large laboratories, in a separate department. In past years, automated coagulation testing systems were used primarily in larger laboratories. However, the availability of small, easy-to-use coagulation analyzers allows even small POLs to have the capability of performing coagulation procedures. **Plasma**, the liquid portion of anticoagulated blood, is the specimen used for most coagulation studies.

Urinalysis.
Like coagulation, urinalysis can be a separate department in a large laboratory or a subdivision of another department, usually hematology or chemistry. In the urinalysis department, physical, chemical, and microscopic examinations of urine specimens are performed. These tests can be performed manually or using automated methods.

Clinical Chemistry

In the **clinical chemistry** department, test procedures are often performed on **serum**, the liquid part of blood remaining after a clot has formed. Tests can also be performed on plasma, urine, and other body fluids such as spinal fluid and joint fluid.

Procedures performed in the clinical chemistry department include blood glucose, cholesterol, assays of heart and liver enzymes, and electrolytes (chloride, bicarbonate, potassium, and sodium).

Clinical chemistry is the largest department in most laboratories and can have one or more subdivisions. Common subdivisions are *special chemistry* and *toxicology*. Procedures such as electrophoresis are performed in special chemistry. In toxicology, blood or urine can be analyzed to determine the drug involved in an overdose, blood levels of prescribed drugs, and hormone levels.

The number of chemistry analyzers has grown rapidly in the last several years (see Lesson 6-3). Most of these analyzers provide a wide range of test procedures yet are simple to operate. Thus, it is possible for even the smallest laboratory to perform some routine chemistry tests.

Immunology

Immunology can be a separate department or, in small laboratories, a part of another department such as blood bank or microbiology. In the past this department was called **serology** because serum was the specimen most often used in the tests. In immunology, many tests are based on antigen-antibody methods. Among tests performed in this section are those for pregnancy, arthritis, and autoimmune diseases. Tests for infectious mononucleosis, HIV infection, influenza, hepatitis, sexually transmitted diseases, and other infectious diseases are also performed.

Blood Bank/Transfusion Services

The **blood bank** department may also be called **immunohematology** or transfusion services. Procedures performed in this department are critical to patient well-being. If a transfusion is required, the patient's ABO group and Rh type are determined by blood bank technologists. Stored units of donor blood are then tested to determine which units would be compatible for transfusion into the patient. The blood bank department might also have the capability to process donated blood into specialized components.

Microbiology

The **microbiology** department is responsible for culturing and identifying microorganisms. **Bacteriology** procedures make up the majority of the work in this department. Bacteria can be isolated from specimens such as sputum, wounds, blood, urine, or other body fluids by inoculating the specimen to culture media. Organisms that grow in the culture are identified, and susceptibility tests are performed to determine the most effective antibiotic treatment. This is done by exposing the bacterial culture to different antibiotics and observing their effect on the organism's growth. Automated systems that can detect growth of an organism, identify an organism, and determine its antibiotic susceptibility are widely used in bacteriology.

Procedures involving **virology**, the study of viruses, and **mycology**, the study of fungi, are usually performed in the microbiology department. Often specimens are cultured in the hospital laboratory, and identification is performed by reference laboratories. Because cultures of pathogenic fungi as well as mycobacteria must be handled with special care, specimens suspected of containing these organisms are usually inoculated to media and then sent to a reference laboratory for identification.

Parasitology.
In **parasitology**, usually a part of the microbiology department, patient specimens are examined for parasites. Fecal samples are examined microscopically for evidence of intestinal parasites such as intestinal amoeba, tapeworms, or hookworms.

Immunological tests are performed to detect parasite antigens in fecal samples. Tests for blood parasites, such as the malarial parasite, are usually performed in the hematology department.

Laboratory Support Services

Laboratory tests begin with the laboratory request form, which must be completed before the test is performed (Figure 1-5). This can be a written request or a computer-generated request. After the request is received, the laboratory will begin the test process—collecting the specimen; performing the test; and interpreting, recording, reporting, and charting results. Most hospital laboratories have a separate department responsible for collecting and processing specimens. This department is called by a variety of names such as support services, phlebotomy, or specimen collection and processing. **Phlebotomists** are the laboratory personnel who collect the blood specimens; sometimes this responsibility is shared by nursing personnel.

In small laboratories, specimens are usually taken directly to the appropriate laboratory department. In larger laboratories, specimens are delivered to a central **accessioning** area where they are processed, logged into the computer, and given a specimen identification code before being distributed to the departments for testing. Many hospitals have pneumatic delivery systems that provide rapid delivery of specimens from the patient room or nursing station, outpatient clinic, surgery, emergency room, or intensive care unit to the clinical laboratory or other department.

Laboratory Information Systems

Large laboratories have computerized laboratory information systems (LIS) that improve efficiency and reduce errors. In hospitals, the LIS can be integrated with the institution-wide computer system. Computerization in the laboratory and hospital has made specimen identification and tracking more error-proof. Specimens are labeled with preprinted bar-coded labels that match bar-coded test requisitions and patient identification bracelets. Data can be entered directly into the computer system using bar-code scanners. Even small laboratories usually have a method to preprint specimen labels with patient data. Advantages of laboratory information systems include:

- Charting errors can be eliminated.
- Efficiency is improved.
- Abnormal or unusual test results are automatically identified.
- Specimens can be matched to test results.
- Unauthorized testing and reporting is prevented.

Point-of-Care Testing

Rapid advancements in technology make possible rapid changes in all aspects of health care. One of the major changes in the clinical laboratory has been the implementation and increased use of **point-of-care testing (POCT)**. POCT brings the laboratory test to the patient rather than obtaining a specimen from the patient and transporting it to the laboratory for testing. This makes laboratory test results available more rapidly, providing improved patient care.

POCT is used in settings such as clinics, health maintenance organizations (HMOs), nursing homes, physician offices, emergency rooms, intensive care units, and surgery suites. POCT is also referred to as bedside testing, near-patient testing, off-site testing, or alternate-site testing.

The evolution of small, simple-to-use analyzers that require only one drop, or less, of specimen has led to widespread POCT implementation. Handheld portable analyzers can measure substances such as hemoglobin, glucose, cholesterol, and electrolytes. Most require only a drop of blood, usually obtained by fingerstick. Most POCT tests are CLIA-waived.

The advent of POCT has created the opportunity for more collaboration between the laboratory and other members of the health care team. Although nonlaboratory personnel from the nursing service or surgery or emergency room teams may perform the tests, the laboratory is usually responsible for selecting instrumentation, training personnel, developing procedure manuals, and monitoring quality assessment procedures and instrument maintenance.

QUALITY ASSESSMENT IN THE LABORATORY

For many years, clinical laboratories have had programs in place to monitor the quality of laboratory results. These program requirements expanded under CLIA '88 and associated legislation. All laboratories now must have comprehensive programs to evaluate and improve the overall laboratory performance. These programs have evolved through many changes, beginning as quality control (QC), progressing to quality assurance and broader programs such as total quality management (TQM) and continuous quality improvement (CQI). The name recommended by CMS is **quality assessment (QA)**, part of a comprehensive quality system (QS).

The QA programs are incorporated into each department's procedure manual and day-to-day operation. One person in the laboratory, usually a supervisory person such as the assistant laboratory manager, may be responsible for implementing the QA programs throughout the laboratory and documenting the results. Every aspect of a test procedure, from ordering the test and collecting the specimen to reporting of results, falls under the QA umbrella. QA responsibilities can also include managing POCT or off-site and satellite laboratory testing; evaluating personnel, training, and providing continuing education; updating procedure manuals; monitoring compliance with regulatory agencies; keeping records; documenting equipment maintenance, calibration, and repairs; and participating in proficiency testing programs.

All institutions receiving Medicare or Medicaid funds are required to develop and maintain a QA program. The intent of this requirement is to improve health care, focusing on patient safety and ways to reduce medical errors. Lesson 1-7 describes in detail how QA is used in the clinical laboratory.

Proficiency Testing

Laboratories performing moderate- or high-complexity testing are required by CLIA '88 to participate in an approved **proficiency testing (PT)** program. Participation in these programs is a part of a laboratory's QA program. PT programs send "unknown" samples to laboratories at regular intervals. The laboratory performs specific tests on the unknowns and reports the results to the PT

LABORATORY ORDER REQUEST

781401 870997

Last Name	First	Middle	Social Security Number	Birthdate
Doe	Jane			

Physician	Date/time drawn	Phlebotomist

ICD-9 code(s)	Bill to: ☐ Insurance ☐ Office ☐ Patient

PROFILES	ICD-9 CODE #	INDIVIDUAL PROCEDURES	ICD-9 CODE #	INDIVIDUAL PROCEDURES	ICD-9 CODE #
☐ BASIC METABOLIC PROFILE		✔ **HEMATOLOGY / COAGULATION**		✔ **CHEMISTRY PROCEDURES**	
Basic Metabolic Profile includes: Calcium Carbon Dioxide Chloride Creatinine Glucose Potassium Sodium Urea Nitrogen		CBC		Potassium (K+)	
		PT (Protime) w/INR		Glucose	
		PTT		BUN (Urea Nitrogen)	
☐ ELECTROLYTE PANEL		Hgb (Hemoglobin)		Calcium	
		HCT (Hematocrit)		Creatinine	
Electrolyte Panel Includes: Sodium Potassium Chloride Carbon Dioxide		ESR (sed rate)		PSA (Prostatic Specific Antigen)	
		Hemoglobin A1-C		PSA Screen	
☐ METABOLIC PANEL COMPREHENSIVE		✔ **SEROLOGY**		TSH	
				T-3 Uptake	
Comprehensive Metabolic Panel Includes: Albumin Chloride Potassium Bilirubin,total Creatinine Protein, total BUN Glucose Sodium Calcium Phosphatase, alkaline ALT/SGPT AST/SGOT		RPR		T4, Free (Free Thyroxine)	
		CRP (C-Reactive Protein)		T4, (Total Thyroxine)	
		ASO (with titer)		CK - Total	
		H. pylori		Troponin	
☐ HEPATIC FUNCTION PANEL		RA (Rheumatoid factor)		Iron	
		ANA (anti-nucleic antibody)		TIBC (Total Iron Binding Capacity)	
Hepatic Function Panel Includes: Albumin Phosphatase, alkaline Bilirubin, total Protein, total Bilirubin, direct ALT/SGPT AST/SGOT		SSA/SBB		Amylase	
		✔ **URINE PROCEDURES**		Vitamin B-12	
		Urinalysis		Folate	
☐ LIPID PROFILE		Urinalysis Culture w/sensitivity		Digoxin Level	
		24-hour Urine Protein		Theophylline Level	
Lipid Profile Includes: Cholesterol Triglycerides HDL LDL		24-hour Urine Creatinine with clearance		**OTHER PROCEDURES**	
MICROBIOLOGY & CULTURES		24-hour Urine, Creatinine		1.	
Culture, Throat		Random Urine, Sodium		2.	
Culture, Sputum		Random Urine, Potassium		3.	
Strep A Screen (swab)		Random Urine, Chloride		4.	
Gram Stain (Note Source)		Random Urine, Myoglobin		5.	
Source:		Random Urine, Osmolality		6.	
				7.	

Physician's Signature: _____ **Date:** _____

Medicare Advanced Beneficiary Notice

Section 1862(a)(1) of the Medicare Law states that Medicare will only pay for services that it determines are "reasonable and necessary." If the service is determined not to be "reasonable and necessary" by Medicare program standards, payment will be denied.

Medical Record - White Copy   Lab - Yellow Copy   Physician's Office - Pink Copy

Form #1258   Revised 6/02

FIGURE 1-5 Example of a laboratory request form

agency, which evaluates them for accuracy and for the laboratory's performance compared to other laboratories in the program.

Participation in a PT program is an important part of a laboratory's QA program and allows the laboratory to have confidence in testing methods and to identify deficient areas. The PT agency provides documentation of performance for accrediting and regulatory agencies.

Accreditation

Accreditation is a voluntary process by which an independent agency grants recognition to institutions or programs that meet or exceed established standards of quality. Most health care institutions seek accreditation because it enhances the institution's reputation and gives the public a way to assess the institution's quality of care.

An institution desiring accreditation invites the accrediting agency to inspect its facility to determine if established standards are being met. Several agencies accredit hospitals and departments within hospitals, including the Joint Commission (JC), College of American Pathologists (CAP), American Association of Blood Banks (AABB), and the Commission on Office Laboratory Accreditation (COLA) (Table 1-5 and Appendix D). These agencies have deemed status with CMS, which means that accreditation by these agencies is recognized as meeting all government standards under CLIA '88.

PRIVACY ISSUES

In 1996, Congress passed the Health Insurance Portability and Accountability Act (HIPAA). From this act, a privacy rule was issued, providing federal protections for personal health information and guaranteeing a patient's right to privacy. This was a response to the potential for loss of privacy created by the increased use and availability of electronic patient records as computers came into wider use in health care recordkeeping. The privacy rule requires health care facilities to use all necessary measures and procedures to ensure that patient information remains private and confidential. At the same time, the rule permits disclosure of information that is needed for patient care. All health care agencies now request that a patient be informed of their privacy rights, and patients must give written permission for health information to be shared, even with family members.

Much communication in laboratories and health care institutions is facilitated by computers. Most laboratories have a central laboratory computer information system through which tests are requested and test results are reported and entered into a database. Use of computers in health care contributes to efficiency and improved patient care. However, it also presents the opportunity for violation of patient privacy, whether intentional or unintentional. Computers with patient information must be password protected so that only authorized persons can access information. Computer monitors should be positioned so that visitors, other patients, and nonauthorized-personnel cannot view the screen. The use of specimen identification codes, instead of patient names, helps protect patient privacy.

It must be emphasized to employees that all patient information must remain private and confidential, and must be shared only with authorized persons to facilitate and improve patient care.

TABLE 1-5. Accrediting agencies with deemed status under CLIA '88.

ACCREDITING AGENCY	ENTITIES ELIGIBLE FOR ACCREDITATION
Joint Commission (JC)	Hospitals
College of American Pathologists (CAP)	Clinical laboratories
American Association of Blood Banks (AABB)	Blood bank departments
Commission on Office Laboratory Accreditation (COLA)	POLs

CRITICAL THINKING

Timothy is a medical assistant working in a small POL. His laboratory operates under a certificate of waiver. The physician requests a microscopic examination of urine for patient Mary Smith. During Timothy's medical assistant training, he learned to perform microscopic examination of urine, classified by CLIA as a moderate complexity test.

1. What is the appropriate action for Timothy to take?
   a. Tell the physician that it is not possible to have the test performed.
   b. Send the specimen to a laboratory approved for performing moderate- to high-complexity testing.
   c. Perform the test and report the results to the physician.

2. Explain your answer.

SUMMARY

Clinical laboratories are found both in hospitals and in nonhospital settings. Laboratories must meet specific qualifications to gain government permission to operate. They are regulated by CLIA '88, which contains standards and regulations designed to protect patients, laboratory personnel and other health care workers, and society as a whole. The aims are to ensure that laboratory tests are done in a manner that assures reliable results and to be sure that laboratory employees work in a safe, healthy environment. Laboratory personnel must also adhere to HIPAA guidelines that guarantee protection of patient privacy.

The clinical laboratory is a dynamic workplace and an important partner on the health care team. As rapid changes continue in medical technology and health care delivery systems, laboratories must be able to adjust to future trends. The increase in POCT and use of computerized accessioning methods are two examples of current laboratory trends.

The organization of a clinical laboratory is determined by the size of the laboratory, the types and number of tests performed, and the qualifications of personnel. Hospital laboratories usually contain several departments, such as hematology, chemistry, microbiology, and blood bank. Each department is responsible for performing specific tests in its area and maintaining a QA program.

The clinical laboratory has a role in fostering good channels of communication in the laboratory and also between the laboratory and physicians, other departments in the hospital, and other health care providers. By educating health care partners about clinical laboratory medicine, such as appropriateness of tests and interpreting and understanding laboratory test results, the best interest of the patient is served.

REVIEW QUESTIONS

1. What is the function of a clinical laboratory?
2. Draw an organizational chart of a typical hospital laboratory.
3. Name five major departments found in a hospital laboratory.
4. Name two procedures performed in the hematology department.
5. Name two tests performed in the chemistry department.
6. How does the HIPAA affect workers in the laboratory?

7. List three locations of clinical laboratory facilities other than in hospitals.
8. Explain the job functions of the laboratory director, technical supervisor, and department head or general supervisor.
9. What is the purpose of CLIA '88?
10. What federal agency is responsible for implementing CLIA '88?
11. What are waived tests?
12. List the five certificates issued under CLIA '88, and state the activities each certificate permits.
13. What is the advantage of proficiency testing?
14. How do laboratories become accredited?
15. Define accessioning, accreditation, American Association of Blood Banks, bacteriology, blood bank, Centers for Disease Control and Prevention, Centers for Medicare and Medicaid Services, Clinical and Laboratory Standards Institute, clinical chemistry, Clinical Laboratory Improvement Amendments of 1988, coagulation, College of American Pathologists, Commission on Office Laboratory Accreditation, Department of Health and Human Services, epidemiology, Food and Drug Administration, Health Care Financing Administration, hematology, HIPAA, immunohematology, immunology, Joint Commission, Laboratory Response Network, microbiology, mycology, National Committee for Clinical Laboratory Standards, parasitology, pathologist, phlebotomist, plasma, point-of-care testing, physician office laboratory, Provider-Performed Microscopy Procedure, proficiency testing, quality assessment, reference laboratory, serology, serum, and virology.

STUDENT ACTIVITIES

1. Complete the written examination on this lesson.
2. Interview an employee of a clinical laboratory. Inquire about the laboratory's organization and the types of tests performed. Obtain various laboratory test report forms and note the types of tests performed in each department.
3. Tour a hospital or reference laboratory in your area.
4. Visit a POL and find out what types of tests are performed there.

WEB ACTIVITIES

1. Select five analytes from Table 1-2. Visit the CMS Web site and list the brands of test kits that qualify as waived for each of the five.
2. Visit the CDC Web site and obtain information about the LRN. Describe the levels of laboratories in the program and the ways in which various laboratories participate.
3. Find Web sites of three clinical laboratories. Note the types of information provided on each Web site.

The Clinical Laboratory Professional

LESSON OBJECTIVES

After studying this lesson, the student will:

- Give a brief history of medical technology.
- List five personal qualities that are desirable in a clinical laboratory professional.
- Describe the educational requirements for clinical laboratory scientists/medical technologists and clinical laboratory technicians/medical laboratory technicians.
- Discuss the relationship between the laboratory professional and the patient.
- Explain the laboratory professional's responsibility in relation to patient privacy.
- Explain the functions of accrediting agencies and credentialing agencies.
- Explain the purpose and benefits of professional societies.
- Discuss rules and importance of ethical conduct for laboratory professionals.
- Name five areas of employment for clinical laboratory professionals other than in hospital laboratories.
- Define the glossary terms.

GLOSSARY

American Association of Medical Assistants (AAMA) / professional society and credentialing agency for medical assistants

American Medical Technologists (AMT) / professional society and credentialing agency for clinical laboratory personnel

American Society for Clinical Laboratory Science (ASCLS) / professional society and credentialing agency for clinical laboratory personnel

American Society for Clinical Pathology (ASCP) / professional society and credentialing agency for clinical laboratory personnel and allied health personnel

American Society of Phlebotomy Technicians (ASPT) / professional society and credentialing agency for phlebotomists

clinical laboratory science / the health profession concerned with performing laboratory analyses used in diagnosing and treating disease, as well as in maintaining good health; the field of medical laboratory technology

clinical laboratory scientist (CLS) / a professional who has a baccalaureate degree from an accredited college or university, has completed clinical training in an accredited clinical laboratory science program, and has passed a national certifying examination; medical technologist

clinical laboratory technician (CLT) / a professional who has completed a minimum of two years of specific training in an accredited clinical laboratory technician program and has passed a national certifying examination; medical laboratory technician

Commission on Accreditation of Allied Health Education Programs (CAAHEP) / agency that accredits educational programs for clinical laboratory personnel; formerly CAHEA

ethics / a system of conduct or behavior; rules of professional conduct

Health Insurance Portability and Accountability Act (HIPAA) / 1996 act of Congress, a part of which guarantees protection of privacy of an individual's health information

medical laboratory technician (MLT) / clinical laboratory technician

medical technologist (MT) / clincal laboratory scientist

medical technology / clinical laboratory science

National Accrediting Agency for Clinical Laboratory Sciences (NAACLS) / agency that accredits educational programs for clinical laboratory personnel

National Credentialing Agency for Laboratory Personnel (NCA) / credentialing agency for clinical laboratory personnel

National Phlebotomy Association (NPA) / professional society and credentialing agency for phlebotomists

INTRODUCTION

Clinical laboratory science, or **medical technology**, is the health profession concerned with performing laboratory analyses. Information gained from the analyses is used in diagnosing and treating disease, as well as in maintaining good health. The analyses are performed by trained, skilled clinical laboratory personnel.

What do these clinical laboratory personnel do? They work as medical detectives. They use microscopes to observe changes in cells. They test blood to find compatible blood for transfusions. They use special stains to identify microorganisms and analyze cells. They measure substances such as glucose and cholesterol in the blood. They discover and identify organisms causing infections. They operate complex instruments. They use standards and controls to ensure reliable results. They work under pressure. They work with speed, accuracy, and precision. They adhere to high ethical standards.

This lesson examines the role the clinical laboratory professional plays in today's health care setting. The personal and educational qualifications required, job responsibilities, employment opportunities, ethics, and professionalism are all discussed.

HISTORY OF MEDICAL TECHNOLOGY

The origins of medical technology can be traced back several centuries. Papyrus writings dating before 1000 B.C. record descriptions of intestinal parasites, an early example of parasitology. Before medieval times, Hindu doctors performed crude urinalyses when they observed that some urine had a sweet taste and attracted ants. With the invention of the microscope in the seventeenth century, the study of biological specimens progressed from simple visual examination to microscopic examination.

Early Clinical Laboratories

The first clinical laboratories in the United States appeared in the late nineteenth century and, by today's standards, were very primitive. Some consisted of only a table and a microscope. They were staffed mostly by doctors who had a special interest in "laboratory medicine." The 1900 U.S. census listed only 100 laboratory technicians, all male.

Modern Clinical Laboratories

After World War I, laboratories grew in size and number. It soon became clear that there was a need for:

- Educating laboratory workers
- Defining educational requirements
- Identifying adequately trained persons

By the 1930s, basic educational requirements had been established and schools of medical technology were training laboratory workers. Certifying examinations were given to measure the knowledge and ability of workers.

Since World War II, rapid changes in technology have been incorporated into testing methods in the clinical laboratory. Laboratory tests have become increasingly sophisticated. Specially trained laboratory workers have come to make up a majority of the laboratory work force. Laboratory tests have come to play an even more essential role in medicine. Tests that were formerly tedious and time-consuming have become obsolete as they have been replaced by more efficient technologies. Laboratory workers no longer have to inoculate laboratory animals to diagnose certain infectious diseases. Tests that once required elaborate, multi-step chemical assays have become streamlined and miniaturized. The introduction of the computer into the laboratory has saved time and decreased errors. The array of analytes that can be tested has increased dramatically.

Clinical Laboratory Science in the Twenty-First Century

The term *clinical laboratory science* has largely replaced the term *medical technology* because it more accurately reflects the profession and the field today. In all health care fields, today's technology provides a level of health care only imagined a few years ago. Changes are continually occurring as the roles of laboratory personnel are redefined and as technology advances. New trends are emerging, such as emphases on wellness, geriatric medicine, and home health care and hospice rather than long hospital stays. Laboratory instruments incorporate state-of-the-art technologies such as micro- and nano-technology components, flow cytometry, and laser imaging. These technologies allow rapid testing and portable testing. The field of clinical laboratory science continues to change and broaden in response to federal regulations, changes in health care needs, and new technologies.

ROLE OF THE LABORATORY PROFESSIONAL IN TODAY'S HEALTH CARE SETTING

The clinical laboratory professional is an integral partner in allied health care. Laboratory workers are found in many types of health care settings, from the local health fair to the sophisticated laboratories of the Centers for Disease Control and Prevention (CDC) where exotic, emerging diseases are studied. The most visible laboratory professional is the worker in the hospital laboratory. These workers daily interact with others on the health care team—physicians, nursing staff, therapists, and various other health care team members—to provide quality patient care.

The work of laboratory professionals is important whether they are employed in a large laboratory or a small one. Personnel staffing large laboratories include highly skilled professionals, such as clinical laboratory scientists/medical technologists or clinical laboratory technicians/medical technicians (Figure 1-6). Smaller laboratories, especially those performing only waived tests, are often staffed by multi-skilled personnel who may be trained to perform some laboratory tests as well as nursing and office procedures. These personnel can be medical assistants or laboratory assistants or have varying levels of nursing training.

REQUIREMENTS FOR CERTIFIED CLINICAL LABORATORY PROFESSIONALS

Completion of an approved course of study and successful completion of a national certifying examination are required to become a certified clinical laboratory professional. Most large clinical laboratories employ clinical workers at several levels, each requiring different education, training, and skill levels. CLIA '88 defines the personnel qualifications required for laboratory workers based

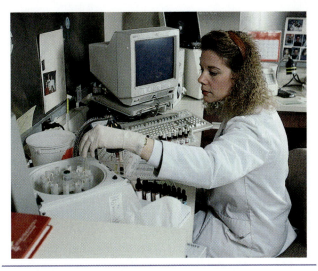

FIGURE 1-6 A clinical laboratory professional at work (*Photo by Marcia Butterfield, courtesy of W. A. Foote Memorial Hospital, Jackson, MI*)

on the job functions associated with the position. Some positions require only a high school education and documented on-the-job training. However, most laboratories performing moderate- to high-complexity testing desire employees who have completed a prescribed program of study in clinical laboratory science.

Educational Programs and Accrediting Agencies

Several types of programs of study are available through hospitals; colleges and universities; technical schools; and private, independent schools. The programs usually consist of an academic component and a clinical component.

Several organizations and agencies are involved in establishing and maintaining the principles and standards of the clinical laboratory profession. Independent agencies such as the **Commission on Accreditation of Allied Health Education Programs (CAAHEP)** and the **National Accreditating Agency for Clinical Laboratory Sciences (NAACLS)**, provide accreditation for clinical laboratory professional programs. Accredited educational programs must meet nationally established standards. Examples of agencies that accredit educational programs are listed in Table 1-6 and Appendix D.

TABLE 1-6. Examples of agencies that accredit programs for clinical laboratory personnel

CAAHEP	Commission on Accreditation of Allied Health Education Programs (formerly CAHEA)
NAACLS	National Accrediting Agency for Clinical Laboratory Sciences
NCCA	National Commission for Certifying Agencies

Educational Requirements for Clinical Laboratory Scientists and Technicians

The two most common levels of professionals working in the hospital or reference laboratory are:

- **Clinical laboratory scientist (CLS) / medical technologist (MT)**
- **Clinical laboratory technician (CLT) / medical laboratory technician (MLT)**

Clinical Laboratory Scientist/ Medical Technologist

The CLS or MT generally has a baccalaureate degree from a college or university and has completed specified clinical training in an accredited clinical laboratory science program. To become certified, the individual must also pass a national examination. Certified CLSs are qualified to perform analyses in all departments of the laboratory. These individuals can also be supervisors or work in other leadership positions in the laboratory.

Clinical Laboratory Technician/ Medical Laboratory Technician

The CLT or MLT generally has an associate's degree from a college or a certificate from an accredited CLT program. Upon passing a national certifying examination, the CLT is certified.

Areas of Specialization

Employees can specialize in one area of laboratory work such as microbiology, hematology, or blood banking. To obtain specialist rank, such as specialist in hematology or specialist in blood bank, the employee must complete appropriate academic work, obtain the required number of years of clinical experience, and pass an examination in the specialty area.

Credentialing and Certification of Clinical Laboratory Personnel

Credentialing or certifying agencies are independent organizations that administer examinations for different levels of laboratory professionals. These include the **American Society for Clinical Pathology (ASCP)**, the **National Credentialing Agency for Laboratory Personnel (NCA)**, and the **American Medical Technologists (AMT)** (Table 1-7).

Agencies differ somewhat in titles used for equivalent training. For instance, the qualifications are the same for CLS (NCA) and MT (ASCP), although the professional designations differ. Table 1-8 gives the designations used by the NCA and the equivalent designations used by the ASCP. Designations are sometimes confusing because there are several certifying agencies. Information about specific eligibility requirements for certification categories can be obtained from the individual certifying agencies. Addresses of these organizations are given in Appendix D.

TABLE 1-7. Some credentialing/certifying agencies for clinical laboratory and other allied health personnel

AAB	American Association of Bioanalysts Board of Registry
AAMA	American Association of Medical Assistants
AMT	American Medical Technologists
ASCP	American Society for Clinical Pathology
ASPT	American Society of Phlebotomy Technicians
NCA	National Credentialing Agency (for Laboratory Personnel)
NPA	National Phlebotomy Association

TABLE 1-8. NCA certification categories and equivalent ASCP certification categories

NCA DESIGNATION	ASCP DESIGNATION
CLS, clinical laboratory scientist	MT, medical technologist
CLT, clinical laboratory technician	MLT, medical laboratory technician
CLSp, clinical laboratory specialist	S, specialist
CLSup, clinical laboratory supervisor	DLM, diplomate in laboratory management
CLPlb, clinical laboratory phlebotomist	PBT, phlebotomy technician

Licensing of Clinical Laboratory Personnel

Although certification is usually sufficient to meet most employment requirements, some states regulate laboratory personnel by requiring workers to obtain a state license. Licensing laws vary from state to state and are nonexistent in some states. Some states require a fee to obtain a license, or that a test be taken before the license is issued; some states require both.

OTHER ALLIED HEALTH PERSONNEL IN THE CLINICAL LABORATORY

Along with the emergence of point-of-care testing (POCT) as an important part of the health care delivery system, a large number of Clinical Laboratory Improvement Amendments of 1988 (CLIA) waived tests have been developed. This has resulted in an expansion of the types of personnel who perform laboratory analyses. Where traditionally mostly CLS/MTs and CLT/MLTs performed these tests, waived testing is now being performed by paramedics, medical assistants, registered nurses, and licensed practical nurses. These individuals provide health care in a variety of settings from the patient's home to the physician's office and the hospital emergency room. Allied health personnel, other than nursing staff, who might perform certain laboratory tests include:

- Phlebotomist/phlebotomy technician (PBT)/clinical laboratory phlebotomist (CLPlb)
- Medical assistant/certified medical assistant/registered medical assistant
- Physician office laboratory technician
- Clinical laboratory assistant
- Biotechnology laboratory technician
- Point-of-care technician

The educational requirements, program of study, and job responsibilities differ for each of these personnel. The programs for phlebotomists and medical assistants are briefly described in this lesson. Information on programs for other categories of personnel may be found by contacting the certifying agency for each career (these are listed in Table 1-7 and Appendix D).

Phlebotomist (Phlebotomy Technician, Clinical Laboratory Phlebotomist)

Phlebotomists are trained to collect blood specimens for laboratory testing. Training programs require a high school diploma or general equivalency diploma (GED) for entrance. After the training program is complete, certification is available through several organizations following successful completion of a national examination. Examples of phlebotomist certifying organizations and professional designations are:

- **AMT (American Medical Technologists)**: registered phlebotomy technician (RPT)
- **ASCP (American Society for Clinical Pathology)**: phlebotomy technician (PBT)
- **ASPT (American Society of Phlebotomy Technicians)**: phlebotomist
- NCA (National Credentialing Agency for Laboratory Personnel): clinical laboratory phlebotomist (CLPlb)
- **NPA (National Phlebotomy Association)**: certified phlebotomy technician (CPT)

Medical Assistant (Certified Medical Assistant, Registered Medical Assistant)

Medical assistants are allied health professionals frequently employed in ambulatory care settings such as physician office laboratories (POLs) and who have been trained in administrative, clerical, nursing, and laboratory skills. They collect blood specimens and perform some waived tests such as hemoglobin, hematocrit, chemical urine testing, pregnancy tests, blood glucose, and fecal occult blood.

Training for medical assistants is available through community colleges and vocational-technical and private schools. A high school diploma or GED is required for entrance. There are two levels of education for medical assistants. One is a diploma program requiring 1 year of post-secondary education; the other is an associate of science degree, consisting of 2 years of post-secondary education. Upon completion of the course of study, certification is obtained by passing a national examination administered by a certifying organization. Two such organizations and their certification designations are:

- **AAMA (American Association of Medical Assistants)**: certified medical assistant (CMA)
- AMT (American Medical Technologists): registered medical assistant (RMA)

ETHICS AND PROFESSIONALISM

Clinical laboratory personnel are expected to subscribe to high ethical standards and to exhibit professionalism in their appearance, behavior, and work.

Ethics and the Clinical Laboratory Professional

Clinical laboratory personnel must observe professional **ethics**, a prescribed code of conduct and behavior. Organizations that credential health care professionals have codes of ethics to which their members are expected to subscribe. One example is the code of ethics for laboratory professionals adopted by the **American Society for Clinical Laboratory Science (ASCLS)**. A portion is shown in Table 1-9.

The principles in this code stress that laboratory professionals have a duty to patients, colleagues, their profession, and society. Laboratory professionals have an obligation to the patient to:

- Provide a high quality of service and maintain high standards of practice

TABLE 1-9. Portion of code of ethics of the American Society for Clinical Laboratory Science (Reprinted with permission of American Society for Clinical Laboratory Science, Bethesda, MD)

As a clinical laboratory professional, I acknowledge my professional responsibility to:

- Maintain and promote standards of excellence in performing and advancing the art and science of my profession;
- Preserve the dignity and privacy of patients;
- Uphold and maintain the dignity and respect of the profession;
- Contribute to the general well-being of the community; and
- Actively demonstrate my commitment to these responsibilities throughout my professional life.

- Exercise sound judgment in establishing, performing, and evaluating laboratory testing
- Maintain strict confidentiality of patient information
- Safeguard the privacy and dignity of patients
- Strive to safeguard the patient from incompetent practice by others

The laboratory professional has an obligation to their colleagues and to their profession to:

- Maintain a reputation of honesty, integrity, and reliability
- Maintain dignity and respect for the profession
- Contribute to the advancement of the profession
- Establish cooperative and respectful working relationships with other health care professionals

They have a responsibility to society to:

- Use their professional competence to contribute to the general well-being of the community
- Comply with laws and regulations pertaining to the practice of clinical laboratory science
- Encourage all in the profession to meet high standards of care and practice

The principles and ideals expressed in the ASCLS code of ethics are applicable to ethical behavior for all health care workers. By adhering to principles such as those given here, the foremost objective—maintaining the safety and well-being of the patient—can be achieved.

Qualities Desirable in Laboratory Professionals

Certain personal qualities are desirable in all health care professionals. These include dedication, dependability, cooperation, competence, discretion, and a caring attitude. Communication skills, honesty, and the ability to relate well to fellow workers are also desirable qualities.

Additional personal qualities and physical capabilities are needed by laboratory personnel to succeed in the clinical laboratory profession. These include physical stamina, good eyesight, manual dexterity, a good intellect, and an aptitude for the biological sciences. Laboratory workers must be observant, motivated, capable of performing precise manipulations and calculations, and also must have good organizational skills.

Personal appearance is important for all health care workers, including laboratory personnel. Workers should present a clean, neat, and professional appearance. This inspires patients' confidence in the worker. Laboratories have rules of dress, and many of the rules relate directly to safety practices. For instance, closed-toed shoes are required—this prevents injury to the feet from accidental spills or breakage. Wearing loose, dangling jewelry is not allowed because it can cause patient injury, harbor microorganisms, or get caught in instruments. Other rules of dress are related to patient welfare; personnel are discouraged from wearing strongly scented personal products to prevent problems for patients who are sensitive or allergic to strong scents. Lessons 1-5 and 1-6 contain further information on appropriate laboratory apparel.

Patient Privacy/Confidentiality

Laboratory professionals carry out their duty to the patient by providing competent service and maintaining high standards. One important principle that *must* be adhered to is that of patient privacy. Patient information is confidential. It must only be discussed with health care employees directly related to the case who have a "need to know" in order to improve patient care. Elevators, cafeterias, or lounges are not appropriate places to discuss patient results or unusual findings.

The reliance on computers in health care has made access to patient information easier for health care workers. However, the use of computers also presents a risk of private information being improperly accessed. Although these advances make information transfer easier, appropriate security measures must be in place to protect patient data from inappropriate access and uses (Figure 1-7).

The privacy rule under the **Health Insurance Portability and Accountability Act (HIPAA)** describes the patient's right to privacy as well as the conditions under which patient information can be shared in order to provide the best possible health care. Each employee must be informed of their employer's privacy policies and procedures and must follow those procedures.

Interactions Between Clinical Laboratory Personnel and Patients

Often, the only contact patients have with the laboratory is through the laboratory assistant, technologist, or phlebotomist who collects a blood sample from them. At best, it is not pleasant to have blood taken from a vein or finger. The laboratory professional needs to be aware at all times of the stress a patient may be

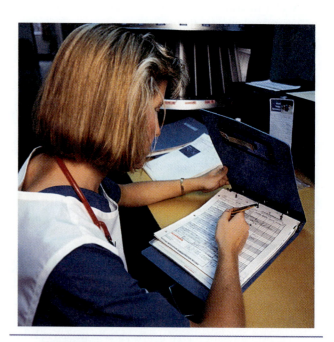

FIGURE 1-7 A patient's right to privacy must be maintained when accessing patient records

feeling when hospitalized or ill. The employee must be professional, courteous, patient, and considerate of patients.

Professional Organizations

Several professional societies for clinical laboratory professionals provide opportunities for professional growth and continuing education by offering workshops and seminars and by publishing journals (Table 1-10). Several journals and journal articles can be found on-line; other journals are available only in print. Some print journals are *Laboratory Medicine, ADVANCE for Medical*

Laboratory Professionals (free subscription), *Clinical Laboratory Science*, and *Medical Laboratory Observer* (free subscription).

Membership in a national society usually also includes membership in that society's state affiliate. A listing of several professional societies can be found in Appendix D. Membership and participation in the activities of a professional society contribute to the continuing competence of the laboratory professional.

Laboratory professionals carry out their duty to colleagues and their profession through professional improvement activities, cooperation, and respect for their colleagues. Through competent practice of their profession, they contribute to the well-being of the community.

Employment Opportunities

Many employment opportunities exist for clinical laboratory professionals. Many of the nation's clinical laboratory workers are employed in hospitals as technologists, supervisors, or laboratory directors or administrators. Other areas of employment include physician offices, clinics, public health agencies, reference laboratories, the military, research, education, veterinary medicine, and pharmaceutics. Laboratory professionals are also employed in sales, product development, and technical service departments of medical suppliers and manufacturers.

SUMMARY

Clinical laboratory professionals are key members of today's health care team. As for all other areas of health care, the field of clinical laboratory science exists for the patient. Every day, nurses, physicians, and other health care workers rely on laboratory professionals to test blood and other body fluids, interpret test

TABLE 1-10. Professional societies for clinical laboratory and other allied health personnel

AAB	American Association of Bioanalysts
AABB	American Association of Blood Banks
AACC	American Association of Clinical Chemistry
AAMA	American Association of Medical Assistants
AMT	American Medical Technologists
APIC	Association of Practitioners in Infection Control
ASCLS	American Society for Clinical Laboratory Science
ASCP	American Society for Clinical Pathology
ASM	American Society for Microbiology
ASPT	American Society of Phlebotomy Technicians
CLMA	Clinical Laboratory Management Association
NPA	National Phlebotomy Association

CASE STUDY

John works in the laboratory at the Bay Regional Hospital. Each work day, before he begins his duties in the laboratory, he helps collect blood from hospital patients. On one occasion, the patient on his collection list was his friend Louis, who had been hospitalized the night before. John collected blood from Louis for several laboratory tests and chatted with him briefly before returning to the laboratory.

After John got home that evening, he received a call from Sally, asking for information about Louis, their mutual friend, who she heard was in the hospital. Sally said she had called the hospital but could get no information about Louis or even confirmation that he had been admitted to the hospital. Sally asked John if he knew if Louis was in the hospital and why.

1. How should John respond to Sally?
2. What are his options?
3. What are his obligations?

Role-play the conversation between John and Sally and/or Louis.

results, and help provide a complete picture of a patient's health. For a patient to receive the best possible care, a correct diagnosis must be made. Physicians rely on these laboratory analyses, along with information gained from the medical history, physical examination, and clinical symptoms to make a diagnosis. Therefore, it is imperative that laboratory analyses be performed carefully and accurately by well-trained, capable laboratory personnel.

Set rules and regulations govern health care in the United States. Health care agencies have very specific standards, rules, and regulations governing the educational requirements and job responsibilities of health care employees. In laboratories performing tests of moderate to high complexity, the personnel performing these tests are clinical laboratory scientists or technicians. These laboratory professionals are required to complete a prescribed program of study and become certified through examination to qualify for this employment. Waived tests can be performed by other allied health personnel such as medical assistants, laboratory assistants, and physician office assistants. All laboratory personnel are expected to strive to provide the best possible patient care, to protect patient privacy, and to exhibit professional and ethical behavior at all times.

Laboratory professionals work in a variety of settings, from hospitals, physician's offices, and community health fairs, to research laboratories. Whatever the setting, the laboratory professionals are working to improve patient care by providing precise and valuable information used in the diagnosis, treatment, and prevention of disease.

REVIEW QUESTIONS

1. What is clinical laboratory science? What is the other term used for this field?
2. Describe the beginnings of medical technology.
3. What are five personal qualities desirable in clinical laboratory personnel?
4. What are the educational requirements for clinical laboratory scientists? For clinical laboratory technicians?
5. List five places of employment for laboratory personnel other than in hospitals.
6. Explain the importance of ethical standards in the practice of clinical laboratory science.
7. Explain the laboratory professional's obligation to the patient.
8. How do laboratory professionals become certified?
9. What is the importance of professional societies to the clinical laboratory professional?
10. Define American Association of Medical Assistants, American Medical Technologists, American Society for Clinical Laboratory Science, American Society for Clinical Pathology, American Society of Phlebotomy Technicians, clinical laboratory science, clinical laboratory scientist, clinical laboratory technician, Commission on Accreditation of Allied Health Education Programs, ethics, Health Insurance Portability and Accountability Act, medical laboratory technician, medical technologist, medical technology, National Accrediting Agency for Clinical Laboratory Sciences, National Credentialing Agency for Laboratory Personnel, and National Phlebotomy Association.

STUDENT ACTIVITIES

1. Complete the written examination for this lesson.
2. Use the interview fact sheet and interview a clinical laboratory professional. Be sure to consider the following areas: job functions, relationship with coworkers and patients, advantages and disadvantages of job, satisfactions, dissatisfactions, salary, and opportunities for advancement. Describe the benefits of talking to the laboratory worker in person rather than reading the information in a book.

WEB ACTIVITIES

1. Visit the Web sites of three agencies or professional societies listed in Tables 1-7 and 1-10. List the programs they certify and the educational requirements of each program.
2. Search the Internet to find a school in your state (or nearby state) that offers training for clinical laboratory scientists. Find out what required courses are listed in the curriculum.
3. Complete a career information fact sheet for the careers of clinical laboratory technician and clinical laboratory scientist. Use this text, other available texts, and the Internet to gather your information. For each, include educational training, cost of program, nature of job, advantages and disadvantages, employment opportunities, and salary range.

Career Information Fact Sheet

LESSON 1-2 The Clinical Laboratory Professional

Name _____   Date _____

Complete this fact sheet using information from this text, other texts, and the Internet.

Job Title:

Legal Requirement:

Name of Program:

    Educational Institution:

    Cost of Program:

    Length of Program:

    Admission Requirements:

Nature of the Job:

    Earnings:

    Advancement:

    Related Occupation(s):

    Advantages:

    Disadvantages:

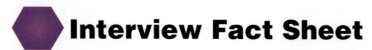

Interview Fact Sheet

LESSON 1-2 The Clinical Laboratory Professional

Name _____ Date _____

Interview a laboratory professional using this sheet as a guide to your questions.

Job Title:

Educational Preparation:

Approximate Cost of Education Program:

Job Functions:

Approximate Salary:

Job Satisfaction:

Job Dissatisfaction:

Opportunities for Advancement:

Options Available to Broaden Employment Opportunities:

1-3

Introduction to Medical Terminology

LESSON OBJECTIVES

After studying this lesson, the student will:

- Discuss the importance of health care workers understanding and correctly using medical terms.
- Define stem words from a selected list.
- Define prefixes from a selected list.
- Define suffixes from a selected list.
- Identify common clinical laboratory abbreviations and acronyms from a selected list.
- Pronounce commonly used medical terms from a selected list.
- Define the glossary terms.

GLOSSARY

abbreviation / the shortening of a word, often by removing letters from the end of the word

acronym / combination of the first letters or syllables of a group of words to form a new group of letters that can be pronounced as a word

prefix / modifying word or syllable(s) placed at the beginning of a word

stem / main part of a word; root word; the part of a word remaining after removing the prefix or suffix

suffix / modifying word or syllable(s) placed at the end of a word

terminology / terms used in any specialized field

INTRODUCTION

Most specialized fields have a unique vocabulary or **terminology**. Medical terminology is the study of terms or words used in medicine. Health care workers must know, understand, and be able to correctly use medical terms to carry out instructions and communicate effectively.

This lesson is only an introduction to the structure of medical terms and to abbreviations and acronyms frequently used in the laboratory. Learning medical vocabulary is a long process. Knowledge and proper use of medical terms

evolve and expand as the terms are used in the workplace. Confidence will be gained by frequently using medical terminology in daily activities.

STRUCTURE OF MEDICAL TERMS

Most medical terms are a combination of three word parts—prefixes, suffixes, and stems. The **stem** or root is the main part of the word. A **prefix** is a word or syllable(s) that modifies the stem and is placed at the beginning of the word. A **suffix** is a word or syllable(s) placed at the end of the word and usually describes what happens to the stem. These word parts are usually connected to the stem by a vowel (such as *a*, *i*, or *o*).

Most of the stems, prefixes, and suffixes used in medical terms are derived from Latin or Greek words and have specific meanings which provide clues to the meanings of the terms. By combining various prefixes, stems, and suffixes, many medical terms with precise meanings may be formed.

Not all terms have all three word parts. Some words have only a prefix and a stem or a stem and suffix. All terms, though, will have a stem, or root, word.

If the meanings of commonly used word parts are known, then a new term can often be analyzed to determine the general idea of its meaning. For example, hyperproteinuria can be divided into three word parts: *hyper*, *protein*, *uria*. *Hyper* means an increased amount. *Uria* refers to in the urine. Therefore, the term refers to a condition in which an increased amount of protein is in the urine. By combining these parts to make a word, a medical shortcut has been created. One word describes a condition that would otherwise require a sentence or perhaps a paragraph.

Medical terms, although shorter than sentences, have precise meanings. Sometimes a slight modification, such as alteration of one or two letters, can change the meaning of a word. For example, a *macrocyte* is a cell larger than normal, while a *microcyte* is a cell smaller than normal. It is very important to spell, pronounce, and use medical terms correctly so the intended meaning is conveyed.

Prefixes

Prefixes placed before stem words give more information about the stem, such as location, time, size, or number. For example, *intra*vascular means inside the vessel and *pre*natal refers to something that happens before birth. Table 1-11 contains a list of commonly used prefixes and the definition of each. A sample term using the prefix is also given.

Stems

The stem or root word gives the major subject of the term. For example, in the term *appendi*citis, the stem is "appendi." Therefore, appendicitis means an inflammation (*itis*) of the appendix. In the term endo*card*itis, the root or stem is "card," referring to heart; the term literally means an inflammation (*itis*) within (*endo*) the heart. Commonly used stem words, their definitions, and examples of usage are listed in Table 1-12.

Suffixes

Suffixes are modifiers attached to the end of a stem word. Suffixes usually tell what is happening to the subject of the stem. They often indicate a condition, operation, or symp-

tom. In the term appendectomy, *ectomy* is a suffix that means to cut out or remove by excision. Therefore, an appendectomy is the surgical removal of the appendix. Commonly used suffixes, their definitions, and examples of usage are listed in Table 1-13.

PRONUNCIATION OF MEDICAL TERMS

It is not enough to just understand written medical terms. You must also be able to pronounce them correctly to communicate effectively with others. Correct pronunciation may be easy for some frequently used or short terms, but is often more difficult for longer terms.

Although most medical terms are derived from Greek or Latin, the Greek or Latin pronunciation is not always used. Your medical dictionary can guide you, but different authors sometimes disagree on pronunciations. By listening to others who work with you, you can learn how words are commonly pronounced in your area. Pronunciation will be improved and confidence gained by practice.

ABBREVIATIONS AND ACRONYMS

An **abbreviation** is a shortening of a word, often achieved by removing letters from the end of the word, and sometimes followed by a period. For example, *diff* is the abbreviation for *differential count*. *Staph* is an abbreviation for *Staphylococcus*. The word *hematocrit* is abbreviated by dropping the first two syllables and using the last syllable *crit*.

An **acronym** is a new pronounceable word created from the first letters or syllables of a group of words. *AIDS* is an acronym for *a*cquired *i*mmuno*d*eficiency *s*yndrome; *SIDS* is an acronym for *s*udden *i*nfant *d*eath *s*yndrome.

Abbreviations and acronyms are used commonly in medicine to avoid having to repeatedly write or say several syllables. Some common abbreviations and acronyms used in the clinical laboratory are listed in Table 1-14. Many of these abbreviations will be used in other lessons in this text. Workers should be familiar with frequently used abbreviations and acronyms so physician's orders or instructions can be carried out correctly and patient records are interpreted correctly.

Because of the wide range of topics in the field of health care, sometimes an abbreviation or acronym can have more than one meaning. Therefore, for proper interpretation, one must be very careful to consider the context of usage. For instance, to laboratory personnel *DAT* usually means *direct antiglobulin test*, while to nursing staff it can mean *diet as tolerated*. Table 1-14 does not include abbreviations or acronyms used in prescriptions, nursing, or other areas of health care.

TABLE 1-11. Selected prefixes commonly used in medical terminology

PREFIX	DEFINITION	EXAMPLE OF USAGE	PREFIX	DEFINITION	EXAMPLE OF USAGE
a, an	absent, deficient	anemia	medi	middle	medicephalic
ab	away from	absent	mega	huge, great	megaloblast
ad	toward	adrenal	melan	black	melanoma
ambi	both	ambidextrous	meta	after, next	metamorphosis
aniso	unequal	anisocytosis	micro	small, one-millionth	microscope, microgram
ante	before	antenatal			
ant(i)	against	antibiotic	milli	one-thousandth	millimeter
auto	self	autograft	mon(o)	one, single	monocyte
baso	blue	basophil	morph	shape	morphogenesis
bi	two	binuclear	necro	dead	necrophobia
bio	life	biochemistry	neo	new	neoplasm
brady	slow	bradycardia	neutro	neutral, neither	neutrophil
circum	around	circumnuclear	olig	few	oliguria
co, com, con	with, together	concentrate	orth	straight, normal	orthopedic
contra	against	contraception	pan	all	pandemic
de	down, from	decay	para	beside, accessory to	paramedic
di	two	dimorphic	per	through	percutaneous
dia	through	dialysis	peri	around	pericardium
dipl	double	diplococcus	phago	to eat	phagocyte
dis	apart, away from	disease	poly	many	polyuria
dys	bad, difficult, improper	dysphagia	post	after	postoperative
			pre, pro	before	prenatal
e, ecto, ex	out from	ectoparasite	pseudo	false	pseudo-appendicitis
end(o)	inside, within	endoparasite			
enter(o)	intestine	enterotoxin	psych(o)	mind	psychoanalyst
epi	upon, after	epidermis	py(o)	pus	pyuria
equi	equal	equilibrium	quad(r)	four	quadrangle
glyco	sweet	glycosuria	retro	backward	retroactive
hemi	half	hemisphere	semi	half	semiconscious
hyper	above, excessive	hyperglycemia	steno	narrow	stenothorax
hypo	under, deficient	hypoventilation	sub	under	subcutaneous
infra	beneath	infracostal	super, supra	above	superinfection
inter	among, between	intercostal	syn	together	synergistic
intra	within	intracranial	tachy	swift	tachycardia
iso	equal	isotonic	therm	heat	thermometer
kilo	one thousand	kilogram	trans	through	transport
macr	large	macrocyte	tri	three	trimester
mal	bad, abnormal	malformation	uni	one	unicellular

TABLE 1-12. Selected stems commonly used in medical terminology

STEM	DEFINITION	EXAMPLE OF USAGE	STEM	DEFINITION	EXAMPLE OF USAGE
adeno	gland	lymphadenitis	lip	fat	lipoma
alg	pain	analgesic	lith	stone	cholelithiasis
arter	artery	arteriogram	mening	membrane covering brain	meningitis
arthr	joint	arthritis			
audio	hearing	auditory	morph	shape, form	morphology
brachi	arm	brachial	myel	marrow	myelogram
bronch(i)	air tube in lungs	bronchitis	myo	muscle	myositis
calc	stone	calcify	nephro	kidney	nephrectomy
carcin	cancer	carcinogen	neur	nerve	neurectomy
card	heart	myocardium	onc	tumor	oncology
caud	tail	caudate	ophthal	eye	ophthalmologist
ceph(al)	head	encephalitis	os	mouth	ostium
chol	bile, gall bladder	cholesterol	os, osteo	bone	osteitis
chondr	cartilage	chondroplasia	oto	ear	otitis
chrom	color	chromogen	path	disease	pathogen
cran	skull	craniotomy	phleb	vein	phlebitis
cut	skin	subcutaneous	phob	fear	phobia
cyan	blue	cyanosis	phot	light	photometer
cyst	bladder, bag	cystocele	pneum	air	pneumonitis
cyt(o)	cell	monocyte	pod	foot	pseudopod
dactyl	finger	arachnodactyly	pulm	lung	pulmonary
dent, dont	tooth	orthodontist	ren	kidney	adrenal
derm	skin	dermatitis	rhin	nose	rhinoplasty
edema	swelling	edematous	scler	hard	sclerosis
erythro	red	erythrocyte	sep	poison	septic
febr	fever	afebrile	soma(t)	body	somatic
gastr(o)	stomach	gastritis	sperm	seed	spermato-genesis
genito	reproductive	genital	stoma	mouth, opening	stomatitis
gloss	tongue	glossitis	thorac	chest	thoracotomy
hem(a), haem	blood	hematology	tome	knife	microtome
hepat(o)	liver	hepatitis	tox(i)	poison	toxicology
histo	tissue	histology	ur(o), uria	urine	hematuria
hystero	uterus	hysterectomy	vas	vessel	intravascular
iatro	physician	podiatrist	ven	vein	intravenous

TABLE 1-13. Selected suffixes commonly used in medical terminology

SUFFIX	DEFINITION	EXAMPLE OF USAGE	SUFFIX	DEFINITION	EXAMPLE OF USAGE
algia	pain	neuralgia	opathy, pathia	diease	adenopathy
blast	primitive, germ	erythroblast	osis	state, condition, increase	leukocytosis
centesis	puncture, aspiration	amniocentesis	ostomy	create an opening	ileostomy
cide	death, killer	bacteriocide	otomy	cut into	phlebotomy
ectomy	excision, cut out	gastrectomy	penia	lack of	leukopenia
emesis	vomiting	hematemesis	phil	affinity for, liking	eosinophil
emia	in the, or of the, blood	bilirubinemia	phyte	plant	dermatophyte
genic	origin, producing	pyogenic	plastic, plasia	to form or mold	hyperplasia
ia	state, condition	anuria	poiesis	to make	hemopoiesis
iasis	process, condition	amebiasis	rrhage	excessive flow	hemorrhage
iole	small	bronchiole	rrhea	flow	diarrhea
itis	inflammation	pharyngitis	scope, scopy	view	arthroscope
lysis	free, breaking down	hemolysis	stasis	same, standing still	hemostasis
oid	resembling, similar to	blastoid	troph(y)	nourishment	hypertrophy
(o)logy	study of	pathology			
oma	tumor	hepatoma			

TABLE 1-14. Abbreviations and acronyms commonly used in clinical laboratories

A	absorbance	diff	leukocyte differential
Ab	antibody	EBV	Epstein-Barr virus
ACT	activated clotting time	EDTA	ethylenediaminetetraacetic acid
AFB	acid-fast bacillus	EIA	enzyme immunoassay
Ag	antigen	EMB	eosin-methylene blue
AHG	anti-human globulin	ESR	erythrocyte sedimentation rate
AIDS	acquired immunodeficiency syndrome	E.U.	Ehrlich units
ALL	acute lymphocytic leukemia	F	Fahrenheit
ALP, AP	alkaline phosphatase	FBS	fasting blood sugar
ALT	alanine aminotransferase (formerly SGPT)	FDP	fibrinogen degradation products
AML	acute myelogenous leukemia	FUO	fever of unknown origin
ANA	anti-nuclear antibody	g	gram
APTT	activated partial thromboplastin time	GC	gonococcus, gonorrhea
ARC	AIDS-related complex	GGT	gamma glutamyl transferase
AST	aspartate aminotransferase (formerly SGOT)	GI	gastrointestinal
BA	blood agar	GTT	glucose tolerance test
bacti	bacteriology	GU	genitourinary
BBP	blood-borne pathogen	HAV	hepatitis A virus
BP	blood pressure	Hb, Hgb	hemoglobin
BSI	body substance isolation	HBV	hepatitis B virus
BT	bleeding time	hCG	human chorionic gonadotropin
BUN	blood urea nitrogen	HCl	hydrochloric acid
C	centigrade, Celsius	HCO_3^-	bicarbonate
CBC	complete blood count	Hct	hematocrit
cc, ccm	cubic centimeter	HCV	hepatitis C virus
CCU	coronary care unit	HDL chol	high-density lipoprotein cholesterol
CFU	colony forming unit	HDN	hemolytic disease of newborn
CGL	chronic granulocytic leukemia	H & H	hemoglobin and hematocrit
chol	cholesterol	HIV	human immunodeficiency virus
CK	creatine kinase	HLA	human leukocyte antigen
Cl	chloride	H_2O	water
CLL	chronic lymphocytic leukemia	HPF	high-power field
CLS	clinical laboratory scientist	HSV	herpes simplex virus
CLT	clinical laboratory technician	ICU	intensive care unit
cm	centimeter	Ig	immunoglobulin
CNS	central nervous system	IgG	immunoglobulin G
CO	carbon monoxide	IgM	immunoglobulin M
CO_2	carbon dioxide	IM	infectious mononucleosis
CPD	citrate-phosphate-dextrose	i.m.	intramuscular
CPK	creatine phosphokinase	ITP	idiopathic thrombocytopenic purpura
crit	hematocrit	IU	international unit
C & S	culture and sensitivity	IV, i.v.	intravenous
CSF	cerebrospinal fluid	K	potassium
cu mm	cubic millimeter, mm^3	kg	kilogram
DAT	direct antiglobulin test	L	liter
DIC	disseminated intravascular coagulation	LD, LDH	lactate dehydrogenase

TABLE 1-14 (Continued). Abbreviations and acronyms commonly used in clinical laboratories

LDL chol	low-density lipoprotein cholesterol		PT	prothrombin time, pro-time
LPF	low-power field		QA	quality assessment
μg	microgram		QC	quality control
μL, μl	microliter		qns	quantity not sufficient
μmol	micromole		qs	quantity sufficient
m	meter		RA	rheumatoid arthritis
M	molar		RBC	red blood cell
MCH	mean cell hemoglobin		RF	rheumatoid factors
MCHC	mean cell hemoglobin concentration		RhIG	Rh immune globulin
MCV	mean cell volume		RIA	radioimmunoassay
mEq	milliequivalent		RNA	ribonucleic acid
mg	milligram		RPR	rapid plasma reagin
MI	myocardial infarction		sed rate	erythrocyte sedimentation rate
MIC	minimum inhibitory concentration		SEM	scanning electron microscope
mIU	milli International Unit		SGOT	serum glutamic oxaloacetic transaminase
mL, ml	milliliter		SGPT	serum glutamic-pyruvic transaminase
MLT	medical laboratory technician		SI	international units (Le Système International d'Unités)
mm	millimeter			
mmol	millimole		SICU	surgical intensive care unit
mol	mole		SP	Standard Precautions
MRI	magnetic resonance imaging		sp. gr.	specific gravity
MRSA	methicillin-resistant *Staphylococcus aureus*		staph	*Staphylococcus*
MSDS	material safety data sheet		stat	immediately
MT	medical technologist		STD	sexually transmitted disease
N	normal, normality		STI	sexually transmitted infection
Na	sodium		strep	*Streptococcus*
NaCl	sodium chloride		STS	serological tests for syphilis
nm	nanometer		TEM	transmission electron microscope
O.D.	optical density		TIA	transient ischemic attack
OGTT	oral glucose tolerance test		TIBC	total iron-binding capacity
O & P	ova and parasites		UA	urinalysis, uric acid
OPIM	other potentially infectious material		UP	Universal Precautions
PCV	packed cell volume		URI	upper respiratory infection
pH	hydrogen ion concentration		UTI	urinary tract infection
PMN	polymorphonuclear neutrophil		UV	ultraviolet
POCT	point-of-care test(ing)		VD	venereal disease
POL	physician office laboratory		VDRL	Venereal Disease Research Laboratory
PP	postprandial		VLDL	very low density lipoproteins
PPE	personal protective equipment		vWF	von Willebrand factor
PPM	parts per million		WBC	white blood cell
PRC	packed red cells		XDP	fibrin degradation products
PSA	prostate specific antigen			

CASE STUDY

On a very busy day, Dr. Martin handed his medical assistant a handwritten preliminary diagnosis and an order for laboratory tests for his patient Mr. Jones. The medical assistant had trouble reading Dr. Martin's handwriting and couldn't decide if the preliminary diagnosis was "temporary arthritis" or "temporal arteritis." Mr. Jones' major symptom was recurring headache and pain in the temple area of the head.

Which preliminary diagnosis is most likely the diagnosis written by Dr. Martin? Discuss the importance of correctly spelling and understanding medical terms.

SUMMARY

Medical terminology encompasses a multitude of special terms with very precise meanings used in the field of medicine. Most medical terms are derived from Greek or Latin. Medical terms are formed by combining prefixes, stems, and suffixes that have specific meanings to produce a term with an exact definition. By learning the meanings of selected prefixes, stems, and suffixes, the worker can deduce the meanings of many medical terms, even if the terms are unfamiliar to the worker.

Clinical laboratory personnel need to understand and be able to use medical terms in both oral and written communications. In addition, personnel should be familiar with several abbreviations and acronyms that are in common use in the laboratory and in laboratory reports. By becoming fluent in medical terminology, personnel will gain confidence in their communication skills.

REVIEW QUESTIONS

1. Why is it important for health care workers to understand medical terminology?

2. What languages are the basis for most medical terms?

3. How can one learn to correctly pronounce medical terms?

4. Name the stems for cell, heart, head, skin, chest, kidney, muscle, liver, and stomach.

5. Name 10 common suffixes and give a meaning for each.

6. Name 10 common prefixes and give a meaning for each.

7. List 10 abbreviations or acronyms frequently used in the clinical laboratory and give the meaning of each.

8. Define abbreviation, acronym, prefix, stem, suffix, and terminology.

STUDENT ACTIVITIES

1. Complete the written examination for this lesson.

2. Practice pronouncing the word parts and medical terms in Tables 1-11 through 1-13. Look up pronunciations of 10 terms from each table and practice saying them out loud.

3. Study the definitions for prefixes, suffixes, and stems listed in the tables. Use each of the prefixes, suffixes, or stems in a word not on the list.

4. Obtain examples of laboratory requisition or report forms. Look for abbreviations or acronyms used on the forms.

WEB 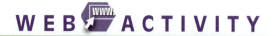 ACTIVITY

Select five terms each from the usage columns in Tables 1-11, 1-12, and 1-13. Write your best definition of the term, using the definitions of stems, prefixes, and suffixes in the tables. Find an online medical dictionary, look up the words, and compare your definitions with the dictionary definitions.

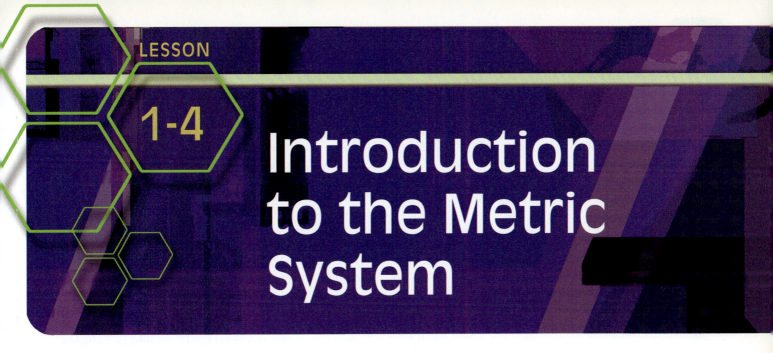

Introduction to the Metric System

LESSON OBJECTIVES

After studying this lesson, the student will:

- Discuss the importance of properly using metric units.
- Name common prefixes used to denote small and large metric units.
- Convert English units to metric units.
- Convert metric units to English units.
- Convert units within the metric system.
- Perform measurements of distance, volume, and weight (mass) using the metric system.
- Make temperature conversions between the Fahrenheit and Celsius scales.
- Define the glossary terms.

GLOSSARY

Celsius (C) scale / temperature scale having the freezing point of water at 0°C and the boiling point at 100°C

centi / prefix used to indicate one-hundredth (10^{-2}) of a unit

deci / prefix used to indicate one-tenth of a unit

English system of measurement / system of measurement in common use in the United States for nonscientific measurements; sometimes called U.S. customary system

Fahrenheit (F) scale / temperature scale having a freezing point of water at 32°F and boiling point at 212°F

gram (g) / basic metric unit of weight or mass

kilo / prefix used to indicate one thousand (10^3) units

liter (L) / basic metric unit of volume

meter (m) / basic metric unit of length or distance

metric system / the decimal system of measurement used internationally for scientific work

micro / prefix used to indicate one-millionth (10^{-6}) of a unit

milli / prefix used to indicate one-thousandth (10^{-3}) of a unit

nano / prefix used to indicate one-billionth (10^{-9}) of a unit

National Institute of Standards and Technology (NIST) / a federal agency that promotes international standardization of measurements; formerly the National Bureau of Standards

pico / prefix used to indicate 10^{-12}

SI units / standardized units of measure; international units

INTRODUCTION

Units of measurements are used frequently in medicine. They are used to measure vital statistics such as height, weight, and body temperature; the amount of fluid intake and output; and dosages of medication. The clinical laboratory uses measurements in almost all aspects of its operations.

Measurements commonly made in the laboratory include:

- Concentration or numbers of substances or cells
- Weight of a substance or object
- Volume of a solution or object
- Size or length of an object
- Temperature
- Time

In the laboratory, time and temperature are most often used to monitor test conditions or procedures. Test results report measurements of concentration, number, weight, volume, and size when indicating numbers and types of cells or indicating quantities of substances in a patient's blood, serum, or other body fluids. These measurements are then compared to reference (normal) values to aid in assessing a patient's condition.

Measurements made in the clinical laboratory can have a direct impact on the quality of patient care. Laboratory results can be a basis for establishing a diagnosis and are also used to follow the course of disease and prescribe appropriate treatment. The measurements must be reliable, accurate, precise, and easily standardized. For this reason, the metric system is used to make laboratory measurements.

SYSTEMS OF MEASUREMENTS

In the United States, two systems of measurements are in common use, the *metric system* and the *English system of measurement,* sometimes called *U.S. customary system.*

English System of Measurement

In everyday life in the United States, the **English system of measurement** is still used for most measurements and observations. Weight is reported in pounds; height, in feet and inches. Cooks use measures such as teaspoon, cup, and pint. Speed is measured in miles per hour. However, the English system of measurement is cumbersome and is not accurate enough for most scientific measurements.

The Metric System

The **metric system** of measurement has been used internationally for scientific work for years. In most countries the metric system is also used in everyday life. Gasoline is purchased by the liter, body weight is measured in kilograms, and distance is expressed in meters or kilometers. Figure 1-8 compares a metric ruler showing centimeters and millimeters with an English style ruler, which shows measurements in inches and fractions of inches.

The metric system is based on a fundamental unit of distance, the **meter (m)**. In this system, the **gram (g)** is the basic unit used to measure mass or weight, and the **liter (L)** is the basic unit used to measure volume. Because the metric system is based on a decimal system, very small quantities can be measured accurately and easily. In the decimal system, units are divided into increments of 10. This means that units larger or smaller than the basic units (meter, liter, and gram) can be obtained by multiplying or dividing by increments of 10.

Although the metric system has been used internationally for laboratory measurements, the units used to report results can differ from country to country or even within countries and among institutions. For example, the concentration of protein can be expressed as grams per liter (g/L) in one laboratory and as grams per deciliter (g/dL) in another. This can be confusing when one is trying to compare laboratory data.

International System of Units (SI Units)

In an effort to standardize scientific measurements worldwide, most countries have adopted the use of **SI units**, from the *International System of Units,* the modern metric system of measurement. The United States adopted this system in 1991, mandating its use in all federal agencies and departments. The **National Institute of Standards and Technology (NIST)**, formerly known as the National Bureau of Standards, is the government agency responsible for assisting in this transition to the uniform use of SI units.

The International System of Units comes from the 200-year old French *Le Système International d'Unités* (hence SI). SI units are derived from the metric system and are based on seven fundamental units, from which commonly used units are derived (Table 1-15). These seven units have internationally agreed-upon values and were selected because they make possible more precise, reproducible measurements.

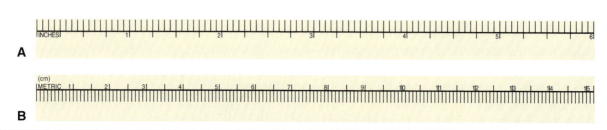

FIGURE 1-8 Comparison of nonmetric or English-style ruler (A) with metric ruler (B)

TABLE 1-15. The seven basic SI units

PROPERTY	UNIT NAME	ABBREVIATION
Length	meter	m
Mass	kilogram	kg
Time	second	s
Electric current	ampere	A
Temperature	Kelvin	K
Luminous intensity	candela	cd
Quantity of substance	mole	mol

TERMINOLOGY OF THE METRIC SYSTEM AND SI UNITS

The SI units most commonly used in medicine are the liter (L), gram (g), meter (m), and mole (mol). By adding prefixes to these terms, one can indicate larger or smaller units (Table 1-16).

For example, **kilo** means 1000. Therefore, a *kilometer* (km) is 1000 meters or 10^3 meters, a *kilogram* (kg) is 1000 grams, and a *kiloliter* (kL) is 1000 liters. Although "kilo" is the prefix most commonly used for large units, "deca" can be used to indicate the unit times 10, as in decaliter. "Hecto" indicates the unit times 100. The prefixes and their definitions are the same for the three basic units.

In laboratory analyses, it is more common to measure units smaller than the basic units. Table 1-16 lists the prefixes and the multiples of the basic unit that each represents. Three common prefixes are **milli**, which means one-thousandth (.001 or 10^{-3}); **centi**, which means one-hundredth (.01 or 10^{-2}); and **deci**, which means one-tenth (0.1). A *milliliter* is .001 liter, or 10^{-3} liter. In chemistry, solutions can be made by adding *milligrams* (mg) of substances to milliliters (mL) of solvent. Analytes can be measured in grams per deciliter (g/dL) or milligrams per deciliter (mg/dL).

Other prefixes commonly used to denote size are **micro**, which denotes one-millionth or 10^{-6}; **nano**, which is 10^{-9}; and **pico**, which is 10^{-12}. Small samples are measured in microliters (μL), which is 10^{-6} liter. Wavelengths of light are measured in nanometers (nm), or 10^{-9} meter.

CONVERSION FACTORS

It is sometimes necessary to convert units within the metric system or to convert English units to metric or metric units to English.

English–Metric Conversions

To make English to metric conversions, it is helpful to have a general idea of the metric equivalents of commonly used English measures. Some of these equivalents are listed in Tables 1-17 and 1-18. To convert units from one system to another, simply multiply by the factor listed. For example, since 1 inch is equal to 2.54 centimeters (cm), 12 inches would equal 12×2.54, or 30.48 cm (Table 1-17). To convert metric units to English units, use Table 1-18 in the same manner. Since 1 kg equals 2.2 pounds, the weight in pounds of a patient weighing 70 kg is determined by multiplying 70×2.2 to equal 154 pounds.

Converting Units Within the Metric System

In laboratory work, it is more common to need to convert units within the metric system. To make these conversions, the worker needs to know equivalents, such as how many milliliters or microliters are in a liter, or how many milligrams are in a gram. These conversions can be made by using the information in Table 1-19.

TABLE 1-16. Commonly used prefixes in the metric system

ABBREVIATION	PREFIX	MEANING	MULTIPLE OF BASIC UNIT	WEIGHT, GRAM (G)	LENGTH, METER (M)	VOLUME, LITER (L)
k	kilo	1000	10^3	kg	km	kL
h	hecto	100	10^2	hg*	hm*	hL*
da	deca	10	10^1	dag*	dam*	daL*
d	deci	.1	10^{-1}	dg*	dm*	dL
c	centi	.01	10^{-2}	cg*	cm	cL*
m	milli	.001	10^{-3}	mg	mm	mL
μ	micro	.000001	10^{-6}	μg	μm	μL
n	nano		10^{-9}	ng	nm	nL*
p	pico		10^{-12}	pg	pm*	pL*

* Units not commonly used in the laboratory

TABLE 1-17. Conversion of English units to metric units

	ENGLISH UNIT	ENGLISH ABBREVIATION		MULTIPLY BY	TO GET METRIC UNIT	METRIC ABBREVIATION
Distance	1 mile	mi	=	1.6	kilometers	km
	1 yard	yd	=	0.9	meters	m
	1 inch	in	=	2.54	centimeters	cm
Mass	1 pound	lb	=	0.454	kilograms	kg
	1 pound	lb	=	454	grams	g
	1 ounce	oz	=	28	grams	g
Volume	1 quart	qt	=	0.95	liters	L
	1 fluid ounce	fl oz	=	30	milliliters	mL
	1 teaspoon	tsp	=	5	milliliters	mL

TABLE 1-18. Conversion of metric units to English units

	METRIC UNIT	METRIC ABBREVIATION		MULTIPLY BY	TO FIND ENGLISH UNIT	ENGLISH ABBREVIATION
Distance	1 kilometer	km	=	0.6	miles	mi
	1 meter	m	=	3.3	feet	ft
	1 meter	m	=	39.37	inches	in
	1 centimeter	cm	=	0.4	inches	in
	1 millimeter	mm	=	0.04	inches	in
Mass	1 gram	g	=	0.0022	pounds	lb
	1 kilogram	kg	=	2.2	pounds	lb
Volume	1 liter	L	=	1.06	quarts	qt
	1 milliliter	mL	=	0.03	fluid ounces	fl oz

TABLE 1-19. Common metric equivalents

Mass	10^{-3} kg	= 1 g	= 10^3 mg	= $10^6 \mu g$
	10^{-3} g	= 1 mg	= $10^3 \mu g$	= 10^6 ng
	10^{-9} g	= 1 ng	= 10^3 pg	
Volume	10^{-3} kL	= 1 L	= 10^3 mL	= $10^6 \mu L$
	10^{-3} L	= 1 mL	= $10^3 \mu L$	= 10^6 nL
	10^{-1} L	= 1 dL	= 10^2 mL	
Length	10^{-3} km	= 1 m	= 10^3 mm	= $10^6 \mu m$
	10^{-3} m	= 1 mm	= $10^3 \mu m$	= 10^6 nm
	10^{-2} m	= 1 cm	= 10 mm	= $10^4 \mu m$
	10^{-3} mm	= 1 nm	= 10 Å	

Converting to Larger Units

To convert metric units to larger units, such as grams to kilograms or milliliters to liters, the decimal in the original unit is moved to the left for the appropriate number of spaces. For example, to con-vert 50 g to kg, multiply by .001, or move the decimal to the left three places: 50 g = .050 kg. To convert centimeters to meters, multiply by .01, or move the decimal two places to the left: 160 cm = 1.6 m.

Converting to Smaller Units

To convert metric units to smaller units, such as grams to milli-grams or liters to microliters, the decimal in the number is moved to the right the appropriate number of spaces. For example, to convert 5 g to milligrams, multiply by 1000, or move the decimal to the right three places: 5 g = 5000 mg. Scientific notation is often used to make the numbers less bulky and easier to compute. For example, 5 g equals 5,000,000 μg or $5.0 \times 10^6 \mu g$.

STANDARDIZED REPORTING OF LABORATORY RESULTS

The Clinical and Laboratory Standards Institute (CLSI, for-merly NCCLS) has published guidelines for uniform reporting of clinical laboratory results using SI units. (The address for CLSI is given in Appendix D.) By phasing out some previously used metric units and using SI units when reporting laboratory values, data are standardized regionally, nationally, and internationally.

Since these previously used units still occasionally appear in older books, manuals, and laboratory reports, it is important to understand the SI equivalents of these units. Tables 1-20 and 1-21 show SI equivalents for formerly used laboratory units.

The correct units of measurement must be included when reporting all laboratory results. This is especially important during the transition from using traditional units to using SI units. A number by itself is meaningless; it must be accompanied by the unit of measure. For example, the normal blood glucose range has traditionally been listed as 70 to 100 mg/dL. However, in SI units, glucose is reported as millimoles per liter (mmol/L), and glucose of 5.6 mmol/L is in the normal range. A glucose reported simply as 5.6 (omitting the mmol/L unit) would alarm someone accustomed to blood glucose measurements reported in mg/dL.

In other examples, blood cell counts have traditionally been expressed as the number of cells per cubic millimeter (cu mm) of blood. In the SI system, however, cell counts are expressed as number of cells per liter of blood. Chemical substances such as bilirubin or protein, which were expressed as mg per deciliter (dL) or per 100 mL, are now expressed as mg or g per liter, or as micromoles (μmol) or millimoles (mmol) per liter.

TIME AND TEMPERATURE

Units of time and temperature are not reported in metric or SI units. In everyday life the time is usually reported using a 12-hour clock (AM/PM). In laboratory reports, time is often recorded in military time (24-hour clock). Twelve-hour clock and equivalent 24-hour clock times are shown in Table 1-22.

Temperature is measured using either the **Fahrenheit (F) scale** or the **Celsius (C) scale** (Figure 1-9). The Fahrenheit temperature scale has a boiling point of 212°F and a freezing point of 32°F. In the United States, the Fahrenheit scale is used for cooking, measuring body temperature, and reporting weather conditions. The Celsius scale has a boiling point of 100°C and a freezing point of 0°C. It is used for making most scientific tem-

TABLE 1-20. SI equivalents recommended for use in the clinical laboratory

OLD USAGE	SI EQUIVALENT
micron (μ)	micrometer (μm; 10^{-6} meter)
cubic micron (μ^3)	femtoliter (fL; 10^{-15} liter)
micromicrogram ($\mu\mu$g)	picogram (pg; 10^{-12} gram)
microgram (mcg)	microgram (μg; 10^{-6} gram)
angstrom (Å)	nm $\times\ 10^{-1}$
millimicron (mμ)	nanometer (nm; 10^{-9} meter)
lambda (λ)	microliter (μL; 10^{-6} liter)

TABLE 1-21. Examples of using SI units in reporting laboratory test results

TEST	OLD UNIT	SI UNIT
Cell counts	cells/mm³ or cells/cu mm	cells/μL or cells/L
Hematocrit	% (ex: 41%)	percentage expressed as decimal (ex: 0.41)
Hemoglobin	g/dL	g/L
MCV	μ^3	fL
MCH	$\mu\mu$g	pg
MCHC	%	g/dL (or g/L)

TABLE 1-22. Comparison of 24-hour clock (military time) with 12-hour clock

TIME	24-HOUR TIME	TIME	24-HOUR TIME
12:30 AM	0030	12:30 PM	1230
1:30 AM	0130	1:30 PM	1330
2:30 AM	0230	2:30 PM	1430
3:30 AM	0330	3:30 PM	1530
4:30 AM	0430	4:30 PM	1630
5:30 AM	0530	5:30 PM	1730
6:30 AM	0630	6:30 PM	1830
7:30 AM	0730	7:30 PM	1930
8:30 AM	0830	8:30 PM	2030
9:30 AM	0930	9:30 PM	2130
10:30 AM	1030	10:30 PM	2230
11:30 AM	1130	11:30 PM	2330
Noon	1200	Midnight	2400

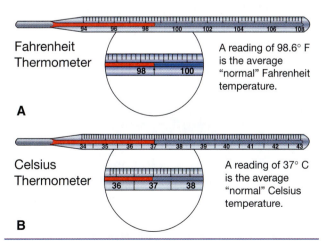

Fahrenheit Thermometer

A reading of 98.6° F is the average "normal" Fahrenheit temperature.

A

Celsius Thermometer

A reading of 37° C is the average "normal" Celsius temperature.

B

FIGURE 1-9 (A) Fahrenheit and (B) Celsius thermometers showing normal body temperature

Problem A: Convert 98.6°F (normal body temperature) to Celsius (C) degrees.

Formula: $C = \dfrac{5}{9}(F - 32)$

Solution: $C = \dfrac{5}{9}(98.6 - 32)$

$C = \dfrac{5}{9}(66.6)$

$C = 36.99$ or 37

Answer: 98.6°F is equal to 37°C

Problem B: Convert 37°C to Fahrenheit (F) degrees.

Formula: $F = \dfrac{9}{5}(C) + 32$

Solution: $F = \dfrac{9}{5}(37) + 32$

$F = 66.6 + 32$

$F = 98.6$

Answer: 37°C is equal to 98.6°F

FIGURE 1-10 Examples of temperature conversions using the formulas. (Problem A) Fahrenheit temperature converted to Celsius, and (Problem B) Celsius temperature converted to Fahrenheit

TABLE 1-23. Temperature conversion chart

°F	=	°C	°F	=	°C	°F	=	°C
23		−5	101		38.3	115		46.1
32		0	102		38.9	116		46.7
70		21.1	103		39.4	117		47.2
75		23.9	104		40	118		47.8
80		26.7	105		40.6	119		48.3
85		29.4	106		41.1	120		48.9
90		32.2	107		41.7	125		51.7
95		35	108		42.2	130		54.4
96		35.6	109		42.8	135		57.2
97		36.1	110		43.3	140		60
98		36.7	111		43.9	150		65.6
98.6		37	112		44.4	212		100
99		37.2	113		45	230		110
100		37.8	114		45.6			

perature measurements such as temperatures of reactions, incubation, and boiling points. Most countries other than the United States use the Celsius scale in everyday life as well as for making scientific measurements.

It is sometimes necessary to convert temperatures from Fahrenheit to Celsius, or vice versa. Although many books contain a temperature conversion table, laboratory workers may not always have access to this information. Two common conversions are body temperature (98.6°F to 37°C) and the freezing point of water (32°F to 0°C). Formulas for temperature conversion and an example of using each are shown in Figure 1-10. A temperature conversion chart is given in Table 1-23.

PROBLEM 1

Jeremy was the only person working the night shift in his town's hospital laboratory. As he prepared to perform a chemistry test, he noticed that the waterbath thermometer was missing. The reagent he needed was frozen and the instructions were to thaw at 30°C to 32°C. He finally located a thermometer, but it was in Fahrenheit scale. What Fahrenheit temperature range would be acceptable for thawing his reagent?

PROBLEM 2

Shirley was on duty when laboratory test results were called in for Dr. Simpson's patient. The results, reported in SI units, were as follows: total protein, 70 g/L; hemoglobin, 150 g/L; and WBC count, 9×10^9/L. Shirley related the test results to Dr. Simpson, but he asked her to give him the results using the "old" units (total protein and hemoglobin in g/dL, and WBC count in cells/μL). Convert the SI units.

Total protein   70 g/L   = _____ g/dL
Hemoglobin   150 g/L   = _____ g/dL
WBC count 9×10^9/L   = _____ cells/μL

SUMMARY

Although English units such as pound, gallon, and mile are used in everyday life in the United States, it is not possible to make accurate measurements using these units, especially when making small measurements. The metric system is used in clinical laboratories because it enables precise, accurate measurements to be made, a requirement for quality laboratory results. The metric system has been in use for years in clinical laboratories, but the reporting methods were not standardized. Laboratories are now transitioning from reporting results using traditional metric units, such as cubic millimeters (cu mm) or milligrams per deciliter (mg/dL), to using standardized SI units.

Laboratory results are used to help assess a patient's condition, establish a diagnosis, and prescribe therapy. Therefore, it is important that all measurements are made correctly and accurately. Laboratory personnel must know, understand, and be able to correctly use the metric system and SI units in making laboratory observations, measurements, and calculations.

REVIEW QUESTIONS

1. What is the basic metric unit of distance or length?

2. What is the basic metric unit of volume?

3. What is the basic metric unit of weight?

4. What are the meanings of deca and hecto?

5. Why is the metric system preferred over the English system for scientific measurements?

6. Use the tables in this lesson to convert the following English measurements to metric units:

    3 inches = _____ cm or _____ mm

    5 qt = _____ L or _____ mL

    64 oz = _____ g or _____ kg or _____ mg

7. Convert the following units:

    12 mg = _____ μg or _____ g

    50 mL = _____ μL or _____ cc or _____ dL

8. Convert the following temperatures using the formulas in Figure 1-10:

    101°F = _____ °C

    25°C = _____ °F

9. Define Celsius scale, centi, deci, English system of measurement, Fahrenheit scale, gram, kilo, liter, meter, metric system, micro, milli, nano, National Institute of Standards and Technology, pico, and SI units.

STUDENT ACTIVITIES

1. Complete the written examination for this lesson.

2. Practice measuring metric volumes, lengths, and weights and converting metric units using Worksheets I, II, and III.

3. Obtain a laboratory report form from a clinical laboratory in your area. Are reference ranges listed? Are SI units used?

WEB ACTIVITIES

1. Search the Internet for information on the International System of Units. Find information about using SI units in reporting laboratory results. Determine what units are used to report results of laboratory tests such as platelet counts, BUN, potassium, and bilirubin.

2. Use the Internet to locate lists of reference ranges for laboratory tests. Examine the lists to determine what system of measurement is used to report results. Are SI units used?

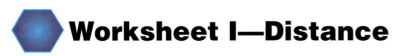 Worksheet I—Distance

LESSON 1-4 The Metric System

Name _____ **Date** _____

Obtain a meter stick or metric ruler and an English ruler from the instructor. Use the information in Tables 1-16 through 1-19 to answer the questions below.

1. Look at the meter stick. Locate the cm and mm divisions. How many centimeters are in a meter? _____ How many mm in a cm? _____ How many mm in a meter? _____

2. Draw the indicated length of line beside each number, beginning at the dot.

   35 mm   .

   6 cm   .

   83 mm   .

   1.2 dm .

3. Measure the lines above using a ruler marked in English units (inches):

   35 mm   =   _____ inches

   6 cm   =   _____ inches

   83 mm   =   _____ inches

   1.2 dm =   _____ inches

   Which of the measurements (English or metric) do you feel is the most accurate? _____

4. How many mm in 1 inch? _____   1 mm = _____ inch

   How many cm in 1 inch? _____   1 cm = _____ inch

   Convert the following units:

   4 inches   =   _____ cm

   0.5 inches =   _____ cm

   38 cm   =   _____ inches

   7 cm   =   _____ inches

   3.5 inches =   _____ mm

   35 mm   =   _____ inches

5. How many inches are in a meter? _____ What English unit of measurement is closest in size to the meter? _____

6. Measure your height or the height of another student using the meter stick. What is the height in cm? _____ in meters? _____ Convert the height in cm to inches: _____ Now measure the height in inches and compare the results.

Worksheet II—Weight

LESSON 1-4 The Metric System

Name _____ **Date** _____

Use Tables 1-16 through 1-19 to answer the questions below.

1. What is the basic metric unit of weight? _____

2. How many mg in a g? _____ How many μg in a g? _____ How many g in a kg? _____

3. Convert the following units:

   300 mg   =   _____ g   =   _____ kg

   50 mg   =   _____ g   =   _____ kg

   4000 mg   =   _____ g   =   _____ kg

   200 μg   =   _____ g

   750 μg   =   _____ mg

   80 g   =   _____ kg

   What decimal rule did you follow to make the conversions? _____

   _____

4. Convert the following units:

   0.4 kg   =   _____ mg   =   _____ μg

   9.2 kg   =   _____ mg   =   _____ μg

   0.6 g   =   _____ μg

   10 mg   =   _____ μg   =   _____ pg

   280 mg   =   _____ μg   =   _____ pg

   What decimal rule did you follow to make the conversions? _____

   _____

5. Weigh yourself or another student. What is the weight in g? _____ in kg? _____

6. A man who weighs 165 pounds would weigh _____ kg.

7. A child who weighs 32 pounds would weigh _____ kg or _____ g.

8. Is a man who is 178 cm tall and weighs 135 kg overweight, underweight, or of normal weight? _____

9. If scales are available, weigh a container, add 10 mL of water, and weigh again. How much does the water weigh? _____ Does 1 mL of water weigh approximately 1 g? Yes_____ No_____

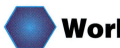 Worksheet III—Volume

LESSON 1-4 The Metric System

Name _____ Date _____

Obtain a medicine cup, a 50-mL graduated cylinder, and a 50-mL beaker from the instructor. Use Tables 1-16 through 1-19 to answer the questions below.

1. What is the basic unit of volume in the metric system? _____

2. How many milliliters in a liter? _____ deciliters in a liter? _____ microliters in a liter? _____

3. Convert the following units:

   45 cc   =   _____ L   =   _____ mL

   550 mL   =   _____ L

   4 dL   =   _____ L

   60 mL   =   _____ L   =   _____ mL

   0.1 dL   =   _____ L

   6,700 mL   =   _____ L

   What decimal rule did you follow to make the conversions? _____
   _____

4. Convert the following units:

   0.3 L   =   _____ dL   =   _____ mL

   5 L   =   _____ mL

   7 mL   =   _____ mL

   3 dL   =   _____ mL   =   _____ mL

   0.1 dL   =   _____ mL

   What decimal rule did you follow to make the conversions? _____
   _____

5. What English unit is closest in volume to the liter? _____

6. Convert the following English units:

   3.5 pints =   _____ mL   =   _____ L

   3 quarts   =   _____ mL   =   _____ L

   5 fl. oz. =   _____ mL   =   _____ L

7. If gasoline is $2.20 per gallon at station A and 60 cents a liter at station B, which has the cheapest gasoline? _____

8. Fill the medicine cup to the 1 fl oz mark with water. Then transfer the water to a 50-mL graduated cylinder. How many milliliters of water are in 1 fl oz? _____

   Fill the medicine cup again with 1 fl oz of water and transfer to a 50-mL beaker. Which gives the most accurate measurement, the beaker or the graduated cylinder? _____

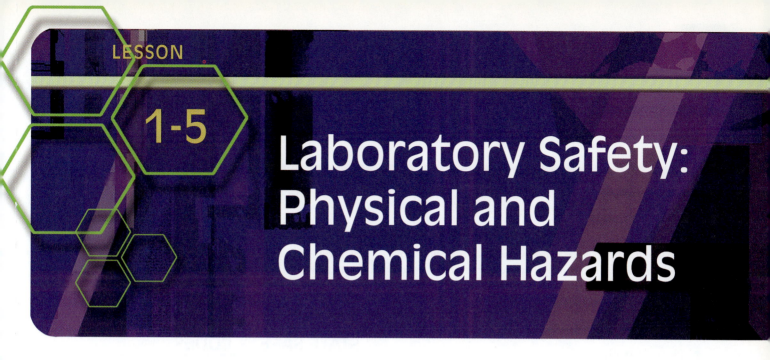

Laboratory Safety: Physical and Chemical Hazards

LESSON OBJECTIVES

After studying this lesson, the student will:

- Describe the evolution of the Occupational Safety and Health Administration (OSHA) safety laws.
- Explain the "right to know" provisions of OSHA.
- Explain why safety rules must be observed.
- List three classifications of laboratory hazards.
- Give two examples of physical hazards and ways to prevent or correct each one.
- Give two examples of chemical hazards and ways to prevent or correct each one.
- List five components of a Chemical Hygiene Plan.
- Use the information on a material safety data sheet (MSDS).
- Describe proper laboratory dress and work habits.
- State 15 safe work practices for the laboratory.
- Define the glossary terms.

GLOSSARY

autoclave / an instrument that uses pressurized steam for sterilization

carcinogen / a substance with the potential to produce cancer in humans or animals

caustic / a chemical substance having the ability to burn or destroy tissue

centrifuge / instrument with a rotor that rotates at high speeds in a closed chamber

Chemical Hygiene Plan / comprehensive written safety plan detailing the proper use and storage of hazardous chemicals in the workplace

fume hood / a device that draws contaminated air out of an area and either cleanses and recirculates it, or discharges it to the outside

material safety data sheet (MSDS) / written safety information that must be supplied by manufacturers of chemicals and hazardous materials

mutagen / a substance with the potential to make a stable change in a gene that can then be passed on to offspring

National Institute for Occupational Safety and Health (NIOSH) / federal agency responsible for workplace safety research and that makes recommendations for preventing work-related illness and injury

Occupational Safety and Health Act (OSH Act) / congressional act of 1970 created to help reduce on-the-job illnesses, injuries, and deaths, and requiring employers to provide safe working conditions

Occupational Safety and Health Administration (OSHA) / the federal agency that creates workplace safety regulations and enforces the Occupational Safety and Health Act of 1970

personal protective equipment (PPE) / specialized clothing or equipment used by workers to protect from direct exposure to blood or other potentially infectious or hazardous materials

radioisotope / an unstable form of an element that emits radiation and can be incorporated into diagnostic tests, medical therapies, and biomedical research; radioactive isotope

INTRODUCTION

Safety in health care should be a priority of all health care providers. Health care employers and employees must provide quality patient care in an environment that is safe for both workers and patients. Creating a safe workplace is not optional, it is required by law.

Clinical laboratory workers encounter unique safety hazards that can be classified in three categories:

- Physical hazards
- Chemical hazards
- Biological hazards

This lesson identifies some physical and chemical hazards that can be present, and outlines safety practices mandatory for safe and legal operation of a clinical laboratory. Safety procedures concerned primarily with biological hazards are addressed in Lesson 1-6.

FEDERAL REGULATION OF SAFETY IN THE WORKPLACE

Although laws to protect workers from biological hazards have been enacted in recent years, rules to protect against physical and chemical hazards have existed for decades. In 1970, Congress enacted the **Occupational Safety and Health Act (OSH Act)** to try to reduce workplace illnesses, injuries, and deaths. The act required employers to provide safe working conditions and to inform and train workers about hazardous conditions present in their workplace. The **Occupational Safety and Health Administration (OSHA)** is the agency that establishes the rules and enforces adherence to the OSH Act.

OSHA's Hazard Communication Rule

In 1983, OSHA issued a rule intended to further protect workers from hazardous chemical exposure. This rule was called the *Hazard Communication* and applied only to the manufacturing industry. However, in 1987, the rule was expanded to include the nonmanufacturing sector. The rule places the burden on the employer to keep workers informed and protected by providing safety training, proper safety apparel, and a safe work environment.

Enforcement of the OSH Act

OSHA has responsibility for general workplace safety. OSHA inspectors can arrive unannounced and conduct an inspection of the safety conditions in a workplace. If safety violations are found, they are noted and managers and/or owners of the facility are fined.

Agencies such as CMS, the Centers for Disease Control and Prevention (CDC), and the **National Institute for Occupational Safety and Health (NIOSH)** are also involved in ensuring that best safety practices are in use. These agencies provide free safety educational materials and/or training, make recommendations for best safety practices, and conduct workplace safety research.

STATE SAFETY CODES

In addition to the OSH Act of 1970, and expanded rules of 1983 and 1987, most states have enacted additional safety codes to ensure that employers provide safe work environments. Under these state laws, the employer, supervisor, or educator has the responsibility to provide safety orientation and training to employees and students.

SAFETY TRAINING

Each laboratory is required to have an up-to-date procedure manual that contains specific safety guidelines. The location of the manual must be posted so that anyone can find it. The manual must include standard operating procedures (SOP); regulations for the safe handling, storage, and disposal of chemicals; and strategies to follow in case of fire. It must also provide general laboratory safety rules and guidelines for employee safety training.

Students and employees must be trained in safe laboratory practices, proper use of safety equipment, and the Hazard Communication. The safety training must be completed and documented in writing before the employee or student is allowed to perform procedures in the laboratory. Both trainer and trainee must sign, verifying that training was given or received and that the trainee understood the training. (An example of a safety agreement form is included in Lesson 1-6, Figure 1-25.)

Refresher safety training sessions must be provided for employees at least once a year to reinforce the importance of using safe practices. It is the responsibility of the employer, supervisor, and educator to monitor employee or student adherence to safety regulations. It is the employee's responsibility to follow safety rules and comply with the institution's safety guidelines and regulations so that the employee or other workers are not endangered.

Personal Protective Equipment

The employer must provide employees or students with **personal protective equipment (PPE)** to protect against identified hazards in the laboratory. Safety equipment appropriate to protect against physical and chemical hazards can include:

- Eye, face, and skin protection such as masks, goggles, or face shield
- Respirator or fume hood to protect against inhalation of fumes
- Gloves to protect skin of hands and arms

In addition, workers must wear uniforms or scrubs and a fluid-resistant laboratory coat or apron.

PHYSICAL HAZARDS

Physical hazards are present in ordinary laboratory equipment and surroundings. Electrical equipment, laboratory instruments, and glassware can all be hazardous if improperly used. Safety signs should be posted in appropriate places throughout the laboratory as a constant reminder to employees to use safe work practices (Figure 1-11). In this textbook, the symbol ⚠ alerts that a physical hazard can be present when performing an activity or using the instrument or equipment.

Electrical Safety

Electricity is a major physical hazard. All electrical equipment must be properly grounded, following the manufacturer's instructions and according to electrical codes. Even minor repairs, such as replacing microscope light bulbs, require that the instrument be disconnected from the power supply before the work is begun. All electrical cords and plugs must be kept in good repair, with no frayed cords or exposed wires. Circuits must not be overloaded; overloading creates a fire hazard and can also cause equipment damage. Extension cords create several safety hazards and should only be used in an emergency.

Fire Safety

Fire is another potential danger in the workplace. Fortunately, laboratory fires are rare.

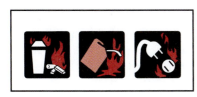
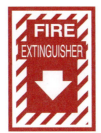
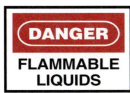

FIGURE 1-11 Examples of safety signs indicating:
(A) classes of extinguishers for different types of fires;
(B) fire extinguisher locator; (C) flammable liquids warning

When possible, open flames (such as from alcohol lamps or Bunsen burners) should not be used in the clinical laboratory. Most clinical laboratory procedures can be modified to use laboratory hotplates, microwave ovens, electric incinerators, and slide warmers instead of open flames. If a flame is required for a procedure, care must be taken to keep loose clothing and long hair away from the flame.

Flammable chemicals should be stored in a flame-proof cabinet, away from heat sources and in a well-ventilated area. In case of fire, a flameproof chemical cabinet protects flammable chemicals from flames until firefighters arrive and also allows workers more time to escape.

Fire extinguishers must be located in several accessible sites in the laboratory. A fire blanket should also be accessible in case clothing ignites (Figures 1-12 and 1-13). All workers must know the locations of fire extinguishers and how to use them. Fire extinguishers must be inspected periodically by the fire department or a certified fire safety company and the date of inspection recorded. Fire drills must be held frequently to be sure that workers know the escape route and the procedure to follow if that exit is blocked (Figure 1-14).

Laboratory Equipment Safety

Laboratory equipment must be used only as the manufacturers' instructions dictate. Any instrument that has moving parts, or

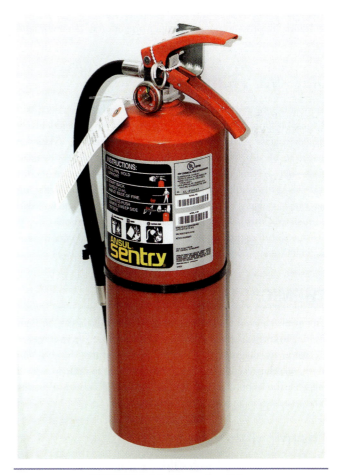

FIGURE 1-12 Fire extinguisher

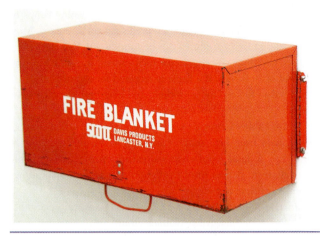

FIGURE 1-13   Fire blanket

operates at high speed, such as a **centrifuge**, must be operated with special attention to safety. Centrifuges should be equipped with safety latches. These latches prevent the centrifuge from being turned on unless the lid is latched, or being opened during operation. Centrifuge lids should not be opened until the rotor has come to a complete stop.

Autoclaves, which use pressurized steam to sterilize surgical instruments, glassware, and other materials, present special hazards. Manufacturers' instructions should be followed carefully to prevent explosions and burns. Insulated gloves should be worn when removing hot items from the autoclave. Lesson 1-9 contains additional information on the proper operation of common laboratory equipment.

Glassware Safety

In most laboratory procedures, glassware has been replaced with disposable polycarbonate, polyethylene, or polystyrene labware. However, glass must still be used for some procedures. Glassware that is to be subjected to heat should be made of heat-resistant glass, such as Kimax or Pyrex. Only glassware that is free of chips and cracks should be used. Damaged glassware is weakened and can break, causing injury. Broken glass should be cleaned up with a brush and dustpan, not with bare hands. Glass should not be discarded into regular trashcans, but into rigid cardboard or plastic containers.

CHEMICAL HAZARDS

Chemicals present a variety of hazards. Chemicals can be flammable, toxic, caustic, corrosive, carcinogenic, or mutagenic. Occasionally, diagnostic or laboratory procedures use radioisotopes, which present the potential of exposure to radioactivity. In this text, the use of the 🔧 symbol alerts that a chemical hazard can be present in a procedure or situation.

Chemical Hygiene Plan

OSHA mandates that a comprehensive, written safety plan for the use of hazardous chemicals be implemented at each workplace. This is often called the **Chemical Hygiene Plan** and must be

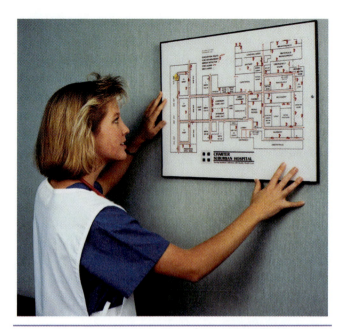

FIGURE 1-14   Workers must be familiar with their institution's fire escape route and emergency plan

readily available to all employees. The plan sets forth specific work practices, procedures, and personal protective equipment that must be used to ensure that employees are protected from the health hazards associated with chemicals used in that particular laboratory. The Chemical Hygiene Plan should include the following components:

- Standard operating procedures for safe use of hazardous chemicals

- Measures to reduce exposure to hazardous chemicals, including the use of personal protective equipment and hygiene practices such as frequent handwashing

- Requirements for proper function of protective equipment and fume hoods

- Specific hazard information about all hazardous chemicals in the laboratory

- Provisions for employee education and training

Material Safety Data Sheets

Manufacturers are required by law to provide a **material safety data sheet (MSDS)** for every chemical. This information describes the hazard(s) of the chemical, the personal protective equipment required, and the body organs that could be adversely affected following exposure to the chemical. Additional information is included for first aid and further medical treatment. These MSDS papers must be kept on file in the laboratory where every employee has access to them.

Chemical Labels

Chemicals must be labeled with detailed hazard information, including exposure symptoms, appropriate first aid procedures on exposure, and spill response procedures (Figure 1-15). The National Fire

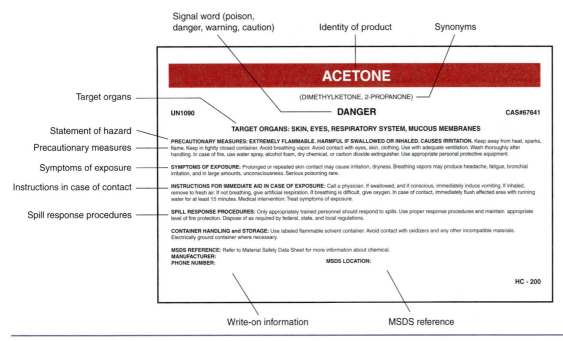

FIGURE 1-15 Chemical label containing hazard information

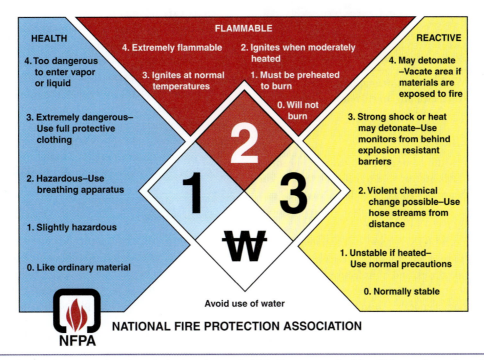

FIGURE 1-16 National Fire Protection Association's color-coded labeling system for identifying and warning of chemical hazards

Protection Association (NFPA) uses four colors on chemical labels to indicate the type of hazard a chemical presents (Figure 1-16). The system is based on a diamond shape that is divided into four smaller diamonds: blue, red, yellow, and white. Each color is associated with a specific class of hazards. The NFPA color codes are:

- Blue indicates health hazards or toxics

- Red indicates fire hazard or flammability

- Yellow indicates reactive or unstable chemicals such as oxidizers

- White indicates reactivity with water or contact hazards

For each blue, red, and yellow color, a number system (0 to 4) rates the relative risk of hazard associated with that category. A *0* means no unusual hazard is present in that category; a *4* indicates the highest hazard level for that category (see Safety Worksheet II p. 59). The white contact hazard category uses a lettering system to denote water reactivity, contact hazard (such as acid, corrosive), or a code for which type of PPE is required when using the chemical. These ratings are also present on the MSDS. Additionally, certain symbols are widely used to warn of specific chemical hazards (Figure 1-17).

FIGURE 1-17 Examples of symbols and signs for chemical hazards

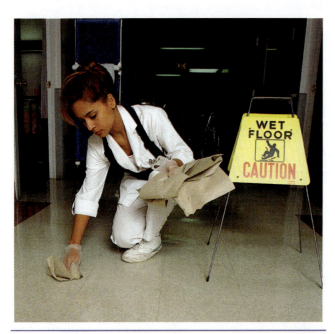

FIGURE 1-18 Workers must wear appropriate PPE and use care when cleaning up chemical spills

Caustic Chemicals

Some chemicals used in the laboratory are **caustic**, meaning they are strong acids or bases capable of causing severe skin burns (Figure 1-17). Fumes or vapors from these chemicals can burn mucous membranes and should be used in a fume hood. Potassium hydroxide (KOH), sodium hydroxide (NaOH), sulfuric acid (H_2SO_4), nitric acid (HNO_3), and concentrated sodium hypochlorite (chlorine bleach) are examples of caustic chemicals. Goggles or a face shield, gloves, and a protective apron should be worn to protect against injury from splashes and spills when working with such strong chemicals. Appropriate PPE must be worn when cleaning up chemical spills (Figure 1-18).

After handling and using chemicals, gloves should be removed carefully, avoiding touching bare skin with the outer glove surfaces (Figure 1-19). Any chemicals that do contact the skin should be washed off immediately with water for at least 5 minutes unless the container label says otherwise. A safety shower should be available in case large quantities of chemicals are spilled on a worker (Figure 1-20). An eyewash station must be accessible for workers who have chemicals splashed into their eyes (Figure 1-21).

Toxic Chemicals

Some laboratory chemicals are toxic or poisonous either through skin contact or by respiratory exposure. When using these chemicals, the worker must follow special safety precautions. Gloves and protective rubber or vinyl sleeves can be used to protect skin from contact. If a chemical produces harmful fumes, it should be used only in a **fume hood**, a special cabinet that draws the fumes away from the worker (see Figure 1-22).

Carcinogens, Mutagens, and Radioisotopes

Most routine clinical laboratory procedures either use chemicals that present few serious hazards, or use chemicals in such dilute concentrations that they represent little danger. When possible, safer chemicals are substituted for hazardous chemicals in laboratory procedures. Even so, is it always wise to avoid direct skin contact with chemicals and inhalation of chemical dust.

Some procedures require the use of hazardous chemicals such as **carcinogens** (cancer-causing substances), **mutagens** (substances that cause birth defects), or **radioisotopes**. These categories of chemicals require special care. Carcinogens must be handled carefully, following all recommended safety precautions and wearing appropriate PPE. Procedures that utilize mutagens must be clearly identified so that females of childbearing age can avoid exposure to mutagens (Figure 1-17). Workers must complete special radiation safety training before working with radioisotopes. Gloves and appropriate radiation shields must be used when handling radioisotopes. Special disposal is required and must be according to state and federal guidelines.

Safe Storage of Chemicals

Flammable liquids, concentrated acids, concentrated bases, and other hazardous chemicals should be stored in proper containers in special chemical cabinets. In the past, chemicals were stored in alphabetical order to make them easier to locate. However, this storage method sometimes placed incompatible chemicals near each other.

Chemical manufacturers offer reliable safety guides that can be used to plan safe chemical storage. Information on color-coded labels on chemical containers also indicates proper chemical storage conditions. Examples of some chemicals that should not be stored near each other are shown in Table 1-24.

Disposal of Chemical Wastes

All chemicals and reagents must be disposed of properly and according to regulations. A few laboratory chemicals can safely be poured down the drain, followed by large amounts of water to dilute them. However, many chemicals, especially those that contain heavy metals such as mercury, lead, or chromium, require special disposal by toxic waste personnel. Therefore, it is very

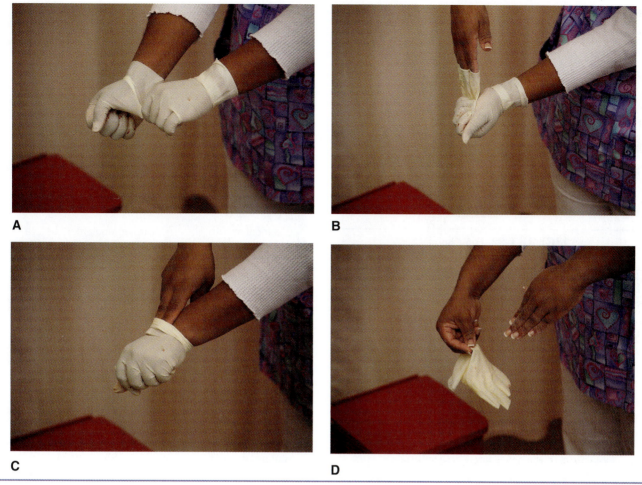

FIGURE 1-19 Proper way to remove gloves. (A–B) Touching only the outside of the glove, grasp the glove cuff and pull the glove down over the hand turning it inside out. (B–C) Hold the removed glove in the palm of the remaining gloved hand and pull the remaining glove off (inside-out) by touching only the inside of the glove with the bare hand. (D) Discard gloves into appropriate container

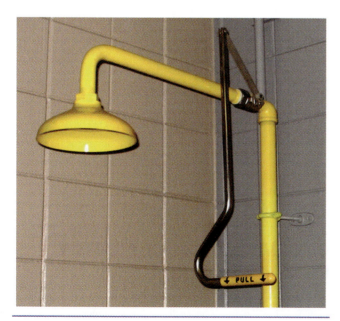

FIGURE 1-20 Safety shower

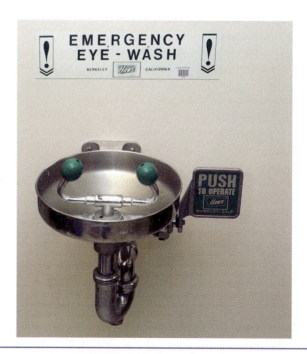

FIGURE 1-21 Eyewash station

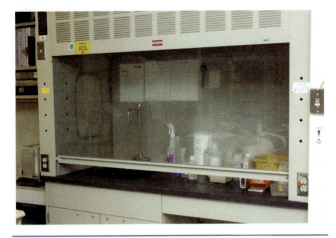

FIGURE 1-22 Fume hood

TABLE 1-24. Examples of some incompatible chemicals

CHEMICAL	DO NOT STORE NEXT TO ANY OF THESE
Acetic acid	Hydroxides (NaOH, KOH), nitric acid
Acetone	Concentrated sulfuric or nitric acids
Flammable liquids	Chromic acid, hydrogen peroxide, nitric acid
Sodium azide	Copper (in plumbing drains)

This is a partial listing; for details, consult a safety handbook and the labels on the chemical containers

TABLE 1-25. Exposure control methods to protect against physical and chemical hazards in the laboratory

HAZARD	EXPOSURE CONTROL METHOD
Spills and splashes on the skin	Wear laboratory coat, apron, gloves
Strong acids	Wear rubberized apron, acid-resistant gloves
Splashes into eyes	Use face shield and/or ANSI*-approved goggles
Toxic fumes or chemical dust	Use chemical fume hood
Electrical shock	Unplug equipment before repairs

* American National Standard Institute

important that laboratory supervisors or instructors provide explicit instructions for chemical disposal.

The types of chemicals used in a method should be considered when adopting laboratory procedures. Efforts should be made to use methods that minimize or eliminate the use of hazardous chemicals when possible or practical, as long as the quality of test results is not adversely affected. The use of safe chemicals eliminates problems associated with disposal of hazardous chemicals.

LABORATORY DRESS

Each employer will have a written policy describing rules and standards of appropriate laboratory clothing, types of PPE, and guidelines for selecting the appropriate PPE for the task (Table 1-25). Because laboratory work has its own particular set of hazards, rules of dress for laboratory personnel are usually slightly different than those for other health care workers.

Some dress rules are intended to reduce risk of injury. Laboratory workers usually are required to wear a uniform or scrubs covered by a buttoned, knee-length, and fluid-resistant laboratory coat to protect skin and clothing from spills and splashes of chemicals, stains, or hazardous material. A rubberized or other special type of apron can be worn when working with strong acids.

If splashes are likely to occur, protective eyewear such as laboratory safety goggles or face shield must be worn (Table 1-25).

Gloves made of the proper material must be worn when hazardous chemicals are handled. MSDSs provide information on the appropriate type of gloves for the chemical, and scientific supply catalogs contain charts to aid in glove selection. Nitrile gloves are nonallergenic, are resistant to most chemicals, and are suitable for routine laboratory use. Latex gloves should not be worn when working with strong chemicals, because chemicals can penetrate latex allowing the chemicals to contact the skin.

Loose jewelry, such as long chains and bracelets, should not be worn because it can get caught in moving equipment and cause serious injury. In addition, metal jewelry can contact electrical parts in equipment and cause injury or death by electrical shock. Shoes should be comfortable and stable and must have closed toes to protect skin from spills or injury from sharp objects. Long hair should be pulled back to prevent contact with moving equipment parts or chemicals.

SAFETY RESOURCES

Official OSHA guidelines must always be consulted to ensure the laboratory is in compliance. A copy of OSHA guidelines can be found in the *Federal Register* in the local library, or on various websites such as those of the CDC, OSHA, and NIOSH. In addition, state universities or state public health laboratories often have a safety consultant who will give advice by phone or send printed information. Additional sources are listed in Appendix D.

GENERAL LABORATORY SAFETY RULES

Despite certain safety hazards, the clinical laboratory can be a safe work environment. Each worker must be responsible, use safe work practices, and observe all safety rules.

CASE STUDY

Michelle, a phlebotomist in the laboratory of a small clinic, arrived at work a few minutes early dressed neatly in scrubs and new sandals. After putting on her laboratory coat and buttoning it, she began work. Within the hour her supervisor told her she was inappropriately dressed. What do you think is the problem?

No set of safety rules can cover every situation that might arise. Also, nothing can replace the use of common sense when working with laboratory equipment and chemicals. General safe work practices to protect against physical and chemical hazards include the following:

1. Report any accident immediately to the supervisor.

2. Do not eat, drink, chew gum, or apply cosmetics in the work area.

3. Wear a laboratory apron, or buttoned laboratory coat, and closed-toe shoes.

4. Pin long hair back to prevent contact with chemicals or moving equipment.

5. Do not wear chains, bracelets, large rings, or other loose jewelry.

6. Use chemical-resistant gloves when working with hazardous chemicals.

7. Clean the work area before and after laboratory procedures and any other time it is needed.

8. Wash hands before and after all laboratory procedures, after removing gloves, and any other time necessary.

9. Wear safety glasses, goggles, or a face shield or use a countertop acrylic shield when working with strong chemicals and when splashes are possible.

10. Wipe up spills promptly, using the appropriate procedure for the type of spill.

11. Use a fume hood or appropriate mask, or respirator, when working with chemicals or other materials that give off dust or fumes.

12. Follow manufacturers' instructions for operating all equipment. Handle all equipment with care and store properly.

13. Report any broken or frayed electrical cords, exposed electrical wires, or damage to equipment.

14. Use a broom or brush and a dustpan to pick up broken glass. Discard into special containers for broken glass.

15. Do not allow visitors into the work area of the laboratory unless they are properly attired and have been instructed in patient confidentiality issues and safety precautions.

SUMMARY

The modern era of workplace safety began with the 1970 OSH Act. This federal legislation and subsequent rules mandated increased attention to safety in workplaces. OSHA is the agency that oversees and enforces workplace safety.

The clinical laboratory has special hazards—physical, chemical, and biological (Lesson 1-6). Physical hazards include fire, electrical hazards, and hazards associated with laboratory equipment. Chemical hazards are associated with the use of chemicals in laboratory procedures. Each laboratory is required to have a comprehensive written safety plan, available to all employees, that explains all hazards and provides specific information about safe work practices. A Chemical Hygiene Plan gives information about the safe handling, storage, and disposal of chemicals. Each laboratory employee must receive documented annual safety training. New employees must complete safety training before being allowed to perform laboratory procedures. Employees are required to use personal protective equipment such as gloves, face protection, and laboratory coats to protect from chemical exposure.

Although laboratory procedures do have associated hazards, the laboratory can be made a safe workplace. It is the employer's responsibility to provide a safe work environment and all necessary safety equipment and supplies. It is each employee's responsibility to follow the safety rules.

REVIEW QUESTIONS

1. What are the three classifications of laboratory hazards?

2. Give two examples of physical hazards, and tell how each might be avoided or corrected.

3. Give two examples of chemical hazards, and tell how each might be avoided or corrected.

4. Why is it important to conduct frequent fire drills?

5. Why must safety rules be strictly observed?

6. What governmental agency is responsible for enforcing safety regulations in the workplace?

7. What type of clothing should laboratory workers wear?

8. State 15 general laboratory safety rules and explain the importance of each.

9. What is the purpose of the safety agreement?

10. Define autoclave, carcinogen, caustic, centrifuge, chemical hygiene plan, fume hood, material safety data sheet, mutagen, National Institute for Occupational Safety and Health, Occupational Safety and Health Act, Occupational Safety and Health Administration, personal protective equipment, and radioisotope.

STUDENT ACTIVITIES

1. Complete the written examination for this lesson.

2. Make a poster warning of a laboratory hazard.

3. Use Safety Worksheet I at the end of this lesson to make a safety check of the laboratory. Check for frayed cords, exposed wires, fire extinguisher, safety posters, and posting of fire exit routes.

4. Practice the procedure to follow in case of fire and the use of the fire extinguisher; learn the fire escape route.

5. Inspect the chemicals in the laboratory and report using Safety Worksheet I. Are chemicals labeled with appropriate information? Do chemical labels contain instructions for accidental exposure? Note the procedure to follow in case of skin contact or chemical spill.

6. Make an inventory of six chemicals in your laboratory, using the inventory form on Worksheet II at the end of this lesson. Consult the MSDS to determine the hazard class and type of PPE required when using each chemical.

WEB ACTIVITIES

1. Use the Internet to find MSDS information for NaOH, HCl, and Clorox. Report on the reactivity, flammability, and health hazard of each chemical. List the PPE that should be worn when working with each of these chemicals.

2. Visit the OSHA or NIOSH Web sites and find out what safety information is available. Look for free safety posters or brochures and order or download and print copies for your laboratory.

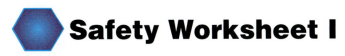

Safety Worksheet I

LESSON 1-5 Laboratory Safety: Physical and Chemical Hazards

Name _____ Date _____

Make a safety check of the laboratory. For each item listed below, determine if the conditions are satisfactory (safe), **S,** or unsatisfactory (unsafe), **U.** If unsatisfactory, recommend correction(s) in the spaces indicated.

I. Safety Check for Physical Hazards

A. Examine all electrical instruments (microscopes, spectrophotometers, etc.) for frayed wires and proper storage conditions (storage away from water and harsh chemicals, use of dust covers, etc.). Evaluate conditions and record recommendations for each instrument examined.

Instrument	S	U	Observation/Recommendation
_____	_____	_____	_____
_____	_____	_____	_____
_____	_____	_____	_____
_____	_____	_____	_____

B. Make a fire safety check of the laboratory.

1. Are fire extinguishers present? _____

   When was the last inspection date? _____

   Do extinguishers have instructions for their use posted with them? _____

   Fire extinguishers: S_____ U_____

2. Is the fire exit route posted? _____

   Is it up to date? _____

   Walk the fire exit route. Was it easy to follow? _____

   Could all exit doors be opened? _____

   Fire exit route: S_____ U_____

Recommendation(s) for improving fire safety: _____

_____

_____

_____

II. Safety Check for Chemical Hazards

A. Examine the chemicals in the laboratory.

1. Are all clearly labeled? _____

2. Do the labels contain information on storage, disposal, and procedure in case of spills or accidental exposure? _____

3. Are chemicals labeled "flammable" stored in a flameproof cabinet? _____

4. Where are concentrated acids and bases stored? _____

Chemical storage: S _____ **U** _____

B. Is a fume hood present? _____

When was it last checked for proper air flow? _____

Fume hood: S _____ **U** _____

C. Is an eyewash station present? _____

Are instructions for its use posted? _____

Eyewash station: S _____ **U** _____

Recommendation(s) for improving chemical safety: _____

_____

_____

_____

III. Laboratory Safety Policy

Inquire about the laboratory's policy regarding employee safety orientation and training.

A. Is a written safety manual available in the laboratory? _____ Is the location of the safety manual posted? _____

B. Does the laboratory administration follow appropriate "employee right-to-know" policies in the safety orientation and training programs? _____

C. Are written records kept of employee safety training sessions? _____

D. Are all employees required to sign safety agreement forms after safety training? _____

E. Is a(n) MSDS on file for each chemical? _____

Laboratory safety policy: S _____ **U** _____

Recommendation(s) for improving safety policy: _____

_____

_____

_____

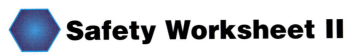

Safety Worksheet II

LESSON 1-5: Laboratory Safety: Physical and Chemical Hazards

Name _____ **Date** _____

CHEMICAL INVENTORY FORM

Location _____ Date _____

Chemical Name	Catalog #	Quantity	Physical State	Hazard Class				Manufacturer	Comments
				H	F	R	P		

(H) Health Hazard
0 - Minimal/None
1 - Slightly hazardous
2 - Hazardous
3 - Extreme
4 - Deadly

(F) Fire Hazard/Flashpoint
0 - Will not burn
1 - Slight, above 200°F
2 - Moderate, below 200°F
3 - Serious, below 100°F
4 - Extreme, below 73°F

(R) Reactivity Hazard
0 - Stable, not reactive with water
1 - Slight, unstable if heated
2 - Water reactive
3 - Shock or heat may detonate
4 - May detonate

(P) Protection Required
A - Goggles
B - Goggles/Gloves
C - Goggles/Gloves/Apron
D - Face shield/Gloves/Apron
E - Goggles/Gloves/Mask
F - Goggles/Gloves/Apron/Mask
X - Gloves

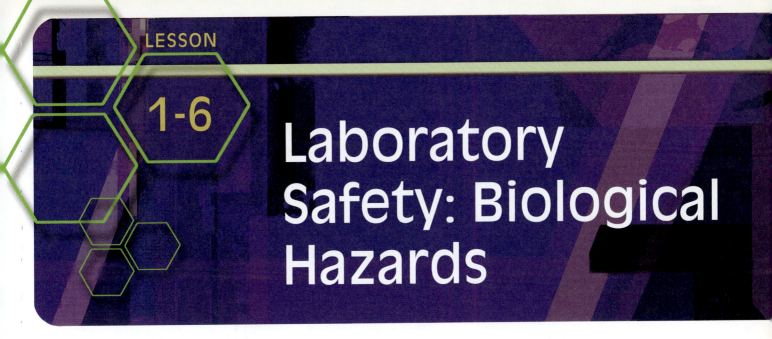

Laboratory Safety: Biological Hazards

LESSON OBJECTIVES

After studying this lesson, the student will:

- Explain the purpose of the Bloodborne Pathogens Standard.
- Explain the reason for issuing Standard Precautions in 1996.
- Explain what is meant by exposure control plan.
- List the components of an exposure control plan.
- Explain the evolution of safety laws and rules since the 1970s.
- Explain the roles of the Centers for Disease Control and Prevention and the Occupational Safety and Health Administration in promoting safety in health care institutions.
- Explain the impact of the Needlestick Safety and Prevention Act of 2000.
- Discuss how work practice controls improve safety.
- Discuss how engineering controls improve safety.
- List types of personal protective equipment commonly used in the clinical laboratory.
- Discuss how sterilization, disinfection, and antisepsis are used in the clinical laboratory.
- Explain the impact of human immunodeficiency virus (HIV) and hepatitis B and C viruses on safety practices in health care.
- List safety precautions that must be observed when handling biological materials.
- List additional safety precautions that must be observed when working in the microbiology laboratory.
- Define the glossary terms.

GLOSSARY

acquired immunodeficiency syndrome (AIDS) / a form of severe immunodeficiency caused by infection with the human immunodeficiency virus (HIV)

aerosol / liquid in the form of a very fine mist

alimentary tract / the digestive tube from the mouth to the anus

antiseptic / a chemical used on living tissues to control the growth of infectious agents

biohazard / risk or hazard to health or the environment from biological agents

biological safety cabinet / a special work cabinet that provides protection while working with infectious microorganisms

bloodborne pathogens (BBP) / pathogens that can be present in human blood (and blood-contaminated body fluids) and that cause disease

Bloodborne Pathogens (BBP) Standard / OSHA guidelines for preventing occupational exposure to pathogens present in human blood and body fluids, including, but not limited to, human immunodeficiency virus (HIV) and hepatitis B virus (HBV); final OSHA standard of December 6, 1991, effective March 6, 1992.

disinfectant / chemical used on inanimate objects to kill or inactivate microbes

engineering control / use of available technology and equipment to protect the worker from hazards

exposure control plan / a plan identifying employees at risk of exposure to bloodborne pathogens and providing training in methods to prevent exposure

exposure incident / an accident, such as a needlestick, in which an individual is exposed to possible infection through contact with body substances from another individual

hepatitis B virus (HBV) / the virus that causes hepatitis B infection and is transmitted by contact with infected blood or other body fluids

hepatitis C virus (HCV) / the virus that causes hepatitis C infection and is transmitted by contact with infected blood or other body fluids

human immunodeficiency virus (HIV) / the retrovirus that has been identified as the cause of AIDS

isolation / the practice of limiting the movement and social contact of a patient who is potentially infectious or who must be protected from exposure to infectious agents; quarantine

nosocomial / hospital acquired; acquired as a result of being hospitalized or institutionalized

other potentially infectious materials (OPIM) / any and all body fluids, tissues, organs, or other specimens from a human source

parenteral / any route other than by the alimentary canal; intravenous, subcutaneous, intramuscular, or mucosal

pathogenic / capable of causing damage or injury to the host

personal protective equipment (PPE) / specialized clothing or equipment used by workers to protect from direct exposure to blood or other potentially infectious or hazardous materials; includes, but is not limited to, gloves, laboratory apparel, eye protection, and breathing apparatus

Standard Precautions / a set of comprehensive safety guidelines designed to protect patients and healthcare workers by requiring that all patients and all body fluids, body substances, organs, and unfixed tissues be regarded as potentially infectious

sterilization / the act of eliminating all living microorganisms from an article or area

Transmission-Based Precautions / specific safety practices used in addition to Standard Precautions when treating patients known to be or suspected of being infected with pathogens that can be spread by air, droplet, or contact

Universal Precautions / a method of infection control in which all human blood and other body fluids containing visible blood are treated as if infectious

work practice controls / methods of performing tasks that reduce the worker's exposure to blood and other potentially hazardous materials

INTRODUCTION

Until the 1980s, clinical laboratory safety training concentrated primarily on using safety measures to protect from chemical and physical hazards and to protect from contagious diseases such as tuberculosis. However, the discovery of **acquired immunodeficiency syndrome (AIDS)**, caused by the **human immunodeficiency virus (HIV)**, and increases in **hepatitis B virus (HBV)** and **hepatitis C virus (HCV)** infections brought about an increased emphasis on biological safety and preventing exposure to and transmission of these agents.

As the modes of transmission of HIV, HBV, and HCV became known, it was realized that more stringent safety measures and work practices must be used to protect health care workers, patients, and the general public from exposure and infection. The Centers for Disease Control and Prevention (CDC) and Occupational Safety and Health Administration (OSHA), as well as other government agencies, have taken the lead in developing safety guidelines to protect health care workers and the public from infectious agents. Over recent years, safety guidelines have been updated, improved, and expanded several times. Educational and training materials are available from several federal and state sources to help clinical sites implement good safety practices.

With this new emphasis on biological safety also came new terminology. The term **biohazard** came into use. A biohazard

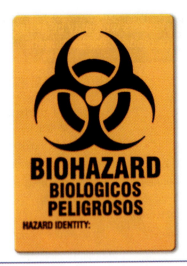

FIGURE 1-23 Biohazard sign

symbol was adopted and is now used widely to indicate the presence of a biological hazard or biohazardous condition (Figure 1-23). The presence of this symbol is used to warn that a risk or hazard to health or the environment from infectious agents exists. In this text, the symbol ☣ alerts that a biological hazard can be present and the worker should use appropriate measures to prevent exposure.

This lesson describes the current status of biological safety regulations and the recommendations to protect individuals from exposure to infectious agents both in the general health care setting and in the microbiology laboratory. By coordinating safety practices for chemical and physical hazards (Lesson 1-5) with the biological safety practices outlined in this lesson, the foundation of a comprehensive safety program can be formed. It should be emphasized that these lessons are merely an introduction to clinical laboratory safety practices. All of the details of safety procedures and practices are too extensive to be covered in full in this text.

EVOLUTION OF BIOLOGICAL SAFETY REGULATIONS AND GUIDELINES

As knowledge about transmission of infectious agents has grown, the guidelines for preventing exposure and infection have evolved. Table 1-26 gives a timeline of the major federal directives calling for improvements in safety practices.

In the first half of the twentieth century, the techniques used for dealing with infectious diseases changed significantly. At one time all infectious patients were quarantined together to try to stop disease from spreading to the public. It was common for infected patients to be sent to infectious disease or tuberculosis hospitals. However, patients infected or reinfected each other, leading to the use of **isolation** rooms or cubicles within these hospitals as a method of controlling disease spread. Also, aseptic procedures, such as handwashing, wearing gloves, and disinfecting patient-contaminated objects, came into wider use.

Isolation Techniques

By the 1960s, tuberculosis hospitals and infectious disease hospitals were closing as the methods of disease transmission became better understood. Infectious patients were placed in isolation rooms in regular hospitals in efforts to contain diseases and prevent their spread. To give guidance in infectious disease management, in 1970 the CDC outlined isolation techniques for hospitals and listed categories of isolation. In 1975 these guidelines were revised to include recommendations for specific safety

TABLE 1-26. Timeline of federal guidelines and laws concerning biological safety

YEAR	ISSUING AGENCY/ENTITY	GUIDELINE/LAW
1970	CDC	Published "Isolation Techniques for Use in Hospitals"
1975	CDC	Revised "Isolation Techniques" to include category-specific precautions and prohibition of recapping needles
1983	CDC	Issued nonbinding guidelines for isolation precautions in hospitals, designating seven isolation categories
1985	CDC	Introduced Universal Blood and Body Fluid Precautions (Universal Precautions or UP), primarily in response to HIV/AIDS epidemic
1987	CDC	Issued Body Substance Isolation guidelines
1988	U.S. Congress	Enacted Clinical Laboratory Improvement Amendments of 1988 (CLIA '88)
1991	OSHA	Issued Bloodborne Pathogens (BBP) Standard, which mandated the use of UP
1996	CDC	Issued Standard Precautions, synthesizing UP and Body Substance Isolation
2000	U.S. Congress	Enacted Needlestick Safety and Prevention Act
2001	OSHA	Revised BBP Standard in response to Needlestick Safety and Prevention Act

precautions for each category. Safe work practices, such as not recapping needles, were emphasized.

Universal Precautions

In 1983, the CDC issued guidelines for isolation precautions in hospitals, which contained specific precautions for each communicable disease or condition. In 1985, in response to the growing HIV/AIDS epidemic, the CDC issued guidelines called *Universal Blood and Body Fluid Precautions,* commonly referred to as **Universal Precautions**. These precautions and practices were designed to protect the health care worker from exposure to blood and to body fluids containing visible blood. UP were to be applied universally to *all* patients, regardless of whether they were suspected of being infectious or not. Universal Precautions were implemented by using **personal protective equipment (PPE)** such as gown, gloves, mask, and eye protection.

Body Substance Isolation and Bloodborne Pathogens Standard

The limitations of the Universal Precautions were that they covered only blood and body fluids visibly contaminated with blood; they did not include all body fluids, secretions, or excretions or the possible need for isolation precautions. In 1987, the *Body Substance Isolation* (BSI) guidelines were issued, recommending the use of precautions for all body fluids and all moist and potentially infectious body substances (and for all patients). However, these guidelines still did not cover all isolation precautions needed to prevent all modes of disease transmission, such as airborne diseases.

In 1991, OSHA issued the **Bloodborne Pathogens (BBP) Standard**, mandating implementation of safety measures with the primary purpose of reducing or eliminating occupational exposure to HIV, HCV, and HBV. The BBP Standard outlined the requirements for protecting workers who could be exposed to **bloodborne pathogens** such as human blood or **other potentially infectious materials (OPIM)**. OPIM included all body fluids, open wounds, and microbiological cultures. The BBP Standard applied to employees in all health care facilities, as well as all other workers who could be at risk of exposure (Table 1-27).

Standard Precautions

Because of some confusion about how to implement Universal Precautions, BSI guidelines, and the BBP Standard, in 1996, the CDC issued **Standard Precautions**, a comprehensive set of safety guidelines for health care workers, which included components of both Universal Precautions and BSI guidelines. Thus, "Standard Precautions" is the current terminology and the fundamental premise employed by health care personnel when rendering care to every patient. The intent of Standard Precautions is to protect the patient, to control **nosocomial** (institution-acquired) infections, and to protect the health care worker. Health care facilities are required to implement Standard Precautions and to insist that all workers comply with them.

The Standard Precautions guidelines also included a section on **Transmission-Based Precautions**, additional prac-

TABLE 1-27. Workers who may be at risk for exposure to bloodborne pathogens*

Physicians	Dentists and other dental workers
Nurses	Laboratory and blood bank technologists
Pathologists	Medical technologists
Phlebotomists	Research laboratory scientists
Dialysis personnel	Emergency medical technicians
Some laundry workers	Morticians
Medical examiners	Some maintenance personnel
Paramedics	Some housekeeping personnel

* Exclusion of a job category here does not denote lack of risk.

tices used with patients known or suspected to be infected with pathogens spread by air, droplet, or contact. Examples of these pathogens include the measles virus, tuberculosis bacterium, meningitis bacterium, and multi-drug resistant bacteria. Lesson 7-2 (in Basic Microbiology) contains a more complete discussion of Transmission-Based Precautions.

Needlestick Prevention

In 2001, OSHA revised the BBP Standard to emphasize safe practices to prevent accidental needlesticks in the workplace. This was in response to the Needlestick Safety and Prevention Act passed by Congress in 2000.

REQUIREMENTS OF STANDARD PRECAUTIONS

The use of Standard Precautions intensifies safety practices by requiring that every patient and every body fluid, body substance, organ, or unfixed tissue be regarded as potentially infectious. Standard Precautions must be applied:

- To *all* patients, regardless of their suspected infection status
- To *all* body fluids, excretions, and secretions
- To nonintact skin
- To mucous membranes
- To organs and unfixed tissue

Standard Precautions includes the use of safe work practices such as handwashing and use of safety needles. The use of protective barriers such as gown, mask, gloves, and eye and mucous membrane protection is required. This added emphasis on exposure prevention is important because, in addition to HIV, other bloodborne viruses such as HBV and HCV can cause severe disease. The safety practices that must be followed using the Standard Precautions guidelines are explained in Figure 1-24.

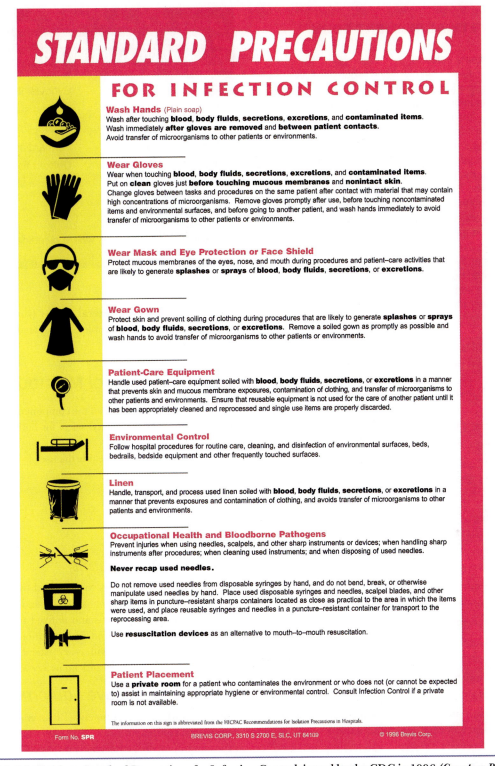

FIGURE 1-24 Guide to Standard Precautions for Infection Control, issued by the CDC in 1996 *(Courtesy Brevis Corp.)*

THE EXPOSURE CONTROL PLAN

Each employer is required to develop an **exposure control plan** (infection control plan) to identify all employees with potential for occupational exposure to human blood or OPIM. A training program must be set up to inform employees of the hazards and the training must be documented. The employer is required to update and document the training yearly. An example of a safety agreement form is shown in Figure 1-25.

The exposure control guidelines deal with safe handling of specimens, contaminated sharps, contaminated laundry, and regulated waste. OSHA guidelines must be followed when the

SAFETY AGREEMENT FORM

Please initial the items below:

_____ I agree to follow all set rules and regulations as required by the instructor or supervisor.

_____ I have been informed about and received training concerning the chemical hygiene plan.

_____ I have been informed of the location of the chemical hygiene plan and the MSDS folder.

_____ I have been informed about and received training concerning the OSHA Bloodborne Pathogens Standard and Standard Precautions.

_____ I understand that biological specimens and blood or blood products are potentially infectious.

_____ I understand that even though diagnostic products and reagents are screened for HIV antibodies and hepatitis B surface antigen (HBsAg), no known test can offer 100% assurance that products derived from human blood will not transmit disease.

_____

Employee/Student Name (Please Print)

_____   _____

Employee/Student Signature   Date

_____   _____

Supervisor   Date

FIGURE 1-25 Example of a safety agreement form

plan is written. Each employee must have access to the plan. For example, a copy should be placed at each nursing station, in the laboratory, and in the housekeeping office.

The employer has several responsibilities to the employee:

- The employee must have access to personal protective equipment appropriate for the tasks they perform.

- Warning labels and signs must be used to identify biohazards.

- The Exposure Control Plan must describe the control methods used to comply with the BBP Standard.

- The employer must provide free HBV immunization to workers at risk of exposure to bloodborne pathogens.

- The employer must provide a confidential, nonpunitive procedure for accident reporting, treatment, and follow-up.

Identifying Employees at Risk

Employers must identify all employees who have occupational risk of exposure to blood or OPIM. Laboratory technicians, nurses, and phlebotomists are not the only workers who require training. Dentists, dental technicians, dialysis personnel, some housekeeping and laundry workers, and others can all be at risk (Table 1-27).

Occupational exposure means reasonably anticipated contact with blood or other potentially infectious materials (Table 1-28). This contact can occur to the eyes, skin, or mucous mem-

TABLE 1-28. Examples of substances recognized by the CDC as having the potential to transmit pathogens such as HBV, HCV, and HIV

Blood	Synovial fluid
Blood products	Vaginal secretions
Semen	Pleural fluid
Peritoneal fluid	Pericardial fluid
Amniotic fluid	Unfixed tissue specimens
Cerebrospinal fluid	Breast milk
Urine	Sweat
Organs	
Saliva in dental settings where bleeding occurs	

branes or through **parenteral** routes (routes other than the **alimentary tract**). An example of parenteral contact would be a needlestick.

Exposure Control Methods

Control methods consist of all the components determined essential for a task to be completed safely for both the patient and the employee (Table 1-29).

These components include the use of:

- Standard Precautions
- PPE
- Engineering controls
- Work practice controls

Standard Precautions

Standard Precautions refers to a method of infection control in which *all* patients and *all* human blood and other body fluids or substances (including organs and unfixed tissues) are treated as if potentially infectious. Standard Precautions must be used each time a worker has contact with *every* patient and *every* specimen, even if the specimen is from a friend or a coworker.

Personal Protective Equipment

Personal protective equipment (PPE) is specialized apparel, devices, or equipment used by workers to protect from direct exposure to potentially infectious materials. This includes, but is not limited to, gloves, fluid-resistant gowns, face shields or masks, goggles, and safety glasses (Figure 1-26).

Engineering Controls

Engineering controls are devices and technology used to isolate the worker from hazards. An example of such a device is the use of an acrylic benchtop shield to protect the worker from aerosols when a tube of blood is being uncapped or serum is being pipetted (Figure 1-27). Biohazard containers, appropriate surface and hand disinfectants, puncture-resistant sharps containers, and safety needles are also engineering controls (Figures 1-27 and 1-28).

TABLE 1-29. Control methods required as part of an exposure control plan

Standard Precautions	Treating all patients, body fluids, unfixed tissue, and organ specimens as if infectious
Personal protective equipment	Specialized clothing or equipment used by workers to protect from direct exposure to blood and other substances
Engineering controls	Devices that eliminate or minimize worker exposure
Work practice controls	Alterations in the manner in which a task is performed to reduce the likelihood of exposure

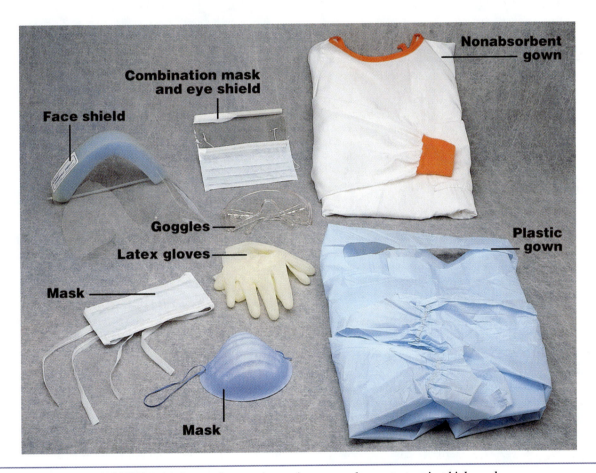

FIGURE 1-26 Personal protective equipment used to protect against biohazards

Work Practice Controls

Work practice controls refer to the manner in which the task is performed. These practices are actually just good, safe work habits. The use of work practice controls should reduce the likelihood of a worker being exposed to hazards (Figure 1-29).

Examples of work practice controls include:

- Handwashing before donning gloves and after glove removal or any other time necessary (Figure 1-29A)

- Wearing appropriate PPE when cleaning up biological spills (Figure 1-30)

- Removal and disposal of PPE when leaving a work area or upon completion of a task

- Regular use of a disinfectant such as 10% chlorine bleach to clean the work area before and after each use, and anytime a spill occurs

One important work practice control is designed to prevent exposure to bloodborne pathogens through accidental sticks with contaminated needles. After the passage of the Needlestick Safety and Prevention Act, OSHA issued a rule prohibiting the recapping or removal of needles from used blood-drawing devices. The rule mandated that engineering controls such as safety needles/devices be used and that used needles immediately be discarded into an accessible sharps container after the safety feature is activated (Figure 1-29B and C). This rule significantly changed phlebotomy practices.

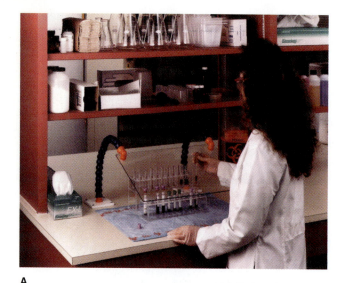

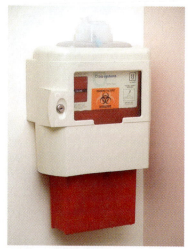

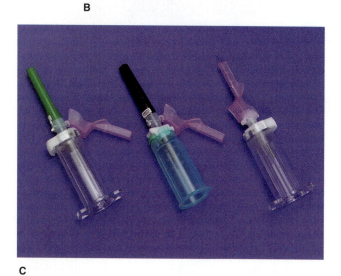

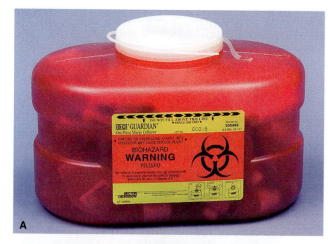

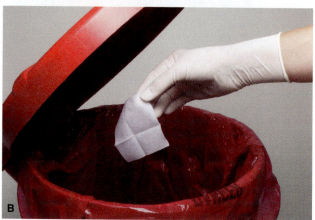

FIGURE 1-28 Engineering controls: (A) rigid container for disposal of contaminated sharps; (B) biohazard container for disposal of non-sharp objects (*Bottom photo courtesy of Roche Diagnostic Corp., Indianapolis IN*)

FIGURE 1-27 Engineering controls: (A) acrylic safety shield to protect worker from splashes; (B) wall-hung sharps collector; (C) vacuum tube holders with safety needles (*Top photo courtesy Mitchell Plastics, Inc.*)

Exposure Incidents

The Exposure Control Plan is designed to eliminate **exposure incidents**, accidental exposure to possible infectious agents through contact with body substances from another individual. Exposure incidents can include needlesticks, splashes onto mucous membranes, and exposure to aerosols of potentially infectious material. If any accident or exposure incident occurs, even if it seems insignificant, the employee should immediately:

- Flood the exposed area with water and clean any wound with antiseptic and water
- Report incident to supervisor, risk control, or infection control
- Seek medical attention

Implementation of an Exposure Control Plan

Implementation of an Exposure Control Plan in the daily routine of the laboratory worker is not as difficult as it may seem. The example in Table 1-30 illustrates how a worker or student would use the plan while performing a venipuncture.

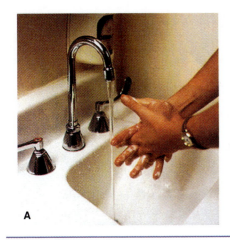
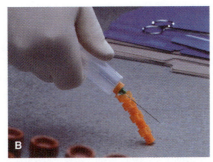
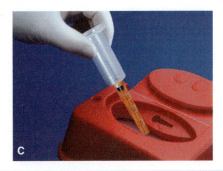

FIGURE 1-29 Work practice controls: (A) wash hands before and after each procedure; (B) engage safety shield on needle immediately after use; (C) discard used blood collecting devices into sharps container immediately after use (*Center and left photos courtesy of Smiths Medical ASD, Inc.*)

BIOLOGICAL HAZARDS OTHER THAN BLOODBORNE PATHOGENS

Clinical laboratory workers are exposed to other biological hazards in addition to bloodborne pathogens. Clinical microbiology specimens can contain a variety of **pathogenic** microorganisms such as bacteria, viruses, fungi, or parasites. Students or workers in the laboratory must know how to protect themselves from these hazards.

Methods of Decontamination

Several methods are used in the clinical and microbiological laboratory to disinfect or decontaminate materials, surfaces, and skin. These can be classified as sterilization, disinfection, and antisepsis.

Sterilization

Sterilization refers to the killing or inactivation of all living organisms and viruses. In the laboratory, this is normally achieved by autoclaving contaminated materials. Autoclaves are used to decontaminate laboratory waste and to sterilize glassware, instruments, media, and reagents used in microbiology and other procedures requiring sterility.

Disinfection

Disinfectants are chemicals used on inanimate objects or surfaces, such as countertops, floors, instruments, or labware, to kill or inactivate microorganisms. Each type of disinfectant has advantages and disadvantages. Disinfectants should be selected that are effective against a wide range of microbes. The appropriate exposure time and dilution for each disinfectant must be followed to achieve maximum disinfection. Some disinfectants can be skin, respiratory, or eye irritants so precautions should be taken when using them. Disinfectants commonly used in the laboratory are:

- Dilute chlorine bleach (hypochlorites), 1:10 dilution
- Alcohols, 70% to 85%
- Iodophors, 75 parts per million (ppm) or 4.5 mL/L of water

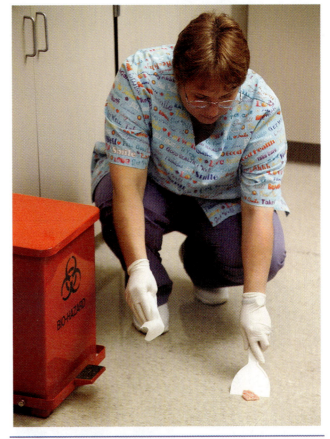

FIGURE 1-30 Work practice control: wear appropriate PPE when cleaning up biological spills

- Phenols
- Quaternary ammonium compounds

Antisepsis

Antiseptics are chemicals used on skin or tissue to inhibit growth and development of microbes. A wide variety of these are available, including alcohols, hydrogen peroxide, triclosan, chlorhexidine (Hibiclens), and iodine. They are used for general skin

TABLE 1-30. Example of using exposure control methods for protecting against biohazards while performing a venipuncture

CONTROL METHOD	MECHANISM
Standard Precautions	Treat all patients and all specimens as infectious
Personal protective equipment	Wear gloves to handle blood and all body fluids; wear fluid-resistant gown or laboratory coat; wear eye protection if splashes are reasonably anticipated
Engineering controls	Use containers for contaminated sharps, containers for biohazardous waste, biohazard containers for contaminated reusable apparel, biohazard containers for disposable apparel, appropriate surface disinfectants
Work practice controls	Always wear gloves when working with blood; never recap, remove, cut, or break needles; use safety needles and needle holders; immediately dispose of contaminated sharps; wash hands with antiseptic after removing gloves or any other time hands are contaminated

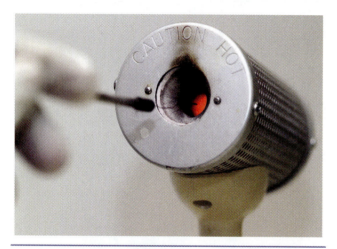

FIGURE 1-31 Work practice control: use an electric incinerator to prevent aerosol formation when sterilizing a loop

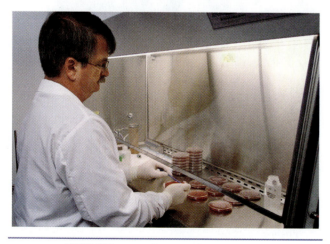

FIGURE 1-32 Biological safety cabinet
(Courtesy CDC, Atlanta, GA)

TABLE 1-31. Exposure control methods to protect against biological hazards in the microbiology laboratory

HAZARD	PROTECTIVE MEASURES
Blood or blood products	Wear gloves and a buttoned, fluid-resistant laboratory coat
Pathogenic microorganisms	Wear gloves and laboratory coat; use biological safety cabinet
Hazardous aerosols	Place acrylic benchtop shield between worker and tubes when removing stoppers; wear mask, goggles, or face shield when disposing of urine
Contaminated work surfaces	Wipe with 10% chlorine bleach solution (or other surface disinfectant) before and after all procedures and any other appropriate time
Needlesticks	Use self-sheathing needles or quick-release holders; never recap, bend, break, or cut used needles

cleaning, cleaning skin prior to injections or surgical procedures, or cleansing wounds.

Microbiology Work Practices

Workers in the microbiology laboratory must follow the guidelines for bloodborne pathogens and Standard Precautions as well as some additional safety practices. Accidents in the microbiology laboratory that can expose the worker to risk include spills of culture material, cuts on fingers and hands, and formation of **aerosols**, fine

CASE STUDY 1

Janie, a laboratory technician in a group practice clinic, frequently collects blood from clinic patients for testing. Janie's friend Bonnie came into the clinic for some blood tests. As Janie prepared to perform the venipuncture, Bonnie became offended when Janie put on gloves before collecting the blood.

How should Janie have handled this situation? Role-play this situation with a fellow student or worker.

CASE STUDY 2

April is preparing serum chemistry control solutions for analysis in her department. She is wearing a laboratory coat and face shield. However, she does not like to wear gloves when handling the small control vials, because she worries about dropping them.

Should she be praised for saving money for the laboratory?

mists that can form anytime a cap is removed from a tube of liquid or when a bacteriological loop is sterilized (Figure 1-31).

Some procedures in microbiology must be performed in a **biological safety cabinet** (Figure 1-32). Positive air pressure in the cabinet keeps infectious materials inside the cabinet. Air inside the cabinet is drawn away from the worker, into a vent or special filter. A Class II biological safety cabinet is the type most commonly used in clinical laboratories.

To prevent exposure to a patient's bacteriological specimen, gloves must be worn when working with the specimen and hands must be washed with antiseptic after the gloves are removed. When a task has been completed, work surfaces must be wiped with a disinfectant, such as 10% chlorine bleach. Examples of measures that can be taken to protect workers from hazards in the microbiology laboratory are illustrated in Table 1-31.

SUMMARY

Adherence to Standard Precautions and other biological safety rules is vitally important when working in the clinical laboratory. All patients and patient specimens present the potential risk of exposure to infectious agents. Laboratories are required to have in place a biological safety program that includes regular biosafety training. As part of the biological safety program, Standard Precautions and many other safety directives and guidelines issued by agencies such as the CDC and OSHA detail precise measures that workers can take to protect themselves and patients from exposure. An exposure control plan outlines specific control measures and work practices that must be used to protect against exposure. Strict adherence to the biological safety plan provides a safe environment for patient and worker.

REVIEW QUESTIONS

1. How have biological safety rules changed in recent decades? Why have they become more stringent?

2. Explain the reason for the Bloodborne Pathogens Standard. Why was it revised in 2001?

3. What is meant by exposure control plan or infection control plan?

4. List the components of an exposure control plan.

5. What is meant by the terms Universal Precautions and Standard Precautions?

6. What additional safety rules and equipment are used in the microbiology laboratory?

7. What class of biological safety cabinet is most commonly used in medical laboratories?

8. Name three work practice controls that should be used in the laboratory workplace.

9. What are the OSHA rules regarding the handling and disposal of used needles?

10. What personal protective equipment is commonly worn when working in the biological laboratory?

11. What action should be taken in case of an exposure incident?

12. Name four common laboratory disinfectants and two antiseptics. Explain when and how antiseptics and disinfectants should be used.

13. Define acquired immunodeficiency syndrome, aerosol, alimentary tract, antiseptic, biohazard, biological safety cabinet, bloodborne pathogens, Bloodborne Pathogens

Standard, disinfectant, engineering control, exposure control plan, exposure incident, hepatitis B virus, hepatitis C virus, human immunodeficiency virus, other potentially infectious materials, parenteral, pathogenic, personal protective equipment, Standard Precautions, sterilization, Transmission-Based Precautions, Universal Precautions, and work practice controls.

STUDENT ACTIVITIES

1. Complete the written examination on this lesson.

2. Make a poster warning of a biological hazard.

3. Design an exposure control plan for performing a capillary puncture.

4. Use the biosafety worksheet at the end of this lesson to evaluate the laboratory's biological hazard safety policy.

WEB ACTIVITIES

1. Visit the OSHA Web site to find information on the Needlestick Safety and Prevention Act. Look for OSHA publications or posters that emphasize safe practices.

2. Search the Internet for engineering controls used to increase safety in the clinical laboratory. Obtain information on engineering controls such as safety needles, sharps containers, and acrylic safety shields.

3. Report on the various types of gloves available for use in the clinical laboratory, using an online health care or laboratory supply catalog. Note which types provide chemical protection and which provide protection from infectious agents.

4. Access the CDC Web site and find the October 25, 2002, *Morbidity and Mortality Weekly Report* (Vol. 51/No. RR-160). Read the "Guideline for Hand Hygiene in Health-Care Settings" and compare the CDC guidelines with your laboratory's written safety plan. Should your laboratory policy be strengthened? If so, how?

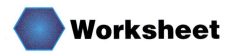 **Worksheet**

LESSON 1-6 Laboratory Safety: Biological Hazards

Name _____ **Date** _____

Use this worksheet to make a biological hazard safety check of the laboratory.

SAFETY CHECK FOR BIOLOGICAL HAZARDS

I. Examine the laboratory for biological hazards

A. Are safety rules posted? _____

B. Where are blood specimens discarded? _____

C. How are contaminated laboratory coats or gowns disposed of? _____

D. Where are needles and other sharps discarded? _____

Is the container puncture-resistant? _____

Are safety needles used? _____

E. Are all sizes of gloves available for workers? _____

F. Are eye protection devices available? _____

faceshields _____ goggles _____ safety glasses _____

G. Are fluid-resistant gowns or coats available for tasks that might involve splashes? _____

H. Is a policy in place to require counters to be wiped at certain intervals and after every spill? _____

Recommendation(s) for improvements: _____

_____

_____

II. Laboratory Safety Policy

Inquire about the laboratory's policy regarding employee orientation and training in the safe handling of hazardous materials.

A. Does the laboratory have a written exposure control plan? _____

B. Are Standard Precautions included in the exposure control plan? _____

C. Have all employees considered at risk of exposure to bloodborne pathogens been offered the hepatitis B vaccination series at no charge? _____

D. Are written records kept of all employee safety training sessions? _____

Do employees sign forms acknowledging the training? _____

E. Is safety training updated yearly? _____

Recommendations or comments concerning the laboratory's safety program: _____

_____

_____

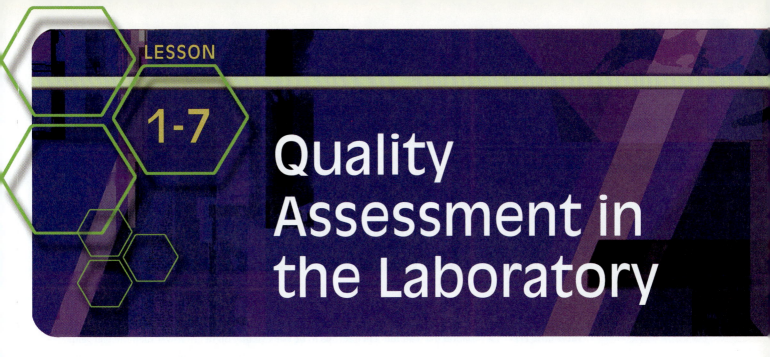

Quality Assessment in the Laboratory

LESSON OBJECTIVES

After studying this lesson, the student will:

- Explain the importance of quality assessment programs in the laboratory.
- Explain the importance of quality assessment programs in point-of-care testing.
- Discuss the use of standards and controls.
- Discuss the role of CLIA '88 in mandating laboratory quality assessment programs.
- Explain the difference between accuracy and precision.
- Determine the mean value for a set of test results.
- Calculate the standard deviation for an analytical method.
- Detect a result that is out of control.
- Explain how to detect the development of a trend in a method.
- Explain coefficient of variation.
- Describe safety procedures that must be followed when performing quality assessment procedures.
- Define the glossary terms.

GLOSSARY

accuracy / a measure of how close a determined value is to the true value

average / the sum of a set of values divided by the number of values; the mean

blind sample / an assayed sample that is sent as an unknown to laboratories participating in proficiency testing programs

calibration / the process of checking, standardizing, or adjusting a method or instrument so that it yields accurate results

coefficient of variation / a calculated value that compares the relative variability between different sets of data

controls / solutions usually made from human serum, and with a known concentration of the same constituents as those being measured in the patient sample

Gaussian curve / a graph plotting the distribution of values around the mean; normal frequency curve

Levey-Jennings chart / a quality control chart used to record daily quality control values

mean / the sum of a set of values divided by the number of values; the average

population / the entire group of items or individuals from which the samples under consideration are presumed to have come

precision / reproducibility of results; the closeness of obtained values to each other

quality assessment (QA) / in the laboratory, a program that monitors the total testing process with the aim of providing the highest quality patient care; a synonym for quality assurance

quality assurance / see quality assessment

quality control (QC) / a system that verifies the reliability of analytical test results through the use of standards, controls, and statistical analysis

quality systems (QS) / in an institution, a comprehensive program in which all areas of operation are monitored to ensure quality with the aim of providing the highest quality patient care

random error / error whose source cannot be definitely identified

sample / in statistics, a subgroup of a population

shift / an abrupt change from the established mean indicated by the occurrence of all control values on one side of the mean

standard / a chemical solution of a known concentration that can be used as a reference or calibration substance

standard deviation / a measure of the spread of a population of values around the mean

statistics / the branch of mathematics that deals with the collection, classification, analysis, and interpretation of numerical data; a collection of quantitative data

systematic error / a variation that can influence results to be consistently higher or lower than the real value

trend / an indication of error in the analysis, detected by increasing or decreasing values in the control sample

variance / the square of the standard deviation; mean square deviation

Westgard's rules / a set of rules used to determine when a method is out of control

INTRODUCTION

Clinical laboratories are required to have programs in place that continually assess the quality of the laboratory's performance. Over the years, programs concerned with quality have been given a variety of names. A few decades ago the common term was **quality control (QC)**. QC programs were mostly concerned with ensuring that the test procedures provided as accurate results as possible. Then the term **quality assurance** came into use. Quality assurance programs included QC programs but also evaluated and monitored a broader range of factors affecting quality, such as specimen collection and results reporting. Other terms, such as Total Quality Management (TQM) and Continuous Quality Improvement (CQI), have also been used to refer to comprehensive quality programs.

In the final CLIA '88 regulations published by the CDC and CMS, which became effective in 2003, more new terminology was introduced. The term **quality assessment (QA)** replaced quality assurance; the term **quality systems (QS)** was designated to be used to refer to all policies, procedures, and processes needed to achieve quality testing. Whatever the names, the purposes of the programs are the same—to ensure performance excellence and reliable results of laboratory tests. For the purposes of this lesson quality assurance and quality assessment are interchangeable.

Under CLIA '88 all laboratories are required to have programs in place to evaluate quality and ensure that laboratories provide the highest quality of patient care. This directive required few operational changes for hospital and larger laboratories, because in order to be accredited they already had QA programs in place. However, some smaller laboratories and those located in physician offices might not have had a QA program. These laboratories are now required to do so and to document the results. The goal of CLIA '88 is to ensure that results from all laboratories, large and small, are as reliable as possible. This lesson describes the basic components of laboratory quality programs and introduces the reader to elementary statistical concepts. In this text, the symbol *QA* is used to call attention to quality assessment components in a procedure or activity.

COMPONENTS OF A QUALITY SYSTEMS PROGRAM

A quality systems program is comprehensive and designed to follow a specimen all the way through the testing process, from the time a test is ordered, through specimen collection and testing to reporting, charting, and delivery of results. The scope of QS programs differs among laboratories, but in general QS programs are broad, ongoing, and encompass evaluation of:

- Personnel qualifications, training, and competency
- Proficiency testing
- QA components
  1. Preanalytical (before test) factors
  2. Analytical factors and QC methods
  3. Postanalytical (after test) factors

Personnel Qualifications and Training

Quality systems programs require that training of testing personnel be up-to-date. Attendance at training sessions, continuing education seminars, and verification of employee competency must be documented and kept on file.

Participation in Proficiency Testing

Proficiency testing (PT) is another component of QS programs. Laboratories that perform nonwaived procedures are required to subscribe to an external PT program. At regular intervals during the year, the PT agency sends **blind samples** to the laboratory. These are samples that have been assayed multiple times by the PT agency. The laboratory analyzes these blind samples and sends its results to the PT agency. The laboratory's results are then compared to the PT agency's assayed values and to the results of peer laboratories in the PT program. A report evaluating their performance is sent to the participating laboratories.

Quality Assessment/ Quality Assurance

Quality assessment is a component of a QS program and is an essential part of every laboratory's daily operations. QA programs are designed to ensure that reliable laboratory results are obtained and reported in the shortest possible time. Errors can occur at many points during a laboratory test procedure, but a QA program is designed to eliminate or minimize this possibility. A comprehensive quality assessment program includes evaluation of preanalytical, analytical, and postanalytical factors that can affect test outcomes. Pre- and postanalytical factors are factors outside of the test procedure that can influence the results. Analytical factors are associated with the actual test procedures.

Preanalytical Factors

Studies have shown that most laboratory errors are due to preanalytical factors. Methods to prevent preanalytical errors include using two patient identifiers, using proper specimen collection and handling techniques, establishing specimen rejection criteria, and maintaining ancillary equipment, such as specimen storage refrigerators and freezers, in good working order. Selecting appropriate test methods, using qualified testing personnel, and regular updating of procedure manuals are also steps that can reduce preanalytical problems.

Postanalytical Factors

Postanalytical errors occur primarily in the reporting and charting of test results. Many postanalytical errors have been eliminated due to the increased use of computers, and improved labeling technology such as barcodes on patient identification armbands, laboratory request forms, preprinted labels, and specimen containers. These same practices also help prevent preanalytical errors. An example of a postanalytical error would be a test that is performed correctly and yields an accurate result, but the result is accidentally written into the wrong patient chart. A postanalytical error could also occur by entering an incorrect patient identification number in the computer. The interfacing of laboratory analyzers and computers with patient records helps eliminate transcription and clerical errors.

Analytical Factors Affecting Laboratory Tests

Quality assessment programs also evaluate analytical factors that can affect the actual test procedure. Many of these factors fall under the umbrella of QC. Analytical factors include:

- Laboratory preparation of samples
- Instrument maintenance and calibration
- Use of standards and procedural controls
- Anything associated with performing the test procedure (reagents, pipetting, timing, etc.)
- Interfering substances or conditions
- Statistical analysis of control results

QUALITY CONTROL COMPONENT OF QUALITY ASSESSMENT PROGRAMS

Quality control procedures are an important part of the QA program and are sometimes the most visible part of the program. The principles and statistics that are part of QC programs can be complicated; this lesson includes just a brief introduction to some statistical concepts that are basic to QC programs. Although every worker may not be required to actually perform statistical calculations as part of their job function, QC terminology and basic QC concepts must be understood and used by all laboratory workers who perform tests. Laboratories are required to have a documented QC program in place.

Safety Precautions

  The laboratory technician can be exposed to bloodborne pathogens while using instrument calibrators and controls. Most controls are of human origin. Although control materials are screened for certain pathogens during the manufacturing process, they should still be considered potentially infectious. Standard Precautions must be followed while performing all control procedures in the same manner as they are followed when working with patient samples.

Controls

A major part of a QC program includes the daily use of controls. **Controls** are solutions that contain the same constituents as those being analyzed in the patient sample. Most controls are commercially produced from pools of human serum; some can be from sheep or pig. The manufacturer analyzes each lot of serum for a variety of components, such as glucose, sodium, cholesterol, and potassium. A listing of the expected range of assay values for each component is included when the controls are shipped to the laboratory, and must be confirmed by each laboratory using their own analytical systems.

The control sera must be analyzed with the patient samples, using identical methods, test conditions, and reagents. At least two levels of controls must be used, and these must be run a minimum of once each day. One control serum must contain constituents that fall within the normal range—this is called the *normal control*. The other control serum must contain constituents that are outside the normal range (either lower or higher than normal), commonly called the *abnormal control*.

A single control serum might contain all the constituents tested on a certain chemistry profile and therefore be suitable to be included in all the chemistry assays the laboratory performs. If a single control does not meet these criteria, the laboratory will have to use a combination of controls to be sure that a control containing each substance that the laboratory tests for is used. In large laboratories, certain controls must be analyzed with each batch of patient samples, at least once per shift, any time patient results seem questionable, after instrument repair or calibration, and when reagents are changed.

Each day's control sera results are used to construct a QC record called a **Levey-Jennings chart** (Figure 1-33). These daily control results are used in laboratory statistics. The records of the control assays must be kept for CLIA and other inspectors.

Calibration and Standards

Standards are also an essential part of a QC program. A **standard** is a substance that has an exact known composition and that, when accurately weighed or measured, can produce a solution of an exact concentration. Standards are also called *reference materials*.

Standards are usually expensive and are not used on a daily basis. Standards are used to calibrate newly purchased instruments and to recalibrate instruments after repair, at manufacturer's recommended intervals, or if a problem is suspected with a test method. **Calibration** refers to the process of checking, standardizing, or adjusting a method or instrument so that it yields accurate results. While some instruments are calibrated with a standard, for others, calibration can be accomplished electronically or by using a calibration strip or cartridge provided by the instrument manufacturer. All analytical instruments must be calibrated at set intervals and controls must be run regularly and these actions documented.

Accuracy and Precision

In any discussion of QC, the terms *accuracy* and *precision* must be considered. The terms have two very different meanings. The worker's goal should be to achieve both precision and accuracy in the laboratory analyses performed.

Accuracy refers to the closeness of a result to the actual, or true, value. Results nearer the true value are more accurate than ones further away. For example, suppose that the true value for an individual's serum protein is 75 g/L. Then suppose that the individual's serum was analyzed three times by one method yielding results of 71, 79, and 75 g/L, and three times by another method yielding results of 66, 69, and 68 g/L. The set of analyses of 71, 79, and 75 g/L would be more accurate than the other set because they are closer to the true value. Imagine that the true value (75 g/L) is the center of a bull's eye target. Accurate values placed on the target would be clustered closely around the true value (target center) as shown in Figure 1-34A.

The term **precision** refers to the reproducibility of results or the closeness of obtained values to each other. Precision can be understood by again examining the two sets of protein values discussed under accuracy. The values 66, 69, and 68 g/L vary little from each other, so they are considered to show precision. However they are not near the true value. These values, if placed on the same bull's eye target (where the true value, or target center, is 75 g/L), would be grouped very closely together but away from the true value (Figure 1-34B).

Test procedures can yield precise results without accuracy. In other words, a test can yield results near in value to each other, but, because of error, the values can be inaccurate, not near the true value. QC procedures are designed to detect errors such as these.

Detection of Analytical Error

One goal of a QA/QC program is to detect errors before test results leave the laboratory. Analytical errors occurring during the test procedure can be random or systematic. **Random errors** are errors for which the source cannot be definitely identified. The possibility of this type of error is always present in any system. Random errors can occur due to variations in voltage, temperature variations, pipetters, dispensers, air bubbles in a reagent line, or differences in technique among workers. Random errors can also be caused by interfering substances in patient specimens because of diet, medication, or disease.

Systematic error is a variation that can make results consistently higher or lower than the actual value. Factors that can cause this type of error are deteriorated or out-of-date reagents,

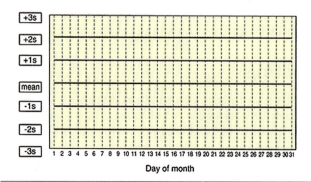

FIGURE 1-33 A form used to construct a Levey-Jennings chart

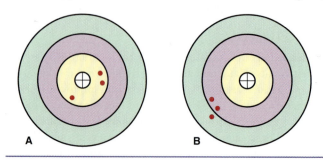

FIGURE 1-34 Illustration of accuracy (A) vs. precision (B)

mechanical trouble in an instrument, or a peculiarity in a worker's technique, such as pipetting.

QUALITY PROGRAMS IN POINT-OF-CARE TESTING

Point-of-care testing (POCT) is also regulated by CLIA '88. A large portion of the total laboratory tests performed in the United States are CLIA-waived tests performed at point-of-care. Waived tests are not subject to the rigorous use of controls required for nonwaived (moderate and high complexity) tests. However, manufacturer's instructions for an instrument or test kit must be kept on file, and their procedural recommendations, including use of controls, must be followed consistently.

Some POCT procedures are moderately complex and are subject to more stringent regulations. Personnel performing these tests must be highly trained, and their training must be documented. Having the test kit and instrument manufacturer's instructions on file is not sufficient—the procedure for each test must be written in a procedure manual. In addition, proficiency testing must be done and records kept of control results.

BASIC STATISTICS

Quality control programs use **statistics**, the branch of mathematics that deals with collecting, classifying, analyzing, and interpreting numerical data. An entire group or collection of observations is called a **population**. In laboratory statistics, a subgroup of the population (a group of specimens) is called a **sample**. The statistics involved in a good QC program can be very complicated; therefore, only the fundamentals will be covered in this lesson.

Calculating the Mean, Variance and Standard Deviation

In a QC program, the mean, variance, and standard deviation for analytical procedures must be calculated. The **mean** is the average of a set of values. The **standard deviation**, a measure of the scatter of the sample values around the mean, is derived from the calculation of the **variance**. Therefore, once the mean of a set of values has been determined, it is possible to determine the acceptable variation in the results of that analytical method.

Calculating the Mean

The mean is calculated by finding the sum of all the values in the set and dividing this by the number of values in the set; in other words, by calculating the **average** of a set of numbers (Figure 1-35). For example, the values obtained in repeated analyses for a glucose control serum were as follows: 82, 85, 89, 85, 91, 90, 81, 85, 93, and 89 (mg/dL). The formula for determining the mean is

$$\overline{X} = \frac{\Sigma X}{n}$$

where $\overline{X}$ = the mean

X = each individual value in the set

ΣX = the sum of all the individual values

n = the number of values in the set

Column One	Column Two	Column Three
Test Value (mg/dL) X	Deviation from Mean $\overline{X} - X$	Deviation Squared $(\overline{X} - X)^2$
82	5	25
85	2	4
89	2	4
85	2	4
91	4	16
90	3	9
81	6	36
85	2	4
93	6	36
89	2	4
sum = 870		sum = 142

mean = $\frac{870}{10}$ = 87

FIGURE 1-35 An example of calculating the deviation from the mean and the deviation squared for a set of 10 values

Substituting into the formula:

$$\overline{X} = \frac{82 + 85 + 89 + 85 + 91 + 90 + 81 + 85 + 93 + 89}{10}$$

$$\overline{X} \text{ (mean)} = \frac{870}{10} = 87$$

Calculating the Variance

The variance (s^2) is calculated by subtracting each value in the set from the mean, squaring this number, and calculating the sum of the squares. That sum is then divided by $n-1$, which is the number of individual values in the set *minus one*. The formula for variance is:

$$\text{Variance } (s^2) = \frac{\Sigma(\overline{X} - X)^2}{n - 1}$$

An example of how to find the deviation from the mean and the deviation squared is shown in Figure 1-35. The values in column two are obtained by subtracting each value in column one from the mean. Therefore, the first entry in column two is negative (–) 5. This is obtained by subtracting 82, the first value in column one, from the mean, 87. It doesn't matter if some of the differences are negative numbers, since squaring them makes them positive numbers. From the example in Figure 1-35, the following substitutions can be made in the variance formula:

$$s^2 \text{ (variance)} = \frac{142}{9} = 16$$

Calculating the Standard Deviation

The standard deviation is obtained by taking the square root of the variance:

$$s = \sqrt{16} = 4$$

Therefore, the standard deviation, $1s$, is 4, $2s$ = 8, and $3s$ = 12 for this particular glucose control.

These calculations may seem complicated, but most analyzers have a statistics program that computes these data automatically.

Using the Standard Deviation in the Laboratory

When a set of values with a normal distribution is plotted on a graph, the distribution of the values around the mean forms a **Gaussian curve** (Figure 1-36). This curve is also known as a normal frequency or normal distribution curve. In a normal distribution, half of the values are greater than the mean, and half are less than the mean. There are also more values close to the mean than values away from the mean.

Once the standard deviation has been determined, the curve can be divided into percentage divisions as shown in Figure 1-36. This figure shows that, in a normally distributed population, 68.2% of all results obtained for this method of glucose analysis will fall between 1s below the mean to 1s above the mean. In other words, 68.2% of the values will fall between 83 (87 − 4) and 91 (87 + 4) in this particular example, which has a mean of 87. In addition, 95.4% of the values will fall between 2s below the mean to 2s above the mean, or between 79 (87 − 8) and 95 (87 + 8). If 3s is used, 99.6% of the values will be between 75 (87 − 12) and 99 (87 + 12).

Clinical laboratories must establish the allowable standard deviation for each analytical method, based on the component being analyzed and the method of analysis. A two-standard-deviation limit is a common choice. This is sometimes called the confidence limit. In this example, using a control with a mean of 87 mg/dL, the laboratory expects the analysis results of that con-trol serum to be within ±2s (between 79 and 95 mg/dL) each time it is analyzed along with patient samples.

QUALITY CONTROL CHARTS

QC charts called Levey-Jennings charts can be constructed for each method based on the calculated mean and standard deviation. Levey-Jennings charts demonstrate a method's precision and allow problems to be detected.

The QC chart shown in Figure 1-37A was constructed using the mean and standard deviation calculated from the glucose data in Figure 1-35. The mean obtained was 87, therefore, the mean line is labeled 87. The lines on either side of the mean represent 1s, 2s, and 3s. As control data are obtained each day, they should be entered on the chart. The chart form has divisions for 31 days, so it can be used for any month. In a hospital laboratory, a control would be plotted at least daily. In an office laboratory, controls might only be run 5 days per week. Figure 1-37B is an example of a quality control chart with control values plotted for 15 days.

Trend

A **trend** occurs when a series of control values consistently increases or decreases (moves away from the mean in the same direction) for several consecutive days (Figure 1-37B). A trend is a signal that something has gone wrong in the procedure—in the

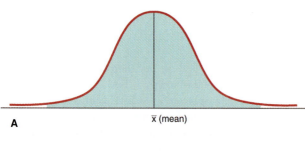

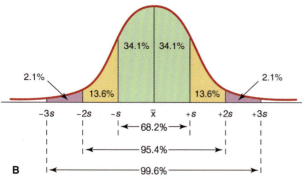

FIGURE 1-36 Normal distribution curves: (A) Gaussian curve showing normal frequency distribution around the mean; (B) Gaussian curve showing the proportion of the population falling between the mean and ± 1s, ± 2s, and ± 3s

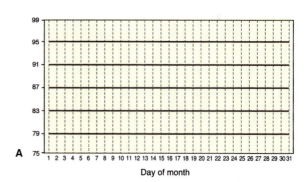

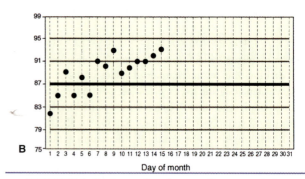

FIGURE 1-37 Levey-Jennings quality control charts: (A) Levey-Jennings chart constructed using the mean and standard deviation obtained from glucose control values; (B) plot of 15 daily control values, showing a normal distribution in values 1–6 and a trend in values 10–15

instrument, the technique, the reagents, or the control sera. The laboratory worker must investigate and find the source of error and correct it. A new lot of control serum can be analyzed; if error is still present, the instrument must be recalibrated.

Shift

Normally, control results randomly alternate above and below the mean. When the control results for several consecutive days are distributed on one side of the mean, but remain at a constant level, a **shift** has occurred. This also signals error; the reagents and the instrument must be investigated for the cause.

Westgard's Rules

When a QC program is established, a set of guidelines must be used to decide whether or not a method is *out of control*. One set of guidelines is called **Westgard's rules**. These rules list specific limits about how much variation is acceptable in control values before patient test results are rejected. To use these rules, the laboratory must analyze two different levels of control sera (normal and abnormal) along with each set of patient samples. A *run* (set of samples) is considered out of control, and the patient results must be rejected if any of the following is true:

1. Both controls are outside the $\pm 2s$ limit
2. The same control level is outside the $\pm 2s$ limit in two successive runs
3. Controls in four consecutive runs have values greater than $\pm 1s$ all in the same direction
4. Ten consecutive control values fall on one side of the mean

Patient test results cannot be reported until the method is considered in control.

COEFFICIENT OF VARIATION

When a laboratory changes from one method of analysis to another, the precision of the new method must be compared to that of the old one. This can be done by calculating the **coefficient of variation (CV)** for each method. The CV is a calculated value that compares the relative variability between two different sets of values by expressing each standard deviation as a percentage of the mean.

If a laboratory was purchasing a new blood glucose analyzer, the means and the standard deviations of the controls using the old and new analyzers would be used to calculate the CV for each instrument. For example, the mean glucose for the normal control using the first (old) analyzer is 98.5 mg/dL with a standard deviation (s) of 2.5 mg/dL. The mean glucose control value using the second (new) analyzer is 96 mg/dL with a standard deviation of 2.3 mg/dL. The CV's for the two methods would be calculated as shown below:

1st method $CV = \dfrac{s}{\bar{x}} \times 100$

$$CV = \frac{2.5 \text{ mg/dL}}{98.5 \text{ mg/dL}} \times 100$$

$$CV = 2.5\%$$

SAFETY Reminders

- Observe Standard Precautions.
- Wear appropriate PPE when handling samples, calibrators, and control sera.

PROCEDURAL Reminders

- Follow the instrument manufacturer's instructions for calibration procedures.
- Be sure to correctly insert values into the statistical formulas.
- Follow the manufacturer's instructions for reconstituting control samples received in dry form.

2nd method $CV = \dfrac{s}{\bar{x}} \times 100$

$$CV = \frac{2.3 \text{ mg/dL}}{96 \text{ mg/dL}} \times 100$$

$$CV = 2.4\%$$

In this comparison, the CVs are about the same, so the precision of the methods is similar. However, if a third analyzer gave a control mean of 95 mg/dL and s of 5.0 g/dL, the CV would be calculated as follows:

3rd method $CV = \dfrac{s}{\bar{x}} \times 100$

$$CV = \frac{5.0 \text{ mg/dL}}{9.5 \text{ mg/dL}} \times 100$$

$$CV = 5.2\%$$

The CV of the third method is 5.2%, indicating that the third analyzer yields less precise results than the first two analyzers.

SUMMARY

Programs for improving the quality of laboratory testing have been in place for years. These programs have gone through many name changes, but the overall goal has not changed—to provide high-quality patient care through performing procedures in a manner that ensures that test results are reliable. CLIA '88 mandates the way in which laboratories accomplish this goal and requires that the laboratory's QA procedures and results must be documented.

Programs that assess quality in the laboratory are an essential part of every laboratory's daily operations. Laboratory workers have the ethical and legal responsibility to perform to their highest level of ability and to ensure that work performed in the

CASE STUDY

Karen was working the day shift in the hematology laboratory. The laboratory's protocol called for three levels of blood cell controls to be run 1) at the beginning of the shift, 2) within each run of patient samples during the day, and 3) any time reagents were changed. The mean for the low (abnormal) control for the red blood cell (RBC) count was given as 2.00×10^{12}/L, the standard deviation was 0.15, and the acceptable control range was 2.0×10^{12}/L $\pm$ 2 s.d. (± 0.3).

The first morning low control result was 2.10 ($\times 10^{12}$/L). In five subsequent runs, the low control results were 2.15, 2.19, 2.20, 2.22, and 2.25.

1. These values represent:
   a. a shift
   b. a trend
   c. neither shift nor trend
2. Should Karen be concerned about these values? Explain.
3. Does Karen need to take any action?

laboratory is of the highest quality. Adherence to a comprehensive QA program by clinical laboratories is important because laboratory results are important to patient care.

REVIEW QUESTIONS

1. What is the importance of quality assessment and quality control in the laboratory?

2. Explain the use of standards and controls in the laboratory's daily operation.

3. Explain how results can be precise but not accurate.

4. How is the mean of a set of values determined?

5. Describe how to calculate the standard deviation.

6. Explain how an out-of-control result can be detected.

7. Explain how to detect a trend in a procedure.

8. How can the coefficient of variation be used to compare methods of analysis?

9. What is the purpose of Westgard's rules?

10. What are preanalytical and postanalytical factors? Give an example of each.

11. What are the differences in systematic error and random error?

12. Define accuracy, average, blind sample, calibration, coefficient of variation, controls, Gaussian curve, Levey-Jennings chart, mean, population, precision, quality assessment, quality assurance, quality control, quality systems, random error, sample, shift, standard, standard deviation, statistics, systematic error, trend, variance, and Westgard's rules.

STUDENT ACTIVITIES

1. Complete the written examination for this lesson.

2. Practice calculating the standard deviation using this group of numbers: 10, 9, 15, 10, 12, 11, 10, 12, 14, 12.

3. Using the results of the calculations from #2, construct a Levey-Jennings quality control chart showing the mean, +1*s*, +2*s*, +3*s*, −1*s*, −2*s*, and −3*s*.

4. Complete the worksheet at the end of this lesson.

WEB ACTIVITIES

1. Use the Internet to find information about quality control. One site is www.westgard.com.

2. Search terms such as Levey-Jennings chart, trend, and shift using the Internet. From the information in your text and on the Web, write a brief set of rules for determining when a control value is "out-of-control" and a list of remedies or checks to perform to identify the problem.

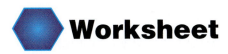 **Worksheet**

LESSON 1-7 Quality Assessment in the Laboratory

Name _____ Date _____

A. Calculating the Mean and the Standard Deviation

Use this worksheet and the data presented below to calculate the mean and the standard deviation. The red blood cell (RBC) counts from an RBC control solution are 3.2, 3.3, 3.5, 3.2, 3.0, 3.4, 3.8, 3.5, 3.4, and 3.3.

1. What is the formula for finding the mean? _____

2. Substitute the values into the formula.

3. The mean of the red cell counts is _____

4. Following the example in Figure 1-35, calculate the deviation squared for each of the values above.

5. What is the formula for variance?

6. Determine the variance using the answer in step 4.

7. What is the formula for determining standard deviation? _____

8. Substitute values from step 6 into the formula.

9. What is the standard deviation? _____ What is ± 2*s*? _____ What is ± 3*s*? _____

B. Constructing a Levey-Jennings Chart

1. Use the mean and standard deviation (*s*) from part A to construct a Levey-Jennings chart. Indicate the mean value, ±1*s*, ±2*s*, and ±3*s* (from part A) on the appropriate lines.

2. Plot these control values obtained for days 1–10 on the chart: Day 1 = 3.2, Day 2 = 3.3, Day 3 = 3.5, Day 4 = 3.2, Day 5 = 3.0, Day 6 = 3.4, Day 7 = 3.8, Day 8 = 3.5, Day 9 = 3.4, and Day 10 = 3.3.

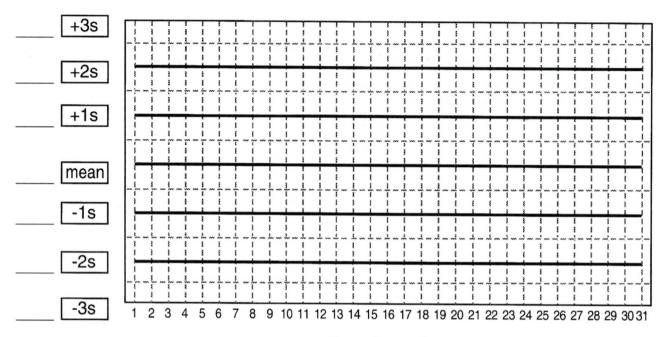

Day of month

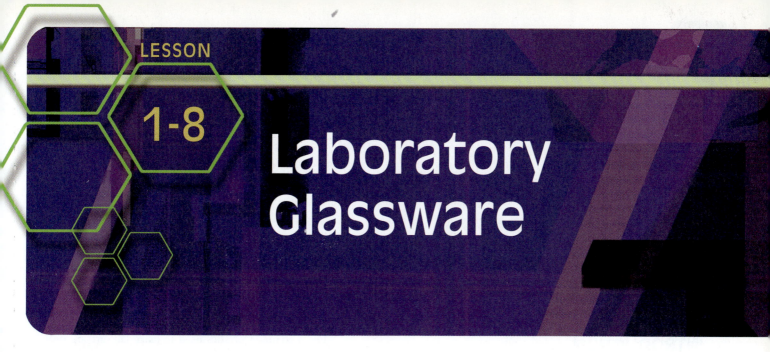

Laboratory Glassware

LESSON OBJECTIVES

After studying this lesson, the student will:

- Identify five basic types of containers used in the laboratory and explain the use of each.
- Explain the differences between critical and noncritical measurements.
- Identify glassware that can be used for critical measurements.
- Identify heat-resistant glassware.
- Identify volumetric pipets and explain their proper use.
- Identify graduated pipets and explain their proper use.
- Measure and transfer liquids using pipets and micropipetters.
- Discuss the advantages and disadvantages of using plastic containers in the laboratory.
- Describe the proper care of and cleaning procedures for laboratory glassware and plasticware.
- List safety precautions to be observed when using labware and plasticware.
- Explain how the condition of labware can affect the outcome of test procedures.
- Define the glossary terms.

GLOSSARY

beaker / a wide-mouthed, straight-sided container with a pouring spout formed from the rim and used to make estimated measurements

borosilicate glass / nonreactive glass with high thermal resistance and commonly used to make high-quality labware

critical measurements / measurements made when the accuracy of the concentration of a solution is important; measurements made using glassware manufactured to strict standards

flask / a container with an enlarged body and a narrow neck

flint glass / inexpensive glass with low resistance to heat and chemicals

graduated cylinder / an upright, straight-sided container with a flared base and a volume scale

labware / article(s) or container(s) intended for laboratory use

meniscus / the curved upper surface of a liquid in a container

micropipet / a pipet that measures or holds one milliliter or less

micropipetter / a mechanical pipetter that can measure or deliver very small volumes, usually less than 1.0 mL

noncritical measurements / estimated measurements; measurements made in containers that estimate volume (such as beakers)

pipet / a slender tube used in the laboratory for measuring and transferring liquids

polyethylene / plastic polymer of ethylene used for containers

polypropylene / lightweight plastic polymer of propylene that resists moisture and solvents and is heat-sterilizable

polystyrene / clear, colorless polymer of styrene used for labware

quartz glass / expensive glass with excellent light transmission; glass used for cuvettes; silica glass

reagent / substance or solution used in laboratory analyses; substance involved in a chemical reaction

solute / the substance dissolved in a given solution

solvent / a dissolving agent, usually a liquid

TC / on pipets, a mark indicating to contain

TD / on pipets, a mark indicating to deliver

INTRODUCTION

Basic laboratory glassware comes in many shapes and sizes. Glassware can be used in a specific test procedure or in preparing or storing **reagents**, solutions used in laboratory analysis.

In recent years, it has become common to use laboratory containers of plastic, as well as glass. Because of this, the term **labware** is sometimes used to include glassware and plasticware. Much of today's labware is designed to be used only once and then discarded. This eliminates the possibility of using labware that is contaminated with residue from a previous use.

This lesson explains the basic types of labware and gives guidelines for proper use, care, and cleaning.

GENERAL LABWARE

General labware includes bottles, beakers, flasks, test tubes, graduated cylinders, and pipets. Labware items are composed of glass or plastic.

Glassware

Laboratory glassware can be made of flint glass, borosilicate glass, or quartz/silica glass.

- **Flint glass** is inexpensive but has a low resistance to heat and chemicals. Disposable test tubes are often made of flint glass.

- **Borosilicate glass** is nonreactive with most chemicals, is usually of high thermal resistance, and can be heat sterilized. *Pyrex* and *Kimax* are brands of borosilicate glass commonly used for beakers, flasks, and other laboratory glassware.

- **Quartz glass,** or silica glass, is an expensive glass that, in the laboratory, is often used when glass must have excellent light transmission without distortion, such as in cuvettes for spectrophotometers.

Plasticware

Plastic containers are useful because they are lightweight and impact- and corrosion-resistant. Plastics are unaffected by most aqueous solutions. Plastics do not release ions as some types of glass do but can bind and release (leach) solutes.

Three common plastics used to make labware are **polyethylene**, **polypropylene**, and **polystyrene**. Containers made of polyethylene and polystyrene are clear, inexpensive, and disposable but are not heat resistant. Polypropylene containers usually have a milky or opaque appearance, are heat resistant, and can be heat sterilized.

TYPES OF LABWARE AND THEIR FUNCTIONS

The function of labware is determined by its design and manufacturing standards. Some labware, such as bottles, beakers, and certain flasks, are used to make **noncritical measurements**, that is, estimated measurements.

Other labware is designed to strict standards to allow measurements to be made that require accuracy; these are called **critical measurements**. This glassware is manufactured and calibrated to standards prescribed by the National Institute for Standards and Technology (NIST), formerly the National Bureau of Standards (NBS). The glassware comes with a certificate of calibration and is marked with capacity tolerance limits.

Bottles

Reagent bottles are available in a variety of sizes and types. Plastic bottles should be used for all reagents that do not interact with plastic. Reagents should not be stored for long periods in low-quality glass containers that can slowly release ions into the reagent solutions. The reagent bottle should be only slightly larger than the volume of reagent. Plastic and glass brown bottles are used for storing light-sensitive reagents.

Beakers

Beakers are wide-mouthed, straight-sided containers with a pouring spout formed from the rim (Figure 1-38). They are used for *estimating* the amount of liquid, mixing solutions, or simply holding liquids. Each beaker is labeled to indicate the approximate capacity in milliliters and the estimated accuracy of the capacity markings. When using a beaker to estimate volume, a beaker with

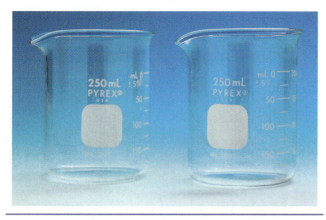

FIGURE 1-38 Beakers with markings

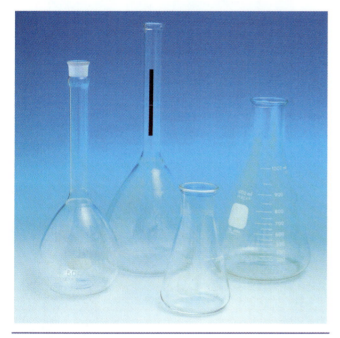

FIGURE 1-39 Flasks: volumetric flasks on left; Erlenmeyer flasks on right

capacity nearest the volume to be measured should be selected. In other words, a 1000-mL beaker should not be used to measure 100 mL. Although beakers have many uses in the laboratory, they should be used only for noncritical measurements. For instance a 250-mL beaker marked ±5% indicates that, when the beaker is filled to the 250-mL line, the actual volume in the beaker could be between 237 mL and 263 mL.

Flasks

A **flask** is a container with an enlarged body and a narrow neck. Two common flasks are Erlenmeyer flasks and volumetric flasks (Figure 1-39).

The *Erlenmeyer flask* has a flat bottom and sloping sides that gradually narrow in diameter so the top opening is bottle-like. The opening can be plain, so it can be stoppered with a cork, or it can have threads for a cap. Erlenmeyer flasks range from 10 mL to 4000 mL capacity. They are used to hold liquids, mix

solutions, or measure noncritical volumes. Markings on the side indicate the capacity in mL. In addition, some also have 50 mL to 100 mL increment marks. These are called "graduated flasks" and are convenient for estimating volumes (noncritical measurements).

The *volumetric flask* is a pear-shaped flask used for making critical measurements, which require accuracy. Volumetric flasks are manufactured to strict standards and guaranteed to contain a certain volume at a particular temperature. A line is etched in the neck of the flask to indicate the proper fill level. The capacity (in mL) is marked on the flask along with the tolerance limit, also usually in mL.

To prepare a reagent using a volumetric flask, water or another **solvent** is placed in the flask. An exact amount of **solute** is measured into the flask. The remaining solvent is then added until it approaches the fill line. The last portion is added slowly until the lowest point of the **meniscus**, or curved liquid surface, is level with the fill line when viewed at eye level (Figure 1-40).

Test Tubes

Test tubes are used in many laboratory procedures. They are available in various types of plastic and glass, and a variety of sizes and shapes (Figure 1-41). Test tubes function as containers for blood, urine, or serum. In some procedures, the analysis is performed in a test tube. Sometimes a test method requires that the contents be heated in the test tube. This should be done with caution, using only a test tube made of heat-resistant glass.

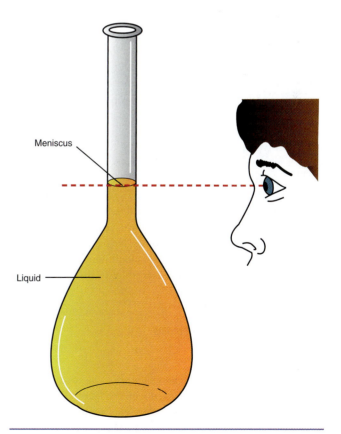

Meniscus

Liquid

FIGURE 1-40 Observing the meniscus at the fill line of a volumetric flask

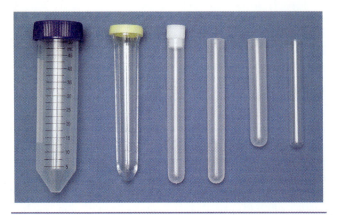

FIGURE 1-41 Test tubes

Graduated Cylinders

A **graduated cylinder** is an upright, straight-sided container with a flared base and a volume scale. Graduated cylinders are commonly used to measure the volume of 24-hour urine specimens (Figure 1-42A). Graduated cylinders are available in capacities ranging from 5 to 2000 mL. Liquids are measured in a graduated cylinder by pouring the liquid into the cylinder and reading the volume at the lowest point of the meniscus (Figure 1-42B).

Glass and Plastic Pipets

Pipets are open-ended glass or plastic tubes used to measure and transfer precise volumes of a liquid. Pipets are manufactured to strict specifications and calibrated to transfer or deliver specified volumes, which are marked on the pipets (Figure 1-43). Many types and sizes of pipets are used in laboratory work. Pipets can range in capacity from 1.0 mL to 50 mL; volumes less than 1.0 mL are delivered by **micropipets** and **micropipetters**. It is important to know the different types of pipets, select the appropriate pipet for the task, and use each type appropriately.

Pipets are filled by suction with the aid of mechanical pipet-aids, bulb-type pipet-aids (Figure 1-44), or hand-held electric or battery-powered pipet filler-dispensers (Figure 1-45). The "mouth" or upper end of the pipet is fitted into the pipet-aid or pipet filler held in the operator's hand. Trigger-type buttons activate a pump that controls aspirating and dispensing in the pipet filler-dispenser. These devices are easy to use and can be used with pipets of various sizes and volumes. No matter which type of pipet is used, it is *never* permissible to mouth-pipet.

Pipets can be categorized according to their design and accuracy as:

- *Volumetric* pipets or
- *Serological* or *graduated* pipets

To Deliver Pipets

Pipets are marked to indicate how they are to be used to deliver liquids. A *to deliver* pipet is marked with the letters **TD** near the suction end of the pipet (Figure 1-43A). This means that when the pipet is emptied by gravity drainage, the pipet is calibrated to deliver the volume marked on the pipet in a specified time and at a specified

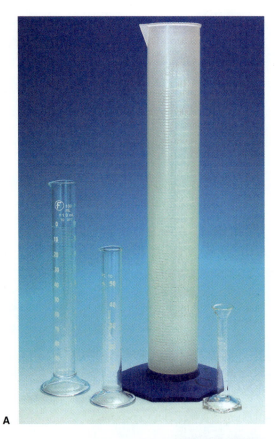

A

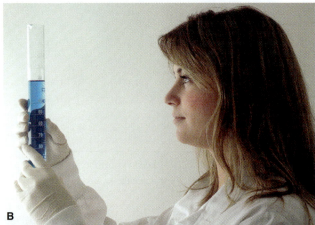

B

FIGURE 1-42 Graduated cylinders: (A) graduated cylinders with markings; (B) observing the meniscus in a graduated cylinder

temperature (Figure 1-43). When used correctly, the TD pipet delivers the specified amount of fluid, leaving a small drop of fluid in the pipet tip.

A TD pipet with a frosted band etched on the pipet neck is called a *blowout* pipet (Figure 1-43B). To correctly deliver the stated volume using a blowout pipet, the last drop remaining in the tip must be expelled or "blown out" using a pipet-aid or pipet filler-dispenser.

To Contain Pipets

A *to contain* pipet has the letters **TC** near the suction end of the pipet, indicating that the pipet is calibrated to contain the volume marked on the pipet. Because liquid will cling to the inner

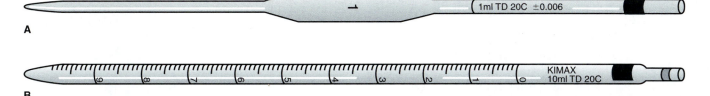

A

B

FIGURE 1-43 Pipets: (A) volumetric pipet; (B) serological pipet. Both pipets are TD and the bottom pipet is blowout type (frosted band)

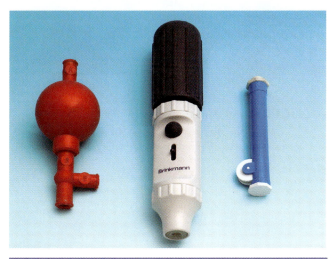

FIGURE 1-44 Pipetting aids

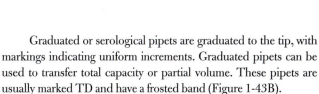

FIGURE 1-45 Using a battery-operated pipet filler-dispenser to transfer a liquid (*Courtesy CDC, Atlanta, GA*)

walls of the pipet it must be rinsed to be sure the stated volume is delivered.

Volumetric pipets

Volumetric pipets have a wide opening on the suctioning end, an oval bulb in the center, and a tapered tip on the dispensing end (Figure 1-43A). Volumetric pipets are usually labeled TD and are used when critical measurements are required, such as preparing a standard solution. Each volumetric pipet is marked and calibrated to deliver only one volume.

Volumetric pipets are used by attaching a suctioning aid or pipet filler to the pipet mouth (Figures 1-44 and 1-45). The liquid is suctioned into the pipet to the marking on the stem above the center bulb. Excess fluid on the outside of the pipet stem is wiped away with tissue, being careful that the tissue does not contact the fluid inside the pipet tip. The pipet is held nearly vertical, and the tip is placed against the inner surface of the container into which the liquid is to be transferred. The suction is released and the liquid is allowed to flow into the container. The tip is left in contact with the container surface a few seconds to completely drain the pipet. A small drop will remain in the pipet tip.

Serological or Graduated Pipets

Graduated pipets have a total capacity marking near the suction end and are usually labeled TD. Graduated pipets that have a frosted band around the opening are used by forcing out the last drop of liquid after the contents are drained.

Graduated or serological pipets are graduated to the tip, with markings indicating uniform increments. Graduated pipets can be used to transfer total capacity or partial volume. These pipets are usually marked TD and have a frosted band (Figure 1-43B).

To use a serological pipet, a suctioning device is attached. The liquid is suctioned up to the line as with the volumetric pipet. The pipet's outside stem is wiped dry with tissue. To deliver the total volume from the pipet, the liquid is allowed to drain out while the pipet is held almost vertically. The last remaining drops are forced out using the pipetting aid. It is more accurate to dispense fluid between two marks on a graduated pipet than to dispense contents in the tip.

Micropipets and Micropipetters

The measuring and transferring of very small volumes (microliter range) requires the use of precisely manufactured pipets or pipetting systems. Calibrated glass capillary tubes that deliver volumes as small as 5 µL are called micropipets. Depending on the design, a micropipet can be the TD or TC type.

Micropipetters are mechanical pipets manufactured by several companies in several designs (Figure 1-46A). Micropipetters are used to perform most manual pipetting tasks in the clinical laboratory. A one-use disposable plastic tip is used for each sampling. The volume is aspirated or delivered when the operator depresses and releases a plunger on the micropipetter (Figure 1-46B). The instructions accompanying each type of micropipette must be followed for pipetting accuracy and precision. Some micropipetters

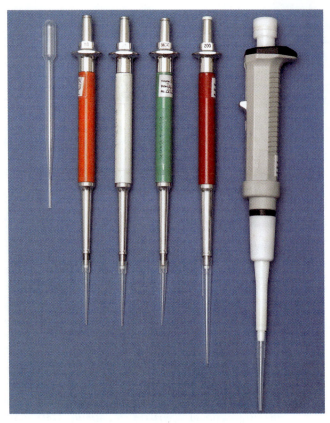

A

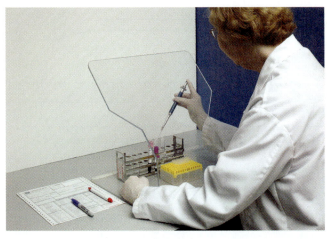

B

FIGURE 1-46 Micropipetters: (A) micropipetters and disposable transfer pipet; (B) using a micropipetter behind an acrylic safety shield

are preset to deliver just one volume while others are adjustable within a narrow range, such as 1 to 20 µL or 20 to 100 µL. The use of micropipetters provides better accuracy than manual pipetting and eliminates the need for pipet-aids or safety bulbs. Many laboratory analyzers aspirate and dispense samples automatically which further eliminates errors due to variation in pipetting techniques.

SAFETY PRECAUTIONS

   The use of labware presents several hazards, such as the potential for spills, splashes, aerosol formation, or injury from broken or chipped glass. Injuries can be prevented by using careful technique and wearing appropriate PPE. Whenever possible, plastic labware should be used to reduce the possibility of injury from broken glass. Each item of glassware should be inspected for chips or cracks before use and should not be used if these are present. If damaged glassware cannot be repaired, it should be discarded into rigid, puncture-proof containers.

Standard precautions must be observed and appropriate PPE must be worn when handling labware containing blood or other body fluids or substances and when repairing or cleaning micropipetters. Disposable contaminated labware and pipet tips must be discarded into appropriate biohazard disposal containers. Reusable labware that has come in contact with any patient specimen, serum control solution, or other potentially infectious materials (OPIM), must be decontaminated by soaking in a disinfectant solution before washing.

Heavy duty gloves and other appropriate PPE must be worn when cleaning glassware. Glassware marked with the Kimax or Pyrex trade name is heat-resistant, can be used for boiling solutions, and can be sterilized by autoclaving. Glassware not manufactured of heat-resistant glass must not be heated over direct heat or autoclaved.

QUALITY ASSESSMENT

Labware must be maintained and used appropriately since the type and quality of labware can affect test outcome. Only certified glassware should be used to make critical measurements. Containers such as beakers and Erlenmeyer flasks should only be used for noncritical measurements. When making volume measurements, containers that have a capacity close to the volume being measured should be used.

Improper pipetting technique can be a source of error in laboratory tests. Practice is required to develop pipetting accuracy and precision. Attention must be paid to the TD and TC markings when using pipets. Manufacturer's instructions for micropipetter maintenance, calibration, and use must be followed to insure that volume delivery with micropipetters is accurate. A regular schedule for maintenance and calibration should be performed and documented, using either micropipette-calibration kits provided by the manufacturer or a micropipette maintenance service, in which a certified technician comes to the laboratory at regular intervals to calibrate and repair the micropipettes.

Whenever possible, disposable labware should be used. For reusable labware, only properly cleaned and dry items free from chemical residues or detergents should be used in test procedures or for reagent storage. Glassware that is not clean will not make accurate measurements and can cause contamination of the solutions that are being measured or stored. Pipets with chipped or broken tips should be discarded because the tip must be intact for the pipet to be accurate.

CARE AND CLEANING OF LABWARE

Good quality glassware is expensive and must be handled with care. Clean labware should be stored protected from dust and accidental breakage.

Routine Cleaning

  Disposable labware is intended to be used once and then discarded. Reusable labware must be cleaned thoroughly after each use. Most cleaning problems, such as dried reagents, can be avoided if labware is rinsed with water immediately after use and soaked in a laboratory detergent solution such as Sparkleen or Cytoclean until it can be washed. Stubborn deposits can usually be removed by soaking the container overnight.

Labware can be washed by hand, using a brush if necessary, and wearing heavy-duty gloves. Washing should be followed by thorough rinsing several times with tapwater, followed by two to three reagent-grade water rinses and a final rinse in Type I reagent water (described in Lesson 1-9). Some sensitive test procedures require using labware that has been rinsed in Type I reagent water several times. After washing, heat-resistant labware can be dried in a drying oven.

Labware can also be washed using an automatic dishwasher. However, some plastics are weakened by frequent washing and drying in automatic dishwashers because of the high heat. Pipets are best washed using a pipet washer.

Cleaning Contaminated Labware

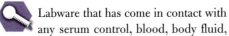 Labware that has come in contact with any serum control, blood, body fluid, patient specimen, or OPIM must be decontaminated before it is washed. This is usually accomplished by soaking the items in a disinfectant solution, such as dilute chlorine bleach, quaternary

ammonium detergent, or a phenolic solution such as Amphyl for at least 1 hour or overnight. Following decontamination, the items should be rinsed of disinfectant and then washed as described earlier for the routine cleaning of glassware. In some cases, labware must be sterilized by autoclaving before it can be washed.

SAFETY Reminders

- Wear appropriate PPE when handling labware containing blood or OPIM
- Disinfect glassware exposed to blood or OPIM before cleaning.
- Inspect beakers, flasks, and cylinders for chips and cracks before using.

PROCEDURAL Reminders

- Review QA section before performing procedure.
- Use the correct glassware for the task.
- Always use clean, dry glassware for measurements.
- Use a clean, dry pipet for each measurement.
- Rinse or soak glassware immediately after use.
- Do not use pipets with broken or chipped tips.

CASE STUDY

Jamie was in training in the Specimen Collection and Processing section of a small hospital laboratory. One of the laboratory employees asked him to measure the volume of a 24-hour urine specimen received in the laboratory that morning. At the work area were a 1000-mL beaker, a 1000-mL Erlenmeyer flask, and a 1000-mL graduated cylinder.

Which item(s) would give the most accurate measurement of volume? Explain your answer.

SUMMARY

Many types of glassware and plasticware having a variety of functions are used in the laboratory. These include bottles, beakers, flasks, test tubes, graduated cylinders, and pipets. Some items, such as bottles and beakers, are used only to hold or contain reagents. Other items such as graduated cylinders, volumetric flasks, and pipets, are used to measure volumes. Test tubes can be used as reaction vessels in laboratory tests. Pipets and micropipetters are used to measure and deliver liquid volumes.

Labware is manufactured to different standards of precision and accuracy, indicated by tolerance markings on the items. Selecting the proper container for the task and using the container properly can be critical to accurate laboratory results. The correct use of mechanical micropipetters with disposable tips increases pipetting accuracy, but these micropipetters require calibration at regular intervals. Disposable labware should be used when possible. Reusable labware must be properly disinfected and cleaned, using special attention to Standard Precautions as well as following safety practices for chemical and physical hazards.

REVIEW QUESTIONS

1. Name five types of containers used to hold liquids.
2. Name two types of laboratory flasks.
3. Which types of glassware are used to make critical measurements?
4. Name two types of glass pipets and explain the differences between them.
5. The last drop is forced out of which type of pipet?
6. Why is it important that damaged glassware not be used?
7. Why should labware be immediately rinsed after use?
8. What are the advantages of micropipetters? How are they used?
9. Why is it important that labware be rinsed until it is free of detergent?
10. How do flint glass and borosilicate glass differ?
11. What types of plastics are commonly used in the laboratory? What are some characteristics of each?
12. What is the procedure for cleaning labware that is contaminated with blood or OPIM?
13. Define beaker, borosilicate glass, critical measurements, flask, flint glass, graduated cylinder, labware, meniscus, micropipet, micropipetter, noncritical measurements, pipet, polyethylene, polypropylene, polystyrene, quartz glass, reagent, solute, solvent, TC, and TD.

STUDENT ACTIVITIES

1. Complete the written examination on this lesson.
2. Measure 100 mL of water in a beaker and transfer it to another beaker or flask. Does it measure 100 mL in the second container?
3. Measure 100 mL of water in an Erlenmeyer flask and transfer it to a 100-mL volumetric flask. Is the volume exactly 100 mL?
4. Practice using pipets, a graduated cylinder, and a volumetric flask following the procedure in the Student Performance Guide.

WEB WWW ACTIVITIES

1. Search the product listing of an online laboratory supply catalog. What types of pipet aids are offered? What types of micropipetters are sold?
2. Visit the NIST Web site. Find information on certified glassware.

Student Performance Guide

LESSON 1-8 Laboratory Glassware

Measuring liquids using a graduated cylinder, volumetric flask, pipets, and micropipetters

Name _____ Date _____

INSTRUCTIONS:

1. Practice using a graduated cylinder, volumetric flask, pipets, and micropipetters following the step-by-step procedure.
2. Demonstrate the procedures satisfactorily for the instructor, using the Student Performance Guide. Your instructor will determine the level of competency you must achieve to obtain a Satisfactory (S) grade.

MATERIALS AND EQUIPMENT

- gloves
- surface disinfectant
- antiseptic
- volumetric flasks
- graduated cylinders, various sizes
- volumetric and serological pipets
- pipet-aids
- pipet filler-dispenser (optional)
- micropipetters and disposable tips (with manufacturer instructions for use)
- large and small beakers
- distilled water or saline solution
- disposable plastic transfer pipets
- laboratory tissue

PROCEDURE ⚠️

Record in the comment section any problems encountered while practicing the procedure (or have a fellow student or the instructor evaluate your performance).

S = Satisfactory
U = Unsatisfactory

You must:	S	U	Comments
1. Clean work surface with surface disinfectant			
2. Obtain assorted glassware and pipetting systems (graduated cylinder, volumetric flask, pipets, pipet-aid and/or pipet filler-dispenser, micropipetter and tips, beaker, disposable plastic transfer pipets) and non-toxic solution such as water or saline			
3. Wash hands and put on gloves			
4. Fill beaker with water or saline			
5. Practice measuring volumes using a graduated cylinder: a. Hold the cylinder so that the desired volume marking is at eye level b. Carefully pour water or saline into the cylinder until it reaches the desired volume marking c. Observe the meniscus holding the cylinder at eye level; the lowest point of the meniscus should be level with the volume marking (Figure 1-42)			

You must:	S	U	Comments
d. Adjust the volume, if necessary, by adding or removing solution dropwise with a disposable pipet until the meniscus is at the proper point e. Pour the solution back into the beaker f. Use a different size cylinder to measure volume, following steps 5a through 5e			
6. Practice measuring volumes using a volumetric flask: a. Examine the flask and find the fill line etched in the flask neck b. Pour water or saline into the flask carefully and slowly until it nears the fill line c. Hold the flask so that the fill line is at eye level d. Use a disposable pipet to deliver solution drop-wise into the flask until the low point of the meniscus is level with the fill line e. Pour the solution back into the beaker f. Practice measuring volumes in volumetric flasks and reading the meniscus			

7. Practice using serological and volumetric pipets to measure and transfer volumes. **NOTE:** *Adjust procedure to fit equipment available. Pipet-aids come in several designs. Consult directions on proper use of pipet-aid*
a. Obtain a pipet and pipet-aid or pipet filler-dispenser
b. Examine the pipet to determine if it is TD or TD blowout (frosted band)
c. Fit the pipet-aid securely to the mouth of the pipet
d. Hold the pipet vertical and insert the pipet tip well below the surface of the fluid in the beaker
e. Draw up fluid into the pipet using the pipet-aid, filling the pipet to slightly above the desired volume marking
f. Remove the pipet from the solution and wipe the outside of the pipet tip quickly with tissue to remove excess fluid, being careful not to allow the tissue to touch the opening in the pipet tip
g. Touch the pipet tip to the inner surface of the beaker and slowly lower the fluid level using the pipet-aid, until the lowest point of the meniscus touches the volume marking
h. Move the pipet to the receiving container and hold it nearly vertical over the container
i. For a TD pipet:
  1) Place the tip against the inner surface of the receiving container
  2) Release the suction on the pipet-aid and allow the liquid to drain from the pipet by gravity drainage
  3) Leave the pipet tip in contact with the side of the container 1 to 3 seconds to allow the correct volume to be delivered
  4) Examine the pipet tip—a small drop of fluid should remain in the tip			

94

You must:	S	U	Comments

j. For a TD blowout pipet:
  1) Follow steps i-1 through i-3
  2) Use the pipet-aid to force out the last drop of solution from the pipet tip into the receiving container			

8. Continue practicing transferring liquids being sure to use both TD and TD blowout pipets			

9. Practice using a micropipetter to deliver liquids following the instructions that accompany the micropipetter
  a. Be sure to seat pipet tip firmly on the micropipetter before pipeting
  b. Be sure to adjust volume correctly before pipetting, if using an adjustable volume micropipetter
  c. Depress and release the plunger slowly so that no bubbles enter the pipet tip
  d. Do not immerse micropipetter into liquid, only a portion of the tip should be in the liquid
  e. Do not allow liquid to be aspirated into the micropipetter shaft
  f. Be sure to correctly use the two dispensing "stops" (if applicable)			

10. Place used glassware in appropriate wash solution or container and put away all equipment			
11. Clean micropipetter and work surface with surface disinfectant			
12. Remove and discard gloves and wash hands with antiseptic			

Evaluator Comments:

Evaluator _____ Date _____

General Laboratory Equipment

LESSON OBJECTIVES

After studying this lesson, the student will:

- Explain the proper use of a centrifuge.
- Explain the function of a pH meter.
- Discuss the operation of an autoclave.
- List four rules for using a laboratory balance.
- Explain how temperature control chambers are used in the laboratory.
- Name three types of reagent water, and explain how they are made.
- Discuss safety precautions that must be followed when using the centrifuge, autoclave, pH meter, and the laboratory balance.
- Explain the importance of performing regular equipment maintenance and keeping maintenance and repair records.
- Define the glossary terms.

GLOSSARY

autoclave / a device that uses pressurized steam for sterilization

centrifuge / an instrument with a rotor that rotates at high speeds in a closed chamber

deionized water / water that has had most of the mineral ions removed

distilled water / the condensate collected from steam after water has been boiled

microfuge / a centrifuge that spins microcentrifuge tubes at high rates of speed; microcentrifuge

pH / a measurement of the hydrogen ion concentration expressing the degree of acidity or alkalinity of a solution

reverse osmosis / purification of water by forcing water through a semi-permeable membrane

rotor / the part of a centrifuge that holds the tubes and rotates during the operation of the centrifuge

serological centrifuge / a centrifuge that spins small tubes such as those used in blood banking; serofuge

INTRODUCTION

Clinical laboratories use several types of general laboratory equipment to prepare and store reagents and specimens. The types of equipment and instruments found in a clinical laboratory are determined by the size of the laboratory and the number of tests performed. A small laboratory may have only a microscope, refrigerator, and centrifuge. Large laboratories have an assortment of general equipment, such as pH meters, autoclaves, balances, incubators, and water baths, as well as several types of analytical instruments. Equipment used in all parts of the testing process must operate correctly. Personnel must know the proper use, care, maintenance, and, sometimes, repair of general laboratory equipment.

This lesson introduces some general guidelines for the use, care, and maintenance of common laboratory equipment. Lesson 1-8 contains information about pipets and micropipetters; Lesson 1-10 contains information about the use and care of the microscope. General laboratory safety rules must be followed (Lessons 1-5 and 1-6) when using laboratory equipment, as well as special safety guidelines required with each particular type of instrument. Manuals provided by equipment manufacturers must be consulted to determine the proper use and limits of each piece of equipment.

LABORATORY EQUIPMENT SAFETY PRECAUTIONS

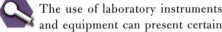 The use of laboratory instruments and equipment can present certain hazards, such as presence of high-voltage electrical current and exposure to moving equipment parts, steam, or hot liquids. Certain instruments can also present the risk of exposure to blood or other potentially infectious materials (OPIM). The hazards differ according to the equipment and how it is used.

All equipment must be operated in a safe manner, following the manufacturers' directions. Preventive maintenance should be performed carefully, adhering to Standard Precautions and other recommended safety practices. Only trained persons should repair equipment. Additional equipment-specific safety information is included in the section describing the function and operation of each type of equipment.

QUALITY ASSESSMENT PROGRAM FOR LABORATORY EQUIPMENT

As part of the overall quality assessment program, regular maintenance, calibration, and performance checks must be performed for all laboratory equipment, including refrigerators, waterbaths, centrifuges, autoclaves, pH meters, and balances. The results of these procedures must be documented. Any problems detected must be corrected before the equipment is used for laboratory work. The laboratory procedure manual will specify the frequency and types of checks that must be performed for each piece of laboratory equipment.

CENTRIFUGES

Centrifuges are instruments that spin samples at high speeds, forcing the heavier particles to the bottom of the container (usually a tube). The part of the centrifuge that holds the tubes and rotates during operation is the **rotor**. The most frequent clinical laboratory use of the centrifuge is for separating the cellular components of blood from the liquid (serum or plasma) so the liquid can be used for testing.

Centrifuges vary in size, capacity, and speed capability. Microcentrifuges, or **microfuges**, are widely used in the clinical laboratory to spin special microtubes (0.5 to 1.5 mL capacity) at high speeds, up to 14,000 rpm (Figure 1-47). The microhematocrit centrifuge is a variation of the microfuge; it spins capillary tubes at high speeds for measuring microhematocrits.

Clinical centrifuge is the name given to models that can be used for urinalysis or serum separation (Figure 1-48). These usually have a speed capacity of 0 to 3,000 rpm (revolutions per minute), and hold tubes ranging in size from 5 to 50 mL depending on the adapters. A **serological centrifuge** is a small centrifuge used in blood banking to spin small tubes (approximately 2–3 mL capacity).

Other types of centrifuges include high-speed refrigerated centrifuges that have speed capabilities up to 20,000 rpm, and ultracentrifuges that are capable of speeds over 50,000 rpm. These centrifuges are specially equipped to keep samples cool

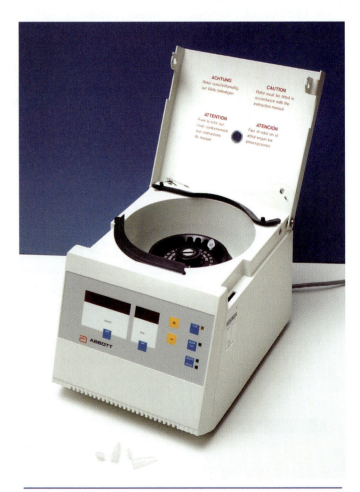

FIGURE 1-47 Microcentrifuge and microtubes (in foreground)

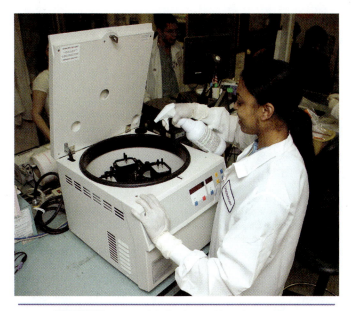

FIGURE 1-48 Disinfecting a clinical centrifuge

during centrifugation. Centrifuges such as these are often used in research laboratories but are not usually required for routine clinical laboratory samples.

Centrifuge Safety

  Centrifuges present several safety hazards. Since they are used to process biological specimens, Standard Precautions must be observed and appropriate personal protective equipment (PPE) must be worn when operating a centrifuge. The centrifuge must be disinfected using surface disinfectant any time spills or splashes occur.

Manufacturer's instructions must always be followed when using a centrifuge. Some general rules to follow include:

1. Load must be balanced before centrifuge operation: A tube of identical size and containing an equal volume of liquid to the specimen tube must be placed opposite each specimen tube in the rotor (Figure 1-49).

2. Tubes should remain capped during centrifugation to prevent aerosol formation.

3. Only tubes rated as appropriate for the particular centrifuge and speed should be used.

4. The centrifuge must not be opened while the rotor is spinning. Centrifuges should be equipped with safety latches (called cover interlocks) that keep the centrifuge lid locked during centrifuge operation.

5. Spills must be cleaned immediately with surface disinfectant (Figure 1-48).

Quality Assessment

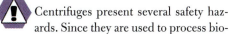 The rotation speeds and accuracy of centrifuge timers must be verified and documented at specific intervals, usually monthly or quarterly.

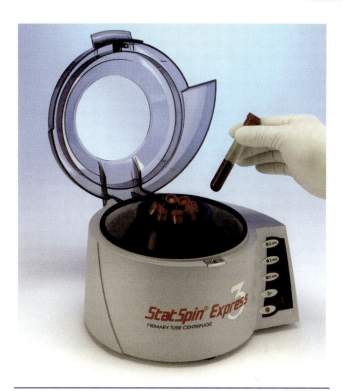

FIGURE 1-49 Proper way to balance tubes in a centrifuge rotor (*Courtesy of Iris Sample Processing, Westwood, MA*)

AUTOCLAVES

Autoclaves use steam under pressure to sterilize items such as dental and surgical instruments, solutions, and materials to be used in microbiology (Figure 1-50). Autoclaves are also used to decontaminate materials such as blood specimens, bacterial cultures, or filled biohazard containers before disposal.

Autoclaves can range in size from large (refrigerator size) to tabletop size. Large autoclaves obtain steam from either an internal steam generator or a pipe connected to the facility's steam plant. Smaller ones create their own steam by heating water.

Items to be sterilized or decontaminated are placed in bags, wrapped in paper, or placed in heat-proof autoclave pans. An indicator such as autoclave tape is used on packages and glassware in each run; this tape changes color when the proper temperature is reached in the autoclave. Items are placed inside the autoclave and the autoclave door is closed and locked. The temperature, length of cycle, and pounds of steam pressure are set. Typical autoclave conditions are 121°C for 15 to 20 minutes at 15 pounds per square inch (psi). Steam is admitted into the chamber and timing begins when temperature and pressure have reached set levels. Autoclaves have temperature and pressure gauges, and most have a chart or digital recorder that records the temperature of each autoclave cycle. At the end of the cycle, the pressure and temperature will drop; the autoclave can be opened when the chamber pressure gauge reads zero (0) psi.

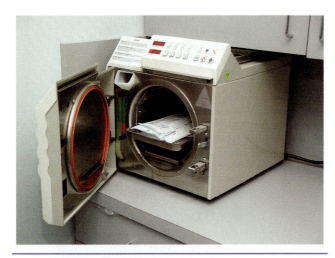

FIGURE 1-50 A tabletop autoclave

Autoclave Safety

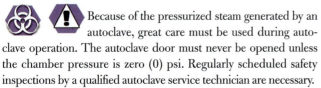 Because of the pressurized steam generated by an autoclave, great care must be used during autoclave operation. The autoclave door must never be opened unless the chamber pressure is zero (0) psi. Regularly scheduled safety inspections by a qualified autoclave service technician are necessary.

To prevent burns, tongs and/or heat-proof gloves must be used to remove items from the autoclave. When liquids are sterilized, they must be in loosely capped, heat-resistant containers that are no more than half full. These containers must be placed in an autoclavable tray or pan to catch overflow. Chamber pressure must be reduced slowly at the end of a "liquid run" to prevent the liquids from boiling over.

Quality Assessment

It is important that autoclaves work properly, since nonsterile items could endanger both worker and patient or could cause problems in a test procedure requiring sterile solutions or components. Indicator strips containing spores from the bacterium *Bacillus stearothermophilus* can be used to check the effectiveness of the steam sterilization process. The strips are autoclaved with a normal load, removed, and then incubated in a tube of bacterial growth medium. Lack of bacterial growth confirms the efficiency of sterilization; growth of bacteria indicates the sterilization method was inadequate and the items in that run are not sterile. Temperature, pressure, and time controls must then be checked to determine the cause of failure.

Daily records must be kept of sterilization times, temperatures, chamber pressures, and indicator strip results. The temperature chart recorder must be changed at specified intervals and the charts maintained in the equipment logbook.

LABORATORY BALANCES

Several types of balances or scales are used in the laboratory. They differ in the maximum amount they can accurately weigh, their sensitivities, and basic design (Figure 1-51).

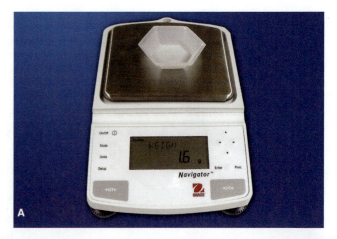

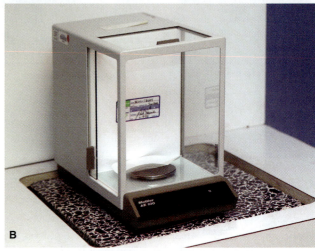

FIGURE 1-51 Laboratory balances: (A) top-loading balance; (B) cabinet balance

Measurements that require sensitivity to 0.10 gram can be made using inexpensive double- or triple-beam balances. Measurements of as little as 0.0001 g (10^{-4} g) or even 0.00001 g (10^{-5} g) can be made using a single-pan balance with sufficient sensitivity. However, most critical weighing is done using electronic top-loading or cabinet balances.

Laboratory Balance Safety

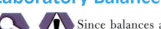 Since balances are used to weigh chemicals, appropriate chemical safety precautions must be used to prevent exposure to the chemical or chemical dust. The technician should observe basic safety rules, know the hazards of the chemical they are working with, and wear appropriate PPE. Care should be taken that chemical dusts are not created during transfer of chemicals. Work practice controls should include:

- Wear eye protection to avoid getting chemicals in the eyes.

- Wear a mask to avoid breathing in chemical dusts that can be respiratory irritants.

- Wear gloves and a laboratory coat to avoid chemical contact with skin and clothing.

■ Clean up spills around the balance so the work area is safe for others.

Quality Assessment

Chemicals must be weighed accurately to prepare reagents correctly. The manufacturer's instruction manual must be followed for the particular balance being used. Some general rules to follow to protect the balance and ensure quality results are:

■ Keep balances clean and wipe up any spills immediately.

■ Protect the balance from jarring, sudden shocks, and temperature extremes.

■ Keep the balance in the same location; do not move it from place to place.

■ Level the balance by adjusting balance legs.

■ Position the balance in a location that is free of drafts and vibrations. Special stabilizing tables are available if vibrations are a problem.

■ Check zero adjustment; scale should read zero (0) when the weigh pan is empty.

■ Always use a container for weighing chemicals; do not place chemical directly on balance pan.

■ Set balance scale to zero (tare balance) with the empty weighing container on the pan.

■ Observe the sensitivity limits of the balance; do not try to weigh 0.001 g on a balance that is accurate only to 0.01 g.

■ Calibrate balances on a regular schedule; perform yearly maintenance or contract to have the services done.

PH METERS

The pH of reagents is critical to many laboratory procedures. The **pH** is a measure of the hydrogen ion (H^+) concentration of a solution. It indicates the acidity or alkalinity of a solution. The pH scale is 0 to 14. A pH of 7 is neutral; at pH 7, the hydrogen ion (H^+) concentration equals the hydroxyl ion (OH^-) concentration. pH values below 7.0 indicate acid solutions; values above 7.0 indicate alkaline solutions. Lemon juice, vinegar, and hydrochloric acid (HCl) are examples of acids; solutions of baking soda, sodium hydroxide (NaOH), and potassium hydroxide (KOH) are examples of alkaline solutions.

A pH electrode connected to the pH meter detects the hydrogen ion concentration of a solution by comparing it to a reference electrode. The meter measures the potential across a membrane inside the electrode. Most meters use a single combination electrode that contains both the detecting electrode and reference electrode in one probe. When an unknown solution is tested, the potential of the unknown solution is compared to the potential created in the reference electrode. The measurement is converted to pH and displayed on the dial or screen of the pH meter (Figure 1-52A). If the pH of a reagent is too low, it can be made more alkaline by adding a few drops of a concentrated alkaline solution, usually NaOH. If the pH is too high, a concentrated acid such as hydrochloric acid or acetic acid can be used to lower the pH.

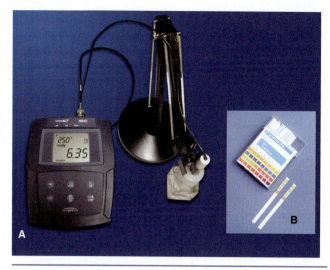

FIGURE 1-52 Measuring pH: (A) pH meter; (B) pH indicator strips for estimating pH (*Courtesy of Alan Estridge*)

pH can be estimated using special papers treated with indicator solutions. These papers are dipped into the solution to be tested, and the color that develops is compared to a color chart to determine the pH (Figure 1-52B). This method is suitable for measuring urine pH, but is not sensitive enough for preparing most laboratory reagents.

pH Meter Safety

Care should be used when performing pH measurements. Caustic or acid solutions to adjust pH must be used carefully. Chemical spills must be wiped up immediately. The pH meter should be disconnected from the electrical source before attempting any repair.

Quality Assessment

Special care must be taken in handling, maintaining, and storing the pH electrode so it will not dry out or be broken. The electrodes must always be rinsed with distilled or reagent water between samples, but never stored in water. Manuals that come with the meters give detailed instructions for use and storage of electrodes.

Electrodes must be calibrated using solutions of known pH values, usually 4.0, 7.0, and 10.0. The electrodes are immersed in the known solutions and the meter is set to that value; the numerical pH values will appear on the dial or digital display.

TEMPERATURE CONTROL CHAMBERS

Most test procedures, specimens, and reagents require testing or storage at specific temperatures. Many reagents must be stored refrigerated or frozen; patient specimens are refrigerated or frozen; and microbiological cultures and some chemistry tests require special incubation conditions. To accomplish these tasks, several types of temperature control chambers are used in the clinical laboratory. These include:

- Ovens for drying labware
- Microbiology incubators
- Water baths
- Refrigerators
- Freezers
- Microwaves

Microbiology incubators are commonly set near body temperature (37°C) for optimum growth of bacterial pathogens. Water baths provide controlled heat above ambient (room) temperature. These can be used as test incubation chambers, or to thaw frozen reagents. Microwaves can be used for thawing or to heat solutions. Refrigerated units are used occasionally for tests that must be performed in the cold, but more commonly refrigerators are used for reagent, blood, and serum storage (Figure 1-53). Freezers are used to store certain reagents and sera. Table 1-32 lists standard permissible temperature ranges for various temperature control chambers.

Temperature Control Chamber Safety

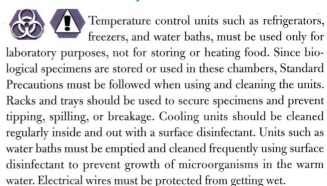 Temperature control units such as refrigerators, freezers, and water baths, must be used only for laboratory purposes, not for storing or heating food. Since biological specimens are stored or used in these chambers, Standard Precautions must be followed when using and cleaning the units. Racks and trays should be used to secure specimens and prevent tipping, spilling, or breakage. Cooling units should be cleaned regularly inside and out with a surface disinfectant. Units such as water baths must be emptied and cleaned frequently using surface disinfectant to prevent growth of microorganisms in the warm water. Electrical wires must be protected from getting wet.

Quality Assessment

All temperature-controlled units must be monitored regularly to be sure they are operating at the proper temperature. The temperature must be recorded daily and checked before each use. Calibrated thermometers must be used for measuring the temperatures; a thermometer should be kept in each unit so that the temperature can be checked frequently. Water baths must be filled to the appropriate level to insure that specimens will heat properly. Freezers and refrigerated units are fitted with alarms to alert when the temperature goes outside the permissible range. They are also usually connected to accessory power in case of power outage.

LABORATORY REAGENT WATER

Several grades of water are used in the laboratory. The Clinical and Laboratory Standards Institute (CLSI) and the College of American Pathologists (CAP) recommend three levels of water purity: type I, type II, and type III, with type I being the most pure. All three types are made from either deionized, distilled or

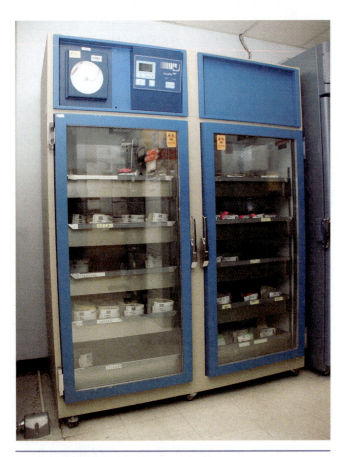

FIGURE 1-53 Temperature control chamber; blood bank refrigerator

TABLE 1-32. Permissible temperature ranges for common laboratory equipment		
EQUIPMENT	**TEMPERATURE (°C)**	**PERMISSIBLE RANGE (°C)**
Refrigerator	6 ± 2	4 to 8
Freezer	−20 ± 5	−15 to −25
Ultracold freezer	−70 ± 5	−65 to −75
Microbiology incubator	36 ± 1	35 to 37
Water bath	36 ± 1	35 to 37

reverse osmosis water. Each type of reagent water has a role in the laboratory. The grade of water used depends on the task. Tap water is used in the laboratory only for the initial washing of labware and never for preparation of reagents.

Distilled, Deionized, and Reverse Osmosis Water

Distilled water is the condensate collected from steam created when water is boiled. This process removes most of the common minerals such as iron, calcium, and magnesium but does not remove volatiles such as carbon dioxide, chlorine, and ammonia.

Deionized water is prepared by passing tap or distilled water through a resin column containing charged particles. The unwanted impurities in the water bind to these charged particles and are removed from the water. However, all organic substances, particulate matter, and microorganisms are not removed.

Reverse osmosis (RO), a process that forces water through a semi-permeable membrane, can also be used as an initial water purification step. RO removes nearly all bacteria, colloidal silica, particulates, organics, and a large percentage of ionic contaminants from water. However, water which passes through the RO membrane still contains small amounts of contaminants and will not meet CLSI/CAP Type I or Type II specifications.

Types of Reagent Water

To make Type I water from RO water, the RO water is passed through a high quality resin to remove remaining ions and through a small pore filter (0.22 μm) to exclude any remaining bacteria from the water. Type I water can also be obtained by processing deionized water using membrane filters to remove microorganisms and insoluble matter, and charcoal absorption to remove organic matter. Distilled water must be passed over resin and membrane filtered to be made Type I.

Type I reagent water is the purest grade and is used to prepare standard and control solutions and buffers for analytical procedures. Many of the standards and controls used in the laboratory are lyophilized (freeze-dried) material. Type I water is used to reconstitute (bring into solution) these materials, since it does not contain substances that can interfere with the analysis being performed.

Type II water can be used when the presence of small numbers of bacteria (≤100 per liter) will not affect results. It can be used for most procedures in hematology, immunology, and qualitative chemistry. It can be used in microbiology if it is sterilized.

Type III water can be used for some laboratory analyses such as routine urinalysis and as a source to prepare Types I and II. It can also be used for washing and rinsing glassware. However, only Type I or Type II should be used as the final rinse for glassware.

Type I water must be used soon after it has been prepared to avoid the absorption of gases such as carbon dioxide. Types II and III can be stored in tightly capped borosilicate glass or polyethylene containers.

EQUIPMENT MAINTENANCE RECORDS

The laboratory procedure manual will outline the required maintenance and performance checks for each piece of equipment. Log sheets are used for recording maintenance, service, repair, and performance checks.

A common schedule of performance checks in a small laboratory would include:

- Monitor and record temperatures of water baths, refrigerators, and incubators daily.
- Check temperature and chamber pressure record of autoclave after each use.
- Measure rpm on centrifuge with a tachometer every three months.
- Calibrate pH meter daily and check with standard solutions before each use.

An example of an equipment maintenance and performance checklist is given at the end of this lesson.

SAFETY Reminders

- Review equipment safety information before attempting any repair.
- Observe all safety rules as stated in your institution's procedure manual.
- Use common sense when operating all equipment.
- Always unplug electrical equipment before attempting any repairs.
- Use care when operating equipment with moving parts.
- Wipe up all spills promptly and appropriately.

PROCEDURAL Reminders

- Follow laboratory procedure and manufacturer's guidelines for routine equipment maintenance.
- Use equipment only according to manufacturer's instructions.
- Record all equipment maintenance and repairs.
- Report any instrument malfunction to the appropriate supervisor.

CASE STUDY 1

Carl is reconstituting clinical chemistry standards. He needs them in a hurry and there is no Type I water in the chemistry department. He sees a full container of Type III water and decides to use it.

What are the possible consequences?

CASE STUDY 2

June was working in clinical chemistry when a blood specimen came in with orders for STAT (immediate) testing. To obtain the serum needed for the test, June used a clinical centrifuge without a lid interlock. To save time, June opened the lid as the rotor slowed and used her hand to stop the rotor.

Since the test was ordered STAT, and the result was needed as soon as possible, did June do the right thing?

SUMMARY

Several types of general equipment are used in clinical laboratories, including refrigerators, freezers, water baths, centrifuges, autoclaves, pH meters, and laboratory balances. Although these types of equipment are not high-tech, they require regular maintenance and performance checks to be sure they are operating optimally. For instance, a refrigerator temperature that is just a few degrees out of the acceptable temperature range can cause reagent failure or specimen degradation, either by accidental freezing or by allowing products or specimens to become too warm and deteriorate.

Each piece of equipment carries its own set of operating procedures, maintenance instructions, calibration methods, and operating hazards. The manufacturer's safety and operating instructions should always be followed for each piece of equipment. These instructions should be incorporated into the laboratory procedure manual. Laboratory equipment such as refrigerators, freezers, and centrifuges may not be directly involved in laboratory analyses, but they do indirectly affect the test results because they are used for reagent preparation, and specimen processing and storage.

REVIEW QUESTIONS

1. Explain the function of a pH meter.
2. What rules should be followed when using a laboratory balance?
3. A solution with a pH of 8.5 is _____ (acidic or alkaline).
4. Give five general rules to follow when operating a centrifuge.
5. Name three types of centrifuges that can be found in a clinical laboratory.
6. Explain how autoclaves operate.
7. What grade of water is used to make laboratory standards and controls?
8. Why is it important to be careful when using an autoclave?
9. What quality control methods are used for temperature control chambers?
10. Why are equipment maintenance records important?
11. Name a hazard associated with: autoclave, centrifuge, pH meter, and laboratory balance.
12. Define autoclave, centrifuge, deionized water, distilled water, microfuge, pH, reverse osmosis, rotor, and serological centrifuge.

STUDENT ACTIVITIES

1. Complete the written examination for this lesson.

Depending on which instruments are available, complete activities 2–5. Read the instruction manual carefully before attempting to use an instrument. Then be sure to follow the instructions carefully when using that instrument.

2. If a pH meter is available, practice measuring the pH of a solution such as saline. Note how the pH changes when a few drops of 0.1% HCl or 0.1% NaOH are added to the solution. Dilute the solution by adding one part water to one

part solution. Now measure the pH. Did it change? How can the result be explained?

3. If a balance is available, practice weighing a nontoxic chemical or a substance such as salt or sugar. Note the capacity of the balance; what is the largest weight that can be measured? What is the smallest increment that can be read (1 g, 0.1 g, 0.01 g, etc.)?

4. If a centrifuge is available, practice centrifuging a sample. Be sure to use appropriate balance tubes. Note the speed scale; what is the maximum rpm the centrifuge can achieve? What size tubes can the centrifuge handle safely?

5. Use the equipment maintenance and performance checklist (at the end of this lesson) to check the performance of any available equipment.

WEB ACTIVITIES

1. Look in online scientific catalogs for calibrators or standards for general laboratory equipment:

   a. Find examples of thermometers for use in clinical refrigerators, freezers, and incubators. List the various designs available. Are the thermometers NIST certified?

   b. Determine what devices are available for calibrating centrifuge speed and how they are used.

   c. Find examples of calibrated weight sets for use with laboratory balances. How are the weight sets used to calibrate a laboratory balance?

   d. Find information on pH standard solutions for calibrating pH meters.

2. Search the Internet for instrument calibration services for clinical equipment such as centrifuges and laboratory balances. What calibration service intervals are recommended?

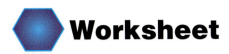 **Worksheet**

LESSON 1-9 General Laboratory Equipment

Name _____ Date _____

Use this form to record general laboratory equipment maintenance and performance. Identify each piece of equipment on the sheet. Locate instruction manuals for the equipment and determine what maintenance and/or calibration procedures are recommended and how often.

I. Temperature-Controlled Chambers

Record the temperatures of any refrigerators, freezers, water baths, or incubators in the laboratory. In a working laboratory, this must be done at least daily. If a thermometer does not stay in the equipment, place one inside for 20–30 minutes, then record temperature. Refrigerator thermometers can be stored with the bulb immersed in water or propylene glycol in a stoppered bottle. If the temperature is not within range, make the proper adjustment and remeasure or inform the supervisor.

Equipment I.D.	Range (°C)	Temperature Observed	Date	Comment/Sign
Freezer _____	-20 ± 5	_____	_____	_____
Refrigerator _____	6 ± 2	_____	_____	_____
Water bath _____	36 ± 1	_____	_____	_____
Incubator _____	36 ± 1	_____	_____	_____

II. Autoclave

During or after each run of the autoclave, check to see that the proper temperature and chamber pressure were reached. Each run should be given a number.

Autoclave: Run # _____   Temp °C _____   Chamber pressure _____

III. pH meter

Calibrate the meter before each use with two calibration solutions, one near the pH of the solution to be measured. (Commercial pH calibration solutions usually are pH 4, pH 7, and pH 10.) Check to see that the pH electrode is always stored in the appropriate solution when not in use.

Date	Calibration Solution	Comment/Sign
_____	_____	_____
_____	_____	_____
_____	_____	_____

IV. Centrifuges

Use a stopwatch to check the timer on the centrifuge. If available, use a tachometer to check rpm. *Do not attempt to check the speed if the centrifuge lid does not have an opening in the center or a see-through cover.*

I.D.	Date	Timer Check	RPM Check	Comment/Sign
Serofuge	_____	_____	_____	_____
Microfuge	_____	_____	_____	_____
Centrifuge	_____	_____	_____	_____

V. Balances

Check balances to see that they are clean and placed on a stable counter in a draft-free location. If available, use standard weights to check the calibration of the balances.

I.D.	Date	Balance Checked	Comment/Sign
_____	_____	_____	_____
_____	_____	_____	_____

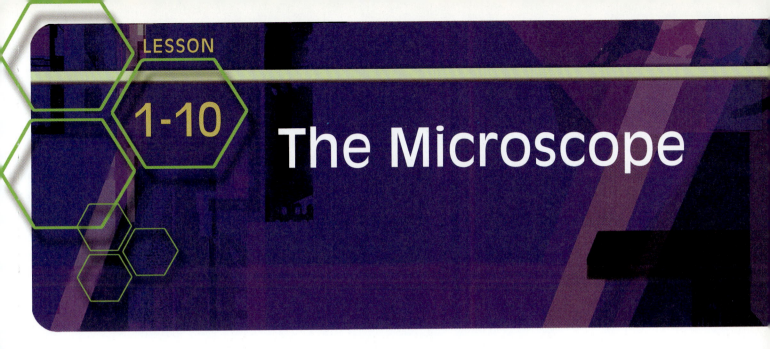

1-10

The Microscope

LESSON OBJECTIVES

After studying this lesson, the student will:

- Locate and name the parts of a light microscope.
- Explain the function of each part of the light microscope.
- Explain the use of coarse and fine adjustments.
- Use the low-power objective to view a specimen.
- Use the high-power objective to view a specimen.
- Use the oil-immersion objective to view a specimen.
- Adjust the condenser and iris diaphragm.
- Use Köhler illumination to align the microscope light path.
- Explain how to perform interpupillary distance and diopter adjustments.
- Explain when Standard Precautions and personal protective equipment should be used while using the microscope.
- Explain how light microscopes differ from electron microscopes.
- Explain how the proper care and storage of the microscope can affect the quality of results.
- Define the glossary terms.

GLOSSARY

binocular / having two oculars or eyepieces

coarse adjustment / control that adjusts position of microscope objectives and is used to initially bring objects into focus

condenser / apparatus located below the microscope stage that directs light into the objective

electron microscope / a microscope that uses an electron beam to create images from a specimen and that is capable of much greater magnification and resolving power than a light microscope

eyepiece / ocular

field diaphragm / adjustable aperture attached to microscope base

fine adjustment / control that adjusts position of microscope objectives and is used to sharpen focus

iris diaphragm / device that regulates the amount of light striking the specimen being viewed through the microscope

Köhler illumination / alignment of illuminating light for microscopy; double diaphragm illumination

lens / a curved transparent material that spreads or focuses light

lens paper / a special nonabrasive material used to clean optical lenses

microscope arm / the portion of the microscope that connects the lenses to the base

microscope base / the portion of the microscope that rests on the table and supports the microscope

monocular / having one ocular or eyepiece

nosepiece / revolving unit to which microscope objectives are attached

objective / magnifying lens closest to the object being viewed with a microscope

ocular / eyepiece of the microscope that contains a magnifying lens

parfocal / having objectives that can be interchanged without varying the instrument's focus

resolving power / the ability of a microscope to produce separate images of two closely-spaced objects

stage / platform that holds the object to be viewed microscopically

working distance / distance between the microscope objective and the microscope slide when the object is in sharp focus

INTRODUCTION

Microscopes are used in many clinical laboratory departments to evaluate stained blood smears and tissue sections, perform cell counts, examine urine sediment, observe cellular reactions, and interpret smears containing microorganisms. The microscopist must be skilled in microscope use if maximum information is to be gained from prepared slides.

This lesson is an introduction to microscopy and includes descriptions of several types of microscopes used in medicine and research. The proper use of the bright-field clinical microscope is described in detail. Because the microscope is a delicate, expensive instrument, special care must be taken in its use, cleaning, and storage.

TYPES OF MICROSCOPES

Microscopes come in various sizes, prices, designs, and capabilities. Microscopes can be divided into two categories based on the type of illumination used. Clinical microscopes are *light microscopes*, meaning that the specimen is illuminated using a light source such as a tungsten, halogen, or mercury lamp. Tungsten and halogen lamps emit a full spectrum of light (white light); mercury lamps emit light in the ultraviolet range. The other major category of microscopes is the *electron microscopes*. These are named because specimens are visualized by focusing an electron beam on the specimen rather than light waves.

Light Microscopes

Modern light microscopes are also called *compound* light microscopes because they have two lens systems, one system in the oculars and one system in the objectives. Common types of light microscopes in the clinical laboratory are the bright-field microscope, phase-contrast microscope, and epi-fluorescence microscope.

Bright-field Microscope

The bright-field microscope is the workhorse of the clinical laboratory (Figure 1-54). The microscope is named bright-field because the object being viewed is seen against a *bright field* of view. All routine clinical laboratory tests requiring a microscope can be performed using the bright-field microscope. Bright-field microscopes are especially well suited for viewing stained specimens, such as stained blood smears. Figure 1-55A shows an image as seen with a bright-field microscope.

Phase-Contrast Microscope

The phase-contrast microscope provides an improved way of viewing unstained cells, which are nearly transparent. By installing special objectives and a phase condenser, bright-field microscopes can be equipped for phase contrast. Phase contrast is useful for viewing specimens such as urine sediments and for performing platelet counts using the hemacytometer. With phase-contrast microscopy, the background (field) appears grey and the specimen is bright. Figure 1-55B shows an image viewed with phase-contrast microscopy.

Epi-fluorescence Microscope

Epi-fluorescence microscopes use ultraviolet light to illuminate the specimen. The epi-fluorescence microscope enables objects that have been stained with fluorescent dyes to be observed. When these dyes are combined with antibodies, it is possible to identify specific areas of reaction within a cell or on a cell surface. The epi-fluorescence microscope can be used to identify microorganisms such as mycobacteria, and to detect the presence of antibodies in certain diseases such as syphilis and lupus erythematosus. Figure 1-55C shows *Borrelia burgdorferi*, the cause of Lyme disease. The bacteria are stained with a fluorescently labeled antibody and viewed with epi-fluorescence microscopy.

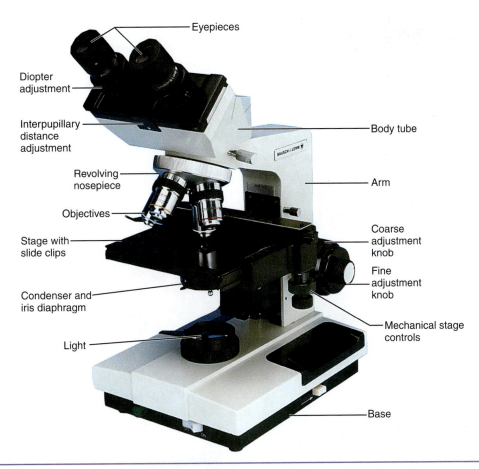

FIGURE 1-54 Binocular bright-field microscope with parts labeled

Labels on microscope: Eyepieces, Diopter adjustment, Interpupillary distance adjustment, Revolving nosepiece, Objectives, Stage with slide clips, Condenser and iris diaphragm, Light, Body tube, Arm, Coarse adjustment knob, Fine adjustment knob, Mechanical stage controls, Base

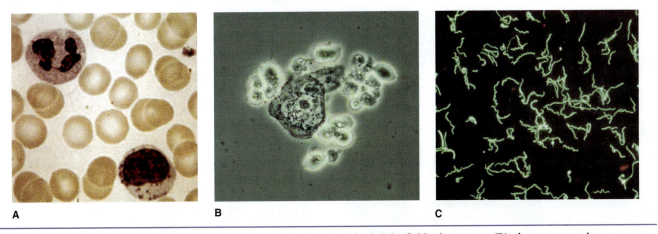

A   B   C

FIGURE 1-55 Microscopy images: (A) stained cells viewed with a bright-field microscope; (B) phase-contrast image; (C) *Borrelia burgdorferi* stained with fluorescent antibody and viewed with epi-fluorescence microscopy
(*Photo A courtesy of Abbott Laboratories, Abbot Park, IL; photo B courtesy of CDC, Atlanta, GA*)

Electron Microscopes

Electron microscopes provide much greater magnification and resolving power than light microscopes. The image from an electron microscope is created by exposing specimens to an electron beam, rather than illuminating them with a light source. Electron microscopes have been used in medical research for several years, but have been limited for the most part to pathology and virology. However, with new knowledge and techniques, their use in clinical medicine is increasing.

With the electron microscope, objects as small as 0.001 μm (too small to be seen with light microscopes) can be viewed. The two types of electron microscopes are the *transmission electron microscope* (TEM) and the *scanning electron microscope* (SEM), shown in Figures 1-56 and 1-57.

Objects are visualized in the TEM by passing an electron beam through the specimen. Minute details inside a cell, such as nuclear structure, can be seen (Figure 1-58A). The image is displayed on a phosphorescent screen and viewed through protective glass or projected onto a monitor (Figure 1-58A). In the

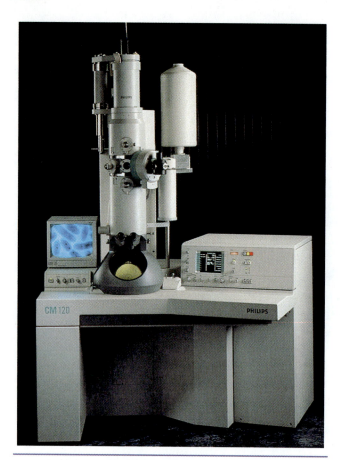

FIGURE 1-56 Transmission electron microscope

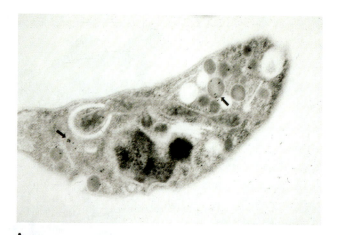

A

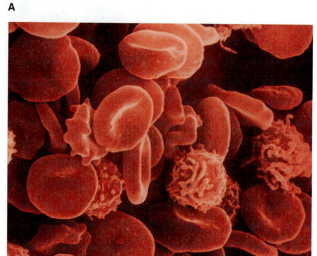

B

FIGURE 1-58 Electron microscopy images: (A) cell viewed with transmission electron microscope (*Courtesy of C.A. Sundermann, Auburn University, AL*); (B) blood cells as seen with the scanning electron microscope (*Courtesy Philips Electronics Instruments Co.*)

Reference laboratories, medical schools, and teaching hospitals are the most likely clinical locations for electron microscopes.

PARTS OF THE MICROSCOPE

Microscope design can differ slightly from one model to another. However, some parts are common to all microscopes. The microscope shown in Figure 1-54 has the parts labeled.

Oculars

A microscope can be **monocular** or **binocular**. Monocular microscopes have only one **ocular**, or **eyepiece**. Because of this, most people find it difficult to use them without eyestrain. Binocular microscopes have two eyepieces to allow viewing with both eyes, resulting in less eyestrain (Figure 1-54).

The oculars, or eyepieces, located at the top of the microscope, are attached to a barrel or tube connected to the **micro-**

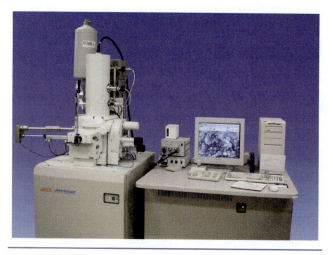

FIGURE 1-57 Scanning electron microscope

SEM, the electron beam is scanned over the surface of a metal-coated specimen, causing electrons to bounce off the specimen. These deflected electrons are measured with a detector and converted into a three-dimensional image similar to an image on a TV screen. Figure 1-58B is a scanning electron microscope image of the surface of blood cells.

Electron microscopes are very expensive and require lengthy specimen preparation and special expertise to operate.

scope arm. Each ocular, through which the object is viewed, contains a magnifying **lens**. The usual magnification is 10 times (10×), but oculars are also available in 15× and 20×.

Objective Lenses

The underside of the microscope arm contains a revolving **nosepiece** to which the **objectives** are attached. Most microscopes have at least three objectives or magnifying lenses: the low-power objective, which magnifies × 10 or × 20; the high-power objective, which magnifies × 40, 43, or 45; and the oil-immersion objective, which magnifies × 95, 97, or 100. Each objective is marked with color-coded bands and the power of magnification (Figure 1-54).

To determine the degree of magnification, the magnification listed on the ocular (usually 10×) is multiplied by the magnification listed on the objective being used (Table 1-33). For example, an object viewed with a 10× ocular and high-power (43×) objective would be magnified 430 times (430×). An object viewed with a 10× ocular and the oil-immersion objective (97×) would be magnified 970 times.

There is a limit to the degree of magnification that can be obtained with a light microscope and still yield a clear image. The ability of a microscope to produce separate images of closely-spaced details in the object being viewed is called its **resolving power**. The resolving power is determined by the quality of the objective lenses.

Light Source, Condenser, and Diaphragm

The microscope arm connects the objectives and eyepiece(s) to the **microscope base**, which supports the microscope. The base also contains the light, which illuminates the object viewed. Located above the light is the moveable condenser and iris diaphragm (Figure 1-54). The **condenser** focuses or directs the available light into the objective as it is raised or lowered and enhances specimen contrast (Figure 1-59). The **iris diaphragm**, located in the condenser unit, regulates the amount of light that strikes the object being viewed (much like the shutter of a camera). The iris diaphragm can be adjusted by a movable lever. Microscopes can also have an adjustable **field diaphragm**, located just over the light source. The field diaphragm is used to help align or focus the light in a procedure called **Köhler illumination**.

Coarse and Fine Focus Adjustments

The two focusing knobs are usually located on the sides of the microscope base. The **coarse adjustment** is used to focus with the low-power objective only. The **fine adjustment** is used to give a sharper image after the object is brought into view with the coarse adjustment (Figure 1-54).

The **working distance** is the distance between the objective and the specimen slide when the object is in sharp focus. The higher the magnification of the objective, the shorter the working distance will be. The coarse adjustment should *not* be used when using the higher magnifications to prevent the objective from accidentally striking the slide and becoming damaged.

Stage

The **stage** of the microscope is supported by the arm and is located between the nosepiece and the light source. The stage serves as the support for the object being viewed and has a stage clip to keep slides stationary. The stage, called a mechanical stage, can be moved by using knobs located just below the stage. These move the stage in a horizontal plane left and right or backward and forward (Figure 1-54).

HOW THE IMAGE IS PRODUCED

To see an image through the microscope oculars, the image must be magnified, focused, and directed into the oculars (Figure 1-59). The light in the microscope base is directed upward through the condenser, which focuses the light beam on the specimen. When light strikes the specimen, some is absorbed, some is deflected, and some is transmitted (passes through the specimen). The transmitted light enters the lens of the objective which magnifies the image. The light then strikes a prism or mirror located between the objective and ocular. This prism deflects or bends the light (image) to direct it into the oculars. The oculars contain magnifying lenses that enlarge the image again and allow the eye to focus on the image. The combination of these two magnifying lens systems is the basis for the compound microscope.

TABLE 1-33. Calculation of total magnification in a compound microscope

OBJECTIVE LENS	MAGNIFICATION STRENGTH	×	OCULAR STRENGTH	=	TOTAL MAGNIFICATION
Low power	10×	×	10×	=	100×
High power	40×	×	10×	=	400×
Oil immersion	100×	×	10×	=	1000×

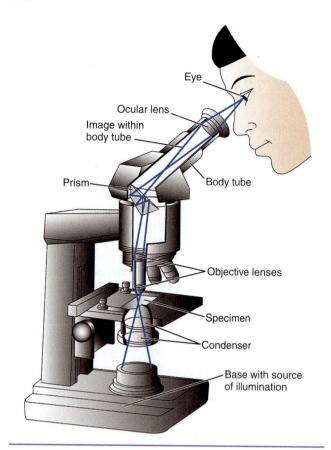

FIGURE 1-59 Light path in a compound microscope

USING THE MICROSCOPE

Much practice is required to become competent and adept at clinical microscopy. Microscopists must be proficient in making all of the adjustments required to achieve an optimal image of various types of biological specimens. They must also use proper safety measures and cleaning and maintenance techniques to keep the instrument operating at maximum capacity. The microscope should be placed on a sturdy table at a comfortable height for the technician. When not in use, the microscope should be left with the low-power objective in position.

Microscope Safety

Appropriate safety rules for electrical equipment must be followed when using the microscope. Electrical cords must not be frayed and should be plugged into a grounded receptacle. Cords must be kept away from liquids. The microscope should be unplugged before attempting to do any maintenance, repairs, or bulb replacement.

Glass slides should be handled carefully to avoid the chance of chipping or breaking. If an unfixed or fluid biological specimen (such as urine sediment) is to be examined, Standard Precautions must be observed and appropriate personal protective equipment (PPE) must be worn. The microscope stage must be disinfected after examining such a specimen.

Quality Assessment

The microscopist should follow good microscopy practice in the care and use of the microscope to avoid damage to the instrument. Patient results should only be reported by experienced technicians who have demonstrated the required level of competency.

Care and Cleaning of Lenses

The amount and quality of information that can be gained from microscopic examination of a specimen is dependent on the condition of the objective lenses. Oculars and objective lenses should be cleaned before and after each use with **lens paper**. Materials such as laboratory tissue, cotton balls, paper towels, or gauze squares must not be used because they can scratch the lenses. Lenses that become damaged or cloudy should be replaced since important information can be missed when viewing a specimen through a cloudy lens.

Immersion Oil

Only immersion oil manufactured for microscopy should be used with the oil-immersion objective. Immersion oil should never be allowed to touch the other (low- or high-power) objectives. After the oil-immersion objective is used, the objective lenses and condenser should be cleaned to remove any residual oil. It is especially important that lenses never be left with oil on them, as oil will soften the cement that holds the lens in place in the objective. Lens cleaner, similar to a glass-cleaning solution, can be used with lens paper to remove oil from objectives.

Focusing with the Low-Power Objective

The low-power objective is used to initially locate objects and to view large objects. The coarse adjustment focus knob is used to bring the objective and the slide as close together as possible. Then, while looking through the ocular, the coarse adjustment is used to move the objective and slide apart until the object on the slide comes into focus. (In some microscopes, the coarse adjustment raises and lowers the objectives. In other microscopes, the stage is raised and lowered when the coarse adjustment knob is turned.) The fine focus adjustment knob can then be used to bring the image into sharp focus. When viewing objects using the low-power objective, the light intensity may need to be decreased.

Adjusting Oculars on Binocular Microscopes

Once the object is in view, the oculars should be adjusted to accommodate each microscopist's eyes. Two adjustments are made, the *interpupillary distance adjustment* and the *dioptic adjustment*.

The interpupillary distance is adjusted by sliding the oculars either closer together or further apart until only one image is seen when looking through both oculars. This adjustment is like the one you would make when adjusting binoculars to your eyes.

Once the interpupillary distance is correct, then the dioptic adjustment should be made. This adjustment compensates for the microscopist's vision. The microscopist should look through the right ocular with the right eye (left eye closed) and use the coarse adjustment to bring the object into sharp focus. Then the microscopist should look through the left ocular with the left eye (right eye closed) and use the knurled collar (Figure 1-54) on the ocular (*not the coarse focus adjustment*) to bring the specimen into focus.

Alignment of Illumination

The path of light through the microscope must be properly aligned to have good resolution. Incorrect alignment causes poor resolution, artifacts, and unevenly lit field of view. The illumination alignment of many student microscopes is pre-set during manufacture and realignment is done periodically by a professional microscope repair and service company. In these cases the microscopist does not perform the alignment procedure; it has been done for them.

Clinical microscopes that have an adjustable field diaphragm built into the light source allow the microscopist to manually align the illumination. The technique of aligning or focusing the light path using the field diaphragm is called Köhler illumination, and must be performed each time the microscope is used before viewing specimens with the microscope.

A specimen slide is placed on the microscope stage (specimen-side up) and positioned so that the specimen is directly beneath the low power objective lens and the microscope light is turned on. The specimen is brought into focus. The field diaphragm is closed as much as possible and the edges of the diaphragm are brought into focus by raising or lowering the condenser. Both the specimen and diaphragm edge should be in focus and the diaphragm outline should be centered in the field of view (Figure 1-60, far left and second from left). The field diaphragm image is centered using the condenser centering knobs. The field diaphragm is then opened so that the edges lie at the edge of the field of view (Figure 1-60, far right). The condenser iris diaphragm is adjusted to produce the desired contrast. The light intensity is adjusted using the voltage control (rheostat). The microscope is now correctly adjusted and ready for viewing specimens.

Using the High-Power Objective

The high-power (40×) objective is used when greater magnification is needed, such as for cell counts and viewing urine

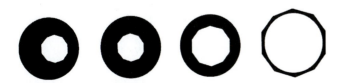

FIGURE 1-60 Köhler illumination. Far left, closed, off-center field diaphragm; second from left, closed, centered field diaphragm; far right, open, centered field diaphragm

sediments. After initial focusing with the low-power objective and illumination alignment (if applicable), the high-power objective is carefully rotated into position. The fine adjustment is used to bring the object into sharp focus. Most microscope objectives are **parfocal** and therefore require only slight changes in the fine adjustment when rotating between objectives.

Because the working distance between the slide and the high-power objective is so small, only the fine adjustment should be used when the high-power objective is in place. This avoids the possibility of the objective striking the slide and possibly damaging the objective or the slide.

To view unstained specimens using the high-power objective, light intensity and iris diaphragm should be adjusted to provide proper lighting and contrast. When viewing most stained preparations with the high-power objective, the condenser should be raised, the diaphragm opened, and light intensity increased.

Using the Oil-Immersion Objective

The oil-immersion objective is used to view stained blood cells, tissue sections, and stained slides containing microorganisms. This objective gives the highest magnification of the bright-field objectives. After initial focusing with the low-power objective, the objective is slightly rotated to the side. A drop of immersion oil is placed on the slide directly over the condenser. The oil immersion objective is then carefully rotated into the drop of oil, taking care that no other objectives contact the oil and that the oil immersion objective does not strike the slide (Figure 1-61A). The object is then brought into sharp focus using only the fine adjustment. *The coarse adjustment should never be used when the oil immersion objective is in position.* When viewing specimens with the oil-immersion objective, the condenser should be raised to its highest position (almost touching the bottom of the slide). The iris diaphragm should be open and maximum light should be used.

After completing examination of the slide, the low-power objective is rotated into position and the slide is removed from the stage. All oil must be cleaned from the oil-immersion objective with lens paper. The stage and condenser should be cleaned if necessary.

Transporting and Storing the Microscope

Microscopes should be left in a permanent position on a sturdy table where they cannot be jarred. However, if a microscope must be moved, it should be held securely, with one hand supporting the base and the other holding the arm (Figure 1-61B). The microscope should be placed gently to avoid jarring.

Microscope Storage

When the microscope is not being used, it should be left with the low-power objective in position and the nosepiece in the lowest position. The stage should be centered so that it does not project from either side of the microscope. The microscope should be stored under a dust-proof cover.

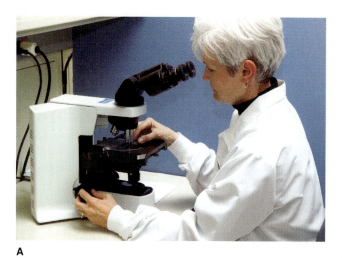

A

FIGURE 1-61 Proper use and care of the microscope:
(A) observe the slide and objectives when changing
from high-power to oil-immersion objective;
(B) proper way to carry a microscope

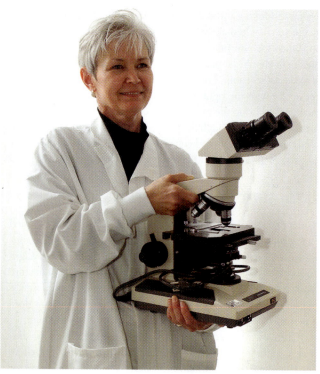

B

SAFETY Reminders

- Use Standard Precautions when examining unfixed biological materials microscopically.
- Clean the microscope stage with a surface disinfectant after examining fluid samples such as urine sediment.
- Unplug the microscope before attempting to replace the bulb or perform any electrical repair.

PROCEDURAL Reminders

Qa

- Clean all oculars and objectives with lens paper before and after each use.
- Use the coarse adjustment with the low-power objective only.
- Use immersion oil with the oil-immersion objective only.
- Adjust interpupillary distance, diopter, and align illumination before using.
- Store the covered microscope in a protected area.
- Avoid jarring or bumping the microscope.
- Transport the microscope with one hand under the base and the other hand gripping the arm.

CRITICAL THINKING 1

Sheila was performing urine microscopic examinations when the light went out on her microscope. She removed the microscope slide, turned the microscope over, and opened up the light compartment. She removed the light bulb with difficulty, saw that the filament was broken, and replaced the bulb. As soon as the bulb was fitted into the holder, the microscope light came on. Comment on Sheila's microscope repair technique.

CRITICAL THINKING 2

Roberta needed to use a microscope to examine a blood smear. She cleaned the oculars and the 10×, 40× and 100× oil-immersion objectives with lens paper, using a clean section of lens paper for each objective. The lens paper used to clean the oil-immersion objective revealed oil on the objective. Roberta mentioned this to Jack, a technician who worked regularly with that microscope, and he replied that it was only necessary to remove oil from the objective once or twice a shift since the objective might be used as many as 10 to 12 times during the day. Is Jack correct? Explain.

SUMMARY

The microscope is a valuable instrument used in many departments in the clinical laboratory. A large clinical laboratory will usually have several bright-field microscopes and also may have phase-contrast and epi-fluorescence microscopes. Electron microscopes are used primarily in research.

Urine sediments, stained blood smears, and bacterial stains are evaluated using the microscope. Specialized tests such as fluorescent antibody techniques also can require microscope use. Microscopists must become skilled in the proper operation of the microscope. Because microscopes are expensive, precision instruments, the technician must use the microscope with care, maintain the microscope in good working order, and be sure that it is cleaned and stored properly after each use. Much practice is required to become a competent microscopist.

REVIEW QUESTIONS

1. Explain the functions of the iris diaphragm and condenser.
2. Name the three objectives commonly used on a clinical microscope.
3. Explain the uses of the coarse and fine adjustments.
4. What is the proper method of cleaning a microscope after use?
5. How should a microscope be stored when not in use?
6. When is the oil-immersion objective used?
7. When is immersion oil used on a slide?
8. Explain how to adjust the interpupillary distance on a binocular microscope.
9. What is the purpose of making a dioptic adjustment? Explain how the adjustment is made.
10. How is total magnification calculated in the compound microscope?
11. How do electron microscopes differ from light microscopes?
12. When must Standard Precautions be used with the microscope?
13. What is Köhler illumination? How is it performed?
14. Define binocular, coarse adjustment, condenser, electron microscope, eyepiece, field diaphragm, fine adjustment, iris diaphragm, Köhler illumination, lens, lens paper, microscope arm, microscope base, monocular, nosepiece, objective, ocular, parfocal, resolving power, stage, and working distance.

STUDENT ACTIVITIES

1. Complete the written examination for this lesson.

2. Obtain a microscope from the instructor. Locate and identify the following parts: oculars, condenser, condenser adjustment knob, condenser centering knobs, field diaphragm, iris diaphragm, light, light intensity control, nosepiece, arm, base, stage, stage controls, coarse and fine adjustment knobs, and diopter adjustment ring. Note which (if any) parts are not found on your microscope.

3. Obtain a stained slide from your instructor. View the specimen with the low-power, high-power, and oil-immersion objectives. Draw the structure(s) you see when using each objective. Observe the specimen when the condenser is raised and when it is lowered, and with the iris diaphragm wide open and closed. Discuss the differences in the image you see in each of these conditions. What adjustments provide the most information from your specimen?

4. If you live near a university or a large research laboratory, find out if they have an electron microscope. If so, try to arrange a visit to the facility.

5. Practice using a microscope following the procedure outlined in the Student Performance Guide.

WEB ACTIVITIES

1. Find images taken with transmission and scanning electron microscopes using the Internet.

2. Use the Internet to find information about various types of light microscopes. Try to find examples of phase-contrast images and fluorescent images. Compare these to the way stained images look with the bright-field microscope in your laboratory.

Student Performance Guide

LESSON 1-10 The Microscope

Name _____ Date _____

INSTRUCTIONS

1. Practice using the microscope following the step-by-step procedure.
2. Demonstrate the proper use of the microscope satisfactorily for the instructor using the Student Performance Guide. Your instructor will determine the level of competency you must achieve to obtain a satisfactory (S) grade.

NOTE: Procedure will vary slightly according to microscope design. Consult operating procedure in microscope manual for specific instructions.

MATERIALS AND EQUIPMENT

- antiseptic
- microscope
- lens paper
- lens cleaner
- prepared slides (commercially available)
- immersion oil
- surface disinfectant

PROCEDURE

Record in the comment section any problems encountered while practicing the procedure (or have a fellow student or the instructor evaluate your performance).

S = Satisfactory
U = Unsatisfactory

You must:	S	U	Comments
1. Wash hands			
2. Assemble equipment and materials			
3. Clean the oculars and objectives with lens paper			
4. Use the coarse adjustment to raise the nosepiece unit			
5. Raise the condenser as far as possible by turning the condenser knob			
6. Rotate the low-power (10×) objective into position, so it is directly over the opening in the stage			
7. Turn on the microscope light			
8. Open the iris diaphragm until maximum light comes up through the condenser			
9. Place slide on stage (specimen side up) and secure with clips. Position the condenser so it is almost touching the bottom of the slide			

You must:	S	U	Comments
10. Locate the coarse adjustment			
11. Look directly at the stage and low-power (10×) objective and turn the coarse adjustment until the objective is as close to the slide as it will go. Stop turning when the objective no longer moves **NOTE:** Do not move any objective toward a slide while looking through the oculars			
12. Look into the ocular(s) and slowly turn the coarse adjustment in the opposite direction (from step 11) to raise the objective (or lower the stage) until the object on the slide comes into focus			
13. Locate the fine adjustment and use it to sharpen the focus of the image			

14. Adjust the oculars for your eyes (steps 14a–14b)
  a. Adjust interpupillary distance by adjusting distance between oculars so one image is seen (as when using binoculars)
  b. Make dioptic adjustment following steps 14b1–14b3
    1) Use coarse and fine adjustments to bring object into focus while looking through the right ocular with right eye (and with left eye closed)
    2) Close the right eye, look into the left ocular with left eye, and *use the knurled collar on the left ocular* to bring the object into sharp focus. (Do not turn coarse or fine adjustment at this time.)
    3) Look into oculars with both eyes to observe that object is in clear focus. If not, repeat the procedure			

15. If field diaphragm is present, perform Köhler illumination, following steps 15a–15g. If field diaphragm is not present, go to step 16
  a. Stop down (close) the field diaphragm located on the microscope base
  b. Bring the edge of the diaphragm into focus using the condenser adjustment knob (which raises and lowers the condenser)
  c. Confirm that both the specimen and the diaphragm edge are in focus
  d. Center the image of the field diaphragm using the condenser-centering knobs
  e. Open the centered and focused field diaphragm so the edges lie just beyond the field of view
  f. Adjust the condenser iris diaphragm to increase or decrease image contrast; the proper position depends on the specimen
  g. Adjust light intensity by adjusting the voltage to the light source with the power supply rheostat			

You must:	S	U	Comments
16. Scan the slide using the stage controls to move the slide in a left and right or backward and forward pattern while looking through the oculars			
17. Rotate the high-power (40×) objective into position while observing the objective and the slide to see that the objective does not strike the slide			
18. Look through the oculars to view the object on the slide; it should almost be in focus			
19. Locate the fine adjustment			
20. Look through the oculars and turn the fine adjustment until the object is in focus. Do not use the coarse adjustment.			
21. Check alignment of Köhler illumination. Repeat steps 15a–15g if necesssary			
22. Scan the slide as in step 16, using the fine adjustment if necessary to keep the object in focus			
23. Rotate the oil-immersion objective slightly to the side			
24. Place one drop of immersion oil on the portion of the slide directly over the condenser			
25. Rotate the oil-immersion objective into position, being careful not to rotate the high-power (40×) objective through the oil. Look to see that the oil-immersion objective is touching the drop of oil			
26. Look through the oculars and slowly turn the fine adjustment until the image is clear. Use only the fine adjustment to focus the oil-immersion objective. Scan the slide as in step 16			
27. Rotate the low-power (10×) objective into position; do not allow high-power (40×) objective to touch oil			
28. Remove the slide from the microscope stage and gently blot the oil from the slide with lens paper			
29. Clean the oculars, low-power (10×) objective, and high-power (40×) objective with clean lens paper			
30. Clean the oil-immersion objective with lens paper to remove all oil			
31. Clean all oil from the microscope stage and condenser			
32. Turn off the microscope light and unplug the microscope			
33. Position the nosepiece in the lowest position using the coarse adjustment			

You must:	S	U	Comments
34. Center the stage so it does not project from either side of the microscope			
35. Cover the microscope and return it to storage			
36. Clean work area; return slides to storage			
37. Wash hands			

Evaluator Comments:

Evaluator _____ Date _____

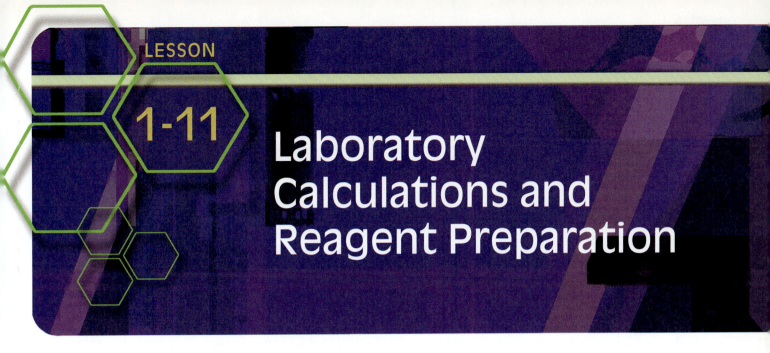

Laboratory Calculations and Reagent Preparation

LESSON OBJECTIVES

After studying this lesson, the student will:

- Prepare percent solutions.
- Prepare a reagent using proportions or ratio.
- Prepare dilutions of a reagent.
- State the formula for preparing a dilute solution from a concentrate.
- Prepare molar or mol/L solutions.
- Perform serial and compound dilutions.
- Discuss safety precautions that must be observed when preparing laboratory reagents.
- Explain the quality assessment procedures that should be used to ensure high-quality laboratory reagents.
- Define the glossary terms.

GLOSSARY

diluent / a liquid added to a solution to make it less concentrated

dilution / a solution made less concentrated by adding a diluent; the act of making a dilute solution; the degree to which a solution is made less concentrated

dilution factor / reciprocal of the dilution

formula weight (F.W.) / weight of the entity represented by a chemical formula; molecular weight

lyophilize / remove water from a frozen solution under vacuum; freeze-dry

molar solution (M) / solution containing one mole of solute per liter of solution

mole / formula weight of a substance expressed in grams

molecular weight (M.W.) / sum of atomic weights of the formula unit; formula weight

percent solution / a solution made by adding units of solute per 100 units of solution

physiological saline / 0.85% (0.15 M) sodium chloride solution

proportion / relationship in number or amount of one portion compared to another portion or to the whole; ratio

ratio / relationship in number or degree between two things

solute / the substance dissolved in a given solution

solution / a homogeneous mixture of two or more substances

solvent / a dissolving agent, usually a liquid

titer / in serology, the reciprocal of the highest dilution that gives the desired reaction; the concentration of a substance determined by titration

INTRODUCTION

Although most laboratory reagents are purchased in the required concentrations, occasionally reagents or solutions must be prepared in the laboratory. To do this correctly, it is necessary to have a knowledge of some basic chemistry terms and simple math.

A **solution** is a homogeneous mixture of two or more substances. Solutions are made by combining a **solute**, the substance being dissolved, with a **solvent**, a dissolving agent. Water is the most familiar and widely-used solvent. Laboratory procedures can also require dilution of a reagent or a serum. A **dilution** is a solution that is made less concentrated by adding a solvent.

Whatever type of laboratory solution is being prepared, math is involved, either directly or indirectly. The calculations required to make reagents are not difficult, but can require step-by-step clarification at first. It is important that reagents be made accurately since worker safety and patient test results can depend on them. This lesson introduces methods of preparing solutions using ratio and proportions, percentage, molarity, and dilution. In this text, the symbol is used to indicate that an activity or procedure requires math skills.

COMMON LABORATORY REAGENTS

Several common laboratory solutions, such as surface disinfectants and dilute acids, are easily prepared by making simple dilutions. *Stock* (concentrated) solutions can be diluted to a *working* concentration. Some tests require that several dilutions of serum be tested. Percent solutions or molar solutions of saline can be made. **Lyophilized** controls and standards can be reconstituted in the laboratory. These are reagents with the liquid removed that are rehydrated by adding either Type I water or a diluting fluid provided by the manufacturer. Examples of lyophilized reagents include positive and negative controls for immunology and serum controls and standards for blood and urine chemistry tests.

PREPARING LABORATORY SOLUTIONS

There are several methods of preparing laboratory solutions, including dilutions, ratios, percent solutions, and molar solutions. When preparing any solution, the technician must follow all safety rules and quality assessment guidelines.

Safety Precautions

 The preparation of laboratory reagents can be associated with potential chemical, physical, and biological hazards. The chemical container label and material safety data sheet (MSDS) must be consulted before using a chemical and the recommended personal protective equipment (PPE) must be used. Chemicals that produce fumes must be used only in a fume hood. (Chemical safety is discussed in detail in Lesson 1-5.)

Standard Precautions must always be observed when making dilutions of patient serum or reconstituting serum controls and standards. Pipet-aids or pipet filler-dispensers must be used when measuring and dispensing liquids using pipets. Mouth pipetting must *never* be done. The use of plastic labware eliminates the possibility of injury due to broken or chipped glass.

Quality Assessment

Formulas for preparing various types of reagents must be used properly and calculations must be correct. Proper pipetting techniques must be used to measure and transfer liquids. The pipet used should be appropriate for the task; volumetric pipets should be used when making critical measurements, such as preparing standards and controls. Pipetting errors in making a reagent can affect all analyses that use the reagent. The measuring container must also be appropriate for the task. Markings on beakers and Erlenmeyer flasks are only approximate; certified glassware such as volumetric flasks must be used for critical measurements.

Reagents should be prepared using chemically clean, dry, non-reactive containers. Standards and controls are usually stored refrigerated; other reagents might be stored at room temperature. Laboratory reagents have a shelf life and should not be used beyond the expiration date. Before using any laboratory reagent, the reagent should be inspected for signs of deterioration, such as color change or turbidity. Fresh reagents should be made before the existing reagent expires; many procedures require that the new reagent be tested along with the one in use to be sure they give equivalent results.

Using Proportion to Make Dilutions

Dilutions are often required in laboratory procedures. A dilution is usually expressed as a ratio, **proportion**, or fraction. For example, if a serum has been diluted 1:5, it means that one (1) part of the serum has been combined with four (4) parts of a

diluent to create five (5) total parts. A simple formula for calculating dilutions is:

$$\frac{(A)}{(A)+(B)} = C$$

where: A = parts or volume of substance being diluted

B = parts or volume of diluent added, and

C = the dilution, expressed as a fraction

(A and B must be in the same units of volume)

An example of using proportion to prepare a reagent is shown in Figure 1-62.

Using a Concentrated Solution to Make a Dilute Solution

Sometimes it is necessary to prepare a dilute solution from a concentrated solution. For instance, 0.1 M HCl solution can be made from a concentrated solution of HCl, such as a 1.0 M solution (Figure 1-63). The general formula is:

$$C_1 \times V_1 = C_2 \times V_2$$

or

$$V_1 = \frac{C_2 \times V_2}{C_1}$$

where: C_1 = concentration of the solution of greater concentration

V_1 = volume required of the solution of greater concentration

C_2 = concentration of final (dilute) solution

V_2 = volume of final (dilute) solution

Solve for V_1, volume of concentrated solution needed to prepare the dilute solution.

Using Ratios to Prepare Dilutions

A **ratio** is the relationship in number or degree between two things. Dilutions, which are ratios, express the relationship between a part of a solution and the total solution. Dilutions are used frequently in the laboratory, especially in hematology and immunology.

One procedure for performing the white blood cell (WBC) count requires that a 1-to-100 (1:100) dilution of the blood sample be made to count the cells. This is accomplished by adding 0.02 mL of blood to 1.98 mL of diluent. The total volume is equal to 2.00 mL. This represents a 1:100 dilution.

The general rule for calculating the concentration of a diluted solution is to *divide* the concentration of the original solution by the **dilution factor**, which is the reciprocal of the dilution. For

Problem:	A buffer is made by adding 2 parts of "solution A" to 5 parts of "solution B." How much of solution A and solution B would be required to make 70 mL of the buffer?
Formula:	$\dfrac{\text{Total volume required (C)}}{\text{parts of "A" + parts of "B"}}$ = volume of one part (V)
Solution:	$\dfrac{70 \text{ mL required}}{2 \text{ parts "A" + 5 parts "B"}}$ = volume of one part $\dfrac{70}{7}$ = 10 mL = volume of one part (V) 2 parts of solution "A" = 2 X 10 = 20 mL 5 parts of solution "B" = 5 X 10 = 50 mL
Answer:	The buffer would be made by mixing 20 mL of solution A with 50 mL of solution B to give a total volume of 70 mL.

FIGURE 1-62 Preparing a solution using proportion

Problem:	Prepare 100 mL of 0.1 M HCl using 1.0 M HCl.
Formula:	$C_1 \times V_1 = C_2 \times V_2$
Solution:	(1.0 M) (V_1) = (100 mL) (0.1 M) $V_1 = \dfrac{100 \text{ mL X } 0.1}{1.0}$ V_1 = 10 mL
Answer:	10 mL of 1.0 M HCl is added to 90 mL of H_2O to make 100 mL of 0.1 M HCl solution.

FIGURE 1-63 Using the formula $C_1 \times V_1 = C_2 \times V_2$ to prepare a solution

instance if a 2.0 M solution is diluted 1:5, the dilution factor is 5, and the concentration of the dilution is 0.4 M:

$$\frac{2.0\ M}{5} = 0.4\ M$$

This rule can also be used to find the original concentration of a diluted solution. For example: the albumin concentration of a 1:10 serum dilution was measured as 4 g/L. By *multiplying* the concentration by the dilution factor, the albumin concentration of the original sample is found to be 40 g/L:

$$4g/L \times 10 = 40\ g/L$$

Using Percentage to Prepare Solutions

One type of expression of concentration is the **percent solution**. A percent solution refers to the weight of solute per 100 weight units or volume units of solution. Percent refers to parts per 100 parts. A penny is 1% of a dollar—one part (cent) per 100 parts (cents). A nickel is 5% of a dollar—5 cents per 100 cents.

In the laboratory, percent solutions usually refer to grams of solute per 100 mL of solution. This is because the solvent used most in the laboratory is water and one mL of water weighs approximately 1.0 gram. So a 1% solution would contain 1 g of solute per 100 mL (or 100 g) of solution. Three ways to prepare percent solutions are weight to volume (w/v), volume to volume (v/v), and weight to weight (w/w).

Weight/Volume (w/v) Solutions

Percent solutions can be made by dissolving a specific weight of a solute (chemical) in 100 mL of solution (water or other liquid). This is called a *weight-to-volume (w/v) solution*.

One example is the 0.85% **physiological saline** solution used for many serological and bacteriological procedures. According to the definition of a percent solution, 100 mL of 0.85% saline contains 0.85 g of sodium chloride (NaCl) in 100 mL of solution. This would be prepared by placing about 50 mL of reagent water into a 100 mL volumetric flask, adding 0.85 grams NaCl, mixing, and then adding reagent water to the flask's fill line. In a similar fashion, 500 mL of 0.85% saline could be prepared as shown in Figure 1-64A.

Volume/Volume (v/v) Solutions

Another type of percent solution is called a *volume-to-volume (v/v) solution*, in which a certain volume of one liquid is added to a specific volume of another. One hundred milliliters of a 10% solution of bleach can be prepared by adding 10 mL of household bleach to 90 mL of water (Figure 1-64B).

Weight/Weight (w/w) Solutions

A percent solution can also be prepared by weighing both the solute and the solvent. In this case, a 5% solution would require that five grams of a chemical be added to about 90 mL of water and, with the flask on a balance, water is added until the total solution weight is 100 grams. This type of percent solution is rarely used in the clinical laboratory.

Problem: Prepare 500 mL of 0.85% saline.

Solution:

1. A 0.85% solution contains 0.85 g of the solute in every 100 mL of solution.
2. Therefore, to prepare 500 mL, 5 X 0.85 g, or 4.25 g, of sodium chloride (NaCl) must be used.
3. To prepare the solution:
   a. Weigh out 4.25 g of NaCl.
   b. Fill a 500 mL volumetric flask approximately half full with water.
   c. Add 4.25 g of NaCl and swirl gently to dissolve.
   d. Add water to the flask's fill line.

A

Problem: Prepare 500 mL of 10% bleach solution.

Solution:

1. A 10% solution of bleach contains 10 mL bleach (hypochlorite) per 100 mL of solution.
2. Therefore, 500 mL of solution would contain 50 mL of bleach (5 X 10 mL).
3. To prepare the solution:
   a. Place 450 mL of water into a flask or bottle.
   b. Add 50 mL of bleach.
   c. Carefully mix; label the container.

B

FIGURE 1-64 Percent solutions: (A) preparing a weight-to-volume (w/v) percent solution; (B) preparing a volume-to-volume (v/v) percent solution

Preparing Molar Solutions

Concentrations of chemical solutions are expressed as moles per liter (mol/L), which is replacing the older term molarity. A solution containing one mole of a substance per liter is a 1.0 **molar solution**. A **mole** of a pure compound is the **formula weight (F.W.)** or **molecular weight (M.W.)** of that compound expressed in grams. For instance, NaCl is composed of sodium atoms and chloride atoms. Sodium has a weight of 23 and chloride has a weight of 35.4, making the formula weight of NaCl = 58.4. A moles per liter solution is made by adding the required weight of chemical to enough solvent to make a total volume of one liter. *Notice that you do not add one liter to the solute, but bring the volume up to one liter after the solute is dissolved.*

A formula for calculating mol/L of a solution is:

$$\frac{\text{Grams (g)}}{1 \text{ liter}} \times \frac{1 \text{ mole}}{\text{F.W. (g)}} = \frac{\text{moles}}{\text{L}} = \text{M}$$

Simplified, to calculate the number of moles, divide the weight of chemical in a solution (the solute) by the formula weight of the chemical. For example: one liter of a solution contains 60 g of NaOH (formula weight 40). The moles per liter of the solution is:

$$\frac{\text{Grams of solute}}{\text{F.W. (g)}} = \frac{\text{moles}}{\text{L}} = \text{mol/L}$$

$$\frac{60 \text{ g NaOH}}{40 \text{ (F.W.)}} = 1.5 \text{ mol/L (or 1.5 M)}$$

An example of preparing a mol/L solution is in Figure 1-65.

Preparing Serial Dilutions

The concept of dilutions was introduced in the section on proportions. In those examples single dilutions were made. However, in some cases laboratory workers have to make *serial dilutions* of a sample to find the **titer** of a particular component in the sample. The titer of a component is the measure of reactivity or strength of the component, and is reported as the reciprocal of the highest dilution giving a reaction. Titers are usually reported when there is not a way to chemically quantitate a component. Most often they are used in immunology to indicate the level of a particular antibody in a serum sample. Dilutions of serum are required for certain tests such as quantitative hCG tests, the test for rheumatoid arthritis, or tests measuring levels of antibodies to infectious agents.

Making a Two-Fold Serial Dilution

In a serial dilution, a sample is diluted a number of times by the same dilution factor. In a two-fold dilution (doubling dilution) series, each dilution is two times as dilute as the previous dilution. Figure 1-66 shows how a nine-tube two-fold serial dilution would be performed. Nine tubes are set up, each containing one mL of diluent. A serum sample is diluted in half (1:2) by adding 1 mL of serum to the one mL of diluent in tube 1 and mixing. Then one mL from tube 1 (1:2 dilution) is transferred to tube 2 and mixed with the one mL of diluent in tube 2. This creates a two-fold dilution in tube 2 (two times more dilute than tube 1). Tube 2 now contains a 1:4 dilution of the original serum. The dilution series is continued by sequentially transferring one

---

Problem:	Prepare one liter of a 2 M solution of NaOH.
Solution:	The gram formula weight of NaOH is 40. A 2 M solution of NaOH contains 40 X 2 g/L. One liter of a 2 M solution contains 80 grams NaOH in one liter of solution

FIGURE 1-65 Preparation of a 2 M solution of NaOH

---

1. Set up 9 tubes, each containing one mL of diluent.
2. Transfer one mL of patient serum to tube 1.
3. Mix the serum and diluent, and transfer one mL of the mixture to tube 2.
4. Repeat the procedure, transferring one mL each time after mixing with diluent.
5. Discard one mL from the last tube.
6. When dilution series is complete, each of the nine tubes should contain one mL.

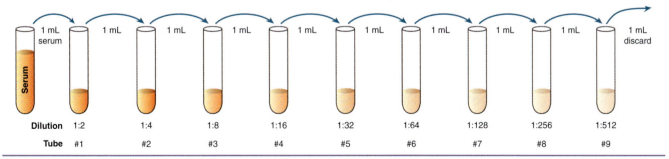

Dilution	1:2	1:4	1:8	1:16	1:32	1:64	1:128	1:256	1:512
Tube	#1	#2	#3	#4	#5	#6	#7	#8	#9

FIGURE 1-66 Setting up a two-fold dilution series

mL to the next tube in the series until the last tube is reached. After the one mL transferred from tube 8 has been mixed with the diluent in tube 9, one mL of the mixture is discarded. This leaves all tubes in the series containing one mL each, and provides serum dilutions ranging from 1:2 in tube 1 to 1:512 in tube 9. This means that in tube 9, only one part in 512 parts is serum from the original sample.

Each tube of the dilution series would then be used as a separate sample in the test procedure. The last tube in the series that shows a reaction is the end-point of the test and determines the titer. For instance, in a test where tubes 1 through 6 were reactive, but tubes 7 through 9 were not, the highest dilution showing a reaction would be 1:64. The titer, the reciprocal of the highest dilution giving the desired reaction, would be reported as 64.

Making a Compound Dilution

Sometimes it is necessary to dilute a concentrated reagent or a patient sample. If the dilution needs to be large, it can be made more accurately by performing a series of small dilutions, rather than just a one-step dilution. For instance, a worker may need to make a 0.001 M solution from a 1.0 M solution. In this example,

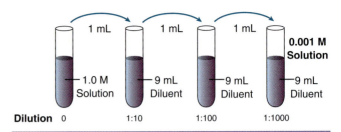

FIGURE 1-67 Making a 10-fold compound dilution

to find the dilution needed, the dilute concentration is divided by the concentrate and the fraction is converted to whole numbers:

$$\frac{0.001}{1} = \frac{1}{1000} = \text{ desired dilution}$$

Therefore, the 1.0 M solution needs to be diluted 1:1000 to make the 0.001 M solution. This can be done more accurately by making a compound dilution—a three-tube, 10-fold dilution series—as shown in Figure 1-67. To determine the final degree of dilution, the rule is to multiply the original concentration by each dilution expressed as a fraction.

SAFETY Reminders

- Observe Standard Precautions when handling standards and controls.
- Consult MSDS information for proper use of chemicals.
- Wear appropriate PPE.
- Clean all spills appropriately.
- Wipe work area with surface disinfectant.
- Wash hands with antiseptic.

PROCEDURAL Reminders

- Weigh and measure chemicals accurately.
- Pipet carefully, using the correct pipets.
- Check mathematical calculations before proceeding with a task.
- Use the correct principles and formulas to make the required solution.

CASE STUDY

Jody, a medical assistant in a small clinic, ran out of surface disinfectant while cleaning the counters in the clinic laboratory. The label of the disinfectant bottle she was using contained instructions for preparing the surface disinfectant from the concentrated stock solution. The instructions read "Dilute the concentrate 1:50 with water." Jody was using a disinfectant bottle with a 500 mL capacity. How should Jody prepare the replacement surface disinfectant? Justify your answer.

a. Add 1 mL of concentrate to 50 mL of water
b. Add 10 mL of concentrate to 500 mL of water
c. Add 10 mL of concentrate to 100 mL of water
d. Add 10 mL of concentrate to 490 mL of water

SUMMARY

Although most analyzers use prepackaged reagents or reagents contained in a reaction cartridge or strip, sometimes reagent preparation is necessary. Preparation of general laboratory reagents such as alcohol solutions or buffers can be required. Specimens may require dilution for accurate measurement of an analyte or for use in an immunological test. Dilute solutions may need to be prepared from concentrates. The technician should be familiar with the principles involved in preparing reagents and making dilutions.

REVIEW QUESTIONS

1. Give an example of a percent solution used in the laboratory.
2. What dilution is created when one part is added to nine parts?
3. What formula is used to prepare a dilute solution from a concentrated solution?
4. How is a 1% (v/v) solution prepared?
5. How is a 5% (w/v) solution prepared?

6. Explain how to prepare one liter of 0.1 M potassium hydroxide (KOH). (Molecular weight = 56).
7. List three safety precautions that must be followed when preparing reagents.
8. In what circumstances must Standard Precautions be used when preparing laboratory reagents?
9. Define diluent, dilution, dilution factor, formula weight, lyophilize, molar solution, mole, molecular weight, percent solution, physiological saline, proportion, ratio, solute, solution, solvent, and titer.

STUDENT ACTIVITIES

1. Complete the written examination for this lesson.
2. Find examples of percent solutions and dilutions or ratios in a chemistry or similar textbook.
3. Practice preparing solutions and serial dilutions as directed by the instructor.
4. Practice the calculations for percentage solutions, proportions, ratios, and molarity using the worksheet.

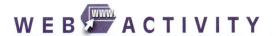

WEB ACTIVITY

Find information about the following chemicals using the Internet: sodium hydroxide, potassium hydroxide, sodium carbonate, ammonium hydroxide, dextrose, and glutamic acid. Find the molecular weights and MSDS information. For each chemical, state the precautions that should be used when working with solutions containing the chemical.

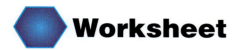

Worksheet

LESSON 1-11 Laboratory Calculations and Reagent Preparation

Name _____ **Date** _____

1. A procedure calls for 200 mL of a 2% glucose solution. A 50% solution is available. How much of the 50% solution is needed? How would the solution be prepared?

2. A 1% solution of hydrochloric acid is required for a procedure. A 5% solution is available. How much of the 5% solution will be required to make 500 mL of a 1% solution?

3. A procedure calls for acetic acid and water, with the proportions being one part acetic acid to three parts water. One hundred milliliters are needed. How much acetic acid and water are required?

4. One liter of 70% alcohol is needed. How much 95% alcohol is required to make the 70% solution?

5. Two hundred milliliters of 2% acetic acid are needed. How many milliliters of 5% acetic acid are required to make the 2% solution?

6. How would 1 L of a 10% solution of chlorine bleach be prepared?

7. How could 250 mL of a 4% solution of hydrochloric acid (HCl) be prepared from a 10% solution of HCl?

8. Give the instructions for preparing a two-fold serial dilution of serum using 0.5 mL serum and 0.5 mL saline in each of five numbered tubes.

9. A 1-to-25 dilution of blood is required for a procedure. How is it prepared?

10. How could a 1:10 dilution of serum be prepared?

11. What is the dilution when 0.5 mL is diluted to a total of 100 mL?

12. If 0.5 mL of serum is added to 4.5 mL of saline, what is the dilution?

13. Give instructions for preparing 500 mL of a 0.5 M solution of $Mg(OH)_2$ (FW = 58).

1-12

Blood Collection: Capillary Puncture

LESSON OBJECTIVES

After studying this lesson, the student will:

- Explain why a capillary puncture might be performed.
- Identify suitable sites for capillary punctures.
- Choose and prepare a site for capillary puncture.
- Perform a capillary puncture.
- Collect a blood specimen from a capillary puncture.
- Discuss how collection procedures affect capillary specimen quality.
- List the safety precautions to be observed when performing a capillary puncture.
- Define the glossary terms.

GLOSSARY

capillary / a minute blood vessel that connects the smallest arteries to the smallest veins and serves as an oxygen exchange vessel

capillary action / the action by which a fluid enters a tube because of the attraction between the fluid and the tube

capillary tube / a slender glass or plastic tube used for laboratory procedures

heparin / an anticoagulant used in certain laboratory procedures and in treatment of thrombosis

lancet / a sterile, sharp-pointed blade used to perform a capillary puncture

lateral / toward the side

INTRODUCTION

Capillary puncture, also called dermal puncture, is a safe, rapid, and efficient means of collecting a blood specimen. In capillary puncture, a small sterile **lancet** or blade is used to puncture the skin and **capillaries** to create a blood flow. Capillary punctures are performed when only a small amount of blood is required, when obtaining blood from infants, or when the patient has a condition that makes venipuncture difficult.

In the clinical laboratory, capillary blood has been used only in special situations, because of the small sample volume and potential for clotting of the sample. However, the increased use of small, portable, easy-to-use instruments that require only a drop or two of blood, has made capillary blood the specimen of choice for these analyzers. The rapid increase in the use of these instruments in bedside testing, physician office laboratories (POLs), and other point-of-care testing (POCT) sites has increased the need to train a variety of medical personnel in correct capillary puncture techniques.

THE CAPILLARY PUNCTURE

Capillary Puncture Sites

The usual site for capillary puncture in adults and children is the fingertip (Figure 1-68). In adults, the ring finger is often selected because it usually is not calloused. Capillary blood can be obtained from the great toe in infants and babies; in newborns, the lateral, or side, portion of the heel pad is used (Figure 1-69).

Lancets

Several types of disposable, sterile safety lancets are available for capillary puncture. These lancets make punctures of uniform depth at the touch of a button and are available in several blade lengths for use in different situations (Figure 1-70). Special pediatric lancets that produce a shallow puncture should be used with infants.

Capillary Collection Containers

Capillary blood can be collected in capillary tubes or collection vials that combine a capillary tube with a microtube, or can be applied directly to a test strip, cuvette, cartridge, or slide.

Capillary Tubes

Capillary tubes are slender tubes about 7 cm long and 1 mm in diameter, used primarily for microhematocrit measurements. Several types of capillary tubes are available: plain, heparinized, precalibrated, flexible, and self-sealing. Tubes coated with the anticoagulant heparin have a red ring on one end. These are used to prevent clotting of the blood during collection of capillary blood samples. Precalibrated tubes are usually heparinized. Nonheparinized (blue ring) capillary tubes are used with venous blood that has been previously collected in an anticoagulant.

In an effort to prevent injury and possible exposure to infectious agents from capillary tube breakage, the Occupational

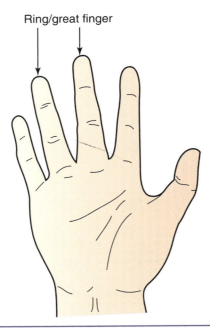

Ring/great finger

FIGURE 1-68 Capillary blood collection sites for adults and children

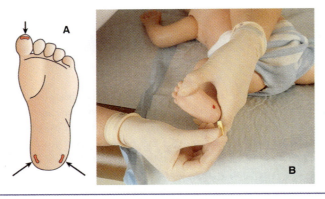

FIGURE 1-69 Pediatric capillary blood collection sites; (A) the heel or great toe can be used for infants and babies; (B) Collecting blood from the heel pad of a newborn

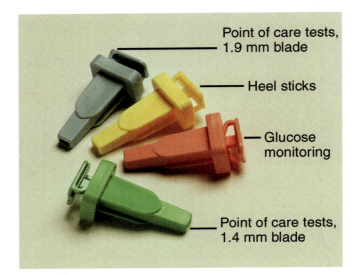

Point of care tests, 1.9 mm blade

Heel sticks

Glucose monitoring

Point of care tests, 1.4 mm blade

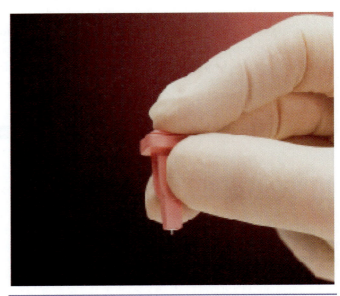

FIGURE 1-70 Single-use lancets of different lengths for capillary puncture (*Photos courtesy of Becton Dickinson and Co.*)

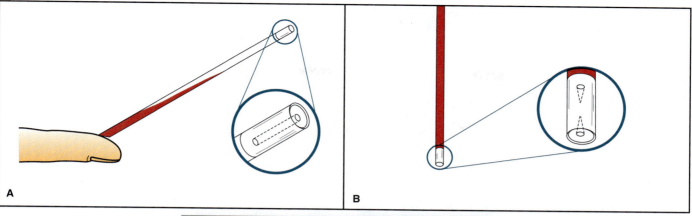

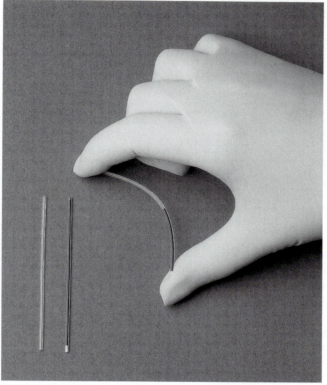

FIGURE 1-71 Hematocrit tubes with improved safety features. Self-sealing, mylar-wrapped capillary tubes:
(A) plug has channel that allows air to escape while the tube is being filled; (B) channel seals automatically
when blood touches plug; (C) Flexible hematocrit tubes (*Photo courtesy StatSpin, Inc., Norwood, MA*)

Safety and Health Administration (OSHA) and National Institute for Occupational Safety and Health (NIOSH) recommended that glass tubes not be used unless sheathed in a plastic protective film. It was also recommended that sealing clay not be used to seal tubes to be centrifuged for microhematocrit. To minimize exposure risk, glass tube alternatives such as flexible plastic tubes or mylar-wrapped tubes with self-sealing plugs should be used when possible. Self-sealing tubes have a plug at one end with a channel that allows air to escape while the tube is filled; the plug expands and seals when blood touches the plug (Figure 1-71).

Capillary Collection Vials

Capillary blood required for tests other than hematocrit can be collected in special vials with a capillary or other extension for directing the blood into the vial (Figure 1-72). These are available plain or with anticoagulant added. Using these tubes, a small quantity of whole blood, plasma, or serum can be obtained, which is particularly useful with pediatric patients.

Procedures that Use Capillary Blood

Several hematology procedures such as blood cell counts, hemoglobin, microhematocrit, and the blood smear can be performed using capillary blood. Many small handheld analyzers require only that a drop or two of capillary blood be applied to the test area, either directly from the puncture or from a capillary tube. These analyzers are widely used in POCT and POLs for hemoglobin, glucose, coagulation, immunology, and chemistry testing.

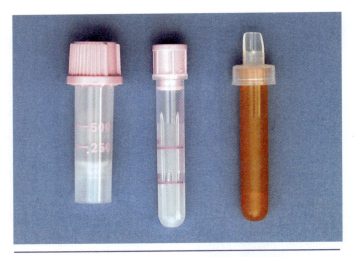

FIGURE 1-72 Capillary collection vials

PERFORMING CAPILLARY BLOOD COLLECTION

Although the capillary blood collection procedure appears to be simple, the technician must consider several factors and use careful technique to collect a quality specimen.

Safety Precautions

Standard Precautions must always be observed when collecting capillary blood. Gloves and other appropriate personal protective equipment (PPE), such as face or eye protection, must be worn by the technician. Plastic or mylar-sheathed tubes should be used to minimize risk of injury and exposure to bloodborne pathogens caused by tube breakage. Used lancets and tubes must be discarded into biohazard sharps container. Other blood-contaminated materials such as cotton or gauze must be disposed of in biohazard containers.

Quality Assessment

Personnel who perform capillary puncture must be adequately trained in correct collection techniques. This includes the use of proper collection equipment, collection procedures, and specimen handling. The capillary puncture should be completed quickly so that blood will not clot during the collection process. Good capillary blood sampling technique is the first step toward obtaining reliable test results.

Selecting the Puncture Site

The capillary puncture procedure should be explained to the patient. The patient's fingertips should be examined for a suitable site that is not calloused and has good circulation. Warm skin indicates adequate circulation; cool skin indicates

decreased circulation. A patient's hands can be gently massaged briefly to enhance circulation. Recent puncture sites should be avoided, especially in pediatric patients.

Preparing the Puncture Site

An alcohol swab should be used to cleanse the puncture site. The site must then be allowed to air-dry or can be wiped dry with sterile gauze. A puncture should not be made on moist skin.

Performing the Puncture

The patient's hand and finger should be held so the puncture site is readily accessible. Using a safety lancet, the puncture is made at the tip of the fleshy pad and slightly to the side (Figure 1-73). If the tips of the fingers are heavily calloused or thickened, a lancet with a longer blade can be used.

Collecting the Blood Sample

The first drop of blood should be wiped away with dry, sterile gauze. This first drop contains tissue fluid, which dilutes the blood drop and can also activate clotting. The second and following drops of blood are used for the test sample. A well-rounded drop of blood should be allowed to form before collection begins (Figure 1-74). Capillary blood should be collected as quickly as possible to avoid clotting.

It may be necessary to gently massage the hand to increase blood flow, taking care not to apply excessive pressure near the puncture site. Squeezing the fingertip should be avoided; this forces tissue fluid into the blood sample.

The capillary tube or blood collecting vial should be held in an almost horizontal position, or tilted slightly downward (Figure 1-75). When the tip of the capillary tube is touched to the drop of blood, blood will enter the tube by **capillary action** because of the attraction between the liquid and the tube. Capillary tubes

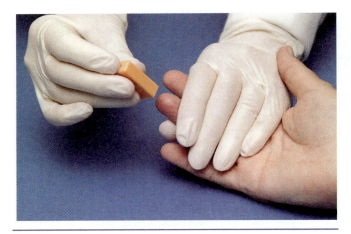

FIGURE 1-73 Proper position of the patient's and phlebotomist's hands during capillary puncture

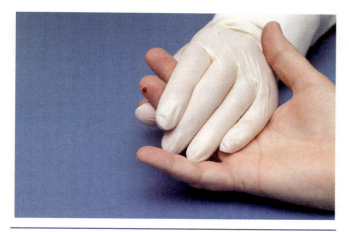

FIGURE 1-74 Well-rounded drop of blood

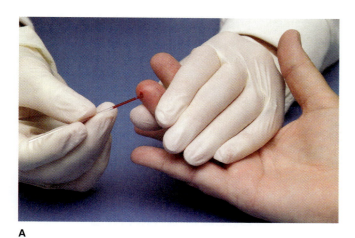

A

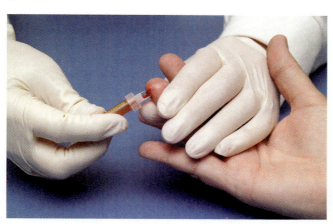

B

FIGURE 1-75 Collecting capillary blood into (A) a capillary tube and (B) a collection vial

should be filled two-thirds to three-quarters full. Test strips or cartridges are filled according to the manufacturer's directions.

Caring for the Puncture Site

After the blood has been collected, sterile gauze or a cotton ball should be placed on the site and pressure applied until bleeding stops.

SAFETY Reminders

- Review safety section before performing puncture.
- Use Standard Precautions when collecting capillary blood.
- Wear gloves when performing capillary puncture.
- Use appropriate face or eye protection.
- Use plastic or mylar-sheathed capillary tubes to minimize risk of breakage, possible injury, and potential exposure to pathogens.

PROCEDURAL Reminders

- Review procedure before performing puncture
- Select a puncture site with adequate circulation.
- Clean the puncture site thoroughly before puncture.
- Dry the puncture site before puncture to get a well-formed drop of blood.
- Do not squeeze the finger excessively.
- Collect capillary samples quickly to prevent the blood from clotting.

CASE STUDY

Mr. Stewart, a construction worker, came into the clinic for a blood test. When Robert, the laboratory technician, performed a capillary puncture on him, he was unable to obtain the amount of blood needed for the procedure ordered. Before Robert repeats the capillary puncture, explain what steps he can take to obtain adequate capillary blood flow.

SUMMARY

Capillary puncture is used to obtain blood when only a small quantity is needed or when blood must be collected from children and infants. Capillary puncture is performed using a disposable lancet, and blood is usually collected into capillary tubes or special capillary collection containers. Although capillary puncture is a relatively easy procedure to perform, much care must be taken to use proper techniques so that a quality sample is obtained. Because capillary blood clots very rapidly, the technician must have the competency to complete the task within a short time period. The quality of the capillary specimen will have a direct impact on the quality and reliability of the test results.

Capillary puncture is quite common because of the increased use of compact analyzers that require only small quantities of blood for testing. These analyzers are used for POCT, such as at the bedside, or in the physician's office, to perform several tests formerly only done in the hematology and chemistry laboratories. Because the tests are usually complete within just 1 or 2 minutes, the health care provider can receive the test results quickly.

REVIEW QUESTIONS

1. What is a capillary puncture?
2. Why are capillary punctures performed?
3. What are the usual puncture sites for adults; for infants?
4. How is a capillary puncture site prepared?
5. What is the procedure if the patient has cold hands?
6. Why is the first drop of blood wiped away?
7. List the safety precautions that must be observed when performing a capillary puncture.
8. When is a capillary tube with a blue band used? When is a tube with a red band used?
9. Why should the blood from capillary puncture be used quickly?
10. What is the advantage of using plastic capillary tubes?
11. Define capillary, capillary action, capillary tube, heparin, lancet, and lateral.

STUDENT ACTIVITIES

1. Complete the written examination for this lesson.
2. Practice performing a capillary puncture as outlined on the Student Performance Guide.
3. Find out how capillary punctures are performed on newborns in a local hospital nursery.

WEB ACTIVITIES

1. Use the Internet to find five analyzers that can use capillary blood in their test procedures. Report on the size of sample required and special requirements of the sample, if any.
2. Search the product listing of an online health care catalog. Find capillary tubes that incorporate safety features, capillary collection vials or containers, and lancets of different blade lengths.

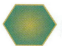 # Student Performance Guide

LESSON 1-12 Blood Collection: Capillary Puncture

Name _____   Date _____

INSTRUCTIONS

1. Practice the procedure for performing a capillary puncture following the step-by-step procedure.

2. Demonstrate the procedure for capillary puncture satisfactorily for the instructor, using the Student Performance Guide. Your instructor will determine the level of competency you must achieve to obtain a satisfactory (S) grade.

NOTE: Follow manufacturer's instructions for the type of capillary tubes used.

MATERIALS AND EQUIPMENT

- safety goggles, glasses, or protective face shield
- gloves
- antiseptic
- sterile, disposable lancets
- sterile cotton balls or gauze squares
- alcohol swabs
- mylar-coated capillary tubes (heparinized and plain, self-sealing)
- precalibrated capillary tubes (optional), sealing caps
- capillary collection vials
- sealing clay (optional)
- surface disinfectant
- biohazard container
- biohazard sharps container

PROCEDURE

Record in the comment section any problems encountered while practicing the procedure (or have a fellow student or the instructor evaluate your performance).

S = Satisfactory
U = Unsatisfactory

You must:	S	U	Comments
1. Assemble equipment and materials			
2. Wash hands and put on gloves and protective facewear			
3. Explain the procedure to the patient			
4. Select and warm the puncture site			
5. Cleanse the puncture site with alcohol			
6. Allow the site to air-dry or wipe dry with sterile gauze or cotton			
7. Position the puncture site, holding the skin taut with one hand and holding the lancet in the other hand			
8. Perform the capillary puncture			

You must:	S	U	Comments
9. Wipe away the first drop of blood with sterile gauze or cotton			
10. Massage the hand gently to produce the second drop of blood			

11. Collect the blood specimen:
  a. For microhematocrit:
    1. Fill a capillary tube two-thirds to three-quarters full using the second and subsequent drops of blood (fill to the line if using precalibrated tubes). Follow manufacturer's directions for the type of tube used
    2. Fill a second tube and seal the tubes
  b. For other point-of-care test:
    1. Apply a free-flowing drop of blood to test strip, slide, or cartridge
    2. Follow directions with instrument to complete the analysis
  c. For blood chemistry, using correct capillary collection vial:
    1. Follow manufacturer's directions for the type of collection vial used
    2. Touch the vial tip to the drop of blood and allow the container to fill, working quickly to prevent clotting
    3. Seal the vial and process the blood to obtain plasma or serum, according to directions			

12. Apply pressure to the puncture site by pressing with dry sterile gauze or cotton. Instruct patient to continue applying pressure			
13. Discard used lancet into a sharps container			
14. Discard used gauze or cotton into biohazard container			
15. Return equipment to proper storage			
16. Clean work area with surface disinfectant			
17. Remove and discard gloves into biohazard container. Wash hands with antiseptic			

Evaluator Comments:

Evaluator _____ Date _____

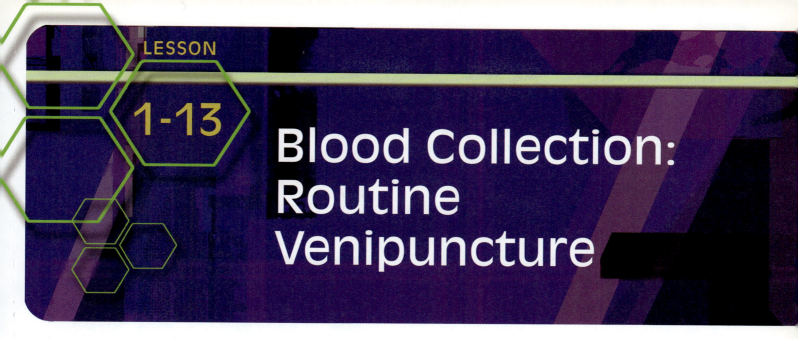

Blood Collection: Routine Venipuncture

LESSON OBJECTIVES

After studying this lesson, the student will:

- Explain the venipuncture procedure.
- Select the equipment necessary to perform a venipuncture.
- Apply a tourniquet.
- Select a proper venipuncture site.
- Perform a venipuncture.
- List the safety precautions to be observed when performing a venipuncture.
- Discuss factors that can affect the quality of the blood sample obtained by venipuncture.
- Name three common anticoagulants in vacuum tubes and state why they are used.
- Define the glossary terms.

GLOSSARY

basilic vein / large vein on inner side ("pinky" side) of arm

cephalic vein / a superficial vein of the arm (thumb side) commonly used for venipuncture

gauge / a measure of the diameter of a needle

hematoma / the swelling of tissue around a vessel due to leakage of blood into the tissue

hemoconcentration / increase in the concentration of cellular elements in the blood

hemolysis / rupture or destruction of red blood cells resulting in the release of hemoglobin

hypodermic needle / a hollow needle used for injections or for obtaining fluid specimens

lumen / the open space within a tubular organ or tissue

median cubital vein / a superficial vein located in the bend of the elbow (cubital fossa) that connects the cephalic vein to the basilic vein

palpate / to examine by touch

phlebotomy / venipuncture; entry of a vein with a needle

syringe / a hollow, tube-like container with a plunger, used for injecting or withdrawing fluids

tourniquet / a band used to constrict blood flow

vein / a blood vessel that carries deoxygenated blood from the tissues to the heart

venipuncture / entry of a vein with a needle; a phlebotomy

INTRODUCTION

The most common method of obtaining blood for laboratory examination is by **venipuncture**. The venipuncture is a quick way to obtain a large sample of blood on which many different analyses can be performed. In a venipuncture, also called a **phlebotomy**, a superficial **vein** is punctured with a **hypodermic needle** and blood is collected into a **syringe** or vacuum tube.

Performing a venipuncture involves several important steps that must be thoroughly understood before the procedure is attempted:

- Observing Standard Precautions and other safety measures throughout procedure
- Selecting the proper equipment
- Preparing the patient for venipuncture
- Selecting and preparing the puncture site
- Applying the tourniquet
- Obtaining the blood
- Caring for the puncture site and observing the patient for adverse reaction

The venipuncture is a safe procedure when performed correctly by a trained worker. The venipuncture must be performed carefully to preserve the condition of the vein. Much observation and practice is required to become skilled and self-confident in the art of venipuncture.

MATERIALS AND SUPPLIES FOR VENIPUNCTURE

Venipuncture can be performed using a vacuum tube safety needle/tube holder assembly (Figure 1-76), a safety syringe and needle (Figure 1-77), or butterfly needle and holder (Figure 1-78). Other materials required for venipuncture include blood collecting tubes, alcohol swabs, sterile gauze, tourniquet, and band-aid or small bandage (Figure 1-79). Venipuncture supplies

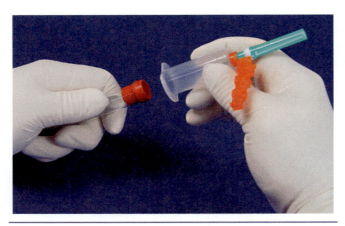

FIGURE 1-76 Vacuum tube system: safety needle, disposable needle holder, and vacuum collection tube
(*Photo courtesy of Smiths Medical ASD, Inc.*)

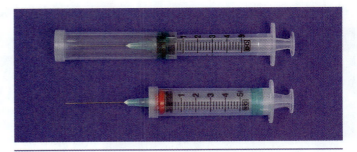

FIGURE 1-77 Safety syringe with sliding plastic sheath covering needle

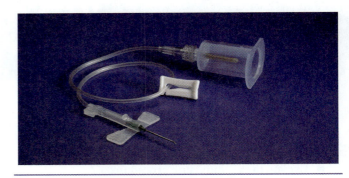

FIGURE 1-78 Butterfly needle
(*Photo courtesy of Smiths Medical ASD, Inc.*)

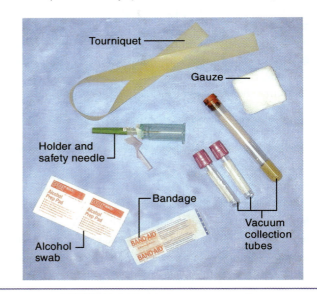

Tourniquet
Gauze
Holder and safety needle
Alcohol swab
Bandage
Vacuum collection tubes

FIGURE 1-79 Venipuncture supplies

should be organized into a portable phlebotomy tray, so that they will be readily available to the phlebotomist.

Needles

The length and **gauge** (diameter) of the needle used for venipuncture varies according to the procedure or preference of the phlebotomist. Venipuncture needles can be from ¾ inch to 1½ inches in length. For routine venipuncture, 21 gauge × 1 inch needles are used. (The higher the gauge number, the smaller the

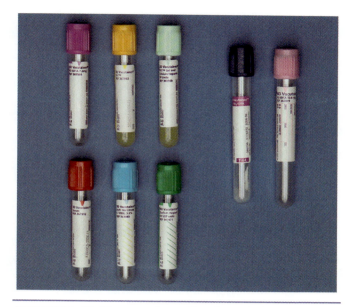

FIGURE 1-80 Vacuum tubes with color-coded tube stoppers

needle diameter.) Larger diameter needles are required for collection of blood donor units.

In response to the mandate to use safer methods to minimize or prevent accidental needlesticks, manufacturers of phlebotomy supplies have modified needle and holder systems to create several *safe* designs. Improved designs are continually being developed. One system uses safety needles that have internal blunting, meaning that the needle is made safe before it is removed from the vein. Other systems use a standard needle and disposable needle holder with a needle guard that snaps or slides over the exposed needle after the venipuncture, covering the needle until the entire unit is discarded (Figures 1-76 and 1-77). Safety needles or needle holders must be used when performing venipuncture.

Vacuum Tubes and Anticoagulants

Vacuum tubes, blood collecting tubes from which most of the air has been evacuated, are made in a variety of types and sizes. Tubes can be sterile or nonsterile, and glass or plastic. Each tube is manufactured to draw a specific volume of blood. Tube sizes commonly used are 3, 5, 7, and 10 mL. Tube stoppers are color-coded to designate which, if any, anticoagulant is present in the tube (Figure 1-80). Tubes with anticoagulant contain the exact amount required for the amount of blood the tube will draw. It is important that tubes be filled to their stated capacities because an improper ratio of anticoagulant to blood can alter cell morphology and cause erroneous test results, especially in coagulation tests. The laboratory procedure manual should include a list of tests performed and the type of vacuum tube that should be used for each.

Table 1-34 is an abbreviated guide to selecting vacuum tubes. Red-stoppered tubes contain no anticoagulant and are used for tests that require serum, such as most blood chemistries. Tubes with red/gray stoppers, called serum separator tubes, contain gel clotting activators that accelerate clotting. After the tubes are centrifuged, the gel is located between the serum and the clot, keeping them separate.

Procedures that use plasma require that blood is collected with a specific anticoagulant. For example, tubes with lavender stoppers contain EDTA, which is the anticoagulant used for most hematology studies, such as cell and differential counts. Light blue-stoppered tubes contain sodium citrate, the anticoagulant used for most coagulation studies. Tubes with dark green stoppers contain heparin and are used for several tests in chemistry and hematology, but these tubes should not be used if stained blood smears are to be prepared from the specimen. Gray-stoppered tubes containing potassium oxalate anticoagulant and sodium fluoride (to inhibit glycolysis) are used for certain glucose tests and legal alcohol.

PERFORMING A VENIPUNCTURE USING A VACUUM TUBE SYSTEM

A widely used method of collecting venous blood is the vacuum-tube system consisting of a double-ended needle, needle holder, and vacuum tubes. The short rubber-sheathed end of the needle is threaded into the needle holder and is used to pierce the stopper in the vacuum tube during blood collection (Figure 1-81). The long end of the needle, covered by a removable plastic cap, is used to puncture the vein.

TABLE 1-34. Guide for selecting vacuum tubes

STOPPER COLOR	ANTICOAGULANT IN TUBE	EXAMPLES OF USE
Red	None	Tests that require serum, such as most blood chemistries and serology tests
Red/gray	None	Serum-separator tube; used for tests that require serum
Lavender	EDTA	Most hematological tests, blood-typing
Green	Heparin	Some special chemistry tests, certain lymphocyte studies, lupus erythematosus test
Light blue	Sodium citrate	Most coagulation studies
Gray	Potassium oxalate	Certain glucose tests, legal alcohol
Black	Buffered sodium citrate	Westergren ESR

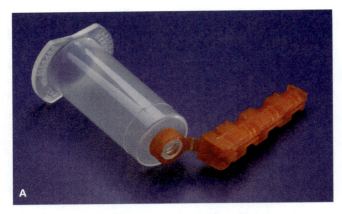

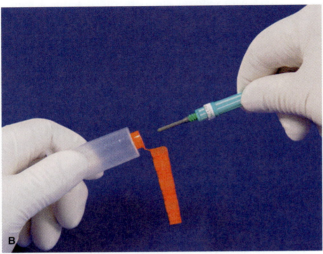

FIGURE 1-81 Vacuum tube blood collecting system:
(A) disposable needle holder with needle safety guard;
(B) inserting sheathed short end of needle into needle holder
(*Courtesy of Smiths Medical ASD, Inc.*)

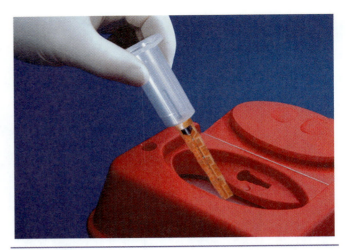

FIGURE 1-82 Disposable of used venipuncture assembly into sharps container (*Courtesy of Smiths Medical ASD, Inc.*)

Safety Precautions

Standard Precautions must be observed and gloves must be worn by the phlebotomist when performing all venipunctures. It is best to use gloves without talc to avoid contaminating collection tubes. The phlebotomist should wear personal protective equipment (PPE) such as a buttoned, fluid-resistant laboratory coat and face protection. Students learning to perform venipuncture must be supervised by a qualified instructor.

Used needles must never be recapped but should be immediately discarded into a biohazard sharps container (Figure 1-82). Venipuncture products with enhanced safety designs should be used. Several types of safety needles, needle holders, and syringes are available (see Figures 1-77 and 1-81). The correct use of engineering controls such as safety needles should decrease the incidence of accidental needlesticks and possible transmission of bloodborne pathogens associated with needlesticks. However, workers must continue to be aware of the potential for injury since no system is 100% safe 100% of the time.

Quality Assessment

Proper specimen collection is the first step in ensuring quality test results on blood samples. The phlebotomist must properly identify the patient, select the correct tubes for blood collection, collect the specimen under the proper conditions, and deliver the specimen to the testing site within the specified time limits. Specimen quality can be compromised because of improper venipuncture technique or the improper handling, transport, or storage of the specimen. Some test procedures require special collection and handling, such as immediate placement of the blood specimen on ice. Specimen collection parameters required for each laboratory test are described in the laboratory procedure manual and must be followed.

Two conditions that can occur as a result of improper blood collection technique are hemolysis and hemoconcentration. Either of these two conditions will adversely affect test results. **Hemolysis**, the rupture of red blood cells, can cause erroneous hematology and blood chemistry results. Hemolysis can be caused by using a small gauge collection needle or when blood flow through the needle is slowed because of improper positioning of needle in vein. **Hemoconcentration** can occur when the tourniquet is left on too long before the venipuncture is performed. This can cause localized stasis in the vein and artificially alter the concentration of blood constituents.

Selecting the Equipment

Phlebotomy supplies should be placed within easy reach of the phlebotomist. A portable phlebotomy tray can hold all supplies (Figure 1-83), including a sharps disposal container, gloves, and face protection. The needle and safety needle holder should be assembled and the correct vacuum tube(s) selected.

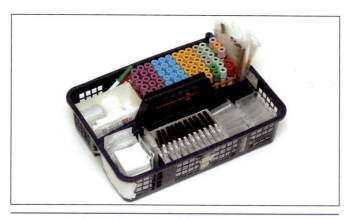

FIGURE 1-83 Portable phlebotomy tray

Preparing the Patient

The patient should be identified by asking the patient name and verifying the name on the laboratory request form. If the patient is hospitalized, the patient identification band must be checked against the request form and any preprinted labels. For some critical procedures, such as collecting blood for pretransfusion testing, the phlebotomist usually places an additional identification wristband on the patient that is coded to the blood-collection tubes.

The venipuncture procedure should be fully explained to the patient to minimize apprehension. The patient should be lying down or seated in a chair that has arm supports. The patient's arm must be fully extended and firmly supported so that it will remain still during the venipuncture (Figure 1-84). The phlebotomist should be trained in first aid procedures to be prepared for the occasional patient who might faint.

Tying the Tourniquet

A **tourniquet** is applied to the arm to make the veins more prominent. Disposable tourniquets are preferred, because they eliminate the need to disinfect ones that come in contact with blood. The tourniquet is placed under the arm 3 to 4 inches above the elbow, and the two ends are stretched and crossed over the top of the arm (Figure 1-85). While tension is maintained on the ends, one side is looped and pulled halfway through. When the tourniquet is tied in this manner, it will release easily with a gentle pull on one end (Figure 1-86). *The tourniquet should never be tied tight enough to compromise circulation.* The tourniquet should be left in place for no more than 1 to 2 minutes.

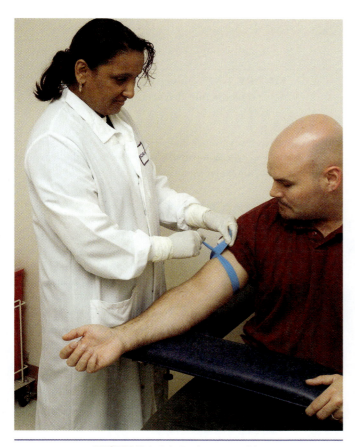

FIGURE 1-84 Patient seated in phlebotomy chair with arm supports

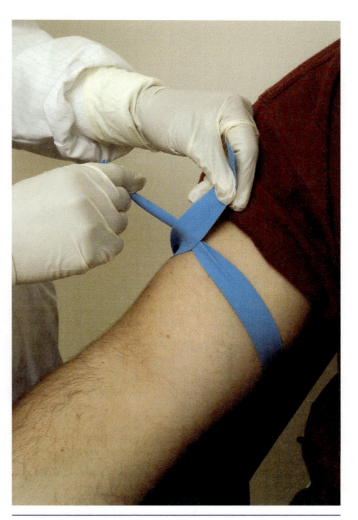

FIGURE 1-85 Tying the tourniquet

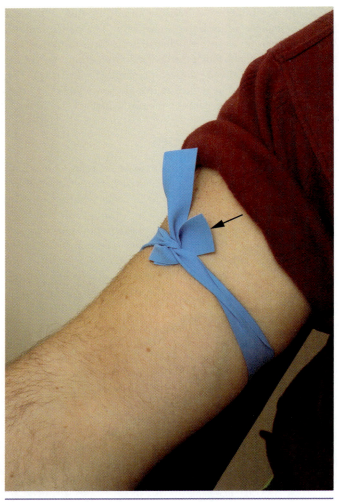

FIGURE 1-86 Release the tourniquet
by pulling on one end (arrow)

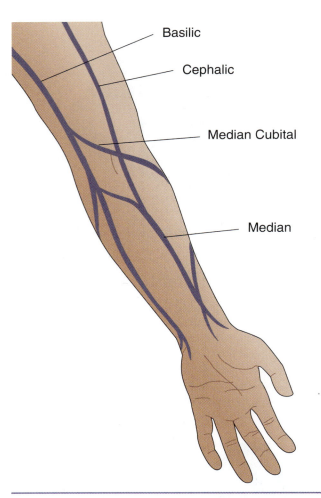

FIGURE 1-87 Veins commonly used for
venipuncture (left arm shown)

Selecting the Venipuncture Site

The puncture site should be selected after inspecting both arms to locate the best vein. The tourniquet can be applied to aid in selection of the puncture site, but it should be released while the site is cleansed, and retied before the puncture is performed. The veins most frequently used are the **median cubital vein** and the **cephalic vein** of the forearm; the **basilic vein** can also be used (Figure 1-87). The phlebotomist should **palpate** the vein by gently pressing the fingertip along the vein to determine its direction and estimate its size and depth (Figure 1-88). The vein will have a *bouncy* feel to it.

Veins that have scarring or bruising, or that have had recent venipuncture should not be used. Blood should not be collected from an arm with an intravenous line or from the arm of a patient who has had a recent mastectomy (breast removal) on that side.

Preparing the Venipuncture Site

The venipuncture procedure is illustrated in Figure 1-89. The area around the puncture site should be cleansed thoroughly in a circular motion from the center outward with a 70% alcohol swab (Figure 1-89A). The site should then be allowed to air-dry or be wiped dry

with sterile gauze. Once the site is cleansed, it should not be touched again except to enter the vein with the sterile needle. If the vein must be palpated again, the skin must be recleansed.

Obtaining the Blood

When the puncture site has been cleansed, the tourniquet should be reapplied to the arm, taking care that it does not touch the cleansed area. The needle/holder assembly should be held in one hand with the needle bevel facing up and the needle shaft lined up with the vein (Figures 1-89B and 1-90A).

The vein should be anchored by grasping the arm, placing the thumb on the vein about 1 inch below the puncture site and pressing and pulling the skin taut toward the phlebotomist. Holding the needle/holder at a 15° to 25° angle, the skin and vein should be entered in one smooth motion until the needle is in the **lumen** of the vein (Figures 1-89C and 1-90B). Penetration of the vein should be at a low angle to prevent piercing the bottom wall of the vein, and possibly causing a **hematoma**, or swelling. *If a hematoma begins to form during the procedure, the tourniquet should be immediately released, the needle withdrawn, and gauze and pressure applied to the puncture site.*

Once the needle is in the vein, the needle holder should be steadied with one hand while the vacuum tube is gently pushed

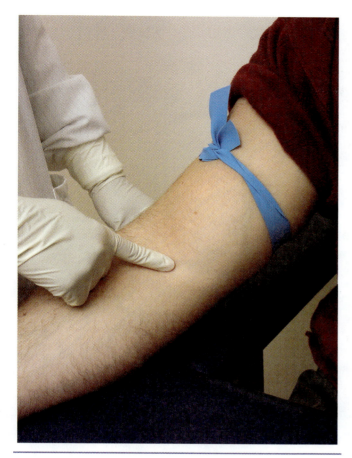

FIGURE 1-88 Palpating a vein

onto the sheathed needle inside the holder, allowing blood to be drawn into the tube by vacuum (Figure 1-89D). When the tube is full, it is removed from the holder. If more than one tube is needed, the second tube is then pushed onto the needle in the holder (1-89E). The rubber sheath on the needle prevents blood leakage between tube changes. If more than one type of tube is to be filled, the *clot tube* (red-stoppered) must be filled first; tubes containing anticoagulant are filled last. Tubes containing anticoagulant should be inverted gently (not shaken) a few times immediately after filling to mix the blood with the anticoagulant. The last tube should be removed from the needle holder before the needle is withdrawn from the vein (Figure 1-89F)

Completing the Venipuncture and Caring for the Patient

When the desired amount of blood has been obtained, the tourniquet should be released. (Or, once the vein is entered and good blood flow is obtained, the tourniquet can be released while the remainder of blood is collected.) The tourniquet is always released before the needle is withdrawn from the vein to prevent hematoma at the venipuncture site. As the needle is withdrawn from the vein, gauze should be immediately placed over the puncture site and pressure applied (Figure 1-87G). The patient should be instructed to press the gauze on the puncture site for 2 to 5 minutes with the arm extended to ensure that bleeding stops and a hematoma does not form.

The needle must not be recapped or removed from the needle holder by hand. The safety device must immediately be used to cover the needle so that an accidental needlestick is not possible. The unit is then discarded into a biohazard sharps container. The phlebotomist should then apply patient labels to the tubes in the presence of the patient. The labels must contain patient information, date and time of collection, and phlebotomist's name or initials. Tubes should not be prelabeled to prevent the possibility of using a prelabeled tube for the wrong patient.

The phlebotomist should check the venipuncture site and be sure that bleeding has stopped before leaving the patient. Most sites will stop bleeding within 2 to 3 minutes. A small bandage or band-aid can be applied to the site if necessary.

PERFORMING A VENIPUNCTURE USING A SYRINGE

Syringes can be used for small, difficult veins that make routine venipuncture with vacuum tubes difficult. When using a syringe to perform a venipuncture, the phlebotomist should use syringes and/or needles designed with safety features to prevent needlesticks. Disposable syringe/needle units are available that have a sliding shield to cover the needle after use. Alternatively a safety needle with a protective sheath can be attached to a disposable syringe.

To use a syringe, the needle should be positioned firmly on the syringe so the bevel and graduations of the syringe face in the same direction. The syringe plunger should be pushed up and down to see that it moves freely. It should then be left pushed completely into the barrel so that no air remains in the syringe.

The syringe venipuncture procedure is the same as with the vacuum tube system except that instead of the vacuum tube drawing the blood automatically, the phlebotomist must steady the syringe with one hand while the other hand gently pulls back on the plunger to draw blood into the syringe. The needle should be observed while the syringe is filling to be sure it is not accidentally pulled out of the vein. After the syringe is filled, the needle is withdrawn from the vein and the blood can be transferred to a vacuum tube using a special safety adapter. The safety feature should then be activated, and the entire unit should be discarded into a biohazard sharps container.

A T T E N T I O N !

ACTION TO TAKE IN CASE OF EXPOSURE INCIDENT

If you receive a **needlestick** or other injury from sharps, or if your eyes, nose, mouth, or broken skin are exposed to OPIM:

1. Immediately flood the exposed area with water, and clean skin with antiseptic soap and water.

2. Report accident immediately to supervisor, risk control officer, or other appropriate person.

3. Seek immediate medical attention.

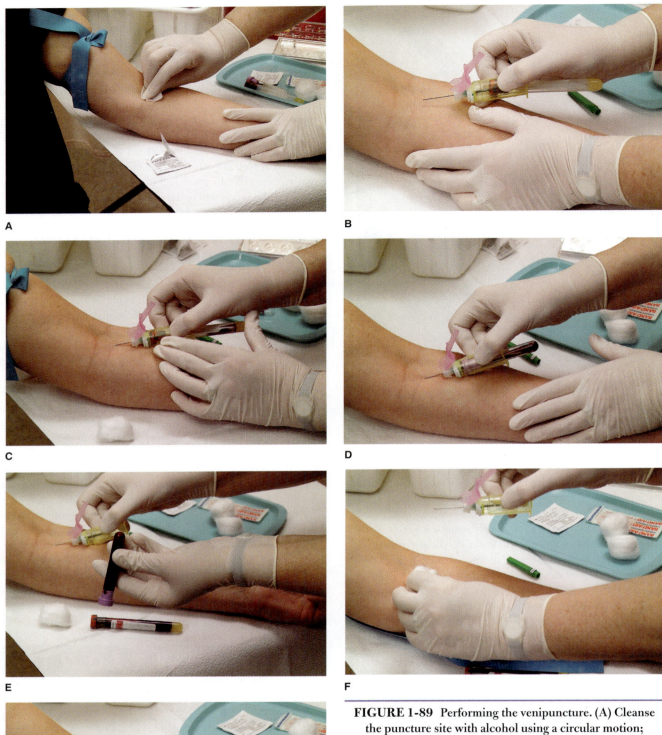

FIGURE 1-89 Performing the venipuncture. (A) Cleanse the puncture site with alcohol using a circular motion; (B) line up needle with vein; (C) pierce skin and vein in one smooth motion and insert tube into holder to puncture cap of vacuum tube; (D) allow tube to fill; (E) fill additional tubes, inverting tubes containing anticoagulant; (F) withdraw tube from needle before withdrawing needle from vein; (G) apply pressure to puncture site

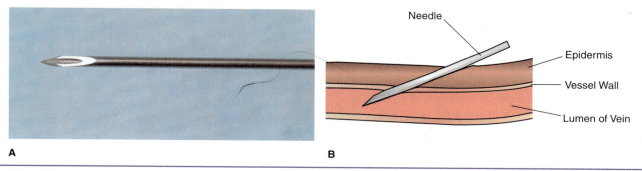

A   B

FIGURE 1-90 Close-up view of bevel of needle (A) and illustration of proper position of needle in lumen of vein (B)

SAFETY Reminders

- Review safety section before performing venipuncture.
- Observe Standard Precautions when performing venipuncture.
- Use safety devices such as self-sheathing needles.
- Never reuse needles or syringes.
- Do not recap needles; discard in appropriate sharps container.
- Check venipuncture site before leaving patient.

PROCEDURAL Reminders

- Review venipuncture procedure before attempting venipuncture.
- Identify patient by asking for a name and checking armband.
- Be sure patient's arm is firmly supported before performing venipuncture.
- Do not allow tourniquet to remain on the arm for more than 1 to 2 minutes.
- Always release the tourniquet before removing the needle from the vein.
- Release tourniquet immediately, withdraw needle, and apply pressure to puncture site with gauze if a hematoma begins to form.
- Label filled tubes as soon as the venipuncture is completed, and before leaving the patient.

C A S E   S T U D Y

Jerry was completing his fourth week of CLT internship at Pleasant Valley Hospital. All interns were required to collect blood each morning from eight to 10 patients before beginning their clinical rotation. Jeremy had completed his phlebotomy rotation the previous week, so he was collecting blood on his own (without supervision). One of the patients on his collection list was 72 years old. Jerry saw only one adequate vein in the patient's left arm but was unable to get blood when he attempted venipuncture.

1. What should Jerry do?
   a. Stick the same vein again
   b. Keep trying other veins until he is successful
   c. Ask for assistance from an experienced phlebotomist
   d. Discretely return the test request form to the stack of collections that are needed and go to his internship rotation assignment
2. Discuss factors that cause venipuncture to be difficult and how these venipunctures can be handled.

SUMMARY

Venipuncture is a common method of obtaining blood for routine laboratory analysis. The procedure is safe when performed by trained phlebotomists. Venipuncture can be performed using a vacuum tube collecting system or a syringe. The phlebotomist must use the proper technique to obtain the blood and must also select and use the correct specimen tubes and handling conditions for each test ordered. This information is provided in the laboratory procedure manual.

The phlebotomist must follow Standard Precautions and wear appropriate PPE when performing venipuncture. The development of safety needles and safety collection devices has increased the safety level for the phlebotomist by decreasing the risk of accidental needlesticks. These safety devices must be used when performing venipuncture.

REVIEW QUESTIONS

1. Why is a venipuncture performed?
2. What is the purpose of a tourniquet?
3. Name five precautions that must be observed when performing a venipuncture.
4. What are the steps in performing a venipuncture?
5. What is the most common venipuncture site?
6. Why must the tourniquet be released before removing the needle from the vein?
7. How should the puncture site be cared for after the needle is removed?
8. Explain briefly the vacuum system of obtaining venous blood.
9. What precautions should the phlebotomist take when performing a venipuncture to avoid exposure to blood?
10. Name three anticoagulants used in collecting blood. Which one is most commonly used in hematology?
11. Why is it important to verify patient identification before performing a venipuncture?
12. Define basilic vein, cephalic vein, gauge, hematoma, hemoconcentration, hemolysis, hypodermic needle, lumen, median cubital vein, palpate, phlebotomy, syringe, tourniquet, vein, and venipuncture.

STUDENT ACTIVITIES

1. Complete the written examination for this lesson
2. Practice applying a tourniquet and locating suitable veins for venipuncture.
3. Practice performing a venipuncture as outlined in the Student Performance Guides.

WEB ACTIVITIES

1. Use the Internet to find information on safety needles and venipuncture devices. Explain how each type protects the worker from accidental needlesticks.
2. Visit Web sites of agencies such as the Centers for Disease Control and Prevention, Occupational Safety and Health Administration, and National Institute for Occupational Safety and Health. Look for information on preventing needlestick or sharps injury. Try to find free brochures, powerpoint presentations, or other safety information that can be downloaded.

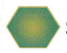 # Student Performance Guide

LESSON 1-13 Blood Collection: Venipuncture—Vacuum Tube Method

Name _____   **Date** _____

INSTRUCTIONS

1. Practice performing a venipuncture using a vacuum tube system and following the step-by-step procedure.
2. Demonstrate the venipuncture procedure using a vacuum tube system satisfactorily for the instructor, following the Student Performance Guide. Your instructor will determine the level of competency you must achieve to obtain a satisfactory (S) grade.

NOTE: If necessary, adjust procedure according to available venipuncture supplies

MATERIALS AND EQUIPMENT

- safety glasses, goggles, or face shield
- gloves
- antiseptic
- tourniquet
- sterile gauze or cotton
- 70% alcohol or alcohol swabs
- vacuum-tube safety needle and holder
- evacuated blood-collection tubes
- sharps container
- surface disinfectant
- biohazard container
- test tube rack

PROCEDURE

Record in the comment section any problems encountered while practicing the procedure (or have a fellow student or the instructor evaluate your performance).

S = Satisfactory
U = Unsatisfactory

You must:	S	U	Comments
1. Assemble equipment and materials			
2. Place venipuncture equipment and supplies within easy reach			
3. Wash hands and put on gloves and face protection			
4. Identify patient			
5. Explain venipuncture procedure to the patient and position the patient			
6. Attach the sterile, capped needle to the needle holder			
7. Insert vacuum-collection tube into needle holder, but do not pierce stopper with needle			

You must:	S	U	Comments
8. Tie the tourniquet around the patient's arm 2 to 3 inches above the elbow. It should be just tight enough so venous circulation is restricted, but not so tight that it is extremely uncomfortable. **CAUTION:** Do not allow the tourniquet to remain on for more than 1 to 2 minutes			
9. Instruct the patient to make a fist to make the veins more noticeable			
10. Inspect the bend of the elbow to locate a suitable vein			
11. Palpate the vein with the fingertips to determine its direction, and estimate its size and depth. **NOTE:** The vein most frequently used is the median cubital vein of the forearm			
12. Release the tourniquet			
13. Cleanse the puncture site in a circular motion from the center out using an alcohol swab			
14. Allow alcohol to dry			
15. Retie the tourniquet, being careful not to touch the sterile puncture site			
16. Instruct patient to straighten the arm and make a fist			
17. Uncap the needle and inspect it to see that the point is smooth and sharp			
18. Hold the needle holder and tube assembly so the bevel of the needle is facing upward (toward ceiling). With the thumb of your other hand, hold the skin below puncture site taut			
19. Hold the needle at a 15° to 25° angle to the arm and insert it into the vein			
20. Push the vacuum tube gently onto the inner needle in the holder while steadying the needle holder with the other hand.			
21. Watch for blood flow into the tube and instruct the patient to open the fist when the tube begins to fill			
22. Release the tourniquet when the desired amount of blood is obtained			
23. Remove the vacuum tube from the needle holder			
24. Place a dry, sterile gauze over the puncture site and withdraw the needle from the vein, taking care not to press down on the needle			

You must:	S	U	Comments
25. Instruct the patient to apply pressure to the puncture site for 3 to 5 minutes keeping the arm extended			
26. Activate the needle safety feature and discard the disposable needle unit into the sharps container. DO NOT RECAP			
27. Label the collection tube properly			
28. Discard other used supplies appropriately			
29. Check patient to be sure bleeding has stopped; apply bandage if necessary			
30. Clean and return equipment to storage			
31. Clean work area with surface disinfectant			
32. Remove and discard gloves in biohazard container			
33. Wash hands with antiseptic			

Evaluator Comments:

Evaluator _____ Date _____

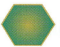

Student Performance Guide

LESSON 1-13 Blood Collection: Venipuncture—Syringe Method

Name _____   **Date** _____

INSTRUCTIONS

1. Practice performing a venipuncture using a syringe and following the step-by-step procedure.

2. Demonstrate the venipuncture procedure using a syringe satisfactorily for the instructor, following the Student Performance Guide. Your instructor will determine the level of competency you must achieve to obtain a satisfactory (S) grade.

MATERIALS AND EQUIPMENT

- safety glasses, goggles, or face shield
- gloves
- antiseptic
- tourniquet
- sterile gauze or cotton
- 70% alcohol or alcohol swabs
- sterile disposable 20 to 22 gauge safety needle
- sterile safety syringe
- collection tubes
- test tube rack
- sharps container
- surface disinfectant (10% chlorine bleach solution)
- biohazard container
- safety adapter for filling vacuum tubes

PROCEDURE

Record in the comment section any problems encountered while practicing the procedure (or have a fellow student or the instructor evaluate your performance).

S = Satisfactory
U = Unsatisfactory

You must:	S	U	Comments
1. Assemble equipment and materials			
2. Place venipuncture equipment and supplies within easy reach			
3. Wash hands and put on gloves and face protection			
4. Identify patient			
5. Explain venipuncture procedure to patient and position patient			
6. Attach the capped needle to the syringe, maintaining sterility			
7. Slide the plunger up and down in the barrel of the syringe to be sure it moves freely			
8. Push the plunger to the bottom of the barrel so no air remains in the syringe			

You must:	S	U	Comments
9. Tie the tourniquet around the patient's arm 2 to 3 inches above the elbow. It should be just tight enough so venous circulation is restricted, but not so tight that it is extremely uncomfortable **CAUTION:** Do not allow the tourniquet to remain on for more than 1 to 2 minutes			
10. Instruct the patient to make a fist to make the veins more prominent			
11. Inspect the bend of the elbow to locate a suitable vein			
12. Palpate the vein with the fingertip(s) to determine its direction, and estimate its size and depth. **NOTE:** The vein most frequently used is the median cubital vein of the forearm			
13. Release the tourniquet			
14. Cleanse the puncture site in a circular motion from the center out using an alcohol swab			
15. Allow alcohol to dry			
16. Retie the tourniquet, being careful not to touch the cleansed puncture site			
17. Instruct the patient to straighten his/her arm and make a fist			
18. Uncap the needle and inspect the needle to see that the point is smooth and sharp			
19. Hold the syringe so the graduations on the syringe and the bevel of the needle are in full view (facing toward the ceiling). With thumb of the other hand, hold skin taut below puncture site, anchoring the vein			
20. Hold the needle at a 15° to 25° angle to the arm and insert it into the vein			
21. Watch for blood flow into the syringe and instruct the patient to open their fist as soon as blood appears			
22. Pull the plunger back slowly with one hand to withdraw the blood, while steadying the syringe and needle with the other hand			
23. Release the tourniquet when the desired amount of blood is obtained			
24. Place a dry, sterile gauze over the puncture site and withdraw the needle from the vein taking care not to press down on the needle			

You must:	S	U	Comments
25. Instruct the patient to apply pressure to the puncture site for 3 to 5 minutes with the arm extended			
26. Fill blood-collecting tube using a safety adapter			
27. Label the tube properly			
28. Activate the safety feature and discard used syringe and needle into biohazard sharps container			
29. Check patient to be sure bleeding has stopped; apply bandage if necessary			
30. Clean and return equipment to storage			
31. Clean work area with surface disinfectant			
32. Remove and discard gloves in biohazard container			
33. Wash hands with antiseptic			

Evaluator Comments:

Evaluator _____ Date _____

UNIT 2

Basic Hematology

UNIT OBJECTIVES

After studying this unit, the student will:

- Explain the functions of the hematology laboratory.
- Identify components of the circulatory system and discuss the formation of blood.
- Perform a hematocrit determination.
- Perform a hemoglobin determination.
- Use a hemacytometer.
- Perform a manual red blood cell count.
- Perform a manual white blood cell count.
- Perform a manual platelet count.
- Prepare and stain a peripheral blood smear.
- Identify normal blood cells from a stained blood smear or visual aids.
- Perform a white blood cell differential count.
- Identify selected abnormal blood cells from stained smears or visual aids.
- Calculate the red blood cell indices and explain their significance.
- Perform an erythrocyte sedimentation rate test.
- Perform a reticulocyte count.
- Discuss the principles of automation in hematology.
- Explain the importance of safety policies in the performance of hematology procedures.
- Discuss quality assessment in relation to the hematology laboratory.

UNIT OVERVIEW

Hematology is the area of medicine involving the study of the cellular elements of blood and the blood-forming tissues. Unit 2 is an introduction to several basic procedures commonly performed in the hematology laboratory. The unit begins with a discussion of the discipline of hematology in Lesson 2-1, including basic information about the circulatory system, the origin of blood cells, blood composition, blood diseases, and analytical methods used in the hematology laboratory.

Information and step-by-step instructions for manually performing the tests comprising the *CBC* (*complete blood count*), one of the most frequently requested hematology tests, are spread over several lessons. The CBC has traditionally included the red blood cell (RBC) count, hemoglobin, hematocrit, white blood cell (WBC) count, and WBC differential count. With the automation now available, many additional parameters can be measured from one blood sample.

Lesson 2-2, Hematocrit, explains the procedure for determining the microhematocrit and discusses the various types of equipment used. A discussion of the theory of hemoglobin measurement and the procedure for using a hemoglobin analyzer are included in Lesson 2-3. In Lesson 2-4, The Hemacytometer, the student learns the principles and procedures of using the hemacytometer before going on to Lesson 2-5, Manual RBC and WBC Counts. The manual platelet count is covered in Lesson 2-6; although platelet count is included on automated analyzers, extremely low counts are often verified by manual count.

Lesson 2-7, Preparing and Staining a Blood Smear, lays the foundation for the next three lessons by teaching the procedure for producing a suitable smear and the importance of the staining technique. Normal blood cell morphology and important points to consider in the identification of blood cells are described in Lesson 2-8. After basic blood cell identification is mastered, the student can proceed to Lesson 2-9, White Blood Cell Differential Count.

Lesson 2-10, Abnormalities in Peripheral Blood Cell Morphology, is included for students who desire more in-depth information on abnormal blood cells. However, the lesson is intended only as an introduction to a complex topic. Lesson 2-10 also includes the formulas for calculating the red blood cell indices using the RBC count and hemoglobin and hematocrit values. The indices estimate the size and hemoglobin content of a red blood cell population and are routinely calculated by most automated cell counters and reported as part of the CBC.

The Reticulocyte Count, Lesson 2-11, gives information about the rate of red blood cell production and is useful in evaluating the response of anemia patients to treatment. In Lesson 2-12 the principles and procedures of the erythrocyte sedimentation rate are presented; the results are used to help the clinician diagnose, prescribe, and evaluate treatment of some inflammatory disease processes. Lesson 2-13, Principles of Automated Hematology, is an introduction to the theory of automated cell counters and hematology analyzers.

Examining blood in the hematology laboratory provides important information used in diagnosing and treating blood diseases such as anemias and leukemias. Hematology tests also aid in diagnosing and managing diseases that originate in other body systems. Practice and skill are required to perform basic hematology procedures in a reliable manner. The tests must be performed with accuracy, precision, and the utmost attention to proper procedure, safety precautions, and quality assessment.

READINGS, REFERENCES, AND RESOURCES

General Hematology

Baker, F. J. et al. (2001). *Baker & Silverton's introduction to medical laboratory technology* (7th ed.). Oxford, UK: Oxford University Press.

Brown, B. A. (1993). *Hematology: principles and procedures* (6th ed.). Philadelphia: Lea & Febiger.

Harmening, D. M. (2006). *Clinical hematology and fundamentals of hemostasis* (5th ed.). Philadelphia: F. A. Davis Co.

Hemocue. Manufacturer's instructions. Lake Forest, CA.

Henry, J. B. (Ed.) (2006). *Clinical diagnosis & management by laboratory methods* (21st ed.). Philadelphia: W. B. Saunders Company.

Lee, R. G. et al. (1998). *Wintrobe's clinical hematology* (10th ed.). Baltimore: Williams & Wilkins.

Lindh, W. Q. et al. (2002). *Comprehensive medical assisting* (2nd ed.). Clifton Park, NY: Thomson Delmar Learning.

Linné, J. J. & Ringsrud, K. M. (1999). *Clinical laboratory sciences: the basics and routine techniques* (4th ed.). Mosby.

McKenzie, S. B. (2003). *Clinical laboratory hematology*. Upper Saddle River, NJ: Prentice Hall.

Miale, J. B. (1991). *Laboratory medicine: hematology* (6th ed.). St. Louis: C. V. Mosby.

Rodak, B. F. (1997). *Diagnostic hematology*. Baltimore: AACC Press.

Scott, A. S. & Fong, E. (2004). *Body structures and functions* (10th ed). Clifton Park, NY: Thomson Delmar Learning.

Simmers, L. (2004). *Diversified health occupations* (6th ed.). Clifton Park, NY: Thomson Delmar Learning.

Stiene-Martin, E. A. et al. (Eds.). *Clinical hematology: principles, procedures, correlations.* Philadelphia: Lippincott-Raven Publishers.

Turgeon, M. L. (1999). *Clinical hematology theory and procedures* (3rd ed.). Hagerstown, MD: Lippincott Williams & Wilkins.

Unopette. Manufacturer's package insert. Becton Dickinson, Rutherford, NJ.

Blood Cell Morphology, Atlases

Bain, B. J. (2002). *Blood cells* (3rd ed.). Ames, Iowa: Iowa State University Press.

Bain, B. J. (2004). *A beginner's guide to blood cells* (2nd ed.). Ames, Iowa: Blackwell Publishing.

Bell, A. & Sallah, S. (2005). *The morphology of human blood cells* (7th ed). Abbott Park, IL: Abbott Laboratories.

Carr, J. H. & Rodak, B. F. (2004). *Clinical hematology atlas.* Philadelphia: W. B. Saunders Co.

Loffler, H. & Rastetter, J. (1999). *Atlas of clinical hematology.* Berlin: Springer-Verlag.

Phlebotomy

Garza, D. & Becan-McBride, K. (2004). *Phlebotomy handbook* (7th ed.). East Norwalk, CT: Appleton and Lange.

Hoeltke, L. B. (2006). *The complete textbook of phlebotomy* (3rd ed.). Clifton Park, NY: Thomson Delmar Learning.

Kalanick, K. (2004). *Phlebotomy technician specialist.* Clifton Park, NY: Thomson Delmar Learning.

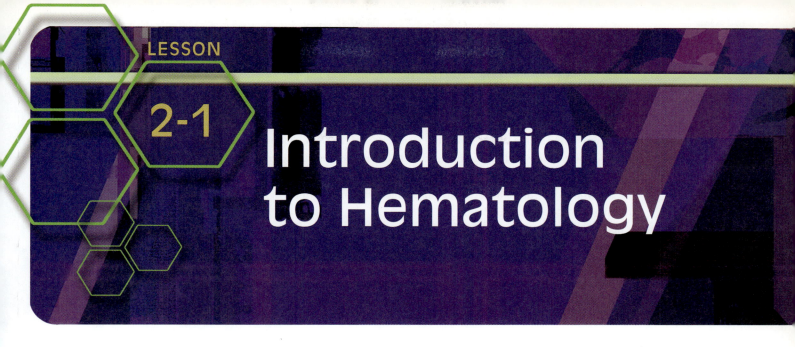

2-1
Introduction to Hematology

LESSON OBJECTIVES

After studying this lesson, the student will:

- Discuss the origin of blood cells.
- Explain the differences among veins, arteries, and capillaries.
- List five plasma components.
- Name the three types of formed elements of blood and state the function of each.
- Name the five types of white blood cells.
- Name the preferred specimens for most hematology tests.
- Name eight tests that are included in the complete blood count (CBC).
- Explain safety precautions that must be observed in the hematology laboratory.
- Explain how quality assessment (QA) procedures in hematology differ from QA in other laboratory departments, such as clinical chemistry.
- Name two inherited hematological diseases.
- Explain what a secondary or acquired hematological disease is.
- Discuss why stem cells may be useful in treating disease.
- Define the glossary terms.

GLOSSARY

anemia / a condition in which the red blood cell count or hemoglobin level is below normal; a condition resulting in decreased oxygen-carrying capacity of the blood

anticoagulant / a chemical that prevents blood coagulation

artery / a blood vessel that carries oxygenated blood from the heart to the tissues

capillary / a minute blood vessel that connects the smallest arteries to the smallest veins and serves as an oxygen exchange vessel

cardiopulmonary circulation / the system of blood vessels that circulates blood from the heart to the lungs and back to the heart

CBC / complete blood count; a commonly performed group of hematological tests

deoxyhemoglobin / the hemoglobin formed when oxyhemoglobin releases oxygen to tissues

EDTA / ethylenediaminetetraacetic acid; an anticoagulant commonly used in hematology

erythrocyte / see red blood cell

granulocyte / a white blood cell containing granules in the cytoplasm; any of the neutrophilic, eosinophilic, or basophilic leukocytes

hematology / the study of blood and blood-forming tissues

hematopoietic stem cell / see hemopoietic stem cell

hemoglobin (Hb, Hgb) / the major functional component of red blood cells that is the oxygen-carrying protein

hemopoiesis / the process of blood cell formation and development; hematopoiesis

hemopoietic stem cell / an undifferentiated bone marrow cell that gives rise to blood cells

hemostasis / the process of stopping bleeding, which includes clot formation and clot dissolution

leukemia / a chronic or acute disease involving unrestrained growth of leukocytes

leukocyte / see white blood cell

megakaryocyte / a large bone marrow cell from which platelets are derived

oxyhemoglobin / the form of hemoglobin that binds and transports oxygen

plasma / the liquid portion of blood in which blood cells are suspended

platelet / a formed element in circulating blood that plays an important role in blood coagulation; a small disk-shaped fragment of cytoplasm derived from a megakaryocyte; a thrombocyte

red blood cell (RBC) / blood cell that transports oxygen (O_2) to tissues and carbon dioxide (CO_2) to the lungs; erythrocyte

stem cell / an undifferentiated cell

systemic circulation / the system of blood vessels that carries blood from the heart to the tissues and back to the heart

thrombocyte / a blood platelet

vein / a blood vessel that carries deoxygenated blood from the tissues to the heart

white blood cell (WBC) / blood cell that functions in immunity; leukocyte

INTRODUCTION

Hematology is the branch of medicine concerned primarily with studying the formed elements of blood (blood cells) and the blood-forming tissues. The formed elements of blood, red blood cells, white blood cells, and platelets, are examined in the hematology laboratory. The tests may be qualitative, such as observing and recording blood cell morphology, or quantitative, such as performing leukocyte or erythrocyte counts or determining the hematocrit. The study of **hemostasis**, the process of stopping bleeding, which includes both clot formation (coagulation) and clot dissolution (fibrinolysis), is included in hematology.

Hematological tests can give important information about a patient's general well-being. The hematology laboratory also performs tests to detect and monitor treatment of anemias, leukemias, and inherited blood disorders such as hemophilia and sickle cell anemia. The effects of radiation or chemotherapy treatments for cancer can also be monitored using hematological tests.

BLOOD VESSELS AND BLOOD CIRCULATION

The Circulatory System

The circulatory system performs several vital functions, including delivery of oxygen (O_2), nutrients, water, and hormones to tissues and cells; removal of carbon dioxide (CO_2) and other waste products from tissues and cells; regulation of body temperature; and protection against infection. These functions are carried out by the *blood*, the fluid that circulates through the vessels of the circulatory system and bathes the tissues.

In the **cardiopulmonary circulation**, blood circulates from the heart to the lungs and back to the heart. Oxygen exchange occurs in the lungs when O_2 is picked up by the blood and CO_2 is released (Figure 2-1). In the **systemic circulation**, blood is carried from the heart to the tissues and back to the heart, providing O_2 to tissues and cells in exchange for CO_2, a waste product (Figure 2-2).

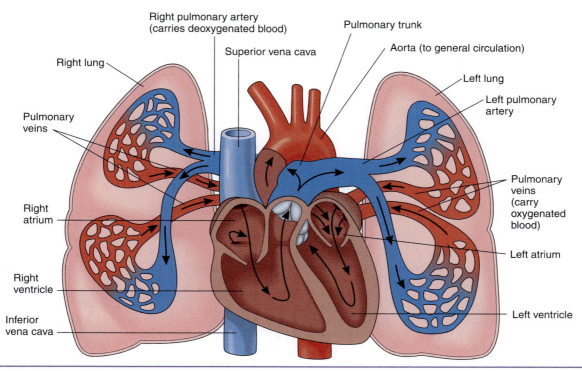

FIGURE 2-1 Diagram of cardiopulmonary circulation

Types of Blood Vessels

Blood is circulated by three major types of vessels: arteries, capillaries, and veins. There are about 60,000 miles of blood vessels in an average adult human. In general, arteries carry oxygenated blood and veins carry deoxygenated blood.

Arteries are thick-walled, elastic, and muscular and are the strongest type of blood vessel (Figure 2-2). The aorta is the largest artery in the body. Blood flows from the heart through the aorta into a series of successively smaller arteries and arterioles (small arteries) that eventually diverge to form a network of capillaries (Figure 2-3).

Capillaries are the smallest of the blood vessels and connect the smallest arterioles with the smallest veins called venules (Figure 2-3). Capillaries have thin walls allowing fluid, nutrients, and waste products to easily pass through these walls to or from the tissue cells. Because capillary beds are the site of O_2–CO_2 exchange, both oxygenated and deoxygenated blood are present.

Veins carry deoxygenated blood from the capillaries to the heart. Capillaries expand into venules and then into veins that eventually converge to larger and larger vessels and form the largest vein, the vena cava. The walls of veins are not as thick, muscular, or elastic as those of arteries (Figure 2-2). Veins have valves that allow blood flow in only one direction—toward the heart.

COMPOSITION OF BLOOD

Blood makes up 6% to 8% of total body weight. A normal adult's blood volume is approximately 5 L, or 10 times the volume of a blood donor unit. Blood is composed of cellular elements suspended in a fluid, plasma. About 50% to 60% of blood volume is plasma; the rest is mostly red blood cells.

Plasma

Plasma is a complex solution in which the blood cells are suspended (Figure 2-4). Plasma is more than 90% water; the remainder is dissolved solids such as proteins, lipids, carbohydrates, amino acids, antibodies, hormones, and electrolytes. Most of these substances are measured in the clinical chemistry department. Plasma also contains fibrinogen and the other blood-coagulation proteins necessary for normal blood clotting. The proteins involved in prevention of unwanted clotting and dissolution of formed clots are also present in the plasma.

Cellular Elements of Blood

The cellular elements of blood are commonly called blood cells. These include **red blood cells**, or **erythrocytes**; **white blood cells**, or **leukocytes**; and **platelets**, also called **thrombocytes** (Figure 2-5). Most hematology tests are designed to evaluate or measure a characteristic or function of one or more of the three blood cell types.

Red Blood Cells

Red blood cells are the most numerous blood cells (Figure 2-5). Each microliter (μL) of blood contains approximately 5 million red blood cells; that means one drop of blood contains about 250 million red cells! Red blood cells live an average of 120 days in the circulation and remain in the circulatory system's vessels for their entire life span.

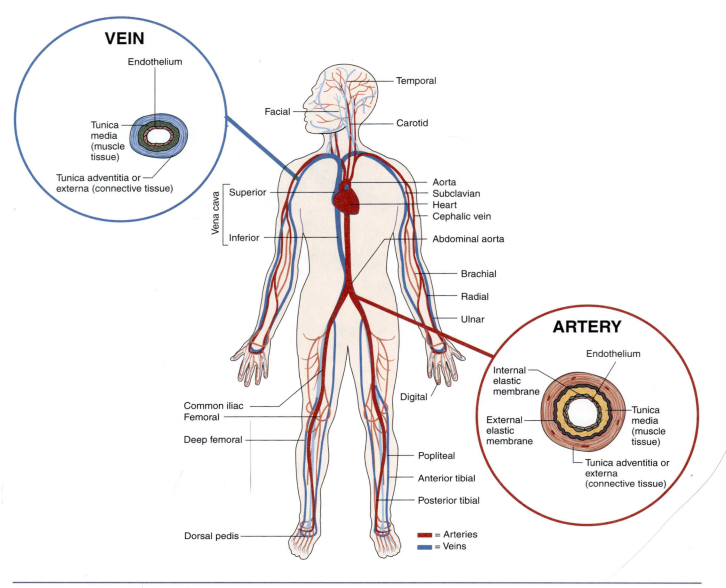

FIGURE 2-2 Systemic circulation showing the differences in the structure of veins and arteries

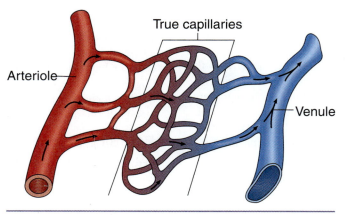

FIGURE 2-3 Capillary bed connecting an arteriole with a venule

The main function of red blood cells is to transport O_2 to the tissues and CO_2 to the lungs. This is actually performed by **hemoglobin** molecules, the major component of erythrocytes. Hemoglobin gives blood its red color. Arterial blood is bright red because of the **oxyhemoglobin**, hemoglobin that has bound O_2. Venous blood is dark red because of the presence of **deoxyhemoglobin**, hemoglobin that has released O_2.

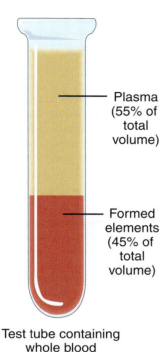

Plasma (55% of total volume)

Formed elements (45% of total volume)

Test tube containing whole blood

FIGURE 2-4 Diagram of a tube of blood showing separation of formed elements from plasma

White Blood Cells

White blood cells are the least numerous blood cells (Figure 2-5). Approximately 5,000 to 10,000 white blood cells are in each microliter of blood, or 5.0 to 10.0×10^9/L.

Five types of white blood cells are present in normal blood: *neutrophils, basophils, eosinophils, lymphocytes,* and *monocytes.* The neutrophils, basophils, and eosinophils are called **granulocytes** because of granules present in the cell cytoplasm.

White blood cells have varied life spans, from a few days to several years. Each type of white cell has unique functions, but all are associated with immunity or defense from infection. White blood cells perform most of their functions in the tissues. White blood cells use blood as a means of transport from one part of the body to another.

Platelets

Platelets, or thrombocytes, are not actually whole cells but are fragments of cytoplasm that have been released into circulating blood from large cells in the bone marrow (Figure 2-5). These large bone marrow cells are called **megakaryocytes**. Platelets average about 200,000 per microliter of blood and remain in the bloodstream about 10 days.

Platelets are important in several stages of hemostasis. They help stop bleeding by forming a plug in injured or damaged vessel walls. They also release chemicals or enzymes that are important in another stage of hemostasis, the coagulation cascade.

ORIGIN OF BLOOD CELLS

Hemopoiesis (hematopoiesis) is the formation and development of blood cells. In the young fetus, blood cells are made in the fetal liver. As the fetus develops, the bone marrow begins to take over this func-

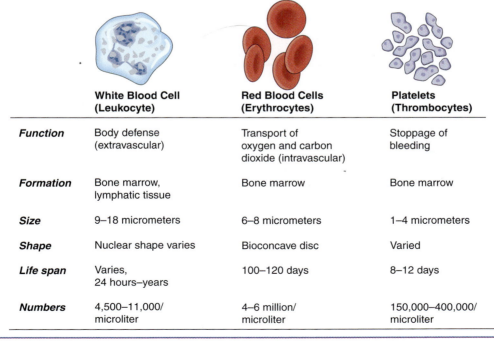

	White Blood Cell (Leukocyte)	Red Blood Cells (Erythrocytes)	Platelets (Thrombocytes)
Function	Body defense (extravascular)	Transport of oxygen and carbon dioxide (intravascular)	Stoppage of bleeding
Formation	Bone marrow, lymphatic tissue	Bone marrow	Bone marrow
Size	9–18 micrometers	6–8 micrometers	1–4 micrometers
Shape	Nuclear shape varies	Bioconcave disc	Varied
Life span	Varies, 24 hours–years	100–120 days	8–12 days
Numbers	4,500–11,000/ microliter	4–6 million/ microliter	150,000–400,000/ microliter

FIGURE 2-5 Characteristics of red blood cells, white blood cells, and platelets

tion. In adults, most of the cellular elements of blood are produced in the bone marrow. Lymphocytes are produced not only in bone marrow but also in secondary lymphoid tissue such as the spleen and lymph nodes. After a period of development and maturation in the bone marrow, mature blood cells are released into the circulating blood, where they function in respiration (erythrocytes), immunity (leukocytes), and hemostasis (platelets). (See Figure 2-6.)

Blood cells require the same basic growth factors for their synthesis as other cell types. In addition, because red blood cells are very specialized, they require iron, vitamin B_{12}, and folic acid for proper formation and maturation.

Blood cells are continuously produced throughout an individual's life. All blood cells are derived from an undifferentiated bone marrow cell called the **hemopoietic**, or **hematopoietic**, **stem cell**. These cells continuously replicate and differentiate into all of the blood cell types, thus replenishing the body's blood cells.

The presence of stem cells in bone marrow is the basis for using bone marrow transplants to treat hematological disorders, such as leukemia and aplastic anemia, and to combat the damaging effects of cancer chemotherapy on blood cell production. The discovery that newborns' umbilical cords are rich in stem cells has provided an additional donor source of stem cells. Because cord blood is routinely collected when the umbilical cord is cut at birth, it is now possible to harvest these cells and use them as substitutes for bone marrow transplants.

HEMATOLOGICAL DISEASES

Many diseases involve primarily the blood cells. Some of these diseases are caused by improper or insufficient production of a cell type. For instance, in **leukemia**, white cell production is out of control and too many cells are produced. In **anemia**, red cell numbers are too low, which could be due to decreased red cell production, such as might be seen when a person has an iron deficiency. Anemia can also result when blood loss is more rapid than blood production by the bone marrow, as when a person has a bleeding ulcer. *Thrombocytopenia*, or low platelet count, which can be caused by viral infections or drug interactions, can result in bleeding tendencies.

Hematological diseases can also be due to defective cell function. Often, a disease can be due to a combination of improper cell production and defective function, as with most anemias and leukemias. For example, in iron-deficiency anemia, the patient has too few red blood cells and these function improperly because they do not contain enough hemoglobin. This causes fatigue, pallor, and shortness of breath, typical symptoms of anemia caused by decreased O_2 available to the tissues. In leukemia, although the patient has many leukocytes, the cells have not matured properly and cannot provide immunity. The patient may then be highly susceptible to infections, even though the WBC count is high.

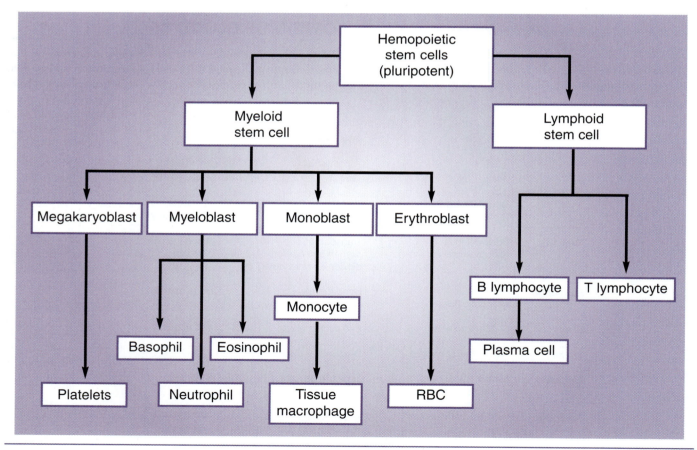

FIGURE 2-6 Origin and maturation of blood cells

Inherited Hematological Diseases

Some hematological diseases, such as *hemophilia*, are inherited. Hemophiliacs have bleeding problems either because they lack one of the coagulation factors required for blood to clot or one of the coagulation factors is defective. In other inherited hematological diseases, patients have abnormal hemoglobin function, such as that caused by the abnormal structure of hemoglobin in *sickle cell anemia*.

Secondary or Acquired Hematological Diseases

Abnormalities in blood cells can also occur because of a condition or disease originating in another organ system. These are called secondary or acquired conditions. For example, abnormal-appearing red blood cells can be present in patients with severe hypertension or renal failure because the cells become damaged as they circulate through small blood vessels. Diabetics may have "lazy leukocytes," which results in slow healing of wounds or infections because some white blood cells function improperly. In infectious mononucleosis, a viral disease, lymphocytes develop an "atypical" appearance that can be observed when a stained blood smear is examined microscopically.

Blood cells are also affected by treatments or medications. High doses of aspirin inhibit platelet function, a temporary condition that corrects itself after aspirin is discontinued. Chemotherapy treatments designed to stop the growth of cancer cells can also inhibit blood cell production. Patients receiving chemotherapy must have regular blood cell counts to be sure their blood cell concentrations do not fall to dangerous levels.

THE HEMATOLOGY LABORATORY

Methods of Analysis in the Hematology Laboratory

Routine hematology tests can be performed manually or using one of the many types of hematology analyzers available. Some are designed for small facilities such as physician office laboratories (POLs) and can perform only a few different tests. Others suitable for large laboratories are designed to perform several analyses on hundreds of samples daily. Lesson 2-13, Principles of Automated Hematology, describes the principles behind the design of hematology analyzers.

All laboratories that use hematology analyzers must also have backup systems for performing analyses in the event of instrument malfunction. Therefore, it is always advisable that personnel be trained in manual techniques for the most frequently requested tests.

Safety Precautions

  Standard Precautions must be observed at all times in the hematology laboratory, as in any other laboratory section. Workers must use proper work practice controls to avoid body fluid spills, splatters, aerosol formation, or other potential exposure to blood and body fluids. Lesson 1-6 contains detailed laboratory biosafety information.

In many facilities, the hematology department is responsible for blood collection as well as hematology testing. Phlebotomists must wear gloves and other appropriate protective clothing such as fluid-resistant laboratory coats, goggles, and masks. Safety shields or face protection can be used in the blood-collecting area, as well as the testing area, to protect against exposure from splashes. Used venipuncture needles must not be recapped but must be discarded into puncture-proof biohazard containers for sharps. The use of safety needles that automatically resheath or enclose the used needle is required and eliminates most needlestick hazards (Lesson 1-6).

Hematology laboratory workers often have greater potential for exposure to bloodborne pathogens than workers in some other laboratory departments. A blood sample tube used to perform a complete blood count (CBC), blood smears, and sedimentation rate, three separate tests, may have to be opened three times, creating three potential exposure events. Instruments capable of sampling specimens by piercing through the tube stoppers can minimize this type of exposure potential.

Quality Assessment

QA In clinical chemistry departments, certified standards for substances such as glucose or sodium are easily obtained. In hematology, however, stable standards are, for the most part, not available. A standard should be as close as possible in composition to the substance being measured and ideally should be stable over a long period. This is not possible with blood cells, since they are living tissues.

The hemoglobin standard is the only true hematology standard. Cell counts and differential counts are standardized using control solutions. Controls for cell counts and automated differentials are made with stabilized cells and have a limited shelf-life of 120 days in the unopened vial but sometimes as short as 5 days once the vial is opened. Controls made with suspensions of latex particles can have a shelf-life of 24 months in the unopened vial but only 30 days once the vial is opened. Hematology controls are available for cell counts, automated differentials, and flow cytometry. Because of the unavailability of true standards, many hematology procedures and instruments require more complex calibration and standardization.

Specimens for Hematology Testing

Both capillary and venous blood are used for routine hematological procedures. Capillary blood obtained by skin puncture is good for procedures such as blood smears because no chemicals are added to the sample to alter cell appearance (Lesson 1-12). However, since only a small sample volume is obtained by capillary puncture, tests usually cannot be repeated unless another sample is obtained.

When a larger sample is required, blood is obtained from a vein by venipuncture (Lesson 1-13). Venous blood samples

CURRENT TOPIC

WHAT ARE STEM CELLS?

Stem cells are often in the news, in relation either to controversy over funding for research or to scientific or medical news about stem cells as a potential cure for a disease or a genetic defect. But what are stem cells, what is their origin, where are they found, and why are they important?

What are stem cells? Stem cells are undifferentiated cells that have the ability to renew themselves by cell division and also have potential to develop into many different types of specialized cells that make up the tissues and organs of the body. The ability of stem cells to replicate themselves means that they can sometimes be grown in the laboratory and studied. Stem cells cannot give rise to a complete organism.

What is the origin of stem cells? Where are they found? Researchers work with two types of stem cells: adult stem cells and embryonic stem cells. These have different sources and different characteristics.

Adult stem cells—Although termed *adult,* adult stem cells are found in low numbers in various tissues and organs of animals and humans of all ages. Typically they can give rise to specialized cells of the organ in which they reside. They are also called *multipotent* cells, meaning they have the potential (potent) to develop into several (multi) cell types. Within our bodies, adult stem cells are our repair systems, replenishing our damaged cells.

The *hematopoietic stem cells* found in the bone marrow are examples of adult stem cells. They can develop into several types of blood cells (such as red cells, white cells, or megakaryocytes) but normally cannot become cells of other tissues, such as kidney or muscle. Bone marrow transplants are successful because the adult stem cells within the transplanted marrow colonize and reproduce to form new blood cells in the transplant recipient. Hematopoietic stem cells can also be harvested from umbilical cord blood and used for transplant. An advantage of cord blood transplant over bone marrow transplant is that cord blood cells are less likely to be rejected by the recipient because cord blood stem cells have not yet developed markers that could stimulate rejection by the recipient.

Embryonic stem cells—When a sperm fertilizes an egg, a single cell is formed, the fertilized egg (see diagram). This single cell has the potential to form an entire organism; that is, the cell is *totipotent.* A few hours after fertilization, this cell divides into several identical cells, any of which still has the potential to develop into an organism. After about 4 days and several cell divisions, the cells become more specialized (pluripotent). A *blastocyst* is formed, with an outer layer of cells (the trophoblast) and an *inner cell mass* of about 30 to 150 cells (see diagram). The cells in the inner mass have the potential to produce a complete fetus if implantation and development proceed normally. Once removed from the blastocyst, they no longer have the potential to form an individual even though they remain *pluripotent*, meaning they have the potential to give rise to all the tissues of the organism. Embryonic stem cells are derived from this inner cell mass of the blastocyst.

In vitro fertilization clinics store fertilized eggs at the blastocyst stage, and blastocysts that are not to be used can be donated to research. Embryonic stem cells obtained from the inner cell mass can be cultured (grown) in the research laboratory under conditions in which the cells continue to divide but do not differentiate or specialize. Cells that survive several months of laboratory growth and replication, and that remain pluripotent and genetically normal, can be used as *embryonic stem cell lines.*

Why are stem cells important? Stem cell researchers foresee almost unlimited possibilities for using stem cells to treat disease, injuries, and genetic disorders—these are called *cell-based therapies.* With further research to learn how to direct the specialization of stem cells, patients who need organ transplants may be able to be treated instead with stem cells. Stem cells could generate new heart tissue when transplanted into a heart; diabetics could grow new insulin-producing cells by receiving stem cell transplants; and Parkinson's disease could be treated by transplants of stem cells that can be induced to become dopamine neurons. Stem cells could also be used as a renewable source of cells to treat diseases and injuries such as spinal cord injury, stroke, Alzheimer's, burns, and arthritis, as well as a way to test new drugs. Stem cells are fascinating and somewhat miraculous in their innate ability to respond to stimulation and develop into a predictable precursor of certain tissues or cells.

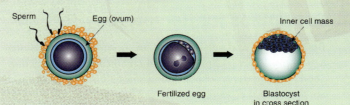

for hematology tests are usually collected in a tube containing an **anticoagulant** to prevent clotting. The anticoagulant most frequently used in the hematology laboratory is **EDTA** (ethylene-diaminetetraacetic acid). Sodium citrate is commonly used as an anticoagulant for coagulation tests.

The Complete Blood Count

One of the most frequently requested procedures in the hematology laboratory is the **CBC**, or complete blood count. The CBC is a combination of tests that usually includes:

- Red blood cell count
- White blood cell count
- Hemoglobin
- Hematocrit
- Red blood cell indices (MCV, MCH, MCHC)
- Differential count
- Platelet count or platelet estimate
- Evaluation of blood cell morphology

An example of a hematology requisition is shown in Figure 2-7. The methods for performing these tests are explained in the remaining lessons of this unit. After completing this unit, the student should be able to perform several tests included in the CBC.

Coagulation Tests and Special Hematology Tests

Many tests other than those included in the CBC are performed in the hematology laboratory. Some of these, such as the erythrocyte sedimentation rate and reticulocyte count, are included in this unit. Basic coagulation tests, such as the prothrombin time and bleeding time, are explained in Unit 3, Basic Hemostasis. Other hematology tests beyond the scope of this book include special stains for blood and bone marrow cells to classify leukemias; identifying hemoglobin variants, such as the hemoglobin that causes sickle cell anemia; assessing iron status; and testing leukocyte function to help diagnose immune deficiencies.

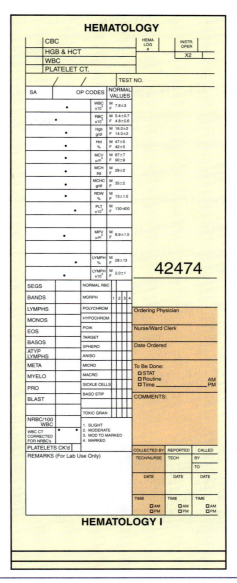

FIGURE 2-7 Hematology requisition form

SUMMARY

Hematology is the study of the formed elements of the blood and the blood-forming tissues. Blood is composed of the cellular elements suspended in plasma, the fluid portion of blood. The cellular elements are commonly called blood cells and include the red blood cells, the white blood cells, and the platelets. The red cells function in respiration, the white cells in immunity, and the platelets in hemostasis.

Hemopoiesis, the formation and development of blood cells, begins in the liver in the early fetus. By the time of birth, the bone marrow has taken over blood cell production. Blood cells, derived from primitive stem cells, continue to be produced throughout an individual's life. Knowledge of the circulatory system, the blood vessels, and the composition of blood is necessary when studying or working in hematology.

Tests performed in the hematology laboratory can be qualitative, such as observation and evaluation of blood cell morphology, or quantitative, such as the red blood cell and white blood cell counts or determination of the hematocrit. The majority of testing is performed using instrumentation. However, manual methods are sometimes required when instrumentation is not available or in cases in which a low white blood cell count or platelet count is expected.

Safety and quality assessment programs are important in hematology. Standard Precautions must always be observed. Hematology personnel can have increased chance of exposure to potentially infectious specimens compared to personnel in some other areas of the laboratory. A comprehensive quality assessment program is essential to ensure that test results are accurate and useful. Hematology tests can give much information about the general well-being of a patient. In addition, hematology test results can be used to monitor the effects of chemotherapy or radiation treatments and to provide information critical to the diagnosis of conditions such as anemias, leukemias, and coagulation disorders.

REVIEW QUESTIONS

1. Where are blood cells produced? What is the most primitive blood cell called?

2. What are the three groups of formed elements in the blood? What are the functions of each group?

3. Name the five types of leukocytes found in the blood. Which are the granulocytes?

4. Name five components of plasma.

5. What two types of blood specimens are used for most hematological tests?

6. What anticoagulant is used for most hematological tests? For most coagulation tests?

7. Name the three major types of blood vessels and explain the differences among them.

8. Name three ways workers can lessen the chance of exposure to blood and body fluids in the hematology laboratory.

9. Which blood component is responsible for oxygen exchange?

10. Name an inherited hematological disease. What is meant by a secondary or acquired hematological condition?

11. What is a CBC?

12. How does hematology quality assessment differ from quality assessment in clinical chemistry?

13. Define anemia, anticoagulant, artery, capillary, cardiopulmonary circulation, CBC, deoxyhemoglobin, EDTA, erythrocyte, granulocyte, hematopoietic stem cell, hematology, hemoglobin, hemopoiesis, hematology, hemopoietic stem cell, hemostasis, leukemia, leukocyte, megakaryocyte, oxyhemoglobin, plasma, platelet, red blood cell, stem cell, systemic circulation, thrombocyte, vein, and white blood cell.

STUDENT ACTIVITIES

1. Complete the written examination for this lesson.

2. Visit a hematology laboratory in the community. Find out what tests are performed there.

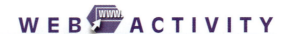

WEB ACTIVITY

Research a hematological disease using the Internet. Report on the cause of the disease, the laboratory tests that can be used for diagnosis, and the appropriate treatment. Possible sources are Web sites of NIH, medical schools, or universities.

2-2

Hematocrit

LESSON OBJECTIVES

After studying this lesson, the student will:

- Explain the principle of the hematocrit test.
- Explain what the hematocrit measures.
- List the reference values for the hematocrit.
- List conditions that affect the hematocrit value.
- Prepare a hematocrit sample.
- Centrifuge a hematocrit sample.
- Determine the hematocrit value.
- Discuss factors that affect the quality of hematocrit results.
- List safety precautions that should be observed in performing the hematocrit.
- Define the glossary terms.

GLOSSARY

buffy coat / a light-colored layer of leukocytes and platelets that forms on top of the red blood cell layer when a sample of blood is centrifuged or allowed to stand undisturbed

capillary tube / a slender glass or plastic tube used in laboratory procedures

hematocrit / the volume of erythrocytes packed by centrifugation in a given volume of blood and expressed as a percentage; abbreviated crit or Hct

microhematocrit / a hematocrit performed in capillary tubes using a small quantity of blood; packed cell volume (PCV)

microhematocrit centrifuge / an instrument that spins capillary tubes at a high speed to rapidly separate cellular components of the blood from the liquid portion of blood

packed cell column / the layers of blood cells that form when a tube of whole blood is centrifuged

INTRODUCTION

The **hematocrit** is a commonly performed test that provides the clinician with an estimate of the patient's red cell volume and, thus, the blood's oxygen-carrying capacity. The hematocrit measurement is useful in screening for anemia, evaluating anemia therapies, estimating blood loss following hemorrhage or trauma, and screening potential blood donors.

There are two methods of determining the hematocrit. The manual method is sometimes called a **microhematocrit**, because only a small volume of blood is required. It is a simple procedure in which whole blood is centrifuged in slender **capillary tubes**. The spun hematocrit is a waived test under CLIA '88.

The hematocrit can also be determined using a hematology analyzer. The complete blood count (CBC) includes the hematocrit which is electronically calculated from the red cell count and red cell volume. Measurements made using hematology analyzers are called hematocrits, while those made using the centrifuge are called microhematocrits. However, in practice, the terms are interchangeable, and both methods provide rapid, reliable results.

PRINCIPLE OF THE HEMATOCRIT TEST

The hematocrit test is based on the principle of separating the cellular elements of blood from the plasma by centrifugation. After the blood is centrifuged in a capillary tube, the red cells are at the bottom of the tube, the white cells and platelets form a thin layer on top of the red cells, and the plasma is at the top (Figure 2-8). This layered arrangement following centrifugation is called the **packed cell column**. The layer containing white cells and platelets has a whitish-tan appearance and is commonly referred to as the **buffy coat** (Figure 2-8).

The hematocrit is determined by comparing the volume of red cells to the total volume of the whole blood sample. This is reported as a percentage. Laboratory personnel often refer to a hematocrit as a *crit* or abbreviate it with the letters *Hct*. Another term sometimes used for hematocrit is *packed cell volume,* or *PCV*.

Microhematocrit Centrifuges

Several types of **microhematocrit centrifuges** are available for performing manual hematocrits (Figure 2-9). Some centrifuges are multifunctional and can spin samples for urinalysis, coagulation, and blood chemistry as well as microhematocrit tubes. Other centrifuges, such as the StatSpin CritSpin (Figure 2-9B) are used only for microhematocrits, and will spin only capillary tubes.

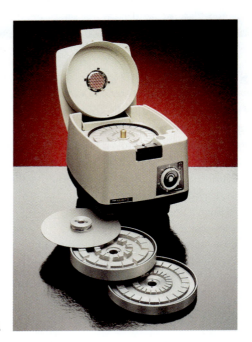

A

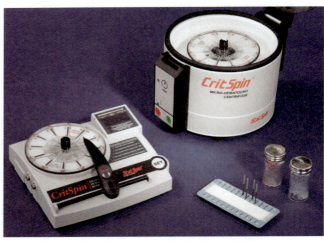

B

FIGURE 2-9 Microhematocrit centrifuges (*Courtesy Becton Dickinson, Franklin Lakes, NJ and StatSpin, Inc., Norwood, MA*)

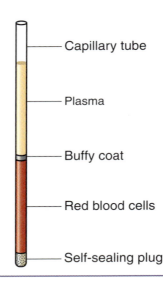

— Capillary tube

— Plasma

— Buffy coat

— Red blood cells

— Self-sealing plug

FIGURE 2-8 Diagram of packed cell column in a microhematocrit tube showing separation of cells and plasma after centrifugation

Hematocrit centrifuges can have built-in hematocrit readers that require the use of precalibrated capillary tubes. For other centrifuges, a separate hematocrit reader that can accept both uncalibrated and precalibrated tubes is used.

The STAT-CRIT, a small, portable instrument, assays blood hemoglobin and hematocrit in 30 seconds. The test is performed by collecting the second drop of blood from a capillary puncture into a disposable blood-sample carrier. The carrier is inserted in the instrument for analysis and the result is displayed digitally.

Microhematocrit Tubes

Several types of capillary tubes are available for manual hematocrit determinations. Heparinized tubes, with a red ring, are used for capillary blood; unheparinized tubes are used for venous blood that already has an anticoagulant added (Figure 2-10). Mylar-wrapped glass tubes or flexible plastic capillary tubes should be used, since they are less likely to break than are unwrapped glass tubes. Self-sealing tubes are available that eliminate the need for sealing clay. Lesson 1-12 on capillary puncture contains additional information about capillary tubes.

Hematocrit Reference Values

The normal hematocrit value varies with the gender and age of the patient and with the test method (Table 2-1). The values range from a low of 32% for a 1-year-old to a high of 61% for a newborn. Hematocrits for females are usually lower than for males. The System of International Units (SI) value for the hematocrit is obtained by multiplying the hematocrit percentage by a factor of 0.01. The result is expressed as liter of packed cells per liter of whole blood (L/L). A hematocrit of 32% would be expressed as 0.32 L/L.

Correlating Hematocrit Results to Patient Health

The hematocrit value is influenced by both physiological and pathological factors (Tables 2-1 and 2-2). A hematocrit value below the normal range can indicate a condition such as anemia

or the presence of bleeding in a patient. A hematocrit value above the normal range can be due to a physical cause such as dehydration or by an uncommon condition such as polycythemia. Since the hematocrit reference ranges are different for males and females and also vary with age, the reference range appropriate for the patient must be considered when determining the significance of hematocrit results. Because of these factors, it is important that identification labels on specimens be complete and include patient age and gender. For instance, suppose a technician performs a hematocrit on a specimen and the results are read as 37%. If the patient were an adult female or a child, this value would be within the reference range and would not require any special attention. However, if the patient were an adult male, the value is well below the reference range, and the result should be identified as below normal on the laboratory report.

The appearance of the blood sample in a spun hematocrit can also give clues to a patient's health. Normal blood samples centri-

TABLE 2-1. Hematocrit reference ranges

	AVERAGE		RANGE	
	Percent (%)	SI Units (L/L)	Percent (%)	SI Units (L/L)
Adults				
Males	47	0.47	42–52	0.42–0.52
Females	42	0.42	36–48	0.36–0.48
Children				
Newborn	56	0.56	51–61	0.51–0.61
1 year	35	0.35	32–38	0.32–0.38
6 years	38	0.38	34–42	0.34–0.42

TABLE 2-2. Conditions affecting hematocrit values

CONDITION	EFFECT ON HEMATOCRIT VALUE
Age	
Newborns	Increased
Children	Less than adult value
Older adults	Decreased from adult value
Gender	Adult female value less than adult male value
Residence at high altitudes	Increased
Severe dehydration	Increased
Anemias	Decreased
Polycythemia	Increased
Leukemias	Decreased
Bleeding, such as bleeding ulcer	Decreased

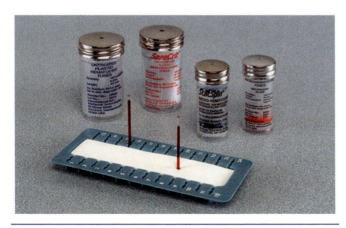

FIGURE 2-10 Microhematocrit tubes (*Courtesy StatSpin, Inc., Norwood, MA*)

fuged in a hematocrit tube will have a characteristic appearance—the plasma portion will be pale yellow and transparent and the buffy coat will be a narrow band above the red cell layer. Plasma that is very yellow could indicate the patient has an elevated bilirubin level; plasma that is opaque could indicate a high fat (triglyceride) level. A prominent buffy coat layer could indicate that the patient has an elevated white blood count. It is the responsibility of the technician to be observant and report unusual findings such as these.

PERFORMING THE MANUAL HEMATOCRIT TEST

Safety Precautions

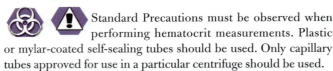 Standard Precautions must be observed when performing hematocrit measurements. Plastic or mylar-coated self-sealing tubes should be used. Only capillary tubes approved for use in a particular centrifuge should be used.

Special care must be taken when operating the centrifuge. Microhematocrit centrifuges operate at more than 10,000 rpm (revolutions per minute). Internal locking lids, as well as outer locking lids, are used to keep tubes in position during high-speed centrifugations. It is unsafe to operate these instruments unless all lids are secured. Lids should never be opened until the rotor has come to a complete stop.

Quality Assessment

Reliable hematocrit tests require proper specimen collection and test setup, properly calibrated centrifuges, and careful reading and reporting of hematocrit values. Although the test is relatively simple, variations in technique and several other factors can affect the results. Measures that should be followed to ensure reliable results include:

■ Hematocrit procedure in the standard operating procedure (SOP) manual must be followed.

■ Hematology controls should be run daily and the results charted.

■ Venous blood specimens should be well-mixed before hematocrit tubes are filled.

■ Proper capillary blood collection techniques should be followed.

■ Heparinized tubes should be used to collect capillary blood for microhematocrit.

■ Microhematocrit tubes should be filled at least three-fourths full.

■ Each patient sample should be run in duplicate; the two results should agree within ± 2%.

■ If results do not agree within ± 2%, the test should be repeated after proper mixing of venous anticoagulated specimens or after re-collection of capillary specimens.

The centrifuge speed and accuracy of the timer must be checked at regular intervals and the results documented. Periodic preventive maintenance must be performed and documented. The centrifugation speed and time directly affect the hematocrit values—failure to spin tubes at the proper speed and for the proper time can cause incorrect hematocrit values. Samples spun at speeds slower than specified or for a shorter time will have falsely increased hematocrit values. Samples spun at speeds higher than specified or for longer times can have falsely decreased values due to excessive cell packing or red cell lysis.

Obtaining and Preparing the Specimen

The blood sample for a microhematocrit can be obtained from a capillary puncture or from a tube of venous blood to which the anticoagulant EDTA (ethylenediaminetetra-acetic acid) has been added (Figure 2-11). Capillary blood should be collected into heparinized capillary tubes. Before sampling from tubes of venous anticoagulated blood, the blood must be gently mixed by either inverting the tube approximately 60 times, or placing it on a mechanical mixer for a minimum of 2 minutes (Figure 2-12).

The blood is drawn by capillary action into microhematocrit tubes (Figure 2-11), which are then sealed. Self-sealing tubes

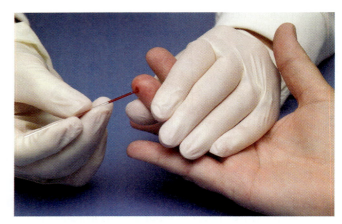

A

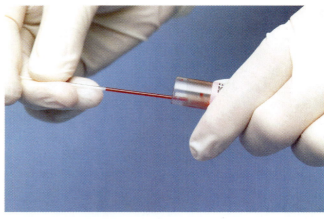

B

FIGURE 2-11 Filling a capillary tube: (A) from a capillary puncture; (B) from a tube of EDTA blood

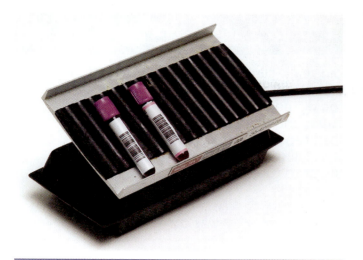

FIGURE 2-12 Mixer for hematology specimens

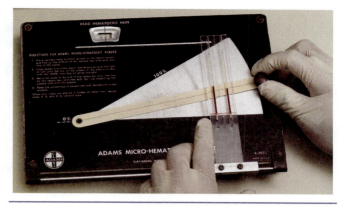

FIGURE 2-13 Using a microhematocrit reader

are preferred. These have a dry plug in one end that expands to form a seal when blood contacts it. However sealing clay is still used (Figure 2-10).

Centrifuging the Samples

The sealed capillary tubes are placed into the rotor of the microhematocrit centrifuge, with the sealed ends against the rubber gasket (toward the outer rim of the rotor). Tubes must be balanced in the rotor. Centrifuge lids must be carefully secured, following all safety precautions of the manufacturer and the laboratory (Figure 2-9). The length of centrifugation is determined by the type of centrifuge, its calibration, and the procedure manual for each facility. Generally, microhematocrit tubes are spun for 2 to 4 minutes at 10,000 rpm.

Reading and Reporting the Hematocrit Value

After tubes have been centrifuged, they should be inspected to see that no leakage occurred during centrifugation and then placed on the hematocrit reader. Some centrifuges have a built-in reading scale, and others have a separate reader (Figure 2-13). The instructions for the type of reader being used must be followed carefully to ensure correct reading of the hematocrit. The percent of red blood cells in the blood sample can be determined using the reader. Only the red blood cell portion of the packed cell column is included in the hematocrit reading (Figure 2-8); neither the buffy coat nor the sealing plug should be included. The hematocrit reading should be observed for each of the duplicate tubes. The values from the two tubes should not vary by more than ± 2%. The average of the two readings is reported.

SAFETY Reminders

- Observe Standard Precautions when performing hematocrits.
- Use plastic or mylar-coated self-sealing tubes.
- Check that capillary tubes are completely sealed before centrifugation.
- Place the sealed end of the capillary tubes against the rubber gasket in the centrifuge.
- Place tubes opposite each other to balance the rotor.
- Close both centrifuge lids securely before operating the centrifuge.
- Never open a centrifuge until the rotor has come to a complete stop.

PROCEDURAL Reminders

- Follow time recommendations for the centrifuge being used.
- Run duplicate tubes for each patient specimen.
- Read the hematocrit value at the top of the red cell layer, not at the top of the buffy coat.
- Mix venous anticoagulated blood well before filling capillary tubes.

CASE STUDY

A hematocrit test was ordered on a 52-year-old male clinic patient during a routine doctor's visit. Following his facility's procedure, Stephen, the laboratory technician, prepared duplicate hematocrit tubes from a tube of the patient's venous blood. During centrifugation the blood leaked out of one tube, and the hematocrit result on the remaining tube was read as 38% (0.38 L/L). Stephen repeated the hematocrit procedure, quickly picking up the patient's tube of blood and filling two capillary tubes. After centrifugation, Stephen read the hematocrit value on both tubes as 32% (0.32 L/L).

1. Which of the following is probably true?
   a. There was no need to repeat the test, the hematocrit of 38 was correct and should have been reported.
   b. Only one tube was required to determine and report the hematocrit value.
   c. The repeat set of hematocrits was from insufficiently mixed blood and thus was probably incorrect.
2. What should Stephen do next?
   a. Report a hematocrit of 32%.   b. Report a hematocrit of 38%.
   c. Perform the procedure a third time after mixing the blood sample well.
3. What conclusions can Stephen make about the patient from the information that is available? Explain your answer.

SUMMARY

The hematocrit is part of the CBC but is also frequently ordered as a single test. The results are relied upon to quickly assess a patient's oxygen-carrying capacity, such as to evaluate magnitude of blood loss and to follow recovery from blood loss. The hematocrit can be performed either manually by centrifugation, or using a hematology analyzer or cell counter. The hematocrit results are influenced by techniques in sample collection, centrifugation, and reading of the results. Standard Precautions must be observed, and all policies of quality assessment must be followed.

REVIEW QUESTIONS

1. What does the hematocrit measure?
2. Give the hematocrit reference values for males, females, and newborns.
3. Name a condition that could cause a decreased hematocrit value.
4. Explain the hematocrit procedure.
5. Blood enters the capillary tube by what action?
6. Why must the capillary tube be sealed securely?
7. What is the usual length of time for centrifugation of the hematocrit tubes?
8. What safety precautions should be observed when performing a hematocrit?
9. What technical factors can affect the quality of hematocrit results?
10. Define buffy coat, capillary tube, hematocrit, microhematocrit, microhematocrit centrifuge, and packed cell column.

STUDENT ACTIVITIES

1. Complete the written examination for this lesson.
2. Practice performing the microhematocrit test on several blood samples as outlined in the Student Performance Guide.
3. Repeat the hematocrit procedure on a blood sample, lengthening or shortening the centrifugation time by 1 to 2 minutes. Record the results and discuss any differences from the previous microhematocrit readings.
4. Demonstrate the importance of using well-mixed blood: perform a microhematocrit on a well-mixed sample; allow the sample tube to stand upright five to ten minutes and perform another microhematocrit without remixing the blood. Compare the results and explain.

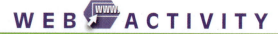

WEB ACTIVITY

Search the Internet for information about hematology analyzer technology. Find out how the hematocrit is performed on a hematology analyzer. Is it centrifuged?

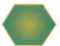

Student Performance Guide

Lesson 2-2 Hematocrit

Name _____   Date _____

INSTRUCTIONS

1. Practice the hematocrit procedure following the step-by-step instructions.
2. Demonstrate the procedure for the hematocrit satisfactorily for the instructor, using the Student Performance Guide. Your instructor will determine the level of competency you must achieve to obtain a satisfactory (S) grade.

NOTE: Consult the instruction manual for the centrifuge being used. Refer to the specific procedure being performed.

MATERIALS AND EQUIPMENT

- gloves
- acrylic safety shield or face protection
- antiseptic
- self-sealing capillary tubes, mylar-coated, heparinized, and plain
- precalibrated capillary tubes (optional)
- microhematocrit centrifuge and reader
- tube of anticoagulated venous blood (or commercially available simulated blood)
- laboratory tissue
- 70% alcohol or alcohol swabs
- gauze or cotton balls, sterile
- blood lancets, sterile, disposable
- surface disinfectant
- biohazard container
- sharps container

PROCEDURE

Record in the comment section any problems encountered while practicing the procedure (or have a fellow student or the instructor evaluate your performance).

S = Satisfactory
U = Unsatisfactory

You must:	S	U	Comments
1. Assemble equipment and materials for capillary puncture and hematocrit; place acrylic safety shield into position or put on face protection			
2. Wash hands and put on gloves			
3. Fill two capillary tubes from a capillary puncture: a. Perform a capillary puncture b. Wipe away the first drop of blood c. Touch one end of a heparinized capillary tube to the second drop of blood d. Allow the tube to fill three-quarters full by capillary action, holding the tube at a slight downward angle. If using precalibrated tubes, fill to the line e. Fill a second tube in the same manner			

You must:	S	U	Comments
f. Wipe the outside of the filled capillary tube with soft tissue, if necessary, to remove excess blood g. Seal the capillary tube. Check to see that the plug has expanded			
4. Fill two capillary tubes using a tube of EDTA antico-agulated blood (If not available, proceed to step 5): a. Mix the tube of blood thoroughly by gently rocking tube from end to end a minimum of 2 minutes by mechanical mixer or 50 to 60 times by hand b. Remove cap from tube (wearing face protection or with an acrylic safety shield placed between worker and tube) c. Tilt the tube so the blood is very near the top edge of the tube d. Insert the tip of a plain capillary tube into the blood and fill three-quarters full by capillary action. If using precalibrated tubes, fill to the line **NOTE:** Wipe the outside of the filled capillary tube with tissue, if necessary, to remove excess blood e. Seal the tube. Check to see that plug expanded f. Fill a second tube in the same manner			
5. Place tubes into the hematocrit centrifuge with sealed ends securely against the gasket. Balance the load by placing the tubes directly opposite each other			
6. Fasten both lids securely			
7. Set the timer and adjust the speed if necessary			
8. Centrifuge for the prescribed time			
9. Allow centrifuge to come to a complete stop and unlock lids			
10. Determine the hematocrit values using one of the following methods: a. A centrifuge that requires calibrated tubes and has a built-in scale: (1) Position the tubes as directed by the manufacturer's instructions (2) Read the hematocrit value b. A centrifuge without a built-in reader: (1) Remove capillary tubes from centrifuge carefully (2) Place tubes on the hematocrit reader provided (3) Follow instructions on the reader to obtain the hematocrit value			
11. Average the values from the two tubes and record the hematocrit. The values must agree within ± 2%			
12. Discard capillary tubes and used lancets into sharps container			

You must:	S	U	Comments
13. Clean and return equipment to proper storage			
14. Clean the work area with surface disinfectant			
15. Remove gloves, discard in biohazard container, and wash hands with antiseptic			

Evaluator Comments:

Evaluator _____ Date _____

Hemoglobin Determination

LESSON OBJECTIVES

After studying this lesson, the student will:

- List the two main components of hemoglobin.
- State the function of hemoglobin.
- Explain the manual and automated methods of hemoglobin determination.
- List the hemoglobin reference values for children and adults.
- Perform a hemoglobin determination using a hemoglobin analyzer.
- List the safety precautions to observe when performing a hemoglobin determination.
- Discuss factors that can affect the quality of a hemoglobin result.
- Define the glossary terms.

GLOSSARY

cyanmethemoglobin / a stable colored compound formed when hemoglobin is reacted with Drabkin's reagent; hemiglobincyanide (HiCN)

Drabkin's reagent / a hemoglobin diluting reagent that contains iron, potassium, cyanide, and sodium bicarbonate

globin / the protein portion of the hemoglobin molecule

heme / the iron-containing portion of the hemoglobin molecule

hemiglobincyanide (HiCN) / cyanmethemoglobin

hemoglobin (Hb, Hgb) / the major functional component of red blood cells that is the oxygen-carrying protein

INTRODUCTION

The measurement of blood hemoglobin is one of the most common clinical laboratory tests. The hemoglobin test is used to indirectly evaluate the oxygen-carrying capacity of the blood. This makes it an important aid in detecting and evaluating blood loss and diagnosing and treating anemia.

The hemoglobin determination can be performed using either capillary or venous blood. It is requested as an individual test or as part of a complete blood count (CBC). The hemoglobin test is precise, simple to perform, and easily standardized. It can be performed manually or using a dedicated hemoglobin instrument or a hematology analyzer.

CHARACTERISTICS OF HEMOGLOBIN

Hemoglobin (Hb or **Hgb)** is the primary constituent of red blood cells, making up over 98% of red blood cell protein content. This molecule gives the characteristic red color to erythrocytes and to the blood. The primary function of hemoglobin is to transport oxygen (O_2) from the lungs to the tissue cells of the body and to carry carbon dioxide (CO_2) from the tissues to the lungs to be expelled (Figure 2-14).

Hemoglobin Structure

The hemoglobin molecule is composed of two parts, heme and globin. The **globin** portion of a hemoglobin molecule contains four protein chains. Hemoglobins are named according to the structure of the protein chains. For example, hemoglobin S (Hb S) present in sickle cell anemia has a different protein structure than normal adult hemoglobin (Hb A).

The **heme** portion of hemoglobin molecules contains iron; therefore, iron is required for hemoglobin synthesis. More than two-thirds of the body's iron is contained in hemoglobin and in the muscle protein, myoglobin. If sufficient iron is not available in the body, hemoglobin production will decrease, causing the red blood cells to be deficient in hemoglobin. When this happens, the oxygen-carrying capacity of the blood is decreased, and the individual will develop symptoms of anemia, such as fatigue and pallor. In situations involving excessive blood loss, such as a bleeding ulcer, anemia may develop because the depletion of iron (in the blood lost) exceeds the intake of dietary iron.

Hemoglobin Reference Values

The hemoglobin value at birth normally ranges from 16 to 23 g/dL. In early childhood, the value declines, and 10 to 14 g/dL is normal. When children begin the rapid growth associated with adolescence, hemoglobin values increase until adult levels are reached. Adult males usually have hemoglobin values in the range of 13 to 17 g/dL, and females have values of 12 to 16 g/dL. Hemoglobin reference ranges are listed in Table 2-3. A rule-of-thumb is that the hemoglobin value should be approximately one-third the hematocrit value. Therefore, an individual with an hematocrit of 45% would be expected to have a hemoglobin of approximately 15 g/dL.

SI Units for hemoglobin are reported as grams per liter (g/L) or as mmol/L. To convert to grams per liter, the Hb (g/dL) is multiplied by a factor of 10. To convert to mmol/L, the Hb (g/dL) is multiplied by a factor of 0.6206.

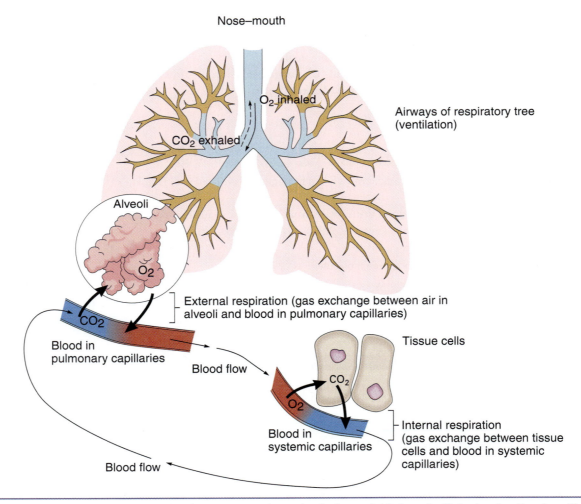

Nose–mouth

O_2 inhaled

CO_2 exhaled

Airways of respiratory tree (ventilation)

Alveoli

O_2

CO_2

Blood in pulmonary capillaries

External respiration (gas exchange between air in alveoli and blood in pulmonary capillaries)

Blood flow

Tissue cells

CO_2

O_2

Blood in systemic capillaries

Internal respiration (gas exchange between tissue cells and blood in systemic capillaries)

Blood flow

FIGURE 2-14 Diagram of lungs showing oxygen exchange by the hemoglobin in red cells in the alveoli and capillaries

CURRENT TOPICS

PHYSIOLOGIC FACTORS AFFECTING HEMOGLOBIN LEVELS

The blood hemoglobin concentration is affected by factors such as diet, age, and gender. The diet must contain adequate amounts of iron for the red blood cells to make hemoglobin. Some foods are higher in iron than others; for example, red meat has more iron than cow's milk. If the diet is deficient in iron, iron deficiency anemia may develop.

The normal hemoglobin value varies according to the age and gender of the individual. Normally, males have higher hemoglobin values than do females. Newborns have higher values than both children and adults.

People who live at very high altitudes have higher hemoglobin values (and red blood cell counts) than people who live at lower altitudes. This is because more red blood cells are necessary to carry sufficient oxygen in the blood, since oxygen pressure is lower in *thin air* than it is at sea level.

TABLE 2-3. Hemoglobin reference ranges

AGE/ GENDER	HEMOGLOBIN REFERENCE RANGE		
	g/dL	(CONVERSION FACTOR)	g/L (SI UNITS)
Newborn	16–23	×10	160–230
Children	10–14	×10	100–140
Adult males	13–17	×10	130–170
Adult females	12–16	×10	120–160

PRINCIPLES OF HEMOGLOBIN DETERMINATION

Various methods of determining hemoglobin have been used over the years. Current methods in use include the specific gravity technique and chemical methods such as the cyanmethemoglobin and azidemethemoglobin methods.

Specific Gravity Technique

The specific gravity method of measuring hemoglobin gives only an estimate of hemoglobin concentration and requires no special instrument. A drop of blood is dropped into a copper sulfate ($CuSO_4$) solution of a particular density (specific gravity). If the drop falls through the solution rapidly, the specific gravity of the blood is greater than the specific gravity of the copper sulfate. Blood with the normal amount of hemoglobin falls rapidly; blood with a low hemoglobin concentration falls slowly or may float (not drop at all).

The specific gravity technique of estimating hemoglobin has primarily been performed in the United States in past years as a hemoglobin-screening method for potential blood donors. Most blood donation centers now measure hemoglobin by hemoglobinometer or estimate hemoglobin indirectly by performing an hematocrit.

Chemical Methods

Measurement of cyanmethemoglobin is a widely used chemical method of determining blood hemoglobin. In this method, blood is reacted with **Drabkin's reagent**, which contains iron, potassium, cyanide, and sodium bicarbonate. The Drabkin's and the hemoglobin combine to form a very stable colored end-product, **cyanmethemoglobin**, also called **hemiglobincyanide (HiCN)**. This product is measured spectrophotometrically using a hematology analyzer or hemoglobinometer.

Some hemoglobin analyzers use a hemoglobin method in which *azidemethemoglobin* is measured. The azidemethemoglobin reagent contains a lysing chemical such as sodium deoxycholate, an oxidizing chemical such as sodium nitrite, and azide. In this method, oxyhemoglobin in the blood (which contains ferrous iron) is oxidized to form methemoglobin (which contains ferric iron). The methemoglobin then combines with azide to form azidemethemoglobin, a stable compound that can be measured spectrophotometrically.

PERFORMING THE HEMOGLOBIN DETERMINATION

Several small analyzers include hemoglobin measurements in their test menus. Other analyzers, sometimes called dedicated hemoglobinometers, measure only hemoglobin and are inexpensive, easy to use, and accurate. Most have been granted waived status under CLIA '88.

Safety Precautions

Standard Precautions must be observed when performing hemoglobin measurements. In addition, because most hemoglobin reagents contain hazardous chemicals such as cyanide or azide, care must be taken when performing the tests and handling the reagents. Work practice controls include wearing gloves, working in a well-ventilated area, properly disposing of used reagents, wiping up all spills, and washing hands after completion of the procedure. Analyzers that

CURRENT TOPICS

VARIATIONS IN HEMOGLOBIN STRUCTURE

Several forms of hemoglobin exist; these forms are determined by differences in the globin structure of the molecule. Red blood cells from a normal adult actually contain three types of hemoglobin:

- Hemoglobin A_1—Hgb A_1 contains two alpha (α) globin chains and two beta (β) globin chains and makes up 95% to 98% of our hemoglobin. It is also called adult hemoglobin.
- Hemoglobin A_2—Hgb A_2 has two α and two delta (δ) chains and makes up 2% to 3% of our hemoglobin.
- Hemoglobin F—Hgb F has two α and two gamma (γ) chains and makes up 2% of our hemoglobin. It is the primary hemoglobin produced by the fetus during gestation and its production usually falls to a low level shortly after birth and to adult levels by 1 to 2 years of age.

Abnormal, or variant, forms of hemoglobin occur when a change such as a mutation occurs in a gene that codes for the globin proteins, causing a change in the amino acid structure of the globin protein. Besides affecting hemoglobin structure, these changes can affect the function, rate of production, or stability of the hemoglobin. The mutation is almost always in the gene for the β globin chain. Hundreds of hemoglobin variants have been discovered, but only a few are common and clinically significant.

We inherit one copy of each globin gene from each parent. If one abnormal gene and one normal gene is inherited, the person is said to be heterozygous for the gene and is considered a carrier. That is, they can pass the gene on to offspring but do not generally have health problems from the abnormal gene themselves—they are usually silent carriers. If two abnormal genes of the same type are inherited, the person is said to be homozygous for the abnormal hemoglobin and will always pass a copy on to offspring.

Three of the more common abnormal hemoglobins are:

- Hemoglobin S—This is the primary hemoglobin in people with sickle cell (Hgb S) disease. Approximately 0.15% of African Americans have sickle cell disease; 8% are heterozygous and are said to have sickle cell trait. In Hgb S disease, individuals have two β^S chains and two normal α chains. The Hgb S causes the red blood cells to deform and assume a sickle shape when oxygen is decreased, such as during exercise. Sickled red blood cells can block small blood vessels, causing pain and impaired circulation. Sickling decreases the oxygen-carrying capacity of the red blood cell and decreases the cell's lifespan, resulting in sickle cell anemia.
- Hemoglobin E—This is one of the most common hemoglobin variants in the world. It is prevalent in parts of southeast Asia and in individuals of southeast Asian descent. People who are homozygous for Hgb E have two copies of β^E and have mild hemolytic anemia, microcytosis (small red blood cells), and slight enlargement of the spleen.
- Hemoglobin C—About 2% to 3% of people of west African descent are heterozygous for Hgb C. Hgb C disease (homozygous for the gene) is rare and relatively mild. It usually causes mild hemolytic anemia and mild to moderate enlargement of the spleen.

There are several other less common hemoglobin variants. Some cause no symptoms, while others affect the way the hemoglobin molecule functions. Hemoglobin H (Hgb H) is an abnormal hemoglobin that is composed of four β globin chains and is created in response to a severe shortage of α chains. Although each of the β globin chains is normal, hemoglobin with four β chains does not function normally. Hgb H has an increased affinity for oxygen, holding onto it instead of releasing it to the tissues and cells. Examples of other variants include Hgb D, Hgb G, Hgb J, and Hgb M.

The role of Hgb F in the fetus is to provide efficient transport of oxygen in a low oxygen environment. Hgb F can remain elevated after birth in several congenital disorders. Hgb F levels are increased in a rare condition called hereditary persistence of fetal hemoglobin (HPFH), in which Hgb F levels are increased with no hematological or clinical features. Different ethnic groups have different mutations causing HPFH.

Thalassemias are a group of inherited disorders in which production of normal hemoglobin is decreased, causing an imbalance of α to β chains. Thalassemia patients often have increased amounts of minor hemoglobins such as Hgb F or Hgb A_2. Thalassemias may have mild to severe symptoms depending on the type of globin affected.

provide through-the-stopper sampling enhance worker safety. (See Lessons 1-5 and 1-6.)

Quality Assessment

QA The use of Drabkin's reagent to form the stable compound cyanmethemoglobin was an important advancement in hematology because it made reliable hemoglobin standards available for the first time. A hemoglobin solution made with Drabkin's is stable for at least 6 months and provides laboratories a reliable standard to use for standardizing hemoglobin assays.

Hemoglobinometers and hematology analyzers used for hemoglobin assays must be calibrated at regular intervals as specified by the manufacturer. Appropriate controls must be run at least daily or when patient samples are run, control results must be recorded, and the records must be maintained. Each instrument used will have its own particular checks that must be performed and documented.

HemoCue Hemoglobin Test System

The HemoCue Hb 201+ is a small handheld analyzer for use in point-of-care testing. The analyzer is simple to use and provides quality results using a very small blood sample. Capillary or venous blood can be used. Hemoglobin determination is CLIA-waived when using both the HemoCue Hb 201+ and the earlier model HemoCue analyzer, the B-Hemoglobin.

The blood sample is collected into a special cuvette that automatically draws up the correct amount of blood (Figure 2-15). Reagents coated inside the cuvette mix with the blood to form azidemethemoglobin. The cuvette is inserted into the analyzer and a dual-wavelength photometer in the analyzer measures the absorbance of the solution (Figure 2-16). The absorbance is converted into units and the hemoglobin result is displayed in g/dL or g/L in less than 1 minute. Because of the dual-wavelength photometers in HemoCue hemoglobin analyzers, blood samples

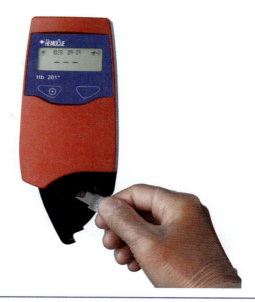

FIGURE 2-16 Inserting cuvette into the HemoCue Hb 201+ analyzer (*Courtesy of HemoCue, Inc., Lake Forest, CA*)

are corrected for lipemia, leukocytosis, and other causes of turbidity which could interfere with the readings.

The Hb 201+ has an internal electronic self-test to automatically verify performance. This feature means that the control cuvette used in the B-Hemoglobin analyzer is not required for the Hb 201+.

STAT-Site M Hgb Meter

The STAT-Site M Hgb test system, by GDS Technology (division of Stanbio Laboratory, Elkhart, IN), is a CLIA-waived system designed to measure hemoglobin in settings such as physician office laboratories (POLs), blood donation centers, health centers, and emergency departments. The system includes a palm-size, battery-operated hemoglobin meter; test cards; and a CODE key (calibration cartridge). The meter can measure hemoglobin from a single drop of blood in just a few seconds. The test method is also based on the azidemethemoglobin method, and either capillary blood or venous anticoagulated blood can be used. A lot-specific CODE key is provided in each package of test cards. When a test card is inserted into the meter, it is prechecked and coded to the CODE key. When a drop of blood is added to the card, the sample is detected by the meter and analyzed. Within a few seconds the hemoglobin result is displayed (in g/dL or mmol/L [SI unit]). This meter can measure hemoglobin in the range of 6 to 21 g/dL and can be used for hemoglobin measurements in infants, children, and adults.

Hgb Pro

The Hgb Pro (ITC, Edison, NJ) is another small handheld hemoglobin meter. The instrument requires a very small blood sample, which is added to the cuvette and inserted into the instrument. The hemoglobin value is read on the display (Figure 2-17).

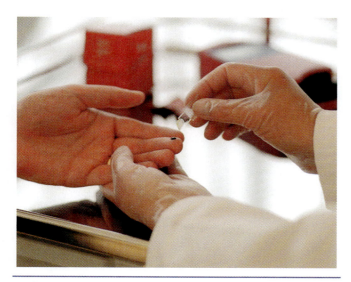

FIGURE 2-15 Filling the cuvette for the HemoCue Hb 201+ analyzer (*Courtesy of HemoCue, Inc., Lake Forest, CA*)

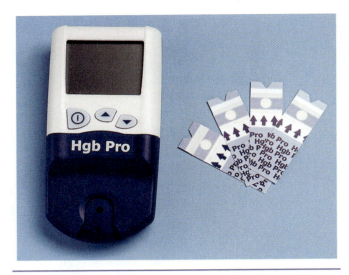

FIGURE 2-17 Hgb Pro (*Courtesy ITC, Edison, NJ*)

Automated Methods

Most cell counters and hematology analyzers also perform hemoglobin determinations. In many of these, the sample is aspirated from the blood collection tube by a probe that penetrates the stopper, offering convenience and safety for the worker. Several clinical chemistry analyzers also are capable of performing hemoglobin assays.

SAFETY Reminders

- Observe Standard Precautions when performing hemoglobin determinations.
- Wear gloves, protective face wear, and a buttoned, fluid-resistent laboratory coat.
- Dispose of hemoglobin reagents according to facility guidelines.

PROCEDURAL Reminders

- Use appropriate controls and standards when performing hemoglobin determinations.
- Store reagent strips, cuvettes, and cartridges as recommended by the manufacturer.
- Do not use reagents beyond the expiration date.
- Perform capillary punctures correctly.

CASE STUDY 1

Jennifer was transferred from her company's Virginia Beach office to Colorado Springs. Before moving, she flew to Colorado Springs for a week of new employee orientation. After being there only a few days, she had to seek medical attention for extreme fatigue and shortness of breath. The physician ordered a hemoglobin test along with other tests.

1. Which of the following is most likely?
   a. Jennifer is depressed because she will be moving away from family.
   b. Jennifer has not had sufficient rest because of stress from the new job.
   c. Jennifer is having problems acclimating to the altitude.
   d. Jennifer does not like her new job.
2. Explain your answer.

CASE STUDY 2

A hemoglobin and hematocrit performed in a pediatric clinic on a 2-year-old gave results of 110 g/L hemoglobin and 0.33 L/L hematocrit.

Do these results agree? What is the boy's general health status based on the hematology results?

SUMMARY

The hemoglobin determination is an essential part of the CBC. The result is used along with the hematocrit to estimate the oxygen-carrying capacity of the blood. The test can be performed either manually using a handheld hemoglobin analyzer, such as the ones described in this lesson, or using a hematology analyzer. All quality assessment steps must be followed to ensure valid results. Standard precautions for safe handling of blood samples must always be observed for the protection of personnel and patients.

REVIEW QUESTIONS

1. What are the two main components of hemoglobin?
2. Explain the function of hemoglobin.
3. What was the significance of the development of the cyanmethemoglobin method?
4. Explain the principle of the specific gravity technique of estimating hemoglobin concentration.
5. Explain the principle of the HemoCue method.
6. Give hemoglobin reference values for children and adults.
7. List safety precautions to be observed when measuring hemoglobin.
8. Define cyanmethemoglobin, Drabkin's reagent, globin, heme, hemiglobincyanide, and hemoglobin.

STUDENT ACTIVITIES

1. Complete the written examination for this lesson.
2. Inquire at physician offices, blood donation centers, or anemia screening clinics in the community about what methods of hemoglobin determination are used.
3. Practice the procedure for determining hemoglobin as listed in the Student Performance Guide.

WEB ACTIVITIES

1. Use the Internet to find information about abnormal forms of hemoglobin (such as Hgb S, E, C, or H). Choose one to research; describe the condition, disorder, or disease associated with it and the laboratory test(s) used to detect and confirm it.
2. Use the Internet to find two brands of hematology analyzers. Look on the Web sites for information about how the instruments measure hemoglobin. Request or download free product information describing the test methods.

Student Performance Guide

Lesson 2-3 Hemoglobin Determination

Name _____   Date _____

INSTRUCTIONS

1. Practice the procedure for determining blood hemoglobin concentration using a hemoglobin analyzer and following the step-by-step procedure.

2. Demonstrate the hemoglobin determination procedure satisfactorily for the instructor, using the Student Performance Guide. Your instructor will determine the level of competency you must achieve to obtain a satisfactory (S) grade.

NOTE: Consult manufacturer's instructions for specific procedure.

MATERIALS AND EQUIPMENT

■ acrylic safety shield or protective face-wear
■ gloves
■ antiseptic
■ surface disinfectant
■ capillary puncture equipment or blood samples collected in EDTA
■ HemoCue Hemoglobin System, or other hemoglobin analyzer with supplies appropriate for the analyzer
■ biohazard container
■ sharps container
■ hemoglobin controls

PROCEDURE

Record in the comment section any problems encountered while practicing the procedure (or have a fellow student or the instructor evaluate your performance).

S = Satisfactory
U = Unsatisfactory

You must:	S	U	Comments
1. Assemble equipment and materials for the hemoglobin analyzer to be used			
2. Put on face protection or position acrylic safety shield. Wash hands and put on gloves			
3. If using the HemoCue 201+, follow steps 4a–4j. If using HemoCue B-Hemoglobin, go to step 5. If using a different brand of hemoglobin analyzer, go to step 6			

4. For the HemoCue 201+:
  a. Turn on instrument to warm up; wait until electronic calibration is completed
  b. Remove a cuvette from vial. Immediately replace the vial cap
  c. Perform a capillary puncture observing Standard Precautions
  d. Wipe away the first drop of blood
  e. Touch the pointed tip of the cuvette to a well-rounded drop of blood and allow the cuvette to fill in one continuous motion			

You must:	S	U	Comments
f. Wipe excess blood from outside of cuvette, being careful not to touch the open end of the cuvette g. Insert the filled cuvette into the holder within 10 minutes of filling the cuvette h. Push the holder into the analyzer to the measuring position i. Read hemoglobin value from display and record j. Repeat steps 4e–4i using the hemoglobin control			

5. For the HemoCue B-Hemoglobin:
  a. Turn on instrument to warm up; the display screen should read "Hb"
  b. Pull out the cuvette holder to the first stop. Within 2–6 seconds, the screen should read "Ready"
  c. Place the control cuvette into the holder and push the holder completely in. The screen should read "Measuring"
  d. Record the control value that appears after 10-15 seconds; the value should be within ±0.3 g/dL of the manufacturer's assigned value. If the value is not within the acceptable range, contact the manufacturer
  e. Remove a cuvette from vial. Immediately replace the vial cap
  f. Perform a capillary puncture observing Standard Precautions
  g. Wipe away the first drop of blood
  h. Touch the pointed tip of the cuvette to a well-rounded drop of blood and allow the cuvette to fill in one continuous motion
  i. Wipe excess blood from outside of cuvette, being careful not to touch the open end of the cuvette
  j. Insert filled cuvette into holder within 10 minutes of filling the cuvette
  k. Push the holder into the analyzer to the measuring position
  l. Read the hemoglobin value from the display and record
  m. Repeat steps 5e–5l using the hemoglobin control			

6. If using another hemoglobin analyzer follow the manufacturer's instructions for calibration and performing a hemoglobin determination			
7. Discard all contaminated materials appropriately			
8. Turn off the instrument, wipe up any spills, and return all equipment to proper storage			
9. Wipe counters with surface disinfectant			
10. Remove and discard gloves into biohazard container			
11. Wash hands with antiseptic			

Evaluator Comments:

Evaluator _____ Date _____

2-4

The Hemacytometer

LESSON OBJECTIVES

After studying this lesson, the student will:

- Identify the parts of a hemacytometer.
- Use the microscope to identify the ruled areas of the hemacytometer used to count red blood cells, white blood cells, and platelets.
- Fill the hemacytometer using a micropipet or capillary tube.
- Use the correct counting pattern.
- Use the boundary rules of the hemacytometer to count blood cells.
- Write and use the general formula for calculating cell counts using a hemacytometer.
- List the safety precautions to observe when using the hemacytometer.
- Discuss quality assessment issues associated with manual cell counts using the hemacytometer.
- Define the glossary terms.

GLOSSARY

hemacytometer / a heavy glass slide made to precise specifications and used to count cells microscopically; a counting chamber

hemacytometer coverglass / a special coverglass of uniform thickness used with a hemacytometer

micropipet / a pipet that measures or holds 1 mL or less

INTRODUCTION

Manual blood cell counts are performed microscopically using the **hemacytometer**, a special glass counting chamber. Hemacytometers are manufactured to meet the specifications of the National Institute of Standards and Technology (NIST). The hemacytometer is used to perform manual cell counts of periph- eral blood cells, bacteria, and cells in cerebrospinal fluid, and to count sperm in fertility testing.

The use of the hemacytometer, explanations of the ruled areas, and the method of calculating cell counts are explained in this lesson. Procedures for performing WBC and RBC counts using the Unopette are outlined in Lesson 2-5. In addition, the use of auto- mated cell counters in hematology is also briefly discussed there.

THE HEMACYTOMETER

The hemacytometer is a heavy, precision-made glass slide with two counting areas. The hemacytometer must be used with a **hemacytometer coverglass** of uniform thickness (0.4 mm) that has been manufactured to meet NIST specifications.

General Features of the Hemacytometer

When viewed from the top, the hemacytometer has two polished raised platforms surrounded by depressions on three sides (Figure 2-18). The depressions surrounding these platforms are called *moats* and form an *H*. Each raised surface contains a ruled counting area marked off by precise lines (rules) etched into the glass. Most hematology laboratories use hemacytometers with Neubauer-type rulings.

The hemacytometer coverglass is positioned so that it covers both ruled areas of the hemacytometer (Figures 2-18 and 2-19). The coverglass creates a chamber, confines the fluid when the chamber is filled, and regulates the depth of the fluid. The chamber depth in the Neubauer-type hemacytometer is 0.1 mm with the coverglass in place.

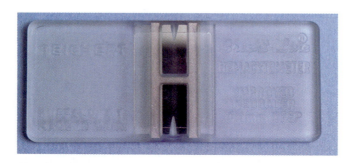

FIGURE 2-18 Top view of hemacytometer with coverglass in place

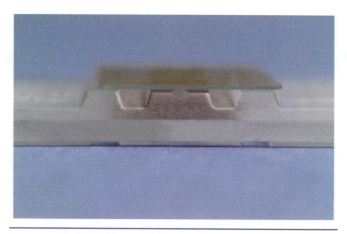

FIGURE 2-19 Side view of hemacytometer with coverglass in place

Hemacytometer Counting Areas

The hemacytometer contains two identical ruled areas composed of etched lines that define squares of specific dimensions. In the Neubauer counting chamber, each ruled area consists of a large square, 3 mm × 3 mm, divided into nine equal squares (Figure 2-20), each 1 mm square (mm²). The total area of the large square is 9 mm².

White Blood Cell Counting Area

The area counted for a white blood cell count is determined by the facility's standard operating procedure. A manual WBC count using the Unopette method requires that all nine large squares are counted (Figure 2-21). Some procedures require that only the four corner squares are counted.

Red Blood Cell Counting Area

The large square in the center is used for RBC counts (Figure 2-22). This center square is subdivided into 25 smaller squares, which in turn are each divided into 16 squares. Of the 25 squares, only the four corner squares and the center square (a through e) within the larger center square in the center are used to perform RBC counts (Figure 2-22).

Platelet Counting Area

The entire large center square is used to count platelets. Platelets in all 25 squares within the large center square (circled) are counted (Figures 2-20 and 2-22).

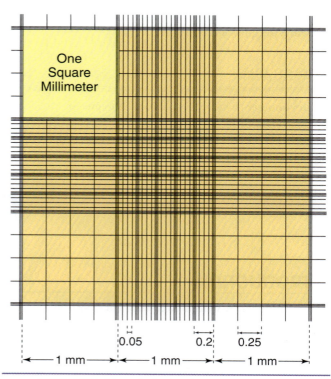

FIGURE 2-20 Ruled area of the hemacytometer showing the dimensions

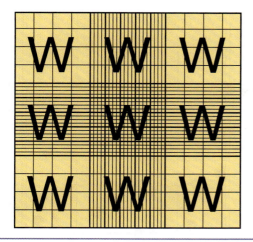

FIGURE 2-21 White blood cell counting area used for Unopette method. All nine large squares are counted

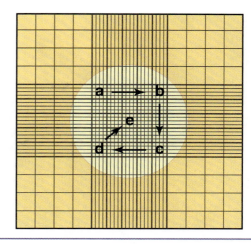

FIGURE 2-22 Red blood cell and platelet counting areas. The four corner squares and center square (labeled a through e) within the large center square are used to count red blood cells. The entire large center square (circled) is used for platelet counts

USING THE HEMACYTOMETER

The worker should be skilled in microscope use before using the hemacytometer. Instructions for using the microscope are in Lesson 1-10.

Safety Precautions

 Standard Precautions must be observed in handling the hemacytometer when counting cells in blood or any other body fluids. Gloves must be worn, and the slide and coverglass must be disinfected after use by soaking in a disinfectant such as a 10% bleach solution for a minimum of 10 minutes. Both can then be gently washed in a solution of laboratory detergent and thoroughly rinsed before being dried and put away. The hemacytometer and coverglass should be handled carefully because they can break and cause cuts.

Quality Assessment

 Because few blood cell standards are available for manual cell counts in hematology, quality assessment for hemacytometer counts is primarily concerned with technique. Specimen collection and preparation, cell counts, and calculations are all areas in which good technique and attention to detail is very important.

The hemacytometer and coverglass are delicate pieces of equipment that must be carefully handled. The hemacytometer and coverglass should be stored covered in a dust-free location to prevent an accumulation of dust and grit that could scratch the surfaces. Before the chambers are filled, the surfaces and the coverglass should be cleaned with lens paper and alcohol to remove fingerprints or debris. This prevents erroneous results caused by counting debris as cells. Care must be taken to avoid overloading the chamber, which would allow the fluid to flow into the moats and alter the cell distribution. If the fluid overflows, the hemacytometer must be cleaned and refilled.

Once the hemacytometer has been filled, the cells must be allowed to settle before counting. Cell counts must be performed using the correct ruled areas. Counting must be completed within 10 minutes of filling the chamber, before evaporation can occur. Calculations must be performed correctly. A variation of more than 10% in the number of cells counted between squares or between the totals of the two sides of the chamber signals that the count should be repeated by filling a clean hemacytometer.

Filling the Hemacytometer

A clean hemacytometer coverglass should be positioned so it covers both ruled areas of a clean hemacytometer. The hemacytometer is then ready to be filled. To do this, a filled capillary tube or **micropipet** is touched to a point where the coverglass and the raised platform meet (Figure 2-23). Approximately 10 µL of fluid from the pipet is allowed to flow into one chamber. The other side is filled in the same manner. Some hemacytometers have a V-shaped groove on each platform to guide the placement of the pipet tip (Figure 2-18).

The fluid should flow into the chamber in a smooth unbroken stream. *It should not be allowed to overflow into the depressions (moats) and there should be no air bubbles.* After the chambers have been correctly filled, the hemacytometer should stand undisturbed for 2 minutes to allow the cells to settle.

Viewing the Ruled Areas

The hemacytometer should be placed on the microscope stage with the low power (10×) objective in place so that a ruled area is located over the light source. The coarse adjustment knob is then used to move the hemacytometer and objective close together so that the objective is almost touching the coverglass. This must be done carefully to prevent the objective from touching the cover-

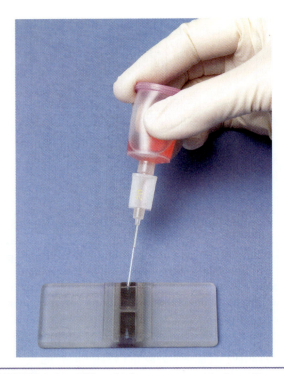

FIGURE 2-23 Filling the hemacytometer using a Unopette

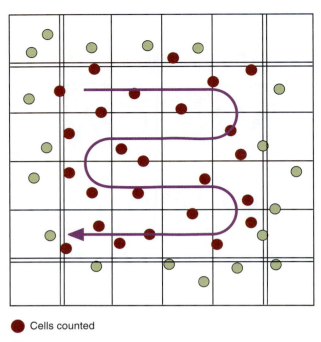

 Cells counted

Cells not counted

FIGURE 2-24 A sample hemacytometer square showing cells to count (red circles) and cells not counted (green circles); the arrow indicates the counting pattern that should be followed

glass. The coarse adjustment is then used to increase the distance between the coverglass and objective while one looks through the oculars. This is continued until the etched lines come into view. The fine adjustment is then used to bring the etched lines into sharp focus. The etched lines are more easily viewed when the microscope condenser is lowered and the light intensity is reduced.

When the ruled area is in sharp focus, the WBC area (all nine large squares) is located by moving the stage. After the WBC area has been observed, the central square used for RBC counts should be located. The high power (40×) objective should be carefully rotated into place. *If the microscope is parfocal, the ruled area will be brought into focus with only a slight rotation of the fine adjustment.* The large center square used for platelet counts and the five small squares used in an RBC count should be located (Figure 2-22).

Once all parts of the ruled area of one side have been located, the low-power objective should be rotated into place, and the stage should be moved to view the second ruled area. *The oil-immersion objective is never used with a hemacytometer.*

Using the Cell Counting Pattern

The counting pattern should be followed to ensure that cells are counted only once. The count should begin in the upper left corner of a square and proceed in a serpentine manner (Figure 2-24).

Single, double, or triple boundary lines divide the squares. When triple lines are present, the center line is the boundary. When double lines are present, the outer line is the boundary. All cells that are completely within the square, and those that touch the left boundary of the square, or touch the top boundary of

the square are considered to be in that square and are counted. Cells that touch the right boundary or lower boundary of a square should not be counted in that square even if they lie mostly within the square (Figure 2-24).

The cells in the appropriate squares should be counted on both sides of the chamber. The results for the two sides are totaled and an average calculated. The average is used in the formula to calculate the cell count.

CALCULATING THE CELL COUNTS

A general formula for calculating hemacytometer cell counts is:

$$\text{Cells}/\mu\text{L} = \text{Cells}/\text{mm}^3 = \frac{\text{avg} \times \text{DF}}{\text{A (mm)}^2 \times \text{D (0.1 mm)}}$$

Where

Cells/μL = Final cell count /μL

Avg = average # of cells counted

D (mm) = depth (always 0.1 mm)

DF = dilution factor

A (mm^2) = area counted

The dilution factor is determined by the blood dilution used for the cell count. The depth is always 0.1 because the chamber is 0.1 mm deep when the coverglass is in place. The area (A) counted will vary according to which cells are being counted and is calculated using the dimensions of the particular ruled area. A sample calculation for a red blood cell count is shown in Figure 2-25.

1. Count the cells:

	Side 1			Side 2	
Square	**Cells counted**		**Square**	**Cells counted**	
a	110		a	105	
b	100		b	115	
c	90		c	100	
d	95		d	106	
e	105		e	94	
	Total	500		Total	520

2. Compute the average:
   A. 500 + 520 = 1020 cells
   B. 1020 ÷ 2 = 510 average

3. Calculate the count:

$$RBC = \frac{\text{Average \# cells counted} \times \text{Dilution factor}}{\text{Area counted (mm}^2) \times D(0.1\text{ mm})}$$

$$RBC = \frac{510 \times 200}{0.2\text{ mm}^2 \times 0.1\text{ mm}}$$

$$RBC = 510 \times 10{,}000/\mu L$$

$$RBC = 5{,}100{,}000/\mu L \text{ (which is } 5.1 \times 10^6/\mu L \text{ or } 5.1 \times 10^{12}/L)$$

FIGURE 2-25 Sample calculation of red blood cell count using a 1:200 dilution

SAFETY Reminders

- Observe Standard Precautions when using the hemacytometer.
- Clean all spills with surface disinfectant.
- Disinfect hemacytometer and coverglass after each use.

PROCEDURAL Reminders

- Clean and polish the hemacytometer and coverglass before use.
- Do not allow fluid to overflow when filling the hemacytometer.
- Refill a clean hemacytometer if bubbles appear while filling.
- Allow cells to settle after filling chamber before performing the count.
- Do not allow microscope objectives to touch the hemacytometer coverglass when viewing the hemacytometer.
- Follow proper counting patterns to avoid counting the same cells twice.
- Complete the count within 10 minutes of filling chamber.
- Use correct calculation methods.
- Store and handle the hemacytometer and coverglass carefully.

CALCULATION PROBLEM

1. Write the formula to use when performing a RBC count with the hemacytometer, showing what area (A) should be counted.
2. A manual red blood cell count was performed using a 1:200 dilution. If 310 cells were counted on side 1 and 332 on side 2, what cell number should be used in the formula to calculate the RBC count?
3. Use the formula and the answer for question #2 to calculate the RBC count. Report it in conventional units (cells/μL) and SI units (cells/L).

CRITICAL THINKING

Melissa had just completed a manual blood cell count. After she reported the result she found that there was also a manual platelet count to be done. The lab had only one hemacytometer. What is the appropriate action?

Melissa should:
a. Wipe the hemacytometer and coverglass with lens paper before using them again
b. Disinfect hemacytometer and coverglass and wash them in detergent before use
c. Wash hemacytometer and coverglass in a laboratory detergent before disinfecting them
d. Wipe the hemacytometer and coverglass with gauze before using them

SUMMARY

The majority of blood cell counts are now performed using hematology analyzers. However, there are instances when it may be necessary to count blood cells manually. This is done using a hemacytometer, a glass counting chamber divided into precise areas for counting blood cells and used with a special coverglass. Exact procedures for diluting the sample, filling the chamber, and counting the cells must be followed for the method being used. A counting pattern must be followed to avoid counting the same cells twice. The chamber and the cover glass must be cleaned correctly to avoid counting dust and dirt as cells. It is important for the laboratory to have a technician who is competent in using the hemacytometer in case the need arises for performing manual cell counts.

REVIEW QUESTIONS

1. How are blood cells routinely counted in the laboratory?
2. Explain the importance of knowing how to perform a manual blood cell count.
3. Name the special slide used to perform manual cell counts.
4. Diagram the hemacytometer and its parts. Indicate the areas used for the WBC count and for the RBC count.

5. List the three functions of the coverglass when it is in place on the hemacytometer.
6. Explain how to position the coverglass on the hemacytometer.
7. Explain how to fill a hemacytometer using a micropipet or capillary tube.
8. Why is it important to ensure that the fluid does not overflow into the moats?
9. What is the proper procedure for disinfecting and cleaning the hemacytometer and coverglass?
10. Write the general formula used to calculate cell counts when using the hemacytometer. Explain A, Avg, D, DF, and C/μL.
11. Define hemacytometer, hemacytometer coverglass, and micropipet.

STUDENT ACTIVITIES

1. Complete the written examination for this lesson.
2. Practice filling the hemacytometer and microscopically viewing the counting areas using the Student Performance Guide.
3. Calculate the cells/μL for the following RBC averages using the general formula: 310, 450, 400.

WEB 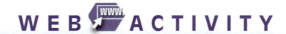 ACTIVITY

Search the Internet for laboratory regulatory Web sites to find out if cell counts performed using the hemacytometer are waived tests under CLIA '88.

Student Performance Guide

Lesson 2-4 The Hemacytometer

Name _____ Date _____

INSTRUCTIONS

1. Practice using the hemacytometer following the step-by-step procedure.
2. Demonstrate the use of the hemacytometer satisfactorily for the instructor, using the Student Performance Guide. Your instructor will determine the level of competency you must achieve to receive a satisfactory (S) grade.

MATERIALS AND EQUIPMENT

- antiseptic
- hemacytometer
- gloves (optional)
- surface disinfectant
- hemacytometer coverglass
- lens paper
- 70% or 95% alcohol
- micropipet (10 to 20 μL capacity)
- micropipetter with disposable tips, or capillary tubes
- microscope
- laboratory tissue
- laboratory detergent
- distilled water (with or without food color)
- biohazard container
- sharps container

PROCEDURE

You must:	S	U	Comments
Record in the comment section any problems encountered while practicing the procedure (or have a fellow student or the instructor evaluate your performance).		S = Satisfactory U = Unsatisfactory	
1. Assemble equipment and materials			
2. Use lens paper and 70% or 95% alcohol to carefully clean hemacytometer and coverglass			
3. Place the coverglass over the ruled areas (chamber) of the hemacytometer			
4. Wash hands (optional: put on gloves)			
5. Draw distilled water into the micropipet (approximately 10 μL will be needed for each side of the chamber). Optional: Use of diluted food color aids in determining if the hemacytometer is correctly filled.			
6. Hold the pipet at a 45° angle and touch the tip to the point where the coverglass and the hemacytometer meet (do not move coverglass)			

You must:	S	U	Comments
7. Allow fluid to flow into one side of the chamber (the chamber should fill in one smooth flow without flooding over into the depressions)			
8. Fill the other side of the chamber in the same manner			
9. Position the low-power (10×) objective in place			
10. Place the hemacytometer on the microscope stage securely with one ruled area over the light source			
11. Look *directly at the hemacytometer* (not through microscope eyepiece) and turn the coarse-adjustment knob to bring the microscope objective and the hemacytometer close together, continuing until the objective is almost touching the coverglass **NOTE:** Use coarse-adjustment knob with care			
12. Look into the eyepiece and slowly turn the coarse-adjustment knob in the opposite direction until the etched lines come into view			
13. Rotate the fine-adjustment knob until the lines are in clear focus			
14. Find all nine squares used for the WBC count on one side of the chamber by moving the stage or the hemacytometer			
15. Scan squares using left-to-right, right-to-left counting pattern and note boundary lines			
16. Locate the center square used for the platelet count			
17. Rotate the high-power (40×) objective carefully into position, and adjust focus using the fine-adjustment knob until the etched lines appear distinct			
18. Locate the four small corner squares and the center square (within the large center square) used for the RBC count			
19. Scan counting area using left-to-right, right-to-left pattern and note boundary lines			
20. Rotate the low power (10×) objective into position and view the second ruled area, repeating steps 14-19			
21. Rotate the low-power objective into position			
22. Remove the hemacytometer carefully from the microscope stage			
23. Clean the hemacytometer and the coverglass carefully using alcohol and lens paper			

You must:	S	U	Comments
24. Dry the hemacytometer and coverglass with lens paper			
25. Clean and return all equipment to proper storage			
26. Clean work area with surface disinfectant			
27. Wash hands with antiseptic			

Evaluator Comments:

Evaluator _____ Date _____

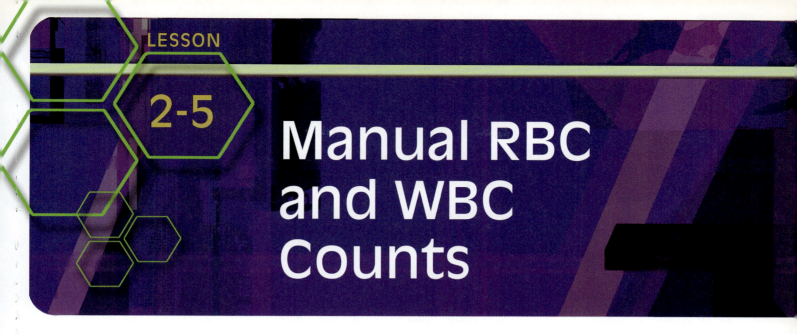

Manual RBC and WBC Counts

LESSON OBJECTIVES

After studying this lesson, the student will:

- Write the general formula for calculating cell counts using the hemacytometer.
- Perform a manual red blood cell count and calculate the results.
- State the important properties of red blood cell diluting fluids.
- List the red blood cell reference values for adult males, adult females, and newborns.
- Name a condition or disease associated with an increased red blood cell count and one associated with a decreased red blood cell count.
- Perform a manual white blood cell count and calculate the results.
- State the important properties of white blood cell diluting fluids.
- List the white blood cell reference values for adults, children, and newborns.
- Name a condition that causes leukocytosis and one that causes leukopenia.
- Discuss the safety issues involved in performing a manual blood cell count.
- Discuss the importance of quality assessment in performing manual blood cell counts.
- Define the glossary terms.

GLOSSARY

anemia / a condition in which the red blood cell count or blood hemoglobin level is below normal; a condition resulting in decreased oxygen-carrying capacity of the blood

aperture / an opening

cell diluting fluid / a solution used to dilute blood for cell counts

erythrocytosis / an excess of red blood cells in the peripheral blood; sometimes called polycythemia

hemolysis / the rupture or destruction of red blood cells, resulting in the release of hemoglobin

immunity / resistance to disease or infection

isotonic solution / a solution that has the same concentration of dissolved particles as the solution or cell with which it is compared

leukemia / a chronic or acute disease involving unrestrained growth of leukocytes

leukocytosis / increase above normal in the number of leukocytes (white blood cells) in the blood

leukopenia / decrease below normal in the number of leukocytes (white blood cells) in the blood; leukocytopenia

INTRODUCTION

The red blood cell (RBC) count and the white blood cell (WBC) count are parts of the routine complete blood count (CBC). Red blood cells are the most numerous of the blood cells. The RBC count approximates the number of circulating red blood cells and thus gives an indirect estimate of the blood's oxygen-carrying capacity. The RBC count is helpful in the diagnosis and treatment of many diseases, especially **anemia**, a condition in which there is a decrease below normal in the RBC count or hemoglobin level. White blood cells are less numerous in the blood than red blood cells. All white blood cells play important roles in **immunity**, the body's ability to resist disease. The WBC count gives general information concerning a patient's ability to fight infection.

Blood cell counts are routinely performed using instrumentation. However, when automated cell counters are not working, or in situations of very low blood cell counts, manual cell counts must be performed. In this lesson Unopette disposable blood collecting and diluting systems are used to perform the cell dilutions. These units consist of calibrated capillary pipets that automatically draw up the correct amount of blood and reservoirs that contain the correct diluting fluid for the type of cells being counted. Manual counts are performed by loading the blood dilution into a hemacytometer (Lesson 2-4) and viewing and counting the cells using the microscope.

UNOPETTE SYSTEMS

For many years, blood dilutions for cell counts were made in *Thoma* pipets, precisely manufactured glass pipets. Counts were performed on the diluted blood using the hemacytometer. Now, the most acceptable manual method of counting blood cells is using self-filling, self-diluting systems such as the Unopette, marketed by Becton Dickinson (Figure 2-26). These systems provide acceptable accuracy and have disposable components. Unopette systems are available for RBC, WBC, and platelet counts, as well as for more specialized tests such as erythrocyte osmotic fragility and some chemistry tests.

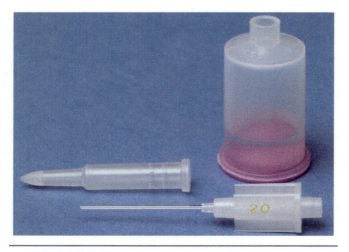

FIGURE 2-26 Parts of a disposable Unopette system

Components of a Unopette System

Each Unopette system for cell counts includes a sealed reservoir containing a premeasured volume of **cell diluting fluid** and a pipet assembly that includes a calibrated capillary pipet and a pipet shield (Figure 2-26). The shield protects the pipet and is used to puncture the diaphragm that seals the reservoir.

Cell Counts Using Unopette Systems

A different Unopette system is used for each type of cell count. Each type of Unopette system is designed to provide a particular dilution of the blood; therefore, different counting methods and calculations are required for each system.

Red Blood Cell Counts

The Unopette system for RBC counts contains 1.99 mL of red cell diluting fluid consisting of a physiological saline (0.85%) solution plus a preservative. The red blood cell diluting fluid is an **isotonic solution**. This is necessary to prevent **hemolysis**, or destruction, of the delicate red cells. The capillary pipet for measuring the blood sample is manufactured to contain 0.01 mL (10 μL). When 0.01 mL is added to the 1.99 mL of diluting fluid, the blood is diluted 1 part blood plus 199 parts diluting fluid. This equals a 1:200 dilution (1 part blood in a total of 200 parts).

White Blood Cell Counts

The Unopette system for WBC counts consists of a sealed reservoir containing 1.98 mL of white blood cell diluting fluid and a 0.02 mL (20 μL) capillary. The white blood cell diluting fluid is a 3% acetic acid solution which lyses (destroys) the red blood cells so the white blood cells are more easily seen using the microscope. When the 0.02 mL of blood is added to the 1.98 mL of diluting fluid, the blood is diluted 1 part blood plus 99 parts diluting fluid (a 1:100 dilution).

PERFORMING MANUAL RED BLOOD CELL AND WHITE BLOOD CELL COUNTS

Safety Precautions

 Standard Precautions must be observed when making blood dilutions, whether a Unopette system or other method is used. Special care must be taken to avoid creating aerosols or breaking capillary tubes. When making blood dilutions, workers must wear gloves and other suitable personal protective equipment. The technician must remember that the blood dilution used to fill the hemacytometer is a biohazardous solution. All contaminated materials must be disposed of in appropriate biohazard containers. The hemacytometer and coverglass must be disinfected by soaking in a 10% bleach solution for at least 10 minutes before being carefully washed and dried.

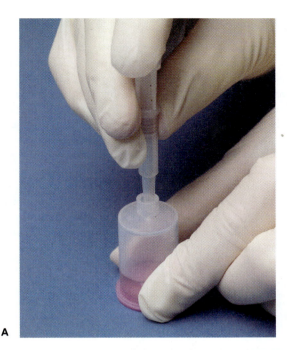

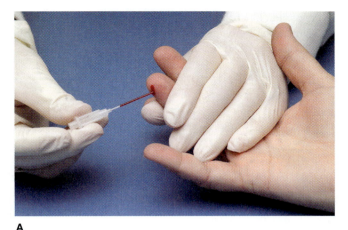

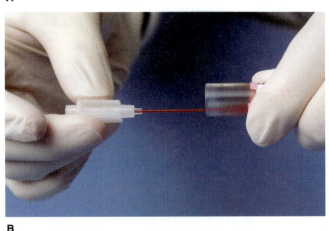

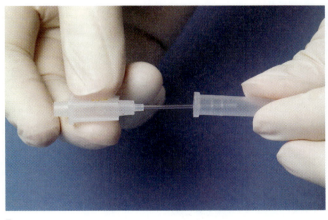

FIGURE 2-28 Unopette procedure: filling the pipet from (A) a fingerstick or (B) a tube of blood

FIGURE 2-27 Unopette procedure: (A) puncture the diaphragm; (B) remove the pipette shield

Quality Assessment

 Manual cell counts will always be less accurate and precise than are counts performed using an automated cell counter. Therefore, when performing manual counts, good technique with attention to detail is very important in specimen collection, preparation of cell dilutions, counting procedure, and calculation of results. Because different Unopette systems use different size capillaries and the reservoirs contain different volumes and cell diluting fluids, care must be taken to use the correct capillary and diluting fluid for the cell type being counted.

Hemacytometers and coverglasses manufactured to precise specifications must be used. They must be carefully cleaned before and after each use. Before the chambers are filled, the ruled surfaces and the coverglass must be inspected for fingerprints or debris.

Any debris present could be mistaken for cells when a count is performed, thus causing erroneous results. Care must be taken to avoid overfilling the chamber, which would allow the fluid to flow into the moats and alter the cell distribution.

A large variation in the number of cells counted among squares on one side of the chamber or between the total cell counts from each side of the chamber signals that the count should be repeated by filling a clean hemacytometer. The total number of cells counted on each side of the chamber should not differ by more than 10%.

Manual RBC Count

Preparing the Unopette

A Unopette RBC system is selected. The pipet shield is used to puncture the diaphragm in the neck of the reservoir, making an opening large enough to accept the capillary pipet (Figure 2-27).

Diluting the Blood Sample

The Unopette 10-μL capillary is filled with blood from a capillary puncture or from a tube of well-mixed EDTA (ethylenediaminetetra-acetic acid) blood (Figure 2-28). The filled capillary pipet is inserted into the reservoir, allowing the blood to mix with the diluting fluid. The resulting blood dilution is 1:200. This blood and diluting fluid mixture is stable for up to 6 hours but can be used immediately (Figure 2-29).

Filling the Hemacytometer

A clean coverglass is positioned on a clean hemacytometer to cover both counting areas. The capillary pipet is removed from the reservoir and reinserted in the reservoir with the pipet extending upward. The reservoir is swirled to mix the contents, and a few drops are expelled from the pipet tip and discarded. The tip of the pipet is touched to the edge of the coverglass, and one side of the chamber is allowed to fill by capillary action (Figure 2-30). The opposite side is then filled in the same manner. If the fluid overflows into the depression around the platforms or if air bubbles occur, the chamber must be cleaned and refilled.

Counting the Cells

The cells are allowed to settle for 2 minutes, and the hemacytometer is placed carefully on the microscope stage. The red blood cell ruled area is located using the low-power (10×) objective. The high-power (40×) objective is then carefully rotated into place to perform the count. Figure 2-31 illustrates the appearance of red blood cells on the hemacytometer using the 40× objective.

The RBC count is performed using the center square of the ruled area as shown in Figure 2-32. Within the center square are 25 smaller squares. Of these 25 squares, the four corner ones and the center square (marked "R" in Figure 2-32) are used for the count. Each of these five squares in turn contains four rows of squares. All cells within each of the small squares are counted using the left-to-right, right-to-left counting pattern. The cells touching either the top or left boundaries of the squares are

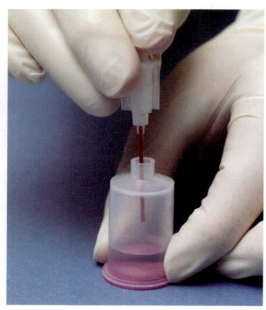

A

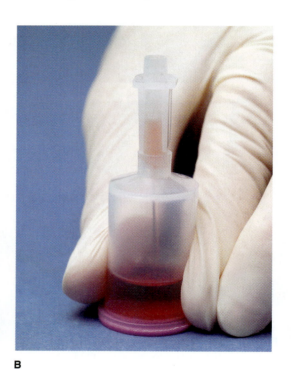

B

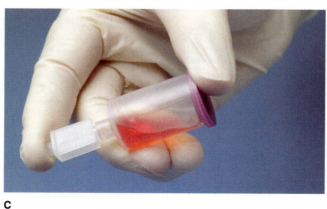

C

FIGURE 2-29 Unopette procedure: dilute the blood sample in the reservoir. **(A) Press gently on sides of reservoir and insert filled pipet; (B) seat pipet in neck of reservoir and release pressure to draw blood into reservoir solution; (C) place gloved finger over pipet opening and mix reservoir contents by inversion**

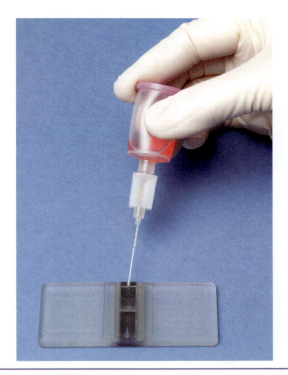

FIGURE 2-30 Filling the hemacytometer using a Unopette capillary

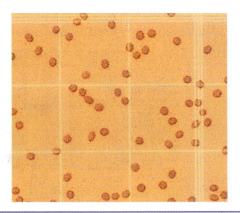

FIGURE 2-31 Photomicrograph of red blood cells as they appear on a hemacytometer

the area is 5×0.04 mm^2 or 0.20 mm^2.) Substitute these numbers into the formula as shown:

$$RBC/\mu L = \frac{\text{Average} \times 200}{0.20 \text{ mm}^2 \times 0.1 \text{ mm}}$$
$$= \text{Average \# cells} \times 10,000$$

When an RBC count is performed this way, the # of cells/μL (or mm^3) can be calculated by simply adding four zeroes to the average number of cells counted (or multiplying by 10,000). A sample calculation is shown in Figure 2-34.

Reference Ranges for Red Blood Cell Counts

The reference values for RBC counts range from approximately 4 million per microliter of blood ($4.0 \times 10^6/\mu L$) to 6 million per microliter ($6.0 \times 10^6/\mu L$), depending on age and gender. Males usually have slightly higher RBC counts than females (Table 2-4). Newborns have elevated RBC counts that slowly decline during childhood, only to increase to adult levels at puberty.

Red blood cell counts can be reported as either the number of cells per microliter (μL) or per liter (L) of blood. For example, a count of 5.6×10^6 red blood cells/μL is 5.6×10^{12} red blood cells/L reported in SI units.

Physiological and Pathological Conditions Affecting the Red Blood Cell Count

The primary function of red blood cells is to facilitate oxygen exchange in the tissues. From the lungs, oxygen (O_2) is carried by the hemoglobin in red blood cells to the tissues and released for use by cells of the body. There, waste carbon dioxide (CO_2) is picked up by the hemoglobin and carried to the lungs where it is exchanged for oxygen. If the RBC count decreases, then less oxygen is available to body tissues. Severe decreases can cause several physical symptoms, such as fatigue, weakness, headache,

included in the count. The cells touching the right boundary and the cells touching the lower boundary of each square are not counted. Cells lying beyond these boundaries are *not* counted (Figure 2-33).

A hand tally counter is used to tabulate the red cells. The cell numbers for each of the squares are recorded and totaled. A count is then performed in the five squares of the second side of the chamber in the same manner. If proper technique was used, the number of cells in a square should not vary from any other square on the same side of the hemacytometer by more than 10%.

Calculating the Red Blood Cell Count

The general formula to use for the hemacytometer is

$$\text{cells}/\mu L = \frac{\text{Avg} \times \text{DF}}{\text{A (mm}^2) \times \text{D (0.1 mm)}}$$

To calculate an RBC count using the UNOPETTE method, the formula is used in the following manner:

1. The average number of cells is obtained by totaling the counts for the five squares on each side of the chamber and dividing the total by two. This gives the average.

2. The dilution using the RBC UNOPETTE system is 1:200. Therefore, the dilution factor is 200.

3. The depth of the chamber is 0.1 mm.

4. The area counted is 0.20 mm^2. (Each square, a to e, has a length of 0.2 mm and a width of 0.2 mm. This gives each square an area of 0.04 mm^2. Since five squares are counted,

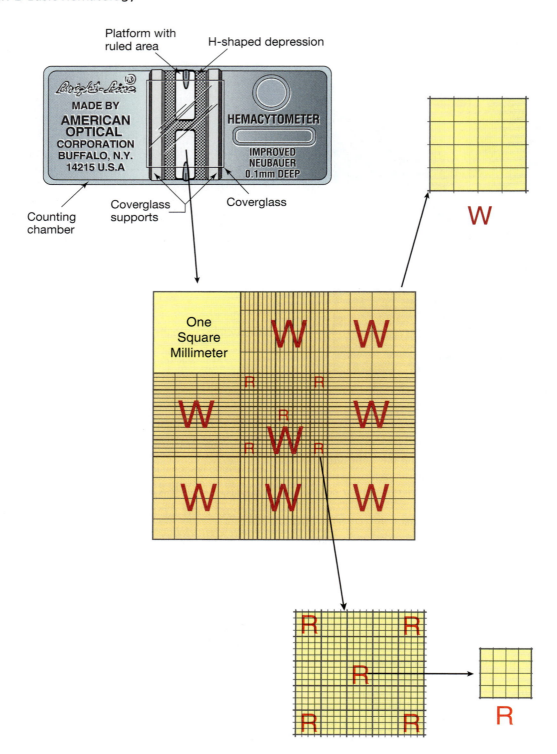

FIGURE 2-32 Ruled area of hemacytometer. The four corner squares and the center square (labeled R) within the large center square are used for RBC counts. All nine large squares (the entire ruled grid) are used for the WBC count

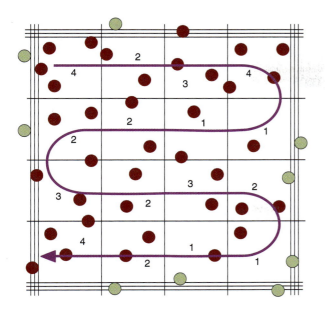

● Cells counted

○ Cells not counted

FIGURE 2-33 A sample hemacytometer square showing cells to count. Red cells would be counted and green cells would not be counted. The count should be performed using the serpentine counting pattern indicated by the arrow

pallor, and increased heart rate. This condition is called **anemia**, and there can be many causes. In order to successfully treat anemia, the cause of the anemia must be discovered.

Two general causes of anemia are:

■ Decreased red blood cell production

■ Increased red blood cell loss or destruction

Anemias caused by decreased red blood cell production can be due to a deficiency in one or more of the substances required to make hemoglobin or red blood cells. For instance, because iron is required for heme synthesis, iron deficiency can cause anemia. The lack of iron can be due to poor diet or poor iron absorption. Vitamins such as B_{12} or folic acid (Table 2-5) are other factors required for red blood cell synthesis, so dietary deficiencies in either of these can result in lower RBC counts and symptoms of anemia.

Anemia caused by increased red blood cell loss or destruction can result from acute or chronic blood loss, such as from a bleeding ulcer. It can also be due to inherited conditions, such as sickle cell anemia, in which the life span of red blood cells is shortened because of the presence of Hemoglobin S in the cells.

At the other end of the scale is **erythrocytosis**—an RBC count above normal. Erythrocytosis can have physiological or pathological causes. People who live at very high altitudes have increased red blood cell levels because the lower O_2 content of the air stimulates red blood cell production. For instance, the red blood cell reference ranges for a population living in a region such

1. Count the cells:

	Side 1			Side 2	
Square	**Cells counted**		**Square**	**Cells counted**	
a	100		a	97	
b	95		b	95	
c	90		c	90	
d	90		d	96	
e	105		e	88	
Total	480		Total	466	

2. Compute the average:
   A. 480 + 466 = 946 cells
   B. 946 ÷ 2 = 473 average

3. Calculate the count:

$$RBC = \frac{\text{Average \# cells counted} \times \text{Dilution factor}}{\text{Area counted (mm}^2) \times D(0.1\text{ mm})}$$

$$RBC = \frac{473 \times 200}{0.2\text{ mm}^2 \times 0.1\text{ mm}}$$

$$RBC = 473 \times 10,000/\mu L$$

$$RBC = 4,730,000 \text{ (or } 4.73 \times 10^6)/\mu L, \text{ or } 4.73 \times 10^{12}/L$$

FIGURE 2-34 Sample calculation of a red blood cell count

TABLE 2-4. Reference ranges for red blood cell counts

	REFERENCE RANGES	
Age/Gender	**Conventional Units**	**SI Units**
Adult male	4.5–$6.0 \times 10^6/\mu L$	4.5–$6.0 \times 10^{12}/L$
Adult female	4.0–$5.5 \times 10^6/\mu L$	4.0–$5.5 \times 10^{12}/L$
Newborn	5.0–$6.3 \times 10^6/\mu L$	5.0–$6.3 \times 10^{12}/L$

as the Andes would be higher than the ranges for a population living near sea level. *Polycythemia vera* is a disease in which the RBC count is greatly increased. Patients with polycythemia vera may require phlebotomy at regular intervals to remove excess red blood cells.

Manual WBC Count

Preparing the Unopette

A Unopette WBC system is selected. The pipet shield is used to puncture the diaphragm in the neck of the reservoir, making an opening large enough to accept the capillary pipet (Figure 2-27).

Diluting the Blood Sample

The Unopette 20 μl (0.02 mL) capillary is filled with blood from capillary puncture or from a tube of well-mixed EDTA blood (Figure 2-28). While pressing lightly on the sides of the reservoir, the filled capillary pipet is inserted into the reservoir, allowing the blood to mix with the diluting fluid but not to overflow from the top of the capillary (Figure 2-29). The 20 μL of blood is mixed with the 1.98 mL of diluting fluid, making a blood dilution of 1:100. The blood-and-fluid mixture must stand for at least 10 minutes before loading the hemacytometer to allow the red blood cells to be destroyed.

Filling the Hemacytometer

After 10 minutes, the reservoir is swirled to mix the contents and the pipet assembly is removed and reinserted in the reservoir with the pipet extending upward. A few drops are expelled from the pipet tip and discarded, the hemacytometer is filled on both sides (Figure 2-30), and cells are allowed to settle for 2 minutes.

Counting the Cells

When the cells have settled, the hemacytometer is placed securely onto the microscope stage for counting. The low-power objective (10×) is used to locate the ruled grid. The white blood cells will be more distinct if the microscope's light level is reduced. This can be accomplished by adjusting the condenser and light.

Cells in all nine of the large ruled areas are counted (as shown in Figure 2-32) using the 10× objective (100× magnification). The white blood cells will appear as refractile round objects with a definite outline (Figure 2-35). The white blood cells lying within each of the nine squares are counted using the left-to-right, right-to-left pattern (Figure 2-33). All cells touching either the upper or left boundary of the square are counted. Cells touching the lower or right boundary of the square are not counted (Figure 2-33). The counts from side 1 are recorded, and the procedure is repeated for side 2. The totals of sides 1 and 2 are added together and divided by two to obtain the average.

Calculating the White Blood Cell Count

The total number of white blood cells per microliter of blood can be calculated using the average number of cells counted, the depth of the counting chamber, the area counted, and the dilution. The dilution made with the Unopette WBC system is 1:100. The total volume counted is 0.9 μL (depth × area = volume; 0.1 mm × 9 mm^2 = 0.9 mm^3 = 0.9 μL). However, the WBC count is reported as cells per μL (or cells/L). To correct for this, the following formula is used:

$$\text{WBC/}\mu\text{L} = \text{average \# cells} + (0.1 \times \text{average \# cells}) \times 100$$

A sample white blood cell calculation is shown in Figure 2-36.

Reference Ranges for the White Blood Cell Count

The reference WBC counts vary according to the age of the individual (Table 2-6). Newborn infants usually have a WBC count of 9,000 to 30,000/μL. Within a few weeks after birth, the count drops rapidly and approaches the children's normal of 6,000 to 14,000/μL. By adulthood, the normal count is in the range of 4,500 to 11,000/μL.

TABLE 2-5. Examples of conditions affecting red blood cell counts	
CONDITION	**EFFECT ON RBC COUNT**
Anemias	Decreased
Iron deficiency	
Sickle cell	
B$_{12}$ deficiency	
Folic acid deficiency	
Acute or chronic blood loss	Decreased
Erythrocytosis	Increased
Polycythemia vera	Increased
Living at high altitude	Increased

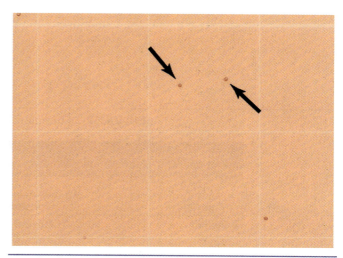

FIGURE 2-35 Photomicrograph of white blood cells as they appear on a hemacytometer (low power)

1. Count the cells:

Square	Side 1 Cells counted		Side 2 Cells counted
1	8		9
2	7		9
3	8		7
4	9		10
5	6		8
6	8		7
7	9		7
8	8		9
9	7		10
	Total 70		Total 76

2. Compute the average:

$$\frac{70 + 76}{2} = 73$$

3. Calculate the count:

WBC/μL = [Average counted + (0.1 × average counted)] × 100

WBC/μL = [73 + (.10) 73] × 100

WBC/μL = (73 + 7.3) × 100

WBC/μL = (73 + 7) × 100

WBC/μL = 80 × 100

WBC/μL = 8000 (8 × 10^3)

WBC/L = 8.0 × 10^9

FIGURE 2-36 Sample calculation of a white blood cell count using a 1:100 dilution

TABLE 2-6. Reference ranges for white blood cell counts

Age	AVERAGE Conventional Units (cells/μL)	AVERAGE SI Units (cells/L)	RANGE Conventional Units (cells/μL)	RANGE SI Units (cells/L)
Newborn	18,000	1.8 × 10^{10}	9,000–30,000	9.0–30.0 × 10^9
One year	11,000	1.1 × 10^{10}	6,000–14,000	6.0–14.0 × 10^9
Six years	8,000	8.0 × 10^9	4,500–12,000	4.5–12.0 × 10^9
Adult	7,400	7.4 × 10^9	4,500–11,000	4.5–11.0 × 10^9

Physiological and Pathological Conditions Affecting the WBC Count

White blood cells play important roles in the body's ability to fight infection. Each type of white blood cell has specific roles. For example, one role of lymphocytes is to respond to viral infections. Eosinophils and basophils increase in response to allergic conditions. Neutrophils and monocytes participate in defense against microorganisms such as bacteria. In response to stimuli such as products of bacterial growth, neutrophils cluster or *marginate* on the walls of venules and capillaries. These marginating neutrophils then migrate through narrow spaces between the endothelial cells in the vessel walls and enter the site of infection in the tissues.

Leukocytosis, an increase in the WBC count, can be caused by many factors. Changes in the WBC count due to disease are called pathological changes and continue until the illness or condition is under control. Bacterial infections usually cause an increase in the WBC count. The increase may be slight, such as in appendicitis, where the WBC count usually does not go above 15 × 10^9/L; or the WBC count may reach 30 × 10^9/L in some other bacterial infections. Physiological factors such as stress, exercise, anesthesia, and even a cold shower can cause the WBC count to increase temporarily (Table 2-7).

Two other conditions accompanied by leukocytosis are **leukemia** and *leukemoid reaction*. In leukemia, an increase in the total WBC count is seen, but it is usually caused by an increase in only one cell line, such as the granulocytes or the lymphocytes. Leukemia patients can have WBC counts of 200 × 10^9/L, and the WBC count can even reach 1,000 × 10^9/L. A leukemoid reaction is a nonleukemic condition in which the total WBC count can be 50 × 10^9/L or higher. The cause for this reaction is unknown.

A decrease below normal in the total number of white blood cells is called **leukopenia** (leukocytopenia). Leukopenia can be caused by certain viral infections, exposure to ionizing radiation, certain chemicals, and chemotherapy drugs. Infection by the human immunodeficiency virus (HIV) is an example of a viral disease that causes a decrease in the WBC count (Table 2-7).

AUTOMATED CELL COUNTERS

The majority of blood cell counts are performed by automation, using instruments that range from relatively simple cell coun-

TABLE 2-7. Some causes of leukocytosis and leukocytopenia

CAUSES OF LEUKOCYTOSIS	CAUSES OF LEUKOCYTOPENIA
Pathological	**Pathological**
Infection	Some viral infections,
Leukemias	including HIV
Polycythemia	Ionizing radiation
	Certain chemicals
Physiological	Chemotherapy drugs
Exercise	
Exposure to sunlight	
Obstetric labor	
Stress	
Anesthesia	

ters to complex hematology analyzers. Small analyzers can be used in a physician office laboratory (POL) or a small hospital (Figure 2-37). More elaborate equipment can be found in large hospitals and reference laboratories. Most instruments perform RBC and WBC counts, hemoglobin, hematocrit, platelet counts, the red blood cell indices, and automated white blood cell differentials.

Automated cell counters operate on one of two principles. In some instruments, the cells to be counted are diluted in a fluid that conducts an electrical current. The cells are aspirated through a special narrow opening called an **aperture**. As the cells are aspirated, they interrupt the flow of the current across the opening. Each interruption is recorded and counted as a cell.

In another type of instrument, the diluted blood sample is aspirated into a special channel so narrow that only one cell can pass through at a time. As the cells pass through the channel, they interrupt a laser beam. Each interruption of the beam is counted as a cell. Lesson 2-13 discusses in more detail the principles of hematology instrumentation.

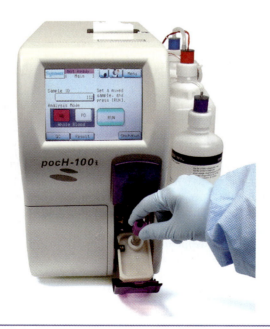

FIGURE 2-37 The pocH-100i is a cell counter suitable for use in small laboratories (*Courtesy of Sysmex America, Inc. All rights reserved.*)

SAFETY Reminders

- Observe Standard Precautions when using the hemacytometer and performing cell counts.
- Clean all spills with surface disinfectant.
- Disinfect the hemacytometer and coverglass after each use.
- Use only gentle pressure on the UNOPETTE reservoir when mixing the blood and diluent to avoid accidentally expelling the mixture through the top.

PROCEDURAL Reminders

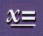

- Clean and polish the hemacytometer and coverglass before use to be sure the surfaces are free of debris and oil.
- Do not allow the microscope objectives to touch the coverglass when viewing the hemacytometer ruled areas.
- Do not allow the fluid to overflow the counting chamber when filling the hemacytometer.
- Follow proper counting and calculation methods as directed by the package insert.
- Repeat the count if variation is greater than 10% from one square to another or between the two sides of the hemacytometer.
- Store and handle the hemacytometer and coverglass carefully to avoid scratching the surfaces.
- Use the correct Unopette system for the type of cell count being performed.

CASE STUDY 1

Hank was performing manual blood cell counts in hematology using the Unopette system. When he performed a WBC count on Mrs. Rodriguez, he counted 78 white blood cells on one side of the hemacytometer and 82 cells on the other side.

1. Calculate the WBC count / L.
2. Is the count within the reference range for an adult female?

CASE STUDY 2

Josh was working alone in the laboratory because Tricia, the other technician, was out on sick leave. The physicians in the practice were very busy that day and were ordering a lot of tests. In addition, the hematology analyzer was not operational. One of the physicians ordered a WBC count on Mr. Morgan (28 years old), who was having abdominal pain. Josh collected Mr. Morgan's blood sample and then looked in the supply room for a Unopette reservoir and a Unopette capillary pipet. He performed the WBC count and got the following numbers:
Side 1: 8, 9, 10, 9, 7, 9, 9, 10, and 7.
Side 2: 8, 6, 6, 8, 7, 8, 7, 9, and 6.

1. Calculate the WBC count. Is it within the normal range?
2. Should Josh report this WBC result? Explain your answer.

SUMMARY

The results of RBC and WBC counts provide valuable information used in the diagnosis and treatment of a patient's disease or condition, as well as important information about the state of a patient's health and wellness. Routinely these two cell counts are performed as part of a CBC. The WBC count is also often ordered separately because it can be used to diagnose and follow the progress of an infection or the effect of certain drug or radiation therapies.

Use of automated cell counters has improved cell count accuracy and laboratory efficiency. Although automated cell counters are essential in most laboratories, sometimes manual counts are required. If an automated cell counter malfunctions and a backup instrument is not available, manual counts must be done. In cases in which a patient's WBC count is depressed by radiation or chemotherapy treatments and is lower than the cell counter's threshold, the WBC count must be performed manually. Therefore, it is important to keep supplies stocked for manual counts and to have employees trained to perform the procedures.

REVIEW QUESTIONS

1. Diagram the hemacytometer and label its parts. Show which areas are counted for a WBC count and for an RBC count.

2. Explain how to prepare a Unopette blood dilution.

3. Explain how to fill a hemacytometer using the Unopette capillary.

4. What is the proper procedure for disinfecting and cleaning the hemacytometer and coverglass?

5. What is the general formula used to calculate cell counts when using the hemacytometer?

6. What is the reference RBC count for a male; a female; a newborn?

7. What are the reference WBC values for newborns, children, and adults?

8. Name three diseases or conditions in which the RBC count is usually abnormal. For each condition listed, state if an increased or decreased RBC count would be seen.

9. What is one requirement of a red blood cell diluting fluid?

10. Name three causes of leukocytosis.

11. Name three factors that may cause leukopenia.

12. Describe how the Unopette systems for RBC and WBC counts differ.

13. What are the functions of the white blood cell diluting fluid?

14. Explain why it is important to know how to perform manual blood cell counts.

15. Define anemia, aperture, cell diluting fluid, erythrocytosis, hemolysis, immunity, isotonic solution, leukemia, leukocytosis, and leukopenia.

STUDENT ACTIVITIES

1. Complete the written examination for this lesson.

2. Practice performing and calculating RBC counts as outlined in the Student Performance Guide, using the RBC count worksheet.

3. Practice performing and calculating WBC counts as outlined in the Student Performance Guide, using the WBC count worksheet.

Student Performance Guide

Lesson 2-5 Red Blood Cell Count

Name _____ Date _____

INSTRUCTIONS

1. Practice performing and calculating an RBC count using the RBC Unopette system.

2. Demonstrate the RBC count procedure satisfactorily for the instructor, using the Student Performance Guide. Your instructor will determine the level of competency you must achieve to receive a satisfactory (S) grade.

NOTE: The following is a general procedure for using a Unopette system. Consult the package insert for specific instructions.

MATERIALS AND EQUIPMENT

- gloves
- antiseptic
- RBC worksheet
- materials for capillary puncture or tube of venous blood anticoagulated with EDTA
- laboratory tissue
- hemacytometer with coverglass
- test tube rack
- Unopette RBC system (reservoir and pipet assembly)
- microscope
- lens paper
- alcohol (70% or 95%)
- hand tally counter
- surface disinfectant
- biohazard container
- sharps container
- acrylic safety shield or face protection
- timer
- calculator

PROCEDURE

Record in the comment section any problems encountered while practicing the procedure (or have a fellow student or the instructor evaluate your performance).

S = Satisfactory
U = Unsatisfactory

You must:	S	U	Comments
1. Assemble equipment and materials. Set up acrylic safety shield or don face protection			
2. Place a clean hemacytometer coverglass over a clean hemacytometer			
3. Wash hands and put on gloves			
4. Puncture the diaphragm of the Unopette reservoir. Hold the reservoir firmly on a flat surface with one hand and use the tip of the pipet shield to puncture the diaphragm. **NOTE:** The opening must be made large enough to easily accommodate the pipet			

You must:	S	U	Comments
5. Remove the shield from the pipet assembly			
6. Fill the capillary pipet from a capillary puncture or from a tube of well-mixed EDTA anticoagulated blood. The pipet will fill by capillary action and will stop filling automatically. (Be sure no air bubbles are present in micropipet) **NOTE:** Keep pipet horizontal or at a slight (5°) upward angle to avoid overfilling			
7. Wipe excess blood from the outside of the capillary pipet with soft laboratory tissue **NOTE:** Do not allow tissue to touch pipet tip			
8. Squeeze the reservoir slightly, being careful not to expel any of the liquid			
9. Maintain the pressure on the reservoir and insert the capillary pipet into the reservoir, seating the pipet firmly in the neck of the reservoir. Do not expel any of the liquid			
10. Release the pressure on the reservoir, drawing the blood out of the capillary pipet into the diluent			
11. Squeeze the reservoir gently 3 to 4 times to rinse the remaining blood from the capillary pipet **NOTE:** Do not allow the blood-diluent mixture to flow out the top			
12. Mix the contents of the reservoir thoroughly by gently swirling the reservoir or turning it side to side			
13. Withdraw the capillary pipet from the reservoir and insert it in the neck of the reservoir in reverse position (the pipet tip should now project upward from the reservoir)			
14. Mix the contents of the reservoir thoroughly. Invert the reservoir and gently squeeze to discard 4 to 5 drops onto laboratory tissue			
15. Fill both sides of the hemacytometer; allow cells to settle for 2 minutes			
16. Place the hemacytometer on the microscope stage carefully and securely			
17. Use the low-power (10×) objective to bring the ruled area into focus			
18. Locate the large central square			
19. Rotate the high-power (40×) objective into position carefully and focus with the fine-adjustment knob until the ruled area is in focus			

2-6

Platelet Count

LESSON OBJECTIVES

After studying this lesson, the student will:

- Discuss the origin and functions of platelets.
- Name two pathological conditions in which the platelet counts may be abnormal.
- Perform a platelet count using the Unopette system.
- Calculate the results of a platelet count.
- List three safety precautions that must be observed when performing a platelet count.
- Discuss the importance of quality assessment in platelet counts.
- Define the glossary terms.

GLOSSARY

petri dish / a shallow, covered dish made of plastic or glass
thrombocytopenia / abnormal decrease in the number of platelets in the blood
thrombocytosis / abnormal increase in the number of platelets in the blood

INTRODUCTION

Platelets are the smallest of the formed elements in the blood. They are not true cells but are fragments of the cytoplasm of megakaryocytes, large cells in the bone marrow. Although platelets are very small, they play an important role in hemostasis. They help initiate blood clotting following injuries to blood vessels. Therefore the platelet count can be used to investigate and assess some bleeding and clotting disorders. Platelets can be counted on most hematology cell counters and the platelet count is often included in the complete blood count (CBC) report.

Some drug and radiation therapies affect the bone marrow and the production of platelets, and the platelet count can be used to monitor the toxic effects of these therapies. In these instances, the platelet count can be very low, and the count must be performed manually, most frequently using a Unopette system. Lesson 3-1 contains more comprehensive material on the function of platelets.

REFERENCE RANGE FOR PLATELET COUNT

The normal platelet count is 150,000 to 400,000 platelets per microliter of blood. This is $1.50 \times 10^5/\mu L$ to $4.0 \times 10^5/\mu L$. In SI units the range would be expressed as $1.5 \times 10^{11}/L$ to $4.0 \times 10^{11}/L$.

CURRENT TOPICS

CLINICAL SIGNIFICANCE OF PLATELET COUNTS

Platelets help control bleeding by forming a sticky plug that seals damaged vessel walls. Platelets also help initiate a series of enzymatic reactions that result in formation of the fibrin clot. Abnormal increases or decreases in the platelet numbers can interfere with the clotting mechanisms and cause either excessive clotting or bleeding.

Thrombocytosis, an increase above normal in platelet numbers, can occur in conditions such as polycythemia or hemolytic anemias or after surgical removal of the spleen (splenectomy). If platelet numbers are extremely high, spontaneous clot formation can occur, which is a dangerous situation.

There are many conditions and diseases that cause thrombocytopenia, a decrease below normal in platelet numbers. Any condition that is toxic to the bone marrow can cause decreased platelets; this is often seen following chemotherapy and radiation therapy. Thrombocytopenia can also occur in some anemias and leukemias, as well as in several other conditions (Table 2-8). If platelet numbers fall to critical levels, 10,000 to 20,000/μL (10×10^9/L to 20×10^9/L), uncontrolled bleeding can occur and can quickly create a life-threatening situation. When this happens, several platelet transfusions may be required to return the platelet numbers to a safe level. Table 2-8 lists examples of conditions that cause thrombocytosis or thrombocytopenia.

PERFORMING A MANUAL PLATELET COUNT

The most acceptable manual method of counting platelets is to use self-filling, self-diluting systems such as the Unopette system. Unopette systems consist of a sealed reservoir containing premeasured diluting fluid, a capillary pipet, and a pipet shield. The Unopette system for platelet counts uses a 0.02 mL (20 μL) capillary pipet to measure the sample and contains 1.98 mL of ammonium oxalate diluting fluid in the reservoir (Figure 2-38).

Safety Precautions

Standard Precautions must be observed when performing all hematology procedures. The worker must wear appropriate personal protective equipment (PPE) such as gloves and a buttoned, fluid-resistant laboratory coat. In addition, the worker should wear protective face wear or work behind an acrylic safety shield when opening vacutainer tubes and pipetting blood. All spills must be wiped up with sur-

TABLE 2-8. Conditions that can cause thrombocytopenia or thrombocytosis

Thrombocytopenia
Bone marrow damage
Sequestration of platelets by enlarged spleen
Disseminated intravascular coagulation (DIC)
Chronic alcoholism
Idiopathic thrombocytopenic purpura (ITP)
Thrombocytosis
Polycythemia vera
Bleeding disorders
Hemolytic anemias
Inflammatory reactions
Chronic granulocytic leukemia

face disinfectant. Contaminated equipment, such as the hemacytometer and coverglass, must be soaked in disinfectant and then washed with laboratory detergent.

Quality Assessment

 Careful attention must be paid to maintaining good technique when performing hemacytometer counts. Since platelets are very small, the hemacytometer must be clean to avoid mistaking dirt particles for platelets. Care must be taken to avoid overfilling the chamber, which would allow the fluid to flow into the moat and alter the cell distribution in the counting chamber.

Because of the tendency of platelets to clump, attention must be paid to distribution of the platelets in the counting chamber. If clumping is seen, the hemacytometer should be cleaned and refilled. If clumping is still seen a new Unopette should be prepared, or the blood sample should be recollected if from a capillary puncture.

After the hemacytometer is filled, the platelets must be allowed to settle for 10 minutes in a moist chamber before performing the count. If cell counts vary by more than 10% between the two sides of the hemacytometer, the count should be repeated.

Collecting the Blood Specimen

Venous blood collected in EDTA is the preferred specimen for platelet counts. Capillary blood can also be used for platelet counts, but venous anticoagulated blood gives better results, because platelets tend to clump rapidly in a capillary sample.

Diluting the Blood Specimen

Using a Unopette system for platelet counts, the diaphragm in the neck of the reservoir is pierced with the pipet shield, making an opening large enough for the capillary pipet. Working behind

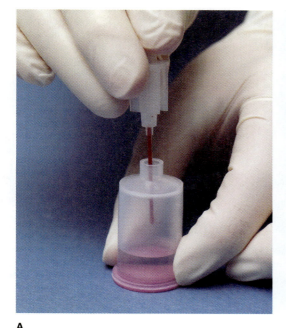

A

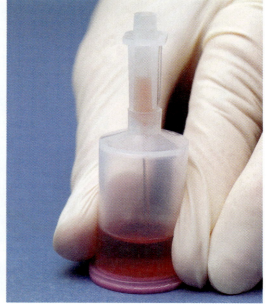

B

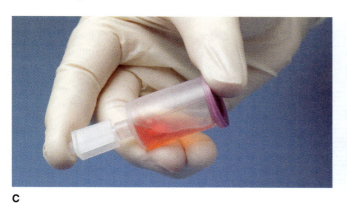

C

FIGURE 2-38 Performing a platelet count using
the Unopette: (A) Press gently on sides of reservoir
and insert filled pipet into reservoir; (B) seat pipet
in neck of reservoir and release pressure to draw blood
into reservoir solution; (C) place gloved finger over pipet
opening and mix reservoir contents by inversion;
(D) remove pipet, reseat pipet in neck of reservoir with
pipet extending upward, and fill the hemacytometer

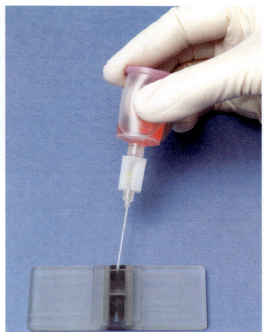

D

an acrylic safety shield, the 20 μL capillary is filled from either a capillary puncture or a tube of well-mixed EDTA blood. The filled capillary pipet is inserted into the reservoir, allowing the blood to mix with the diluting fluid (Figure 2-38). The resulting dilution is 1:100 (20 μL added to 1.98 mL). The reservoir is inverted to mix the contents and then allowed to stand for at least 10 minutes, but no longer than 3 hours, to allow the red blood cells to be lysed (destroyed). After 10 minutes, the reservoir is again swirled to mix the contents, and the pipet assembly is removed and reinserted in the reservoir with the pipet extending upward.

Filling the Hemacytometer Chamber

A clean hemacytometer coverglass is placed on a clean hemacytometer so both sides of the chamber are covered by the coverglass. A few drops of the well-mixed sample are expelled onto laboratory tissue through the capillary pipet. Both sides of the hemacytometer are then filled (Figure 2-38D).

The filled hemacytometer is placed into a covered **petri dish** with moistened filter paper for 10 minutes (Figure 2-39). This provides a moist chamber to prevent evaporation of the

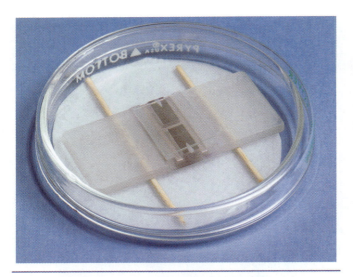

FIGURE 2-39 Hemacytometer in moist chamber (covered petri dish containing moistened filter paper)

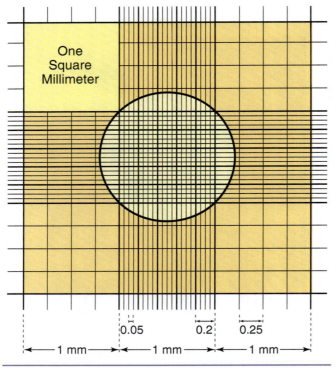

FIGURE 2-40 Platelet counting area. Count platelets in all 25 squares inside the large center square (circled)

solution in the counting chamber while allowing time for the platelets to settle so they can be more accurately counted.

Counting the Platelets

To perform the platelet count, the hemacytometer is removed from the moist chamber and placed on the microscope stage. The low-power (10×) objective is used to locate the counting area. In a platelet count, the entire center square (1 mm²) is counted (Figure 2-40) using the high-power (40×) objective.

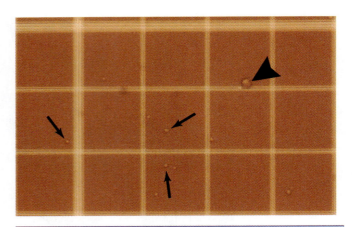

FIGURE 2-41 Photomicrograph of platelets (arrows) as they appear on a hemacytometer (arrowhead points to a WBC)

Manual platelet counts are best performed using a phase-contrast microscope. If a brightfield microscope is used, the platelets can be seen more easily by adjusting the condenser and the light level. The platelets will appear as shiny refractile objects that darken when the fine-adjustment knob is rotated (Figure 2-41). The platelets in *all 25 small squares of the large central square* are counted. The count is performed on both sides of the chamber, and the average of the two sides is calculated. The number of platelets counted on each side should not differ by more than 10%.

Calculating the Platelet Count

The number of platelets per μL of blood is calculated using the general formula:

$$platelets/\mu L = \frac{Avg \times DF}{A\ (mm)^2 \times D\ (0.1\ mm)}$$

To simplify, use the following figures:

1. The platelet average is computed using counts from both sides of the chamber.
2. The dilution factor (DF) is 100.
3. The area (A) counted is 1 mm².

These numbers are substituted into the formula as follows:

$$platelets/\mu L = \frac{Average\ \#\ of\ platelets \times 100}{1 \times 0.1}$$

$$platelets/\mu L = Average\ \#\ of\ platelets \times 1000$$

Therefore, the platelet count can be calculated by simply multiplying the average number of platelets by 1000 (or by adding three zeroes). A sample calculation of a platelet count is shown in Figure 2-42.

AUTOMATED PLATELET COUNTS

Although manual platelet counts are still performed in some laboratories, instruments that perform platelet counts have been used for years. Most hematology analyzers perform platelet counts along with other tests included in the CBC. Lesson 2-13 contains more information on hematology automation.

1. Count the platelets in the entire large center square (1 mm²):

   Side 1 = 166   Side 2 = 170

2. Compute the average:
   A. 166 + 170 = 336 platelets
   B. 336 ÷ 2 = 168 average

3. Calculate the count:

   $$\text{Platelets/}\mu L = \frac{\text{Average \# platelets} \times \text{Dilution factor}}{\text{Area counted (mm}^2) \times D\ (0.1\ \text{mm})}$$

   $$\text{Platelets/}\mu L = \frac{168 \times 100}{1 \times 0.1}$$

   $$\text{Platelets/}\mu L = 168 \times 1000$$

   $$\text{Platelets/}\mu L = 168{,}000\ (\text{or}\ 1.68 \times 10^5)$$

   $$\text{Platelets/L} = 1.68 \times 10^{11}$$

FIGURE 2-42 Sample calculation of platelet count

SAFETY Reminders

- Standard Precautions must be observed when performing manual platelet counts.
- The worker should wear face protection or work behind an acrylic safety shield.
- The hemacytometer and coverglass must be disinfected after each use.

PROCEDURAL Reminders

- The platelet count must be performed within 3 hours of diluting the sample.
- The hemacytometer must be free of dirt and debris before being filled.
- The fluid must not be allowed to overflow into the moats when filling the hemacytometer.
- The high-power (40×) objective must be used to count platelets.
- The microscope condenser, iris diaphragm, and light intensity must be adjusted to provide good contrast when observing and counting platelets.
- If clumps or uneven distribution of platelets are observed, the sample should be remixed and the chamber should be cleaned and refilled. If clumps are still present, a new sample should be obtained.

CASE STUDY

Dr. Jones ordered a manual platelet count on Mrs. Rogers, who reported being frequently and easily bruised. Marco, the technician, counted the platelets in five small squares within the large center square of the hemacytometer and got the following numbers on one side: 13, 14, 12, 15, and 14. On the second side he counted: 13, 12, 16, 14, and 15. Using the standard formula for counting platelets, Marco determined the patient's platelet count was 6.9×10^{10}/L.

Because of the results of the count, Marco reviewed the platelet count procedure in his facility's standard operating procedure manual, and then he immediately repeated the platelet count. His total from side one was 350, and the total from side two was 346.

1. Is the first count normal, high, or low?
2. Calculate the repeat platelet count.
3. Explain why the two counts are different. Which is the correct count? Is the correct count low, normal, or high?

SUMMARY

The platelet count is important because of the role of platelets in stopping bleeding. Although platelet counts are included on hematology cell counters, very low counts can require verification by manual counting. Quality assessment policies must be followed to ensure accurate results. It is important that the technician use a clean hemacytometer and coverglass to avoid having debris counted as platelets. All Standard Precautions for handling blood must be observed. Several factors can affect platelet numbers, causing either increases or decreases in the counts. An extremely low platelet count may create a life-threatening situation, making the accuracy of such counts critical.

REVIEW QUESTIONS

1. Where do platelets originate? What is the function of platelets?
2. Name a condition in which thrombocytosis can occur.
3. Name a cause of thrombocytopenia.
4. Why is it important to thoroughly clean the coverglass and hemacytometer before performing the platelet count?
5. What is the purpose of the moist chamber?
6. What area of the hemacytometer is used to count platelets?
7. State the formula for calculating a platelet count.
8. What blood dilution is used for a platelet count using the Unopette system?
9. What PPE must be worn while performing manual platelet counts?
10. Define petri dish, thrombocytopenia, and thrombocytosis.

STUDENT ACTIVITIES

1. Complete the written examination for this lesson.
2. Practice performing a platelet count as outlined in the Student Performance Guide.
3. Read more about the function of platelets in Lesson 3-1.

WEB 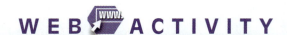 ACTIVITY

Research thrombocytopenia using the Internet: Select a condition listed in Table 2-8 and prepare a report on it. Include cause, symptoms, laboratory findings, treatment, and prognosis. Or find a condition causing thrombocytopenia that is not listed in Table 2-8 and prepare a report on it.

Student Performance Guide

Lesson 2-6 Platelet Count

Name _____ Date _____

INSTRUCTIONS

1. Practice performing a platelet count following the step-by-step procedure.

2. Demonstrate the platelet count procedure satisfactorily for the instructor using the Student Performance Guide. Your instructor will determine the level of competency you must achieve to obtain a satisfactory (S) grade.

NOTE: The following is a general procedure for the use of the Unopette system. Consult the package insert for specific instructions.

MATERIALS AND EQUIPMENT

- gloves
- antiseptic
- capillary puncture supplies
- blood sample, anticoagulated with EDTA
- test-tube rack
- acrylic safety shield or face protection
- hemacytometer with coverglass
- Unopette for platelet count (reservoir and pipet assembly)
- microscope
- materials for moist chamber:
  - petri dish
  - moist cotton ball or moistened filter paper and wooden applicator stick
- lens paper
- alcohol (70% or 95%)
- hand tally counter
- surface disinfectant
- biohazard container
- sharps container
- timer
- laboratory tissue

PROCEDURE

Record in the comment section any problems encountered while practicing the procedure (or have a fellow student or the instructor evaluate your performance).

S = Satisfactory
U = Unsatisfactory

You must:	S	U	Comments
1. Assemble equipment and materials			
2. Place a clean hemacytometer coverglass over a clean hemacytometer			
3. Wash hands and put on gloves			
4. Put on face protection or work behind acrylic safety shield			

229

You must:	S	U	Comments
5. Puncture the diaphragm of the Unopette reservoir. Hold the reservoir firmly on a flat surface with one hand, and use the tip of the pipet shield to puncture the diaphragm. Remove the shield from the pipet assembly **NOTE:** The opening must be made large enough to easily accommodate the pipet			
6. Fill the capillary pipet from a capillary puncture or from a tube of well-mixed EDTA anticoagulated blood. The pipet will fill by capillary action and will stop filling automatically. Be sure no air bubbles are in capillary pipet **NOTE:** Keep pipet horizontal or at a slight (5°) upward angle to avoid overfilling			
7. Wipe excess blood from the outside of the capillary pipet with soft laboratory tissue **NOTE:** Do not allow tissue to touch pipet tip			
8. Squeeze the reservoir slightly, being careful not to expel any of the liquid			
9. Maintain the pressure on the reservoir and insert the capillary pipet into the reservoir, seating the pipet firmly in the neck of the reservoir. Do not expel any of the liquid			
10. Release the pressure on the reservoir, drawing the blood out of the capillary pipet into the diluent			
11. Squeeze the reservoir gently 3 to 4 times to rinse the remaining blood from the capillary pipet **NOTE:** Do not allow the blood-diluent mixture to flow out the top			
12. Mix the contents of the reservoir thoroughly by gently swirling the reservoir or tilting it from side to side			
13. Let reservoir stand at least 10 minutes but no longer than 3 hours			
14. Prepare a moist chamber using a petri dish and a slightly moist cotton ball or moist filter paper			
15. Withdraw the capillary pipet from the reservoir, and place it in the neck of the reservoir in reverse position (the pipet tip should now project upward from the reservoir)			
16. Mix the contents of the reservoir thoroughly. Invert the reservoir and gently squeeze to discard 4 to 5 drops onto laboratory tissue			
17. Fill both sides of the hemacytometer using the capillary pipet, using care not to overfill			
18. Place the hemacytometer in the petri dish. If using a moist cotton ball, do not allow it to touch the hemacytometer			

You must:	S	U	Comments
19. Place the cover on the petri dish and allow the preparation to stand 10 minutes (this permits the platelets to settle in the chamber). Do not wait longer than 30 minutes to complete the platelet count			
20. Place the hemacytometer on the microscope stage carefully and securely			
21. Use the low-power (10×) objective to bring the ruled area into focus			
22. Locate the large central square			
23. Rotate the high-power (40×) objective into position carefully and focus with the fine-adjustment knob until the ruled lines are in focus			
24. Lower the condenser and reduce the light by partially closing the diaphragm for best contrast. Platelets should appear as round or oval particles that are refractile and smaller than red blood cells			
25. Count the platelets in the entire center square of the ruled area (all 25 small squares) using the left-to-right, right-to-left counting pattern and record results			
26. Repeat the count on the other side of the hemacytometer			
27. Average the results from the two sides			
28. Calculate the platelet count: $$\text{platelets}/\mu L = \frac{\text{Avg} \times \text{DF}}{A\,(\text{mm}^2) \times D\,(0.1\,\text{mm})}$$ or $$\text{platelets}/\mu L = \text{average \# platelets} \times 1000$$			
29. Record the results			
30. Disinfect hemacytometer and coverglass with surface disinfectant and then wash them			
31. Discard specimen as directed by instructor and Unopette assembly into sharps container			
32. Return equipment to proper storage			
33. Clean work area with surface disinfectant			
34. Remove and discard gloves in biohazard container			
35. Wash hands with antiseptic			

Evaluator Comments:

Evaluator _____ Date _____

Preparing and Staining a Blood Smear

LESSON OBJECTIVES

After studying this lesson, the student will:

- Explain the purpose of staining blood smears.
- Explain what information can be obtained from a stained blood smear.
- List the blood components that can be observed in a stained blood smear.
- Prepare a blood smear.
- Preserve a blood smear.
- Stain a blood smear.
- List five features of a properly prepared blood smear.
- List the safety precautions to observe when preparing and staining a blood smear.
- Explain how the preparing and staining of blood smears can affect the quality of blood smears.
- Define the glossary terms.

GLOSSARY

buffer / a substance that lessens change in the pH of a solution when acid or base (alkali) is added

cytoplasm / the fluid portion of the cell surrounding the nucleus

eosin / a red-orange stain or dye

fixative / preservative; a chemical that prevents deterioration of cells or tissues

methylene blue / a blue stain or dye

morphology / the form and structure of cells, tissues, and organs

nucleus (pl. nuclei) / the central structure of a cell that contains DNA and controls cell growth and function

polychromatic / having many colors

Wright's stain / a combination of eosin and methylene blue in methanol; a polychromatic stain

INTRODUCTION

The examination of a stained blood smear is a routine part of the complete blood count (CBC). Stains are applied to blood smears so the formed elements—red blood cells, white blood cells, and platelets—can be viewed, identified, and evaluated using the microscope, as in the differential count. A properly prepared blood smear enables the technologist to view the cellular components of blood in as natural a state as possible. The **morphology**, or structure, of the cellular components can be studied.

Careful examination of a well-prepared stained blood smear can provide valuable information to the physician for diagnosing and treating diseases as diverse as infectious mononucleosis, leukemia, sickle cell anemia, and malaria.

Information gained during routine evaluation of blood smears may lead the physician to order special blood stains for further study. These special stains are used to identify specific components of cells such as iron granules or nucleic acids.

PREPARING A BLOOD SMEAR

Safety Precautions

  Standard Precautions must be observed when preparing and staining blood smears. Gloves, protective eye wear, and a fluid-resistant laboratory coat must be worn when making and staining smears. Since most blood stains contain methanol, which is toxic, care should be taken to avoid skin contact or inhalation of fumes. Slides should be handled with care to prevent accidental cuts. Injury from glass slides can be avoided by using beveled-edge, rounded-corner slides. Once used, slides must be discarded in sharps containers.

Quality Assessment

  Blood smears must be prepared in a manner that minimally alters the distribution and morphology of the cells. Specimens must be collected properly. Anticoagulated blood must be well mixed before smears are made. Only EDTA anticoagulant should be used because other anticoagulants can alter the morphology and staining characteristics of the cells. Smears should be made within 2 hours of blood collection. Smears should be stained when dry or at least within 1 hour of being prepared. Exact staining times for the method being used must be followed.

Slides

Slides used for blood smears must be free of grease and dust. Slides can be purchased precleaned or washed with soap and water, rinsed thoroughly in hot water and then distilled water, dipped in 95% ethanol, and polished with a clean, lint-free cloth. Clean slides can be stored in 95% ethanol and should be handled by the edges only. Slides with frosted ends are preferred because they are easily labeled.

Collecting the Blood Specimen

The preferred specimen for blood smears is capillary blood that has no added anticoagulant. Capillary blood can be applied directly to the slide from the puncture site or can be collected in plain capillary tubes and then dispensed onto the slides. A satisfactory smear can also be made from venous blood that has the anticoagulant EDTA added to it, provided the smear is made within 2 hours of collection.

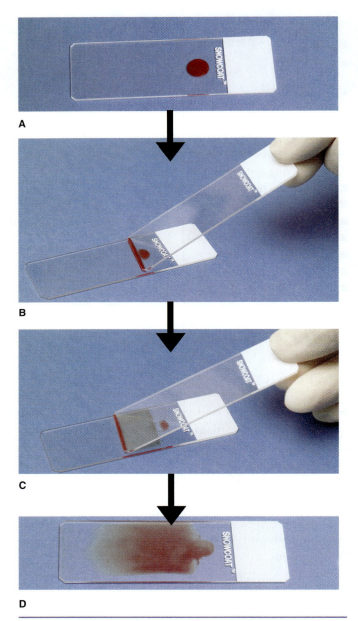

A

B

C

D

FIGURE 2-43 Making a blood smear: (A) dispense one drop of blood onto end of slide; (B) using a spreader slide, gently bring the back edge of the spreader slide into contact with the drop of blood; (C and D) quickly and gently push the spreader slide forward to make the smear

Making the Smear

Several methods of spreading blood on a slide can result in good smears. Each individual needs to find the technique that is least awkward and provides good results. Tubes of anticoagulated blood must be mixed for at least 2 minutes by mechanical mixer or inverted gently 60 times by hand before the smear is made.

Two-Slide Method (Wedge Method)

The blood smear can be prepared by placing a small drop of well-mixed blood about one-half to three-quarters of an inch from the right end (left end for left-handed) of a precleaned slide placed on a flat surface (Figure 2-43A). The end of a second "spreader" slide is brought to rest at a 30° to 35° angle in front of the drop of blood (Figure 2-43B). The spreader is then brought back into the drop of blood until the drop spreads along three-quarters of the edge of the spreader slide (Figure 2-43C). As soon as the blood spreads along the edge of the spreader, the spreader is pushed to the left (right for left-handed) with a quick, steady motion (avoiding pressure on the slide) to spread the blood into a thin film (Figure 2-43D).

Each end of the spreader slide should be used only once, and then the slide should be discarded in a sharps container. The smear is placed in a slide-drying rack and allowed to air-dry as quickly as possible. It is then ready for staining or preserving.

DIFF-SAFE

Devices such as DIFF-SAFE by Alpha Scientific eliminate the need to remove the stopper from a tube of blood to make a blood smear (Figure 2-44). When used properly, the dispenser deposits an appropriately sized drop of blood onto the slide, without the necessity of opening the blood-collection tube.

DiffSpin Method

The DiffSpin Slide Spinner is a centrifuge that produces uniform, monolayer blood smears that can be stained for differential counts (Figure 2-45). This method eliminates differences in smear quality due to technique and allows all personnel to make quality smears. Because the cells on these smears are uniformly distributed, cell distribution may be slightly different from that obtained when making smears using the two-slide (wedge) technique.

Preserving the Smear

If a dried smear cannot be stained immediately, it can be preserved by immersing in methanol for 30 to 60 seconds and then air-dried. The methanol is a **fixative**, or preservative, that prevents changes or deterioration of the cellular components. Slides preserved in this way can be stained at a later date.

Features of a Good Blood Smear

A well-prepared smear is illustrated in Figures 2-43D and 2-46A. The smear should cover about one-half to three-fourths of the slide and should show a gradual transition from thick to thin. It should have a smooth appearance, with no holes or ridges, and should have a feathered edge (about 1.5 cm long) at the thin end. When the smear is examined microscopically, the cells should be distributed evenly, and there should be an area at the thin end where red blood cells are not overlapping.

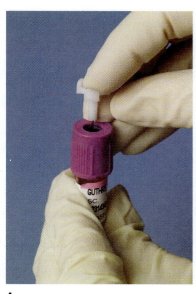
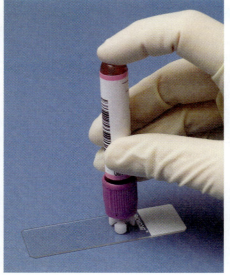
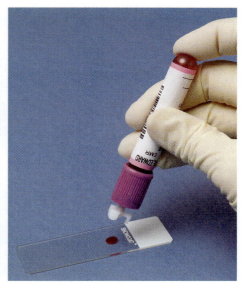

A   **B**   **C**

FIGURE 2-44 DIFF-SAFE blood dispensing device: (A) insert DIFF-SAFE cannula through rubber stopper; (B) invert tube and press against slide; (C) a drop of blood is dispensed onto slide

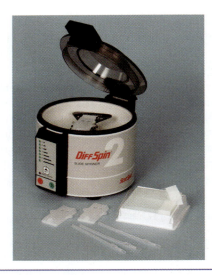

FIGURE 2-45 DiffSpin 2 Slide Spinner produces a monolayer blood smear in seconds (*Courtesy of StatSpin, Inc., Norwood, MA*)

Factors Affecting Blood Smear Quality

Several factors can affect the quality of the blood smear (Table 2-9). The length and thickness of the smear are affected by:

- The size of the drop of blood
- The angle at which the spreader slide is held
- The speed at which the blood is spread

Thick, short smears occur when the angle of the spreader is too high or the drop of blood is too large. Thin smears occur when the blood drop is too small, the angle of the spreader slide is too low, or too much pressure is applied to the spreader. In the latter case, the smear may also be uneven. In general, the more rapid the spreading procedure, the thinner the smear. Too much pressure on the spreader slide can also push most of the white blood cells to the end of the slide. This affects the distribution of the types of white blood cells and decreases the number of white blood cells seen in the rest of the smear.

Drying time can affect the appearance of the cellular elements. If high humidity causes slow drying, the cells can appear abnormal. For example, the red blood cells may appear to have holes in them.

STAINING A BLOOD SMEAR

The **Wright's stain** commonly used for the routine microscopic examination of blood is a **polychromatic** stain. It contains a combination of **methylene blue**, a basic dye that gives a blue stain; **eosin**, an acid dye that gives a red-orange stain; and methanol, a fixative.

Some structures, such as cell nuclei, attract the basic dyes and stain blue or purple. Other cell structures attract the acid dyes and stain pink-red. The cells and structures are thus more

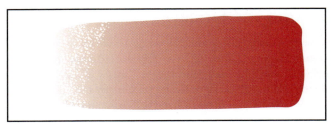

A

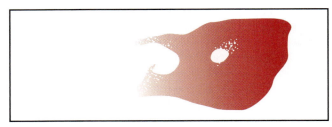

B

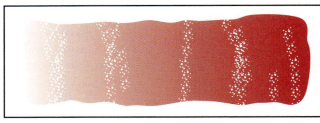

C

FIGURE 2-46 Properly prepared smear (A) versus improperly prepared smears (B and C)

easily visualized and differentiated (hence the name differential count). The two most commonly used blood stains in the United States are Wright's stain and Giemsa stain.

Staining Procedures

Smears can be stained by a quick stain method, two-step method, or an automatic stainer. A quick-stain is adequate for most routine work, but the two-step method (or automatic stainer) should be used to evaluate cell abnormalities and bone marrow cells.

Quick Stains

Quick stains are available in kits from several companies. These stains are modifications of Wright's stain. The kits contain three separate components: a fixative, a red dye such as eosin, and a blue dye such as methylene blue (Figure 2-47).

To perform a quick stain, the smear is dipped sequentially into the staining solution(s) for a specified length of time and then it is rinsed and air-dried. The entire quick-staining method takes only 2 to 5 minutes. It may be easier for the inexperienced technician to obtain an adequate stain with quick methods, but

TABLE 2-9. Common problems in preparing blood smears and the possible causes

PROBLEM	POSSIBLE CAUSE(S)
Smear too thin or too long	Drop of blood too small Spreader slide at too low an angle Improper speed in making smear
Smear too thick or too short	Drop of blood too large Spreader slide at too high an angle Improper speed in making smear
Ridges or waves in smear	Uneven pressure on spreader slide Hesitation in pushing spreader slide
Holes in smear	Slides not clean Uneven or dirty edge of spreader slide
Uneven cell distribution	Uneven pressure during spread of blood Delay in spreading blood Uneven or dirty edge of spreader slide
Artifacts or unusual cell appearance	Smear dried too slowly Smear not fixed within 1 hour after preparation High humidity

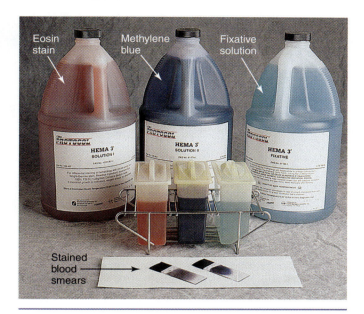

FIGURE 2-47 A quick stain kit for staining blood smears

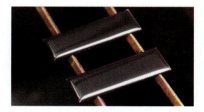

FIGURE 2-48 Staining blood smears on a simple slide-staining rack

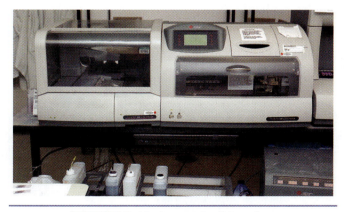

FIGURE 2-49 Automatic slide stainer

experienced technicians can achieve superior results using the two-step method.

Two-Step Method

In a two-step method, a smear is placed on a staining rack and flooded with Wright's stain (Figure 2-48). Fixation occurs in this step because of the methanol in the stain. After approximately 1 to 3 minutes, an equal volume of **buffer** is added dropwise to the stain, mixing the stain and buffer together. A buffer is a substance that prevents changes in the pH of a solution when acid or alkali is added. A green metallic sheen appears when the solutions mix, usually within 2 to 4 minutes. Times may vary according to the stain and buffer used. The slide is rinsed gently, allowed to air-dry, and can then be examined using the microscope.

Automatic Stainers

There are two basic types of automatic slide stainers. In one type, the slides are placed on a moving belt, which carries them through the staining reagents (Figure 2-49). Another type of stainer is the "basket" or "batch" type, in which baskets of slides are taken stepwise through the staining process. One basket of slides is fixed, then dipped into the stain solution, and so on. This is continued throughout the complete staining process.

Automatic stainers are helpful when large numbers of slides must be stained or staining must be performed frequently during a workday. A disadvantage of automatic stainers is that if the stain solutions are not working correctly, many slides may be processed before the technician becomes aware of the problem.

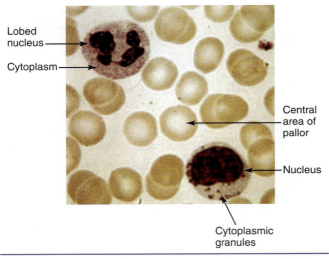

Lobed nucleus

Cytoplasm

Central area of pallor

Nucleus

Cytoplasmic granules

FIGURE 2-50 Stained blood cells neutrophil (top left), lymphocyte (bottom right), red blood cells, and platelet (top right) (*Courtesy of Abbott Laboratories, Abbott Park, IL*)

Evaluating Stain Quality

A properly stained smear should appear pinkish-blue to the naked eye. When viewed microscopically, the red blood cells should appear pink-tan. The **nucleus**, or central structure, of the leukocytes should appear purple. The leukocyte **cytoplasm**, or area surrounding the nucleus, will vary from pink to blue or blue-gray, depending on the cell type (Figure 2-50). Inconsistencies in color or staining intensity can be caused by variations in pH, timing, or characteristics of the stain or buffer and are best evaluated using the oil-immersion objective.

- Smears that are too pink may be due to the stain time being too short, the wash time being too long, or the pH of the stain or buffer being too acidic.
- Smears that are too blue may be due to overstaining, wash or buffering time being too short, or the pH of the stain or buffer being too alkaline.

STORAGE OF BLOOD SMEARS

Stained (or preserved) smears should be stored in the dark in a dust-free slide box or container. If protected from light and moisture, stained smears will last for years, with little fading. The smear can be protected from scratches by mounting a permanent coverglass over it. For routine work, however, this is not necessary.

SUMMARY

A properly prepared and stained peripheral blood smear can contribute valuable information toward diagnosis and treatment of a patient. It is essential that the smear is made and stained correctly. Blood smears can be made by a variety of methods, but the two-slide method is most frequently used. Capillary blood is the best specimen, but venous blood collected in EDTA can be used if the smear is made within 2 hours of collection. The most common blood stain is Wright's stain, a polychromatic stain combining eosin and methylene blue in the fixative, methanol. Instructions for the particular stain being used must be followed exactly. The physician can use the information from a blood smear report for diagnosis and treatment of a patient. Therefore, the smear must present an accurate representation of cells in the peripheral blood.

PROCEDURAL Reminders

- Use a spreader slide with a clean, polished end.
- Use the proper size drop of blood to make the slide.
- Use proper angle on spreader slide.
- Spread capillary blood immediately to avoid clotting.
- Avoid hesitation or jerky motion when spreading the blood.
- Preserve or stain smears within 1 hour after preparation.
- Store stains tightly capped to prevent evaporation or absorption of moisture.
- Do not allow stain to dry on the slide before rinsing.
- Rinse slides thoroughly after staining.
- Observe proper staining and/or buffering times.

SAFETY Reminders

- Observe Standard Precautions when preparing and handling blood smears.
- Handle products containing methanol with care; do not inhale fumes or allow skin contact.
- Wear gloves and fluid-resistant laboratory coat and handle slides with forceps.
- Use beveled-edge, rounded-corner slides.
- Handle glass slides carefully to prevent accidental cuts.

CASE STUDY

Vidya worked in the hematology laboratory of a small hospital. The laboratory's hematology procedure manual contained instructions for staining blood smears by the two-step method, and called for applying the stain for 2 minutes and the buffer for 2 minutes. Vidya stained three patient blood smears, but the smears appeared bluer than normal. When she examined the smears microscopically, the cells also appeared blue, making it difficult to identify them.

1. What can cause blood smears to stain too blue?
2. Discuss factors that could have affected the stain results.

REVIEW QUESTIONS

1. What is the purpose of staining blood smears?

2. What specimen(s) can be used to prepare blood smears?

3. What blood components can be viewed on a stained smear?

4. Explain the two-slide method for making a blood smear.

5. What are some errors to avoid when making a blood smear?

6. Describe and diagram the appearance of a properly prepared blood smear.

7. How can unstained blood smears be preserved?

8. Explain what is meant by polychromatic stains.

9. Name two commonly used blood stains.

10. How should a properly stained smear appear?

11. What is the proper method of storing preserved or stained slides?

12. Name three factors that can affect staining results.

13. Define buffer, cytoplasm, eosin, fixative, methylene blue, morphology, nucleus, polychromatic, and Wright's stain.

STUDENT ACTIVITIES

1. Complete the written examination for this lesson.

2. Practice preparing and staining blood smears by the two-step and/or quick-stain method as outlined in the Student Performance Guide.

3. Compare smears stained by the two-step and quick-stain methods. Which method produced the most desired effect?

4. Experiment with variations in staining and buffering times using the two-step method. Explain the results.

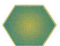

Student Performance Guide

Lesson 2-7 Preparing and Staining a Blood Smear

Name _____ Date _____

INSTRUCTIONS

1. Practice preparing and staining a blood smear following the step-by-step procedure.

2. Demonstrate the procedure for preparing and staining a blood smear satisfactorily for the instructor, using the Student Performance Guide. Your instructor will determine the level of competency you must achieve to receive a satisfactory (S) grade.

NOTE: Stain characteristics may vary with stain lot. Follow manufacturer's instructions for best results.

MATERIALS AND EQUIPMENT

- face protection or acrylic safety shield
- gloves
- antiseptic
- slide storage box
- pencil or pen for labeling slides
- microscope slides (1" × 3"), beveled-edge, rounded corners, frosted-end optional
- 95% ethanol
- laboratory tissue
- plastic or mylar-sheathed capillary tubes (plain and heparinized)
- slide-drying rack
- DIFF-SAFE (optional)
- methanol in covered staining (Coplin) jar
- EDTA anticoagulated blood specimen
- capillary puncture supplies
- surface disinfectant
- biohazard container
- sharps container
- blood stain reagents: Wright's stain and buffer, or commercial blood stain kit (quick stain)
- staining rack
- immersion oil
- microscope
- lens paper
- lens cleaner
- forceps
- staining jars for quick stains
- timer

PROCEDURE

Record in the comment section any problems encountered while practicing the procedure (or have a fellow student or the instructor evaluate your performance).

S = Satisfactory
U = Unsatisfactory

You must:	S	U	Comments
1. Assemble equipment and materials			

You must:	S	U	Comments

2. Obtain several clean slides:
  a. Use precleaned slides, or
  b. Clean slides with 95% ethanol, and polish dry with clean lint-free cloth			

3. Prepare blood smears following steps 3a through 3l:
  a. Place a clean slide on a flat surface (be sure to touch only the edges of the slide with fingers). Write patient identification on slide
  b. Wash hands and put on face protection and gloves
  c. Obtain an anticoagulated blood sample (provided by the instructor)
  d. Mix blood well and fill a plain capillary tube with blood or use DIFF-SAFE
  e. Dispense a small drop of blood onto the slide about one-half to three-quarters of an inch from the right end (if left-handed, reverse instructions)
  f. Place the end of a clean, polished, unchipped spreader slide in front of the drop of blood at a 30° to 35° angle. Spreader should be lightly balanced with fingertips
  g. Pull the spreader slide back into the drop of blood by sliding it gently along the slide until the blood spreads along three-fourths of the width of the spreader
  h. Push the spreader slide forward with a quick steady motion (use other hand to keep slide from moving while spreader is pushed)
  i Examine the smear to see if it is satisfactory
  j. Repeat steps 3a–3i until two satisfactory smears are obtained
  k. Perform a capillary puncture, wipe away the first drop of blood, and fill one or two capillary tubes
  l. Prepare two blood smears from capillary blood, repeating steps 3e–3j			

4. Allow the smear(s) to air-dry quickly (stand slides on end in slide-drying rack)			
5. Place the dried smears in absolute methanol for 30 to 60 seconds			
6. Remove the slides from the methanol and allow to air-dry			
7. Store slides for staining or proceed to step 9			
8. Discard blood specimens appropriately or store for later use. Place contaminated materials in biohazard or sharps container			

You must:	S	U	Comments

9. Stain blood smears by the two-step method (9a) and/ or quick stain method (9b)
  a. Stain a blood smear by the two-step method:
    (1) Place the dried smear on the staining rack, blood side up
    (2) Flood the smear with Wright's stain, but do not let stain overflow the sides of the slide
    (3) Leave stain on slide 1 to 3 minutes (get exact time from instructor)
    (4) Add buffer drop by drop to the stain until buffer volume is about equal to that of the stain
    (5) A green metallic sheen should appear on the surface
    (6) Allow buffer to remain on slide for 2 to 4 minutes (do not allow mixture to run off slide); get exact time from instructor
    (7) Rinse thoroughly and continuously with a gentle stream of tap or distilled water
    (8) Drain water from slide
    (9) Wipe the *back* of the slide with a laboratory tissue to remove excess stain
    (10) Stand smear on end to dry
  b. Stain a smear using quick stain:
    (1) Dip dried smear into solutions as directed by manufacturer's instructions (do not allow slide to dry between solutions)
    (2) Rinse slide (if instructed to do so)
    (3) Remove excess stain from the *back* of the slide with laboratory tissue
    (4) Allow slide to air-dry by standing on end			

10. Observe stained smears microscopically:
  a. Place thoroughly dried slide on microscope stage, stain side up. Be sure objectives and eyepieces are clean
  b. Focus with low-power (10×) objective
  c. Scan slide to find area where cells are barely touching each other (in feathered edge of smear)
  d. Place a drop of immersion oil on the slide
  e. Rotate oil-immersion lens carefully into position
  f. Focus with fine-adjustment knob only
  g. Observe erythrocytes; color should be pink-tan
  h. Observe leukocytes; nuclei should be purple; neutrophil granules should be pink-lavender
  i. Observe platelets; they should appear purple and granular			

You must:	S	U	Comments
11. Rotate the low-power (10×) objective into position			
12. Remove slide from microscope stage			
13. Clean oil objective thoroughly with lens paper and lens cleaner			
14. Blot oil from slide gently with soft tissue			
15. Clean equipment and return to proper storage			
16. Discard slides as instructed or store in slide box for use in Lesson 2-8			
17. Clean work area with surface disinfectant			
18. Remove and discard gloves in biohazard container and wash hands with antiseptic			

Evaluator Comments:

Evaluator _____ Date _____

Normal Blood Cell Morphology

LESSON OBJECTIVES

After studying this lesson, the student will:

- State the importance of blood cell identification.
- List three features of cells that are evaluated during blood cell identification.
- Use the microscope to identify five types of white blood cells from a stained, normal blood smear.
- Identify platelets microscopically.
- Identify red blood cells microscopically.
- Discuss safety precautions involved in the microscopic examination of blood smears.
- Explain how quality assessment affects the results of blood cell identification.
- Define the glossary terms.

GLOSSARY

band cell / an immature granulocyte with a nonsegmented nucleus; a "stab cell"

basophil / a leukocyte containing basophilic-staining granules in the cytoplasm

basophilic / blue in color; having affinity for the basic stain

eosinophil / a leukocyte containing eosinophilic granules in the cytoplasm

lymphocyte / a small basophilic-staining leukocyte having a round or oval nucleus and playing a vital role in the immune process

megakaryocyte / a large bone marrow cell from which platelets are derived

monocyte / a large leukocyte usually having a convoluted or horseshoe-shaped nucleus

neutrophil / a neutral-staining leukocyte; usually the first line of defense against infection

platelet / a formed element in circulatory blood that plays an important role in blood coagulation; a small disk-shaped fragment of cytoplasm derived from a megakaryocyte; a thrombocyte

vacuole / a membrane-bound compartment in cell cytoplasm

INTRODUCTION

Hematology technologists must be experienced in identifying normal blood cells and in detecting abnormal blood cells. Much information can be gained from the observation of the cellular components of the blood on a stained peripheral blood smear. The report on blood cell morphology combined with results from the red blood cell counts and white blood cell counts can often provide the physician the information needed to aid in diagnosis and treatment of the patient.

The examination of the stained blood smear, including the evaluation of cellular components, and the determination of the relative numbers of white blood cells is called the *white blood cell differential count*. The student or technician must become proficient in identifying normal blood cells and abnormal blood cells before being permitted to report a differential count. The procedure for the differential count is outlined in Lesson 2-9.

STUDYING BLOOD CELL MORPHOLOGY FROM A STAINED BLOOD SMEAR

The feathered edge of the stained smear should be located using the low power (10×) objective of the microscope (Figure 2-51). In this area the cells are not overlapping and the red blood cells are just touching each other. The feathered edge of the smear is then examined using the oil-immersion objective. The condenser of the microscope should be raised until it almost touches the bottom of the slide being examined. With the diaphragm open, the light should be bright enough to allow the features of the stained cells to be visible. In the feathered edge, the cells are slightly flattened and cellular structures are more easily seen.

Safety Precautions

Stained dry blood smears are not a biological hazard. However, microscope slides must be handled carefully to avoid accidental cuts on hands and fingers. Used slides must be discarded into a sharps container.

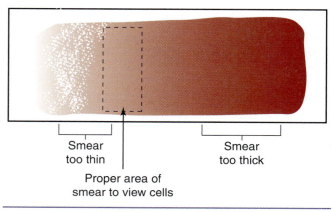

Smear too thin   Smear too thick

Proper area of smear to view cells

FIGURE 2-51 Proper area of the smear to view for identification of blood cells

Quality Assessment

It is important that blood smears be properly prepared and stained in order to be able to study blood cell morphology and easily identify cells. The smear must be allowed to air-dry completely before the stain is applied to avoid distorting the cell morphology. The stain should be free of precipitate that could obscure cellular features and cause confusion in identification. The smear must have a feathered edge and an area where the red cells are just touching each other. The cells in this area must be evenly distributed to represent the actual distribution of cell types in the blood. The feathered edge of the smear should be examined to be sure that a large number of white blood cells were not pushed to the end of the smear because of use of excessive pressure on the spreader slide. Good smear preparation and staining techniques along with competency in cell morphology can ensure that blood cells are correctly identified.

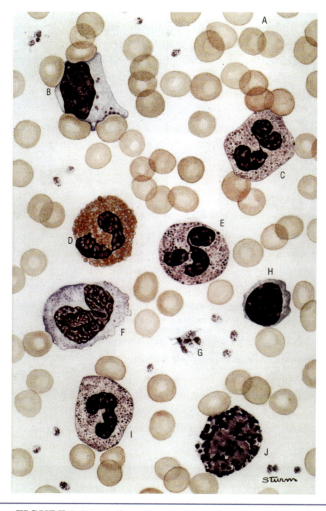

FIGURE 2-52 Cells present in normal peripheral blood
(A) red blood cells; (B) large lymphocyte; (C) neutrophil;
(D) eosinophil; (E) neutrophil; (F) monocyte; (G) platelets;
(H) small lymphocyte; (I) band cell; (J) basophil
(*Courtesy of Abbott Laboratories, Abbott Park, IL*)

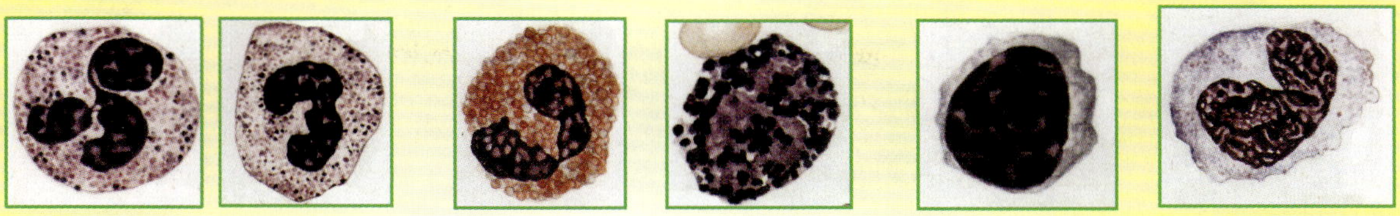

	Neutrophilic Series		Eosinophil	Basophil	Lymphocyte	Monocyte
	Segmented (mature)	Band or Stab (immature)				
Cell Size (μm)	10–15	10–15	10–15	10–15	8–15	12–20
Nucleus						
Shape	2–5 lobes	Sausage or U-shaped	Bilobed	Segmented	Round, oval	Horseshoe
Structure	Coarse	Coarse	Coarse	Difficult to see	Smoothly stained, velvety	Folded, convoluted
Cytoplasm						
Amount	Abundant	Abundant	Abundant	Abundant	Scant	Abundant
Color	Pale pink-tan	Pale pink-tan	Pale pink-tan	Pale pink-tan	Blue	Gray-blue
Inclusions	Small, lilac granules	Small, lilac granules	Coarse, orange-red granules	Coarse, blue-black granules	Occasional red-purple granules	Ground-glass appearance

FIGURE 2-53 White blood cell identification guide

BLOOD CELL MORPHOLOGY

The formed elements of the blood normally seen in a stained blood smear include the red blood cells (erythrocytes), white blood cells (leukocytes), and platelets (Figure 2-52). By careful evaluation of the staining characteristics of these formed elements in a stained blood smear, blood cell morphology can be learned.

Identification of Blood Cells in a Normal Blood Smear

The cells usually seen in a normal blood smear are described in the following sections. The descriptions are for cells as they would appear in a Wright's-stained smear using the oil-immersion objective. A white blood cell identification guide with abbreviated descriptions is given in Figure 2-53.

Cellular Features Evaluated in Identification

Red blood cells and platelets are relatively easy to identify on a stained smear. However, the white blood cells are more difficult to identify and classify; they can be classified by evaluating three features:

- Relative cell size
- Nuclear characteristics
- Cytoplasmic characteristics

The size of white blood cells can be estimated by comparing them to the size of red blood cells. The nucleus is observed for shape, size, structure, and color. The cytoplasm is evaluated by noting the color, amount, and type of granules. When the information from these three observations is combined, most normal white blood cells can be identified (Figure 2-53).

Beginners will find it necessary to consciously consider each of the cell properties as they try to identify cells. As experience is gained, the process becomes almost automatic for normal cells. Much practice is required to be able to recognize and classify abnormal cells that may be seen in various disease states.

Red Blood Cells

Red blood cells are the most numerous of the blood cells. Red blood cells in the peripheral blood do not have a nucleus. Normally, a red blood cell loses its nucleus before it enters the peripheral blood, causing it to have a flattened disk-like appearance, often called a biconcave disk. Normal mature red blood cells stain pink-tan, have no nucleus, and are 6 to 8 μm in diameter (Figures 2-52, 2-54B, and 2-55). The pink-tan color is due to the staining of hemoglobin within the cells. Because red blood cells are thin in the center, the central area of the cells stain lighter than the margins. This is called the "central area of pallor."

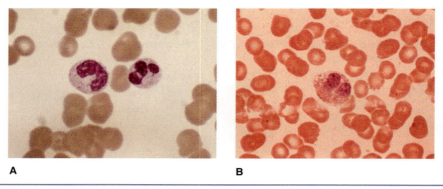

A   B

FIGURE 2-54 Photomicrographs of cells in peripheral blood: (A) band cell (left) and neutrophil (right); (B) eosinophil

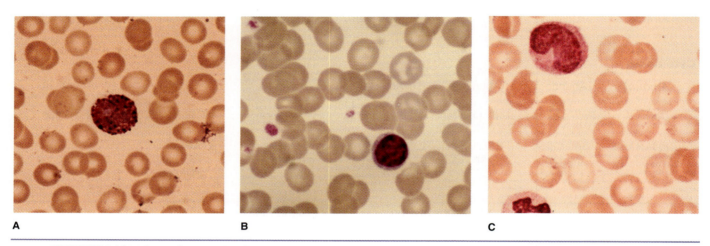

A   B   C

FIGURE 2-55 Photomicrographs of cells in peripheral blood: (A) basophil; (B) small lymphocyte; and (C) monocyte

Platelets

Platelets (thrombocytes) are the smallest of the formed blood elements, being about 2 to 3 μm in diameter, or about one-third the diameter of a red blood cell. Platelets are not cells but are fragments of cytoplasm from a larger cell, the **megakaryocyte**, found in the bone marrow. The platelet cytoplasm stains bluish and usually contains small reddish-purple granules (Figure 2-52). Platelets can be round or oval or can have spiny projections.

White Blood Cells

White blood cells are the largest of the normal blood components. Their sizes range from just slightly larger than a red blood cell (8 μm) to a diameter of 20 μm. Each of the five types of white blood cells has a characteristic appearance (Figure 2-53). The granular white blood cells—neutrophil, eosinophil, and basophil—contain many distinctive cytoplasmic granules, and each usually has a segmented nucleus. The lymphocyte and monocyte have few, if any, easily visible cytoplasmic granules and each has a nonsegmented nucleus.

Neutrophil

The granular white blood cell with neutral-staining cytoplasmic granules is called a **neutrophil**. The neutrophil nucleus is usually segmented into two to five lobes, each connected by a strand or filament. The nucleus stains a dark purple and has a coarse, clumped appearance. The cytoplasm is pale pink to tan and contains fine pink or lilac granules. The neutrophil is about twice the diameter of an erythrocyte and is the most numerous leukocyte in normal adult blood (Figures 2-53 and 2-54A). Other names for the neutrophil are *PMN* (polymorphonuclear neutrophil), *poly*, or *seg*.

A younger, or more immature stage, of the neutrophil is called a **band cell**. The staining characteristics are similar to that of the neutrophil. However, the nucleus is not segmented but is shaped like a curved sausage (Figures 2-53 and 2-54A).

Eosinophil

The **eosinophil** is the white blood cell with granules that have an affinity for the eosin portion of the stain. The nucleus of the eosinophil is usually divided into two or three lobes and stains purple. The cytoplasm is pink-tan but may be difficult to see because it is filled with large red-orange (eosinophilic) granules (Figures 2-53 and 2-54B). Eosinophils are approximately the size of **neutrophils** but are much less numerous in the peripheral blood.

Basophil

The **basophil** is the white blood cell with granules that have an affinity for the basic portion of the stain. The basophil nucleus is segmented and stains light purple. The nuclear shape is often difficult to see because numerous coarse blue-black granules often obscure the nucleus and the cytoplasm (Figures 2-53 and 2-55A). Basophils are only seen occasionally in smears from normal blood.

Lymphocyte

The **lymphocytes** are the smallest of the white blood cells. Although most lymphocytes are only slightly larger than a red blood cell, some can be twice the diameter of a red blood cell and are called large lymphocytes. The lymphocyte nucleus usually has a rather smooth appearance, a round or oval shape, and stains purple. The cytoplasm is **basophilic** (blue) and varies in amount. Occasionally, a few red-purple (azurophilic) granules are present in lymphocyte cytoplasm (Figures 2-53 and 2-55B).

Monocyte

The **monocyte** is the largest circulating white blood cell. The monocyte nucleus can be oval, indented, or horseshoe-shaped and can have brain-like convolutions or folds. The cytoplasm is gray-blue and often has an irregular outline. Very fine granules are distributed throughout the cytoplasm, giving it a dull, ground-glass appearance. **Vacuoles,** membrane-bound compartments in the cytoplasm, can also be present (Figures 2-53 and 2-55C).

PROCEDURAL Reminders

- Observe cells in an area of the smear where red blood cells are just touching.
- Raise the microscope condenser and open the iris diaphragm for maximum light.
- Consult an experienced technologist for assistance in identifying cells.

SUMMARY

The identification of cells in normal peripheral blood is an important requirement of laboratory work. Much valuable information can be learned from the examination of a blood smear. Learning to identify the various types of blood cells and to recognize the differences between normal and abnormal cells can be an interesting and absorbing process. Many visual aids are available to help with blood cell identification, but nothing replaces the experience gained from examining many well-prepared, stained smears of peripheral blood. The basic requirements for learning blood cell morphology are a well-prepared and stained blood smear, a good color atlas of blood cells, an experienced technician to teach and guide, and a strong desire to learn.

REVIEW QUESTIONS

1. Why is it important to identify blood cells?
2. What three features of cells are evaluated during cell identification?
3. List the five types of white blood cells.
4. What is the source of platelets?
5. Describe the area of the smear used to identify blood cells.
6. Describe the microscopic appearance of stained red blood cells.
7. What features of platelets should be noted on a stained blood smear?
8. What color granules are present in neutrophils? Eosinophils? Basophils?
9. Define band cell, basophil, basophilic, eosinophil, lymphocyte, megakaryocyte, monocyte, neutrophil, platelet, and vacuole.

STUDENT ACTIVITIES

1. Complete the written examination for this lesson.
2. Practice blood cell identification as outlined in the Student Performance Guide, using the worksheet.
3. Practice identifying blood cells on additional stained smears, from atlases, or from unlabeled colored illustrations of blood cells.

WEB 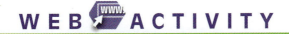 ACTIVITY

Look on the Internet for resources such as online blood cell atlases and other aids to help in learning normal blood cell identification.

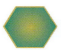

Student Performance Guide

LESSON 2-8 Normal Blood Cell Morphology

Name _____ Date _____

PROCEDURE

Record in the comment section any problems encountered while practicing the procedure (or have a fellow student or the instructor evaluate your performance).

S = Satisfactory
U = Unsatisfactory

You must:	S	U	Comments
1. Wash hands			
2. Assemble materials and equipment			
3. Place stained blood smear on microscope stage and secure with clips			
4. Use the low-power (10×) objective to locate the feathered edge of the smear			
5. Bring the cells into focus using the coarse adjustment			
6. Scan the smear to find an area where the red blood cells are barely touching			
7. Place one drop of immersion oil on the smear			
8. Rotate the oil-immersion objective (97× or 100×) carefully into position			

You must:	S	U	Comments
9. Focus, using the fine adjustment, until cells can clearly be seen			
10. Raise the condenser and open the iris diaphragm to allow maximum light into the objective			
11. Scan the slide to observe the leukocytes			
12. Study the smear; find and identify all five types of white blood cells. Use the Worksheet to describe and sketch each cell type as it is found; label the nucleus and cytoplasm			
13. Scan the smear to find platelets; sketch several platelets			
14. Scan the smear to observe red blood cells; sketch several			
15. Repeat steps 11 to 14 until cells can readily be identified			
16. Repeat steps 3 to 15 using a different smear			
17. Rotate the low-power (10×) objective into place			
18. Remove the slide from the stage			
19. Clean the oil-immersion objective thoroughly, using lens paper			
20. Check the microscope stage and condenser for oil and clean with laboratory tissue			
21. Place the slide in slide box or discard slides as instructed			
22. Clean remaining equipment and return it to proper storage			
23. Wipe work counter with surface disinfectant			
24. Wash hands with antiseptic			

Evaluator Comments:

Evaluator _____ Date _____

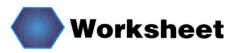 **Worksheet**

LESSON 2-8 Normal Blood Cell Morphology

Name _____ **Date** _____

Specimen I.D. _____

Examine stained blood smears and identify the white blood cells present. Draw two cells from each category below and describe their appearance, commenting on nuclear size and shape, cytoplasm color, and relative cell size.

Segmented neutrophil:

Lymphocyte:

Monocyte:

Eosinophil:

Basophil:

Platelets:

Red blood cells:

Comments: _____

_____

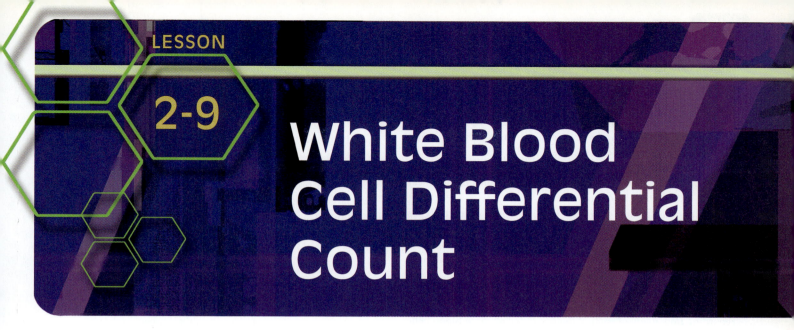

White Blood Cell Differential Count

LESSON OBJECTIVES

After studying this lesson, the student will:

■ Explain the purpose of the white blood cell differential count.
■ State the importance of the white blood cell differential count.
■ List the reference ranges for white blood cells in a differential count.
■ Identify the five types of white blood cells microscopically on the stained smear.
■ Perform a white blood cell differential count and report the results.
■ Evaluate and report the morphology of red blood cells on a smear.
■ Observe the morphology of platelets and estimate the platelet count from a blood smear.
■ List the safety precautions to be observed when performing a differential count.
■ Discuss the role of quality assessment in performing a differential count.
■ Define the glossary terms.

GLOSSARY

anisocytosis / marked variation in the sizes of erythrocytes when observed on a peripheral blood smear
atypical lymphocyte / lymphocyte that occurs in response to viral infections and that is common in infectious mononucleosis; reactive lymphocyte
differential count / a determination of the relative numbers of each type of leukocyte; leukocyte differential count; white blood cell differential count
hypochromic / having reduced color or hemoglobin content
macrocytic / having a larger-than-normal cell size
microcytic / having a smaller-than-normal cell size
normochromic / having normal color
normocytic / having a normal cell size
phagocytosis / the ingestion of a foreign particle or cell by another cell
poikilocytosis / significant variation in the shape of erythrocytes
reactive lymphocyte / see atypical lymphocyte

INTRODUCTION

Much useful information can be gained from the microscopic examination of a stained blood smear. Many situations arise in which the physician requires more knowledge than is provided by a cell count alone. By viewing a blood smear microscopically, the technologist or physician can identify blood cells and evaluate any abnormalities present. Many hematologists (blood specialists) believe that more information is obtained from a blood smear than any other single laboratory test.

The classification of white blood cells into different types and determination of their relative numbers is a **differential count**. The *diff*, as it is often called, is usually a part of a complete blood count (CBC). However, the *WBC count and diff* combination is also a common laboratory request.

The procedure for the differential count involves counting 100 to 200 white blood cells on a stained blood smear and recording how many of each of the five types of white blood cells are seen. Information is also obtained concerning the red blood cells and platelets. The red blood cells are evaluated for morphology and hemoglobin content. The platelets are evaluated for morphology and an estimation of platelet numbers.

The differential count can be used to diagnose and monitor the treatment of leukemias, anemias, and other diseases. For example, the viral infection that causes infectious mononucleosis produces a characteristic white blood cell differential. In iron deficiency anemia, a characteristic red blood cell morphology with small red blood cells that have a reduced amount of hemoglobin is seen. The student should be proficient in blood cell identification (Lesson 2-8) before attempting this lesson.

ORIGIN AND FUNCTION OF WHITE BLOOD CELLS

The white blood cells, as well as the red blood cells and platelets, originate from hemopoietic stem cells. All white blood cells are involved in the body's immune response in some way. Any condition or disease that damages or decreases the body's ability to produce normal functioning white blood cells will also cause a compromised immune response.

The Granulocytes

The granulocytic (myeloid) blood cells—*neutrophils, eosinophils,* and *basophils*—develop in the bone marrow (Figure 2-56). They are derived from a common precursor cell called a promyelocyte or progranulocyte. As a granulocyte matures, its nucleus changes from a round shape to a segmented shape. When granulocytic cells reach the stage where the nucleus is either band-shaped or segmented, they migrate out of the bone marrow into the peripheral circulation (Figure 2-56). Mature granulocytes have a life span of only a few days.

The neutrophilic granulocytes are especially active in **phagocytosis**, the ingestion of foreign particles or cells, including bacteria. Normally, in bacterial infections the number of neutrophilic granulocytes is increased. Eosinophils, and basophils to a lesser extent, are increased in allergic reactions.

The Lymphocytes

The lymphocytes are produced in the bone marrow and other lymphoid tissue, such as lymph nodes. These cells are involved in the immune response by producing antibodies to foreign antigens and by producing messenger molecules called *cytokines* that help target foreign cells and cells such as tumor cells for removal. Lymphocytes can have a lifespan of a few days to months or years.

The Monocytes

Monocytes also arise from stem cells in the bone marrow and are influenced by *colony stimulating factors* (CSFs) to become monocytes instead of neutrophils, eosinophils, or basophils. They often have vacuoles visible in their cytoplasm. Along with the neutrophils, the monocytes are a primary defense against invading pathogenic organisms. Phagocytosis and antigen-processing are two major roles of monocytes.

REFERENCE RANGES FOR THE WHITE BLOOD CELL DIFFERENTIAL COUNT

The reference ranges for the differential count vary with age. Normal values for adults and children are listed in Table 2-10. In a normal differential count, neutrophils and lymphocytes comprise 85% to 95% of cells, with monocytes, eosinophils, and basophils making up the remaining 5% to 15%. Children normally have a higher percentage of lymphocytes than adults.

PERFORMING THE DIFFERENTIAL COUNT

The purpose of a differential count is to determine the percentage of each type of white blood cell in peripheral blood. This is done by counting and identifying 100 white blood cells and reporting the percent of each type. The stained blood smear should always be examined using immersion oil on the slide and the oil-immersion objective (97× or 100×). The condenser of the microscope should be raised until it almost touches the bottom of the slide. The iris diaphragm should be open, and the light should be bright enough so the stained cell features can be easily seen.

The feathered edge of the smear is examined in the area where the red blood cells are barely touching each other (Figure 2-57). Cells are easiest to identify in this area of the smear because of their slightly flattened shape, which allows better viewing of cell structures. The white blood cell identification guide in Figure 2-58 shows examples of white blood cells that are present in normal peripheral blood and lists characteristics important in cell identification.

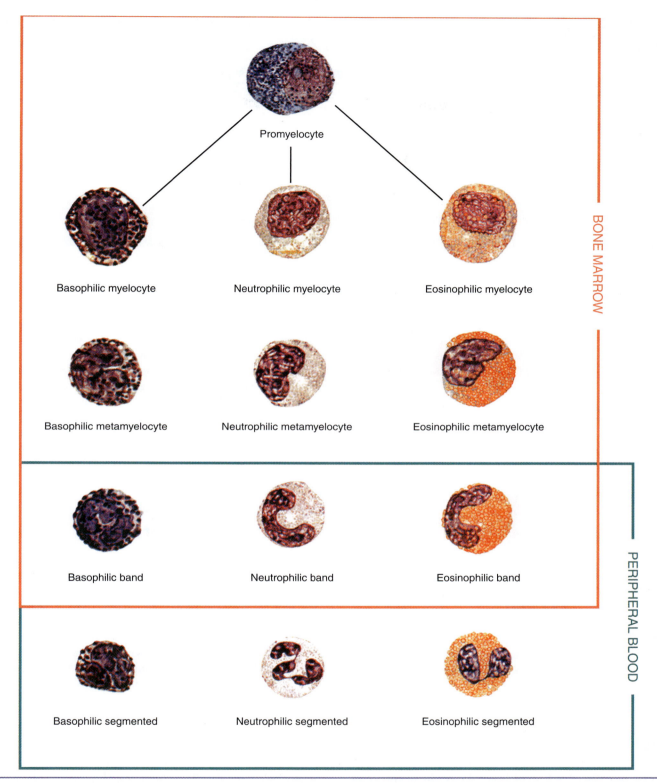

FIGURE 2-56 Origin and development of the granulocytic (myeloid) blood cells (*Courtesy of Abbott Laboratories, Abbott Park, IL*)

TABLE 2-10. Reference ranges for the white blood cell differential count and absolute white blood cell counts

Type of Cell	DIFFERENTIAL COUNT REFERENCE VALUES (%)				ABSOLUTE COUNT REFERENCE VALUES (CELLS/μL)
	1-month-old	6-year-old	12-year-old	Adult	Adult
Neutrophil (seg)	15–35	45–50	45–50	50–65	2250–7150
Neutrophil (band)	7–13	0–7	6–8	0–7	0–770
Eosinophil	1–3	1–3	1–3	1–3	45–330
Basophil	0–1	0–1	0–1	0–1	0–110
Monocyte	5–8	4–8	3–8	3–9	135–990
Lymphocyte	40–70	40–45	35–40	25–40	1125–4400
Platelets	An average of 7-20 platelets per oil immersion field is considered normal				

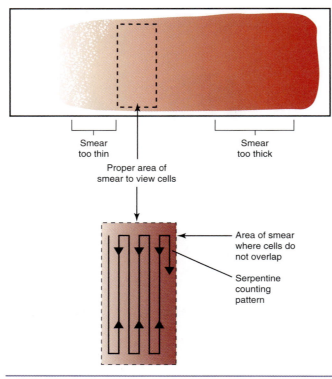

Smear too thin

Smear too thick

Proper area of smear to view cells

Area of smear where cells do not overlap

Serpentine counting pattern

FIGURE 2-57 Proper area of a blood smear to view and illustration of counting pattern for the white blood cell differential count

Safety Precautions

⚠ Performing a white blood cell differential should be a safe routine laboratory procedure if all safety policies are followed. Glass slides should be handled carefully to avoid cuts. Before the microscope is connected to an electrical source, the cord and plug should be inspected to be sure there are no frayed or exposed wires.

Quality Assessment

QA The differential count report can give rise to a variety of actions, treatments, and further testing. Therefore, it is imperative that great care and thoroughness are used when examining the cells and reporting the differential results.

Because there are no controls for white blood cell differential counts, it is important that only qualified personnel perform differential counts and report the results. The written policy and procedure in each laboratory's standard operating procedure manual will identify qualified persons and the exact counting and reporting procedure. The staining procedure must be carefully followed so that cell components are properly stained. In addition, the count must be performed in an area of the smear where the red blood cells are just touching, but not overlapping each other, when viewed microscopically. The appropriate supervisor should always be consulted when abnormal cells are seen or when there is difficulty identifying cells.

White Blood Cell Differential and Absolute Counts

When an area of the slide has been located in which the stain appears satisfactory and the cells are not crowded or distorted, 100 white blood cells are counted. A definite pattern, such as the one shown in Figure 2-57, must be followed to avoid counting the same cells twice. The numbers of each type of white blood cell observed are recorded using a differential counter (Figure 2-59) or a tally counter. Any abnormalities of the cells are also noted.

It is often beneficial to the physician to be able to correlate the differential count with the white blood cell count. This is done by calculating the *absolute count*, the number of a particular white blood cell type per μL or L of blood. The absolute counts are obtained by multiplying the WBC count by the differential percentage of each cell type. For example, a patient who has a WBC count of 9,000/μL and 60% neutrophils, has an absolute neutrophil count of 5,400 neutrophils/μL (calculated by multiplying 9,000 times 60%). The adult reference ranges for absolute white cell counts are listed in Table 2-10.

Red Blood Cell Observations

After the differential count has been completed, the red blood cells and platelets are observed and evaluated. Normal red blood cells and platelets are shown in Figure 2-60. With some experi-

	Neutrophilic Series					
	Segmented (mature)	**Band or Stab (immature)**	**Eosinophil**	**Basophil**	**Lymphocyte**	**Monocyte**
Cell Size (μm)	10–15	10–15	10–15	10–15	8–15	12–20
Nucleus						
Shape	2–5 lobes	Sausage or U-shaped	Bilobed	Segmented	Round, oval	Horseshoe
Structure	Coarse	Coarse	Coarse	Difficult to see	Smoothly stained, velvety	Folded, convoluted
Cytoplasm						
Amount	Abundant	Abundant	Abundant	Abundant	Scant	Abundant
Color	Pale pink-tan	Pale pink-tan	Pale pink-tan	Pale pink-tan	Blue	Gray-blue
Inclusions	Small, lilac granules	Small, lilac granules	Coarse, orange-red granules	Coarse, blue-black granules	Occasional red-purple granules	Ground-glass appearance

FIGURE 2-58 White blood cell identification guide

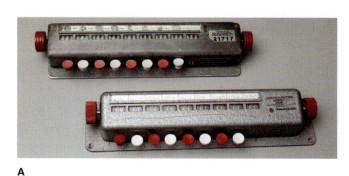

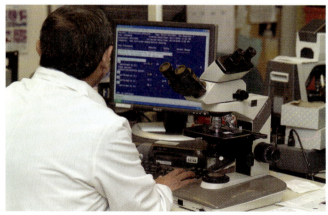

A   B

FIGURE 2-59 Differential cell counters: (A) manual counters; (B) performing differential count using computer keyboard and computer screen for display

ence, one can estimate the red blood cell size as **normocytic** (normal), **microcytic** (small), or **macrocytic** (large). The condition in which markedly different sizes of red blood cells are present is called **anisocytosis**.

The hemoglobin content of red blood cells can also be estimated. Red blood cells with the normal amount of hemoglobin are called **normochromic**. These cells stain evenly, with only a small pale area in the center of the cells. A **hypochromic** red blood cell is one that has less than the normal amount of hemoglobin, with only a ring of hemoglobin around the outer edge and a large central pale area. Normal red blood cells are round or slightly oval. The condition in which there is a significant variation in the shape of red blood cells is called **poikilocytosis**.

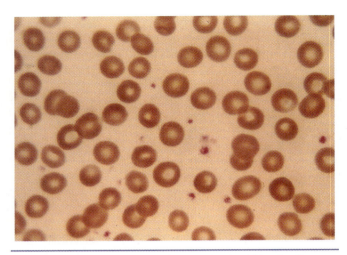

FIGURE 2-60 Photomicrograph of red blood cells and platelets in peripheral blood

Platelet Observations

Platelets are observed for any abnormalities in their morphology, and an estimate of platelet numbers is made. The total number of platelets counted in 10 oil-immersion fields is divided by 10 to give the average number per field. Seven to 20 platelets per oil-immersion field indicates a normal platelet count.

Factors Affecting the White Blood Cell Percentages

Many disease states can change the percentages of the different types of white blood cells (Table 2-11). Bacterial infections usually cause an increase in the bands and segmented neutrophils. Viral infections can increase the number of lymphocytes or change their morphology, causing them to appear atypical. The number of eosinophils is increased in parasitic infections and allergies. The number of monocytes is usually not affected by infections but occasionally will increase in tuberculosis. In leukemias, there is usually an increase and abnormality in one type of cell. The leukemia is named according to the predominant cell present. For example, an increased ratio of lymphocytes is found in lymphocytic leukemia.

Factors Affecting Red Blood Cells

Normal production and development of red blood cells requires certain factors such as vitamins and minerals. Iron deficiency is one cause of microcytic, hypochromic red blood cells. Deficiencies of vitamins such as B_{12} and folic acid cause the cells to be macrocytic. Table 2-12 lists conditions that affect red cell morphology.

Factors Affecting Platelets

The platelets can be affected by several factors. In some leukemias, the number of platelets is below normal. Exposure to chemicals, radiation, or drugs used in cancer therapy can also reduce platelets. If there is a delay in making a smear from a capillary puncture, the platelet distribution may be uneven; this may cause the platelet estimate from a blood smear to be erroneous.

AUTOMATED DIFFERENTIALS

Most hematology blood cell counters, even the smaller units for point-of-care testing (POCT), can perform automated differentials. The automated differential can be either a three-part or five-part. In a three-part differential, the blood is subjected to a

TABLE 2-11. Examples of conditions affecting white blood cell percentages

CONDITION	EFFECT ON WHITE BLOOD CELLS
Bacterial infections	Increased total white blood cells, increased percentage of neutrophils and bands
Viral infections	Decreased total white blood cells, increased percentage of lymphocytes
Infectious mononucleosis	Increased total white blood cells, increased lymphs, increased atypical lymphs
Parasitic infections, allergic reactions	Increased eosinophils
Leukemias	Total white blood cells usually increased, increase in type of leukocyte involved

TABLE 2-12. Examples of conditions that affect red blood cell morphology

CELL MORPHOLOGY	CONDITIONS
Size	
Normocytic	Normal
Microcytic	Iron deficiency anemia, thalassemias
Macrocytic	Vitamin B_{12} deficiency, folate deficiency
Shape	
Round, biconcave disk	Normal
Sickle (drepanocyte)	Sickle cell disease
Spherical	Hereditary spherocytosis
Hemoglobin Content	
Normochromic	Normal
Hypochromic	Iron deficiency anemia
Hyperchromic	Appearance caused by thickness of cells in spherocytosis

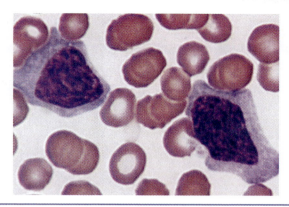

FIGURE 2-61 Photomicrograph showing two atypical lymphocytes (*Courtesy of Abbott Laboratories, Abbott Park, IL*)

Most atypical lymphocytes are characterized by a large nucleus and a large amount of blue cytoplasm easily indented by red blood cells. The indentations cause the lymphocytes to have a holly-leaf appearance (Figure 2-61). In most laboratories the technologist is allowed to report atypical lymphocytes, but all smears with abnormal cells reported are later reviewed by the supervisor or pathologist. Lesson 2-10 contains more information on abnormal cells.

In performing a differential count, it is important to know what is normal so that it becomes easy to recognize the abnormal. If suspicious cells are seen, the differential can be repeated, counting 500 cells to increase the chances of finding more abnormal cells. Whenever there is doubt about identification of a cell, more experienced personnel should be consulted.

special reagent that shrinks the cytoplasm of each type of white blood cell in a specific way. The analyzer then sorts the cells by size and classifies them as either lymphocytes, granulocytes, or mononuclear cells. Five-part differentials in which neutrophils, lymphocytes, eosinophils, basophils, and monocytes are classified and counted, are available on many hematology analyzers. The majority of hematology analyzers use impedance technology (electrical interruption) or a combination of impedance and light scatter to classify cells. Details about hematology automation are found in Lesson 2-13.

ABNORMAL OR ATYPICAL CELLS

Recognition and identification of atypical or abnormal white blood cells requires much study and practice. The reporting of such cells should be left to the hematology supervisor or the pathologist. One exception to this is the **atypical** or **reactive lymphocyte** seen in infectious mononucleosis (Figure 2-61).

PROCEDURAL Reminders

Qa

- Observe and count cells in an area of the smear where red blood cells are just touching.
- Always use the oil-immersion objective to perform counts.
- Do not count cells near the edges or end of the smear.
- Raise the microscope condenser and open the iris diaphragm.
- Consult a more experienced technologist or hematology supervisor if there is difficulty in identifying cells.

CASE STUDY 1

Keisha is a technician in a physician office laboratory that has a cell counter for performing red blood cell counts and white blood cell counts. The physician ordered a WBC count and differential count on a patient who came in complaining of pain and fever. Keisha performed the WBC count using the cell counter and prepared a stained blood smear to be sent to a reference laboratory for the differential count. The WBC count was 16×10^9/L. When checking the quality of the blood smear and stain before sending it to the reference laboratory, Keisha saw few white blood cells on the smear.

1. Is the patient's WBC count low, normal, or high?
2. Should Keisha have expected to see many white blood cells on the smear?
3. Should the WBC count and/or smear be repeated?
4. Give your interpretation of this situation and state what you think Keisha's next step(s) should be.

CASE STUDY 2

Antonio, a technician who had completed school 3 weeks previous, was working alone in the laboratory when Dr. Moore ordered a WBC count and differential count. While examining the smear, Antonio noticed several blood cells he could not readily identify. The physician insisted on receiving a report on the WBC count and the differential count. Discuss the appropriate action(s) for Antonio to take.

SUMMARY

The white blood cell differential count gives the relative numbers of each type of white blood cell in the peripheral blood. The reference ranges for the differential count vary according to age.

The white blood cell differential count can provide much valuable information to the physician. When used along with the physical examination of the patient, it can aid in diagnosis and treatment. The technologist must have a thorough knowledge of blood cell morphology and be willing to ask a more experienced person for help in identifying difficult cells. In larger laboratories, white blood cell differential counts are routinely performed on hematology analyzers. These instruments *flag* abnormal results so a technologist can verify the abnormality. To ensure quality results that are helpful to the physician and to the patient, care must be exercised in all stages of the performance of the white blood cell differential count.

REVIEW QUESTIONS

1. Why is it important to correctly identify blood cells?

2. Describe the area of the smear where the differential count should be performed.

3. What is the purpose of a white blood cell differential count?

4. What three characteristics of white blood cells are evaluated in cell identification?

5. List the five types of white blood cells, and state their reference ranges in percentages.

6. Describe the appearance of normochromic red blood cells and hypochromic red blood cells.

7. How many platelets should be noted per oil-immersion field if the platelet count is normal?

8. What could cause the number of band cells to be increased above normal?

9. Describe the appearance of atypical lymphocytes and give one condition that causes them.

10. What are the functions of neutrophils; of monocytes; of lymphocytes?

11. What safety hazards are associated with performing the white blood cell differential count?

12. Why is it important that differential counts only be performed and reported by experienced, qualified personnel?

13. Define anisocytosis, atypical lymphocyte, differential count, hypochromic, macrocytic, microcytic, normochromic, normocytic, phagocytosis, poikilocytosis, and reactive lymphocyte.

STUDENT ACTIVITIES

1. Complete the written examination for this lesson.

2. Practice performing a differential count as outlined in the Student Performance Guide, using the worksheet or CBC report form.

3. Perform differential counts on additional smears provided by the instructor.

4. If an automated cell counter is available to perform differentials, compare the results of a manual differential count with the instrument result.

Student Performance Guide

LESSON 2-9 White Blood Cell Differential Count

Name _____ **Date** _____

INSTRUCTIONS

1. Practice identification of red blood cells, white blood cells, and platelets from a stained smear.
2. Practice the procedure for performing the differential count following the step-by-step procedure.
3. Demonstrate the differential count procedure satisfactorily for the instructor, using the Student Performance Guide and the worksheet. Your instructor will determine the level of competency you must achieve to receive a satisfactory (S) grade.

MATERIALS AND EQUIPMENT

- gloves (optional)
- antiseptic
- stained normal blood smears
- microscope with oil-immersion objective
- immersion oil
- lens paper and lens cleaner
- laboratory tissue
- blood cell atlas; drawings or photographs and descriptions of stained blood cells
- tally counter or differential counter
- worksheet
- sharps container
- surface disinfectant
- slide storage box

PROCEDURE

Record in the comment section any problems encountered while practicing the procedure (or have a fellow student or the instructor evaluate your performance).

S = Satisfactory
U = Unsatisfactory

You must:	S	U	Comments
1. Wash hands and put on gloves (optional)			
2. Assemble materials and equipment			
3. Place stained blood smear on microscope stage and secure with clips			
4. Use the low-power (10×) objective to locate the feathered edge of the smear			
5. Bring the cells into focus using the 10× objective and coarse adjustment			

You must:	S	U	Comments
6. Scan the smear to find an area where the red blood cells are barely touching			
7. Place one drop of immersion oil on the smear			
8. Rotate the oil-immersion objective (97× or 100×) carefully into position			
9. Focus, using the fine adjustment, until cells are in focus			
10. Raise the condenser and open the iris diaphragm to allow maximum light into the objective			
11. Scan the slide to observe the white blood cells			
12. Count 100 consecutive white blood cells, moving the slide so that consecutive microscopic fields are viewed; use the counting pattern illustrated in Figure 2-57			
13. Record on the worksheet how many white blood cells of each type are seen			
14. Observe the red blood cells in at least 10 fields. Note the hemoglobin content; record as normochromic or hypochromic			
15. Observe the red blood cell size. Record as normocytic, microcytic, or macrocytic. If present, estimate number of microcytic or macrocytic red blood cells by using a grading system of 1+ to 4+			
16. Observe platelets in at least 10 fields: a. Note morphology b. Estimate the number of platelets per oil-immersion field: Count platelets in 10 fields and divide by 10 to obtain the average number per field c. Record as adequate, decreased, or increased, using the guide on the worksheet			
17. Rotate the low-power (10×) objective into place			
18. Remove the slide from the stage			
19. Clean the oil-immersion objective thoroughly, using lens paper			
20. Check the microscope stage and condenser for oil and clean with tissue if necessary			
21. Place the slide on its edge in slide box or discard slides as instructed			
22. Clean remaining equipment and return it to proper storage			

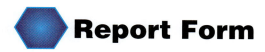 **Report Form**

LESSON 2-9 Hematology CBC Report Form

Name _____ Date _____

Specimen I.D. _____

WBC/L _____ $4.5\text{--}11.0 \times 10^9/\text{L}$ ($4.5\text{--}11.0 \times 10^3/\mu\text{L}$)

RBC/L _____ Male: $4.5\text{--}6.0 \times 10^{12}/\text{L}$ ($4.5\text{--}6.0 \times 10^6/\mu\text{L}$)
Female: $4.0\text{--}5.5 \times 10^{12}/\text{L}$ ($4.0\text{--}5.5 \times 10^6/\mu\text{L}$)

Platelets/L _____ $1.5\text{--}4.0 \times 10^{11}/\text{L}$ ($1.5\text{--}4.0 \times 10^5\mu\text{L}$)

Hgb (g/L) _____ Male: 130–170 g/L (13–17 g/dL)
Female: 120–160 g/L (12–16 g/dL)

Hct _____ Male: 0.42–0.52 (or 42%–52%)
Female: 0.36–0.48 (or 36%–48%)

Differential Count:

_____% segmented neutrophils 50%–65%

_____% lymphocytes 25%–40%

_____% monocytes 3%–9%

_____% eosinophils 1%–3%

_____% basophils 0%–1%

_____% bands 0%–7%

_____% other

Red Blood Cell Morphology:

Cell size: ❏ normocytic normocytic

❏ microcytic

❏ macrocytic

Cell color: ❏ normochromic normochromic

❏ hypochromic

Platelet Estimate: ❏ appear adequate 7–20/oil-immersion field

❏ appear decreased <7/oil-immersion field

❏ appear increased >20/oil-immersion field

Comments: _____

_____

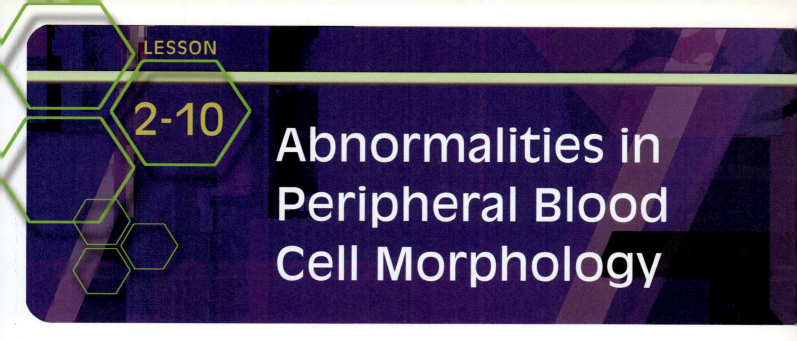

Abnormalities in Peripheral Blood Cell Morphology

LESSON OBJECTIVES

After studying this lesson, the student will:

- State the importance of differentiating between normal and abnormal blood cells on a peripheral blood smear.
- List two conditions in which anisocytosis is found.
- List two conditions in which poikilocytosis is found.
- List two conditions in which hypochromic red blood cells can be found.
- Discuss the relationship of the red blood cell indices to red blood cell morphology.
- Discuss the significance of RBC inclusions.
- List two causes of leukopenia.
- List two causes of leukocytosis.
- Discuss neutrophilia and a shift to the left.
- Discuss the characteristics of leukemias.
- List conditions in which abnormal thrombocytes can be found.
- List safety precautions to be observed when examining a blood smear.
- Discuss the importance of quality assessment when examining blood smears that contain abnormal cells.
- Define the glossary terms.

GLOSSARY

basophilia / abnormal increase in the number of basophils in the blood

basophilic stippling / remnants of RNA and other basophilic nuclear material remaining inside the erythrocyte after the nucleus is lost from the cell and which appear as small purple granules in red blood cells stained with Wright's stain

blast cell / an immature blood cell normally found only in the bone marrow

codocyte / target cell

crenated cell / a shrunken red blood cell with scalloped or toothed margins

drepanocyte / sickle cell

elliptocyte / elongated, cigar-shaped red blood cell

eosinophilia / abnormal increase in the number of eosinophils in the blood

femtoliter (fL) / a unit of volume; 10^{-15}L

folic acid / a member of the B vitamin complex

269

Howell-Jolly body / nuclear remnant remaining in red blood cells after the nucleus is lost, commonly seen in pernicious anemia and hemolytic anemias

keratocyte / a red blood cell deformed by mechanical trauma

leukemia / a chronic or acute disease involving unrestrained growth of leukocytes

mean cell hemoglobin (MCH) / mean corpuscular hemoglobin; average red blood cell hemoglobin expressed in picograms (pg)

mean cell hemoglobin concentration (MCHC) / mean corpuscular hemoglobin concentration; comparison of the weight of hemoglobin in a red blood cell to the size of the red blood cell, expressed in percentage or g/dL

mean cell volume (MCV) / mean corpuscular volume; average red blood cell volume in a blood sample, expressed in femtoliters (fL) or cubic microns (μ^3)

neutrophilia / abnormal increase in the number of neutrophils in the blood

nucleated red blood cell (NRBC) / a red blood cell that has not yet lost its nucleus

picogram (pg) / micromicrogram; 1×10^{-12}g

red blood cell indices / calculated values that compare the size and hemoglobin content of red blood cells in a blood sample to reference values; erythrocyte indices

schizocyte / a fragmented red blood cell; formerly schistocyte

shift to the left / the appearance of an increased number of immature neutrophil forms in the peripheral blood

sickle cell / crescent- or sickle-shaped red cell; drepanocyte

sickle cell anemia / inherited blood disorder in which red blood cells can form a sickle shape due to the presence of hemoglobin S

stomatocyte / red blood cell with an elongated, mouth-shaped central area of pallor

target cell / abnormal red blood cell with target appearance; codocyte

thalassemia / an inherited condition in which abnormal hemoglobin is produced, resulting in anemia

vitamin B$_{12}$ / a vitamin essential to the proper maturation of blood and other cells in the body

INTRODUCTION

The information gained from a complete blood count (CBC) with a differential count can be very valuable to the physician in making or confirming a diagnosis. Several conditions can be indicated by the presence of abnormal red or white blood cells observed while performing a differential count.

Occasional abnormal red and/or white blood cells can be observed on a peripheral blood smear that is considered to be normal. The finding might be as simple as finding a few hypochromic red cells in the smear of a patient with mild iron deficiency anemia or observing a small number of atypical lymphocytes associated with a viral infection. However, there are also times when examination of a smear expected to be normal yields unexpected results, such as the observation of immature white blood cells. These abnormal cells could be few in number and might only be recognized by an experienced technologist, or they could be numerous but difficult to classify. Becoming proficient in identification of abnormal

cells comes only after much practice in the identification of normal cells.

Some conditions and diseases present very characteristic cellular changes in blood cells that can be observed on a Wright's-stained smear. Conditions such as iron deficiency anemia, **folic acid** deficiency, **vitamin B$_{12}$** deficiency, and **sickle cell anemia** produce characteristic changes in the red cell morphology. Abnormalities in the white blood cell count, percentages of white blood cells, and/or white blood cell morphology can result from conditions such as viral or bacterial infections, hematological diseases, allergic reactions, stress, or recent exercise. Certain conditions also cause abnormalities in platelet numbers and/or morphology.

Evaluation of red and white blood cell morphology is an important part of the white blood cell differential count. The information can aid in diagnosis or treatment of disease. Correct identification of cells and accurate evaluation of cell morphology requires much knowledge and practice. The technologist must be proficient in identifying normal cells before studying abnormal morphology. The student should successfully complete Lessons 2-8 and 2-9 before attempting this lesson.

Safety Precautions

  Standard Precautions must be observed during the preparation and staining of blood smears. Chemical and physical hazards are present when using blood stains, handling glass slides, and operating electrical equipment. Appropriate personal protective equipment (PPE) must be worn. The methanol used in the staining process is toxic; splashes onto the skin or into the eyes must be avoided. Glass slides should be handled carefully to avoid cuts. The microscope cord and plug should be inspected before the microscope is connected to power.

Quality Assessment

All personnel who perform white blood cell differential counts and evaluate white and red blood cell and platelet morphology should follow the written procedure of the facility. This will describe the area of the slide to be examined, the pattern of counting, and a standardized method of grading any abnormal morphology that is observed. The quality of the smear, the staining technique, and the method of examining the smear influence the quality of the results.

A smear can contain abnormal cells, even though the patient seems normal, or healthy. Technologists performing differential counts must be experienced and conscientious. A more experienced worker, laboratory supervisor, or pathologist must be consulted if there are questions regarding cell identification.

ABNORMAL ERYTHROCYTE MORPHOLOGY

Disorders that affect the red blood cells can cause *poikilocytosis*, variations in shape, or *anisocytosis*, variations in size. Increase (erythrocytosis) or decrease (anemia) of the red blood cell numbers from the normal reference range and changes in the hemoglobin content of red blood cells can also occur (Table 2-13).

Anisocytosis

Red blood cells of normal size, 6 to 8 μm in diameter, are said to be *normocytic*. Red blood cells that are smaller than 6 μm are *microcytic* (Figure 2-62). Patients with conditions such as iron deficiency anemia and inherited conditions such as **thalassemia** have microcytic red blood cells. Thalassemias are caused by defects in the synthesis of the globin portion of the hemoglobin molecule. Iron deficiency anemia can be due to conditions such as inadequate intake of dietary iron, an increased iron demand in pregnancy, or chronic blood loss.

Red blood cells with a diameter greater than 8 μm are *macrocytes*, also called *megalocytes*. Macrocytes are produced in deficiencies of vitamin B_{12} or folic acid (folate) and in liver disease. Deficiency of vitamin B_{12} or folic acid prevents proper maturation

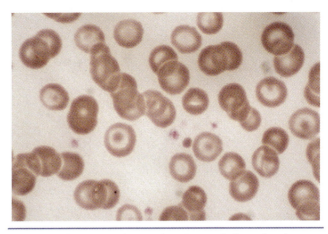

FIGURE 2-62 Abnormal RBC morphology showing target cells and hypochromic microcytes

of blood cells in the bone marrow, causing the cells to remain larger than normal. Vitamin B_{12} deficiency was formerly known as pernicious anemia because it was a fatal disease until its cause and treatment were discovered in the mid-1950s.

Poikilocytosis

Many conditions can cause poikilocytosis, variations in the shape of red blood cells.

Sickle Cells—Drepanocytes

Sickle cell disease is an inherited condition in which hemoglobin S causes the red blood cells to have a characteristic *sickle* shape when exposed to decreased levels of oxygen (Figures 2-63 and 2-64A). Another name for a **sickle cell** is a **drepanocyte**. Because of their abnormal shape, they block the smaller blood vessels, cutting off oxygen to tissues in that area. The lowered oxygen level then causes more red blood cells to change to the sickle shape. This is called a crisis, a serious and painful event for the patient because of damage to vital organs.

Spherocytes

Spherocytes are red blood cells that have lost their biconcave shape (Figures 2-63 and 2-64B). Anemia develops because the spleen recognizes these cells as abnormal and destroys them prematurely.

Elliptocytes

Elliptocytes are elongated, cigar-shaped red blood cells (Figure 2-63). In hereditary elliptocytosis, the patient has large numbers of these abnormal cells. Anemia develops because the spleen destroys these red blood cells and only a small number of normal red blood cells remain.

Stomatocytes

Red blood cells with a linear area of pallor through the center are called **stomatocytes** because the pale area is shaped like a mouth. These cells occur in the condition known as hereditary stomatocytosis.

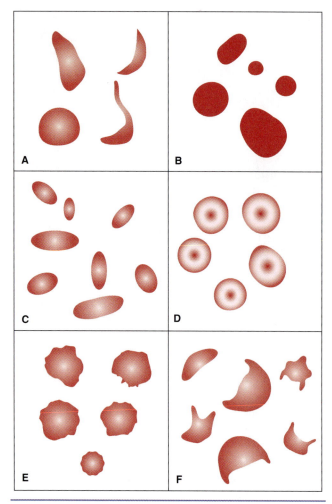

FIGURE 2-63 Morphology of selected abnormal red blood cells: (A) drepanocytes (sickle cells); (B) spherocytes; (C) elliptocytes; (D) codocytes (target cells); (E) crenated cells; and (F) keratocytes including helmet cells

Target Cells—Codocytes

In thalassemia, sickle cell disease, and other hemoglobin abnormalities, red blood cells called **codocytes** are produced. They are also called **target cells** because they resemble a bull's eye target (Figures 2-62 and 2-63).

Keratocytes—Schizocytes

Fragmented red blood cells are called either keratocytes or schizocytes. The **keratocytes** are red blood cells that have been deformed by some mechanical trauma, such as passing through an artificial heart valve or being cut by a fibrin strand in a blood clot (Figures 2-63 and 2-64). When cells are actually sheared into fragments, as may happen in severe burn patients, they are called **schizocytes**.

Crenated Cells

Crenated red blood cells have bumpy projections on the cell surface (Figure 2-63). These are caused by prolonged exposure of the blood sample to anticoagulant or incorrect blood-to-anticoagulant proportions in the collection tube. These cells should not be confused with pathological cells. When using anticoagulated blood, it is important to make blood smears within

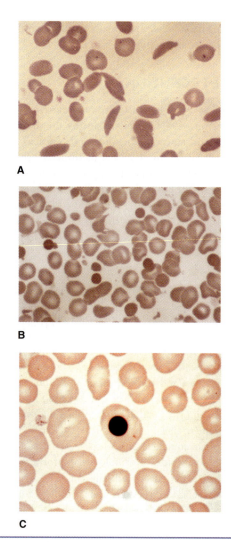

FIGURE 2-64 Photomicrographs of red blood cells found in various conditions: (A) sickle-shaped cells in smear from patient with sickle cell anemia; (B) spherocytes and schizocytes in smear from burn patient; and (C) nucleated red blood cell

2 to 4 hours of the blood being drawn to prevent alterations in blood cell morphology.

Variations in Hemoglobin Content

Red blood cells containing the correct amount of hemoglobin for their size are *normochromic*. A deficiency of hemoglobin due to lack of iron, or another condition, causes the red blood cells to have a large central area of pallor with only a small outer rim of hemoglobin; these cells are *hypochromic* (Figure 2-62). Red blood cells that appear to be completely filled with hemoglobin (have no central area of pallor) are called *hyperchromic*.

Red Blood Cell Inclusions

Basophilic Stippling

Basophilic stippling is caused by the fine granular remnants of RNA and other basophilic substances remaining in the red blood cell when it loses its nucleus. On a Wright's-stained smear, the RNA remnants cause cells to have a diffuse blue color (diffuse basophilia), orange and blue mottled appearance (polychromatophilia), or punctate fine and coarse granules (basophilic stippling.) These red blood cells are also known as reticulocytes when stained with New Methylene Blue stain.

An occasional stippled cell is normal. An increased number in the peripheral blood smear can indicate certain toxic conditions such as lead poisoning. Stippled cells are also increased in response to increased production of red blood cells due to acute hemorrhage, or after treatment for iron, vitamin B_{12}, or folate deficiency.

Howell-Jolly Bodies

Howell-Jolly bodies are DNA remnants remaining in the red blood cell after the nucleus is lost. They appear on Wright's-stained smears as intense dark blue-purple bodies inside the cell and are common in pernicious anemia and hemolytic anemias.

Cabot Rings

Cabot rings are found in red blood cells in certain anemias and in lead poisoning. They appear as dark blue-purple ring-like structures.

Nucleated Red Blood Cells

Nucleated red blood cells (NRBCs), normally found only in bone marrow, can be seen in peripheral blood in severe anemia. The metarubricyte is the form most commonly seen (Figure 2-64). These cells are also present in small numbers in the peripheral blood of normal newborns.

THE RED BLOOD CELL INDICES

The red blood cell (erythrocyte) indices are calculations that estimate the:

- Mean cell volume (MCV)
- Mean cell hemoglobin (MCH)
- Mean cell hemoglobin concentration (MCHC)

These calculations are performed using the red blood cell count and hemoglobin and hematocrit values to define cell size and concentration of hemoglobin within the cell (Figures 2-65, 2-66, and 2-67). Although some information about size and hemoglobin content of red blood cells can be obtained from microscopic examination of the stained smear, the red blood cell indices provide a quantitative measurement of red cell volume and hemoglobin concentration that can be compared to normal reference values.

The indices can be used to classify anemias. However, the validity of the indices is dependent on the accuracy of the RBC count and the hemoglobin and hematocrit determinations. Laboratories with hematology analyzers rely on the instrument to automatically calculate the indices. There may be occasions when the indices must be calculated manually, such as in a smaller laboratory or in research. The formulas for calculating the red cell indices are given in Figures 2-65, 2-66, and 2-67.

$$MCV = \frac{Hematocrit\ (percent)}{RBC} \times 10$$

Using a hematocrit of 36% and an RBC of 4.0×10^{12}/L:

$$MCV = \frac{36}{4.0} \times 10$$

$$MCV = 90\ fL\ (or\ \mu^3)$$

FIGURE 2-65 Calculation of mean cell volume (MCV)

$$MCH = \frac{Hemoglobin\ (grams)}{RBC} \times 10$$

Using a hemoglobin value of 15 g/dL and an RBC of 5.2×10^{12}/L:

$$MCH = \frac{15.0}{5.2} \times 10$$

$$MCH = 28.8\ pg$$

FIGURE 2-66 Calculation of mean cell hemoglobin (MCH)

$$MCHC = \frac{Hemoglobin\ (grams)}{Hematocrit\ (percent)} \times 100$$

Using a hemoglobin value of 15 g/dL and a hematocrit of 44%:

$$MCHC = \frac{15}{44} \times 100$$

$$MCHC = 34\%$$

FIGURE 2-67 Calculation of mean cell hemoglobin concentration (MCHC)

Mean Cell Volume

The mean cell volume (MCV) is the volume of an average red blood cell in a blood sample. The MCV is calculated by using the hematocrit value and the RBC count (Figure 2-65). It is reported in femtoliters (fL). (The MCV was formerly reported in cubic microns.) The normal reference range for MCV is 86 to 98 fL (Table 2-13). An MCV above 98 fL indicates macrocytes; a value below 86 fL indicates microcytes.

Mean Cell Hemoglobin

The mean cell hemoglobin (MCH) estimates the average weight of hemoglobin in a red blood cell. The unit of weight is the picogram (pg), which is equivalent to 10^{-12} g. The MCH is calculated using the hemoglobin value in grams/dL and the RBC count (Figure 2-66). The normal MCH is 27 to 32 pg (Table 2-13). Since the MCH is calculated without using the hematocrit, it is not useful in classifying anemias.

TABLE 2-13. Reference ranges for the red blood cell indices

	REFERENCE RANGE
MCV	86–98 fL
MCH	27–32 pg
MCHC	32%–37%

Mean Cell Hemoglobin Concentration

The **mean cell hemoglobin concentration (MCHC)** expresses the concentration of hemoglobin in the red blood cells in relation to their size and volume. The MCHC is obtained from calculations using the hemoglobin and the hematocrit (Figure 2-67). The result is expressed in percentage. A value within the reference range of 32% to 37% (Table 2-13) indicates *normochromia*, while a decreased value indicates *hypochromia*.

WHITE BLOOD CELL DISORDERS

Diseases or conditions affecting white blood cells can be detected from the presence of abnormal white blood cells on the peripheral blood smear or from the total white blood cell count (Table 2-14). A white blood cell (WBC) count increased above the normal range is called *leukocytosis*; a count below the normal range is called *leukopenia*. The total WBC count and the types of cells present are usually characteristic for a particular condition.

Leukopenia

Leukopenia is usually defined as a WBC count less than 4×10^9 WBCs/L. A reduction in all white blood cell types is called *balanced leukopenia*; however, in most cases, only one white blood cell type is decreased.

Neutropenia, a reduced number of neutrophils, may be inherited or caused by certain infections, antibiotics, sulfa drugs, and chemotherapy treatments. *Lymphopenia*, a reduced number of lymphocytes, can be caused by exposure to radiation or by

conditions such as lupus erythematosus, cardiac failure, or even stress.

Leukocytosis

Many factors can cause an increase in circulating white blood cells (leukocytosis). Bacterial infections, exercise, anxiety, or pain usually cause leukocytosis and neutrophilia. A *leukemoid reaction* is an excessive response of the white blood cells in which the count can be 50×10^9/L or higher. The reason for the heightened response is not understood.

In leukemias, the white blood cell increase is almost always an increase in percentage and total number of just one cell line, such as lymphocytes or granulocytes.

Neutrophilia

Neutrophilia is a type of leukocytosis that involves an abnormal increase in the number of the neutrophils. Bacterial infection is the most common cause of neutrophilia (Table 2-14).

In acute infections, neutrophilia is accompanied by an increase in immature neutrophils in the peripheral blood. This is called a **shift to the left**, in which immature forms known as bands, *metamyelocytes* (juveniles), or *myelocytes* enter the peripheral blood prematurely to help fight the infection (Figure 2-68A). The reference values for these cells in normal adult peripheral blood is one to five bands and zero metamyelocytes and myelocytes (Table 2-15). In mild infections, only the neutrophils and band cells are usually increased. In more severe infections, the WBC count and the neutrophil count can increase, or more bands and metamyelocytes may appear in the peripheral blood. Vacuoles may be present in the cytoplasm of the neutrophils and can indicate a serious infection.

Eosinophilia

Eosinophilia is an abnormal increase in the percentage of eosinophils in the peripheral blood. Eosinophils increase in allergic conditions, parasitic infections, and certain skin diseases.

Basophilia

The number of basophils in the peripheral blood is usually constant and is not affected by exercise, time of day, etc. **Basophilia**, an abnormal increase in the number of basophils, is usually associated with an

TABLE 2-14. Conditions that affect white blood cell counts and percentages

CONDITION	EFFECT ON WBC COUNTS
Bacterial infections	Increased total white blood cells, increased percentage of neutrophils
Viral infections	Decreased total white blood cells, increased percentage of lymphocytes
Infectious mononucleosis	Increased total white blood cells, increased lymphs, increased atypical lymphs
Parasitic infections, allergic reactions	Increased eosinophils
Leukemias	Total white blood cells usually increased, increase in type of leukocyte involved

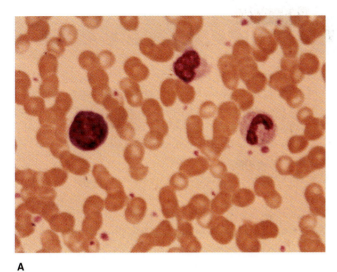

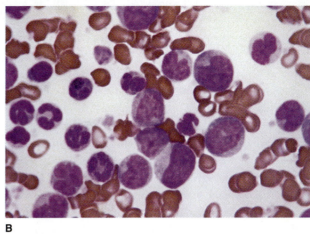

A   **B**

FIGURE 2-68 Photomicrographs showing (A) Neutrophilic shift to the left and (B) myelocytic leukemia

TABLE 2-15. Reference ranges for the white blood cell differential count

TYPE OF CELL	REFERENCE VALUES (%)			
	1 month	**6-year-old**	**12-year-old**	**Adult**
Neutrophil (seg)	15–35	45–50	45–50	50–65
Neutrophil (band)	7–13	0–7	6–8	0–7
Eosinophil	1–3	1–3	1–3	1–3
Basophil	0–1	0–1	0–1	0–1
Monocyte	5–8	4–8	3–8	3–9
Lymphocyte	40–70	40–45	35–40	25–40
Platelets	An average of 7–20 platelets per oil-immersion field is considered normal			

increase in the granulocytes and can be caused by conditions such as ulcerative colitis, chronic sinusitis, and viral infections such as small-pox and chickenpox. Increases in basophils are also seen in *chronic myelogenous leukemia* and *polycythemia vera*.

Monocytosis

Monocytosis, an increase in circulating monocytes, is rare but can occur in tuberculosis, subacute bacterial endocarditis, typhus, and rickettsial infections.

Lymphocytosis

The total lymphocyte count is normally higher in infants and young children than in adults. In adolescents and adults, an increase can be due to acute viral infection, especially infectious mononucleosis. The predominant cell in infectious mononucleo-sis is the atypical lymphocyte, also called a reactive or variant lymphocyte. Most atypical lymphocytes are characterized by a large nucleus and large amount of blue cytoplasm easily indented by red blood cells; the indentations may cause the lymphocytes to assume a holly-leaf shape (Figure 2-69).

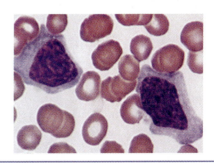

FIGURE 2-69 Photomicrograph showing two atypical lym-phocytes (*Courtesy of Abbott Laboratories, Abbott Park, IL*)

Leukemias

Leukemias are distinguished by unrestrained production of leu-kocytes in the bone marrow, causing the production of red cells and platelets to be literally "crowded out" by the leukemic white blood cells. Leukemias can be classified as chronic or acute. In general, the survival rates are better for chronic leukemias than for acute leukemias.

CURRENT TOPICS

CHARACTERISTICS OF LEUKEMIAS

In earlier times leukemia was known as *cancer of the blood* or a condition in which the white blood cells were crowding out the red blood cells. Today leukemia, a type of cancer, is defined as an acute or chronic disease characterized by unrestrained growth of the white blood cells and their precursors and with unknown etiologies or causative factors.

Most of the symptoms of leukemia are related to the inability of the bone marrow to produce normal numbers of red blood cells and platelets due to the large numbers of white blood cells in the bone marrow. As a result, the patient develops anemia, fatigue, increased infections, and bleeding problems. In addition, the leukemic white blood cells infiltrate the liver, spleen, lymph nodes, and nervous system, disrupting their normal functions. Blood flow in the smaller vessels such as capillaries can be slowed or stopped due to the large numbers of white blood cells.

The leukemias are classified according to the severity of the disease and the dominant cell involved. *Chronic* leukemias worsen slowly. The total numbers of white blood cells and of abnormal cells are small, the abnormal cells can still function to some extent, and the bone marrow is not affected to a large degree. *Acute* leukemias worsen rapidly and are characterized by abnormal cells that cannot carry out normal immune functions. Leukemias are further classified by the type of white blood cells affected. Leukemia can arise from the *myeloid* line or the *lymphoid* line. Leukemia that arises from the myeloid cells is called *myelogenous*; when it arises from the lymphoid line it is called *lymphocytic*.

The four common types of leukemia are:

- *Chronic lymphocytic leukemia* (CLL)—This type of leukemia affects mostly people over 55 years of age, almost never affects children, and accounts for about 7,000 new cases each year.
- *Chronic myeloid leukemia* (CML)—Also called chronic granulocytic leukemia, this type accounts for about 4,400 new cases each year and mainly affects adults.
- *Acute lymphocytic leukemia* (ALL)—ALL is the most common type in young children and accounts for about 3,800 new cases each year. Adults can also have ALL.
- *Acute myeloid leukemia* (AML)—Also called acute nonlymphocytic leukemia, AML accounts for about 10,000 to 12,000 new cases each year and affects both children and adults. Other rarer types of leukemia account for about 5,200 additional new cases each year.

Some causes of leukemia are known, such as exposure to ionizing radiation that caused leukemia in many Japanese exposed to atomic bomb fallout at the end of WWII. Heredity has also been shown to play a part in developing leukemia; the siblings and twins of leukemia patients have a greater chance of developing leukemia than the general population. However, other possible causes of leukemia have yet to be proven. Usually, the cause of an individual case cannot be pinpointed.

Factors that have been identified as possible causes of leukemia include:

- Therapeutic radiation for treatment of another type of cancer
- Exposure to chemicals such as benzene or formaldehyde
- Drugs such as chloramphenicol, phenylbutazone, and certain chemotherapy agents
- Viruses, especially retroviruses

New treatments for leukemia are constantly being developed. What works for one patient may not work for another. Treatment consists of four basic types:

- Chemotherapy is a mainstay of leukemia treatment. Chemotherapy agents kill leukemic cells but also damage or kill normal cells. Improvements in chemotherapy include *targeted therapy* in which drugs target only the leukemic cells.
- Radiation therapy uses high-energy rays directed at specific organs such as the spleen or brain to kill leukemia cells.
- Biological therapy is one of the newer forms of treatment in which monoclonal antibodies or interferon is used. Monoclonal antibodies are used against the abnormal cells in CLL; interferon has been found to be an effective treatment in CML.
- Stem cell transplants have been used for several years and have several variations. The patient is treated with high doses of drugs or radiation (or both), resulting in the destruction of both leukemic cells and normal cells in the bone marrow. The patient then receives a stem cell transplant from which new blood cells can develop. These stem cells can come from bone marrow transplantation, peripheral stem cell transplantation, or umbilical cord blood transplantation. Of the three, the public is probably most familiar with bone marrow transplants. The donated marrow usually comes from a donor whose tissue has been matched to the patient by tissue typing. In other cases, the patient's own blood cells can be harvested before the patient is subjected to whole body radiation. These harvested cells are treated to kill the leukemia cells, then frozen and stored until transfused back into the patient after radiation or chemotherapy is completed.

Although leukemia continues to cause many deaths each year, much progress has been made in the diagnosis, classification, and treatment of the disease. The hope is that, once specific causes are identified, the cause can be avoided or eliminated, and improved treatments will result in leukemia simply being another curable disease.

In acute leukemias, immature blood cells called **blast cells** and other immature forms of white blood cells are the predominant cells in the peripheral circulation (Figure 2-68B). Blast cells are the earliest identifiable blood cell precursors and are normally found only in the bone marrow. The total WBC count is usually, but not always, elevated in acute leukemia. Usually, the platelet count is decreased and anemia is present because leukemic cells affect the production of other cells in the bone marrow.

Chronic leukemias are characterized by leukocytosis with WBC counts of $50,000 \times 10^9$/L or greater. In the peripheral circulation, the predominant cells are mature cells along with some immature forms of the same cell type as well as some blast cells.

Diagnosing leukemias is a task for pathologists and hematology specialists. However, many cases are first noticed by a technologist performing a differential or because a hematology analyzer flags a sample as abnormal. It is critical for the technologist to carefully perform every differential and to closely examine all the characteristics of any cells that appear different. Sometimes it is necessary to count 200 to 500 leukocytes to find more of the abnormal cells.

PLATELET DISORDERS

Platelets can be abnormal in number or in function. In *thrombocytopenia*, platelet numbers fall below the reference range. Many factors can cause decreased platelets, including radiation exposure, certain drugs, chronic alcoholism, platelet destruction by the spleen, and the effect of diseases such as leukemia on bone marrow.

Elevation of platelet numbers above the reference range is called *thrombocytosis*. Some causes of thrombocytosis include a reaction to inflammatory conditions, a secondary reaction to other blood disorders, and removal of the spleen. Platelet disorders are discussed in Lesson 3-2.

SAFETY Reminders

- Observe Standard Precautions when preparing and staining peripheral blood smears.
- Take care to avoid cuts from the sharp edges of the glass slides
- Use appropriate PPE to avoid skin, eye, or mucus membrane exposure to stains and methanol.

PROCEDURAL Reminders

- Follow the institution's written procedure for reporting differential counts.
- Follow the institution's written procedure for reporting abnormal cells.
- Follow all policies related to patient identification and sample collection.
- Only technologists competent in blood cell identification should perform and report differential counts.
- Abnormal findings should be verified by the appropriate supervisor.

SUMMARY

The technologist must remember that any smear being examined may contain abnormal blood cells even though the patient seems in good health. The peripheral blood smear must be properly prepared and stained. The technologist must be very familiar with normal and abnormal blood cell morphology to accurately identify and evaluate the morphology of cells observed during the differential. A more experienced and knowledgeable technologist or the laboratory director must be consulted before certain types of abnormal cells are reported, depending on the particular healthcare facility's policy.

This lesson is only an elementary introduction to the morphology of abnormal blood cells. It is not possible to adequately cover the subject in this space; complete books have been written about each of these cell lines and the disorders associated with their abnormalities. It is hoped that this lesson will stimulate students and instructors to have the desire to know more about disorders of the white blood cells, red blood cells, and platelets.

REVIEW QUESTIONS

1. Why is it important to recognize an abnormal blood cell?
2. List three conditions in which abnormal red blood cell morphology can be found.
3. Why is it important to report red blood cell inclusions?
4. How can red blood cell indices be used to classify anemias?
5. List three conditions in which abnormal white blood cell morphology can be found.
6. What is leukemia?

7. Discuss the differences between acute and chronic leukemias.

8. Why do leukemia patients develop anemia?

9. List one cause of thrombocytosis and one cause of thrombocytopenia.

10. Define basophilia, basophilic stippling, blast cell, codocyte, crenated cell, drepanocyte, elliptocyte, eosinophilia, femtoliter, folic acid, Howell-Jolly body, keratocyte, leukemia, mean cell hemoglobin, mean cell hemoglobin concentration, mean cell volume, neutrophilia, nucleated red blood cell, picogram, red blood cell indices, schizocyte, shift to the left, sickle cell, sickle cell anemia, stomatocyte, target cell, thalassemia, and vitamin B_{12}.

STUDENT ACTIVITIES

1. Practice recognizing and identifying abnormal blood cells as outlined in the Student Performance Guide.

2. Practice calculating the red blood cell indices.

WEB 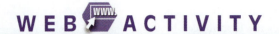 ACTIVITY

Search the Internet for information on treatments for leukemia. Prepare a short report on the latest treatment regimen for one of the leukemias.

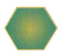

Student Performance Guide

LESSON 2-10 Abnormalities in Peripheral Blood Cell Morphology

Name _____ Date _____

INSTRUCTIONS

1. Practice calculating the red blood cell indices and identifying abnormal blood cells.

2. Demonstrate the recognition and identification of abnormal blood cells on peripheral smears or other visual learning aids using the Student Performance Guide. Your instructor will determine the level of competency you must achieve to receive a satisfactory (S) grade.

MATERIALS AND EQUIPMENT

- antiseptic
- microscope with oil-immersion objective
- microscope immersion oil
- microscope slides of various blood disorders: iron deficiency anemia, B_{12} or folate deficiency, infectious mononucleosis, leukocytosis, leukemias, and sickle cell disease are especially recommended
- blood cell atlas
- lens paper and lens cleaner
- slide storage box

PROCEDURE

Record in the comment section any problems encountered while practicing the procedure or have a fellow student or the instructor evaluate your performance.

S = Satisfactory
U = Unsatisfactory

You must:	S	U	Comments
1. Wash hands			
2. Assemble appropriate equipment and materials to view blood smears using the microscope			
3. Observe the slide or visual aid of iron deficiency anemia. Look in several oil-immersion fields and identify microcytic red blood cells			
4. Observe the slide or visual aid of B_{12} or folate deficiency: a. Look in several oil-immersion fields and locate macrocytic red blood cells b. Observe the white blood cells and identify any that are larger than normal			

You must:	S	U	Comments

5. Observe the slide or visual aid of infectious mono-nucleosis or other viral infection:
  a. Scan the differential counting area of the smear. Observe the white blood cells for an increase in total number of lymphocytes
  b. Locate several reactive lymphocytes and note the characteristics of the cytoplasm and the nucleus			

6. Observe the slide or visual aid of sickle cell disease:
  a. Identify any sickled red blood cells present
  b. Identify microcytic red blood cells
  c. Look in several fields; identify codocytes			

7. Observe the leukemia slide:
  a. Locate and identify the predominant white blood cell type present
  b. Observe the red blood cell morphology
  c. Observe the platelets for an increase or decrease in number			

8. Blot the immersion oil from the slides and replace them in their storage containers or return visual aids to storage			
9. Clean the microscope objectives and return the microscope to proper storage			
10. Wash hands with antiseptic			

Evaluator Comments:

Evaluator _____ Date _____

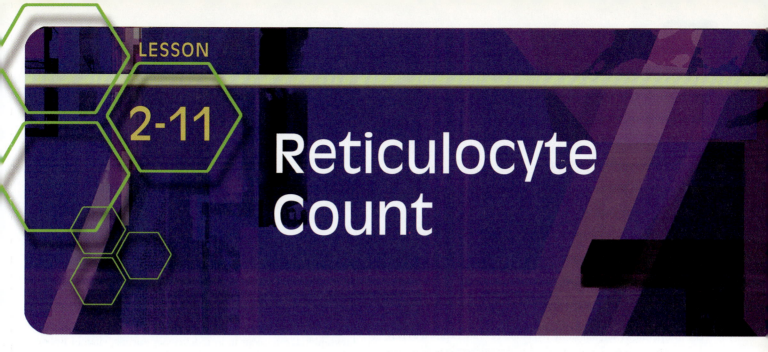

Reticulocyte Count

LESSON OBJECTIVES

After studying this lesson, the student will:

- Explain the purpose of performing a reticulocyte count.
- Name two dyes that can be used in the reticulocyte procedure.
- Prepare a reticulocyte smear.
- Perform a reticulocyte count.
- Calculate a reticulocyte percentage.
- Name two conditions in which the reticulocyte count would be low.
- Name two conditions in which the reticulocyte count would be elevated.
- List the normal reticulocyte reference ranges for adults and newborns.
- Discuss the safety precautions to be observed when performing the reticulocyte count.
- Discuss quality assessment policies that must be followed when performing the reticulocyte count.
- Define the glossary terms.

GLOSSARY

reticulocyte / an immature erythrocyte that has retained RNA in the cytoplasm

reticulocytopenia / a decrease below the normal number of reticulocytes in the circulating blood

reticulocytosis / an increase above the normal number of reticulocytes in the circulating blood

reticulum / a network

RNA / the nucleic acid that is important in protein synthesis and that is found in all living cells; ribonucleic acid

supravital stain / a dye that stains living cells or tissues

INTRODUCTION

The reticulocyte count is a method of estimating the number of immature red blood cells in the circulating blood; therefore, it is an indirect method of estimating the rate of red blood cell production. The test is most commonly used to determine the cause of a low red blood cell (RBC) count or anemia. It is also used to monitor the course of treatment for anemia.

PRINCIPLE OF THE RETICULOCYTE COUNT

Red blood cells are produced in the bone marrow. After a maturation process, red blood cells enter the blood circulation. For the first 24 hours in the circulation, they are still slightly immature and can be identified by the presence of **RNA** (ribonucleic acid) in the cell cytoplasm. When immature red blood cells are exposed to certain stains, the RNA forms stained granular aggregates or filaments called a **reticulum** (Figure 2-70). For this reason, these immature red blood cells are called **reticulocytes**.

The staining technique for reticulocytes is called supravital staining, a procedure in which living cells are stained. Two common dyes used for **supravital stains** are New Methylene Blue and Brilliant Cresyl Blue. With these stains, reticulocytes appear as blue-tinged red blood cells containing dark bluish-purple granules or filaments. Mature red blood cells appear uniformly bluish-green.

Reference Values for Reticulocyte Counts

The normal reticulocyte count varies with age (Table 2-16). Newborn infants have high counts that decrease to adult levels by 2 weeks of age. In a healthy adult, approximately 1% of the red blood cells will stain as reticulocytes when a supravital stain is applied to a blood sample.

Reticulocyte counts above 3% in an adult indicate that red blood cells are being produced at an increased rate.

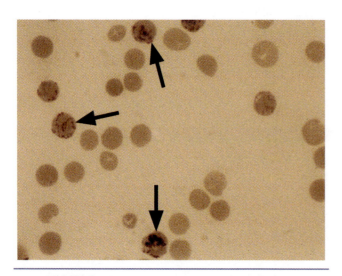

FIGURE 2-70 Photomicrograph of reticulocytes stained with New Methylene Blue (1000×)

TABLE 2-16. Reference values for reticulocyte counts

	REFERENCE VALUE (%)	UPPER LIMIT OF NORMAL (%)
Adults	0.5–1.5	3
Newborns	2.5–6.5	10

Reticulocytosis, an increased number of reticulocytes, can occur in response to acute blood loss from hemorrhage, chronic blood loss such as from a bleeding ulcer, or treatment for anemia.

Reticulocyte values below 0.5% indicate a decreased rate of red blood cell production. A decrease in reticulocytes, **reticulocytopenia**, can occur in iron deficiency anemia, vitamin B_{12} or folic acid deficiencies, or aplastic anemia.

PERFORMING THE RETICULOCYTE COUNT

The reticulocyte count can be performed manually using either capillary or venous blood. A few drops of blood are mixed with equal parts of New Methylene Blue stain in a small test tube and the mixture is allowed to stand for 15 minutes. The blood-stain mixture is then used to prepare blood smears.

Safety Precautions

  Standard Precautions must be observed when performing the reticulocyte count to protect the worker from potential exposure to bloodborne pathogens. In the reticulocyte procedure, cells are stained in the living state and no fixative is used. Therefore, the stained cells still represent a biological hazard. Appropriate personal protective equipment (PPE) must be worn while obtaining the blood sample, staining the cells, making the smears, and performing the counts.

Quality Assessment

   The reticulocyte procedure must be performed within 4 hours of blood collection, because immature red blood cells continue to mature as blood stands. If the procedure is delayed, the reticulocyte count will be falsely decreased.

When performing the reticulocyte count, the technician must be careful to distinguish reticulum from artifacts and debris. Frequent filtering of the stain will eliminate debris and precipitate. Smears must be examined carefully, so that faintly-stained fine reticulum is not overlooked. A definite counting pattern must be used to avoid counting the same cells twice.

Reticulocyte control solutions are available for manual or automated counts. One control is Retic-Chek from Streck Laboratories, Inc., which is manufactured from human red blood cells and meets federal and state regulations for a positive control.

Reticulocyte Counting Procedure

After the blood smears air-dry, they are examined microscopically using the oil-immersion objective. A total of 1,000 red blood cells are counted (500 per slide), and the number of reticulocytes seen per 1,000 red blood cells is recorded. (A reticulocyte is also counted as a red blood cell.) The percentage of reticulocytes is then calculated.

Calculating the Reticulocyte Percentage

A reticulocyte count is reported as the percentage of red blood cells that are reticulocytes. The percentage of reticulocytes is calculated using the following formula:

$$\frac{\text{\# Reticulocytes counted}}{\text{Total \# RBCs counted}} \times 100 = \% \text{ Reticulocytes}$$

or

$$\frac{\text{\# Reticulocytes}}{1000} \times 100 = \% \text{ Reticulocytes}$$

or

$$\frac{\text{\# Reticulocytes}}{10} = \% \text{ Reticulocytes}$$

A sample calculation is shown in Figure 2-71.

Correction for Anemia

In order for the reticulocyte count to give valuable information about red blood cell production, it should be correlated with the RBC count or the hematocrit. For example, the normal reticulocyte count is approximately 1%. An individual with an RBC count of 5×10^6 RBC/μL and a reticulocyte count of 1% would have approximately 50,000 reticulocytes/μL of blood. However, another individual with a 1% count and 3×10^6 RBC/μL would have only 30,000 reticulocytes per μL.

Although the reticulocyte percentages are the same in these two individuals, the total numbers of reticulocytes are not. For this reason, reticulocyte counts are often corrected for anemia to give the physician a more accurate reflection of the status of red blood cell production in the patient. The reticulocyte count can be corrected by calculating the *absolute reticulocyte count* or by calculating the *corrected reticulocyte count*.

Absolute Reticulocyte Count

The *absolute reticulocyte count* is a calculation that estimates the number of reticulocytes per volume of blood. This is done by multiplying the reticulocyte percentage by the patient's RBC count.

For example, if a patient has a reticulocyte count of 2% and an RBC count of 4×10^6 RBC/μL, the absolute reticulocyte count would be calculated as follows:

$$
\begin{aligned}
\text{Absolute} \\
\text{reticulocyte count} &= \text{RBC count} \times \% \text{ Reticulocytes} \\
&= 4 \times 10^6/\mu\text{L} \times 2\% \\
&= 8 \times 10^4/\mu\text{L or} \\
&= 80{,}000 \text{ reticulocytes}/\mu\text{L}
\end{aligned}
$$

Corrected Reticulocyte Count

Another way of correcting the reticulocyte percentage for anemia is to calculate the *corrected reticulocyte count*. This is done by multiplying the reticulocyte count (in %) times the patient's hematocrit divided by 45 (the normal hematocrit). For example, if a patient has a reticulocyte count of 3% and a hematocrit of 35%, the corrected reticulocyte count would be calculated as follows:

$$
\begin{aligned}
\text{Corrected retic count} &= \text{Retic count (\%)} \times \frac{\text{Patient Hct}}{45} \\
&= 3\% \times \frac{35}{45} \\
&= 2.3\%
\end{aligned}
$$

Automated Reticulocyte Counts

Instrumentation makes it possible to count reticulocytes with more precision than provided by manual counts. Most instruments that perform reticulocyte counts use the principle of flow cytometry (see Lesson 2-13 for detailed discussion). These instruments use RNA-specific stains to identify reticulocytes in a blood sample as it flows through a special electronic counting chamber. In automated methods, large numbers of cells are counted, which results in increased accuracy.

I. Count the reticulocytes using two smears:

	Erythrocytes counted	Reticulocytes seen
Smear 1	500	7
Smear 2	500	5
Total	1000	12

II. Calculate the percentage of reticulocytes:

$$\% \text{ Retics} = \frac{\text{\# Reticulocytes counted}}{\text{\# RBC counted}} \times 100$$

$$\% \text{ Retics} = \frac{12}{1000} \times 100$$

$$\% \text{ Retics} = \frac{12}{10}$$

$$\% \text{ Retics} = 1.2$$

FIGURE 2-71 Sample calculation of a reticulocyte percentage

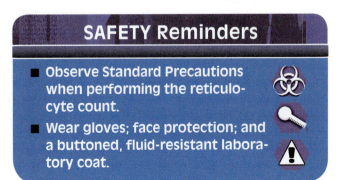

SAFETY Reminders

- Observe Standard Precautions when performing the reticulocyte count.
- Wear gloves; face protection; and a buttoned, fluid-resistant laboratory coat.

CRITICAL THINKING

Mary Beth was preparing to perform a reticulocyte count when she noticed sediment in the bottom of the stain bottle. Time was of the essence because the blood had been drawn 3 hours previously. However, Mary Beth decided not to use that stain.

1. What is the reason Mary Beth decided not to use the stain?
2. What should she do to make the stain usable?
3. Why was the time important?

PROCEDURAL Reminders

- Examine cells carefully to avoid overlooking reticulum.
- Do not confuse artifacts with reticulum.
- Use a definite counting pattern to ensure cells are not counted twice.
- Perform the reticulocyte count within 4 hours of blood collection.
- Filter stain to remove precipitate.

SUMMARY

The reticulocyte count is an indicator of red blood cell production. It is an important tool for assessing the bone marrow's ability to produce red blood cells. The reticulocyte reference range is 0.5% to 1.5% for adults and 2.5% to 6.5% for newborns. The count is usually performed by a hematology analyzer but can also be performed manually. The manual method is subject to several errors, such as inadequate mixing of the blood before making the slides and improper counting procedures. The reticulocyte count is useful in the diagnosis of certain anemias and to measure the response to treatment of anemia. An increase in the reticulocyte count can indicate blood loss, such as chronic bleeding from an ulcer.

REVIEW QUESTIONS

1. What is a reticulocyte?
2. Why would a reticulocyte count be performed?
3. What is the normal reticulocyte reference range for adults; for newborns?
4. What are two dyes (stains) used to stain reticulocytes?
5. What conditions can cause a high reticulocyte count?
6. Why must Standard Precautions be observed during the reticulocyte count?
7. What conditions can cause a low reticulocyte count?
8. State the formula for calculating a reticulocyte count.
9. Calculate the absolute reticulocyte count and the corrected reticulocyte count from the following values: Hct = 32%; RBC = $3.8 \times 10^6/\mu L$; Retic count = 3%.
10. Define reticulocyte, reticulocytopenia, reticulocytosis, reticulum, RNA, and supravital stain.

STUDENT ACTIVITIES

1. Complete the written examination for this lesson.
2. Practice performing reticulocyte counts and calculating reticulocyte percentages as outlined in the Student Performance Guide, using the worksheet.
3. Repeat a reticulocyte count on a specimen that has been stored at 4° C for 1 to 2 days after the initial reticulocyte count. Compare the two counts and explain the results.

WEB 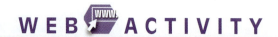 ACTIVITY

Use the Internet to find information about hematology analyzers and report on the technology used to perform automated reticulocyte counts.

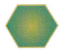 # Student Performance Guide

LESSON 2-11 Reticulocyte Count

Name _____ Date _____

INSTRUCTIONS

1. Practice the procedure for performing a reticulocyte count following the step-by-step procedure.

2. Demonstrate the procedure for the reticulocyte count satisfactorily for the instructor using the Student Performance Guide and the worksheet. Your instructor will determine the level of competency you must achieve to receive a satisfactory (S) grade.

MATERIALS AND EQUIPMENT

- gloves
- face shield or face protection
- antiseptic
- microscope
- microscope slides
- lens paper
- acrylic safety shield
- timer
- immersion oil
- disposable transfer pipets
- New Methylene Blue stain, freshly filtered, or commercial reticulocyte kit
- 70% alcohol or alcohol swabs
- sterile cotton or gauze
- sterile lancet
- capillary tubes, heparinized and plain
- test tube 10 × 75 mm
- tally counter
- surface disinfectant
- biohazard container
- sharps container
- commercially available stained reticulocyte slides (optional)
- reticulocyte count worksheet

Optional:

- freshly collected EDTA blood specimen
- materials for RBC count and microhematocrit
- reticulocyte controls

PROCEDURE

Record in the comment section any problems encountered while practicing the procedure (or have a fellow student or the instructor evaluate your performance).

S = Satisfactory
U = Unsatisfactory

You must:	S	U	Comments
1. Assemble equipment and materials. Put on face protection or position acrylic safety shield			
2. Wash hands and put on gloves			
3. Perform a capillary puncture and wipe away the first drop of blood with dry sterile cotton or gauze (or use freshly collected, well-mixed venous anticoagulated blood to perform the test)			

You must:	S	U	Comments
4. Fill one or two heparinized capillary tubes with blood (use plain capillary tubes if using anticoagulated blood)			
5. Dispense two to three drops of blood into the bottom of a small test tube			
6. a. Add an equal amount of New Methylene Blue stain to the test tube and mix b. Allow mixture to stand for 15 minutes at room temperature			

7. a. Remix contents of test tube and fill a plain capillary tube with the blood-stain mixture
  b. Prepare two blood smears from the blood-stain mixture and allow smears to air-dry
  c. Follow manufacturer's guidelines if using a kit such as Retic-Set			

8. Place one slide on the microscope stage and secure it			
9. Use the low-power (10×) objective to find a good area of the smear			
10. Place one drop of immersion oil on the slide and carefully rotate oil-immersion objective into position			
11. Count all erythrocytes in one oil-immersion field and record the number of reticulocytes in the field. **NOTE:** Any reticulocytes seen are counted twice—once as a reticulocyte and once as a red blood cell			
12. Move the slide to an adjacent microscopic field			
13. Count all erythrocytes in the (adjacent) field and record the number of reticulocytes in the field			
14. Continue steps 12 and 13 until 500 erythrocytes have been counted. Record count on worksheet			
15. Repeat steps 8 to 14 using the second slide			
16. Calculate the reticulocyte percentage using the worksheet: $$\frac{\text{\# of retics counted}}{1000 \text{ red blood cells}} \times 100 = \% \text{ reticulocytes}$$			
17. Record the results on the worksheet			
18. Clean the oil-immersion objective carefully and thoroughly with lens paper			
19. Clean any oil from the microscope stage with laboratory tissue			

You must:	S	U	Comments

20. Optional: If specimen used for reticulocyte count is from a tube of anticoagulated blood, perform an RBC count and microhematocrit from the same specimen. Record results on worksheet. (If anticoagulated specimen is not available, go to step 21)
   a. Calculate the absolute reticulocyte count using the worksheet
   b. Calculate the corrected reticulocyte count using the worksheet			

21. Return equipment to proper storage			
22. Store or discard slides as instructed			
23. Clean work area with surface disinfectant			
24. Remove and discard gloves in biohazard container			
25. Wash hands with antiseptic			

Evaluator Comments:

Evaluator _____ Date _____

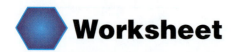 **Worksheet**

Lesson 2-11 Reticulocyte Count

Name _____ Date _____

Specimen I.D. _____

I. Perform the reticulocyte count and record the results

A.   Red blood cells counted   Retics counted

Slide 1   _____   _____

Slide 2   _____   _____

Total   _____   _____

B. Write the formula for the reticulocyte count:

C. Calculate the reticulocyte count:

_____ = % reticulocytes

II. Optional: If available, perform RBC count and hematocrit on the same blood specimen used for the reticulocyte count and record the results.

A. RBC/μL = _____ Hct (%) = _____

B. Calculate the absolute reticulocyte count:

   1. Write the formula for the absolute reticulocyte count:

   2. Calculate the absolute reticulocyte count:

      The absolute retic count is _____.

C. Calculate the corrected reticulocyte count:

   1. Write the formula for the corrected reticulocyte count:

   2. Calculate the corrected reticulocyte count:

      The corrected retic count is _____.

III. Comment / Interpretation

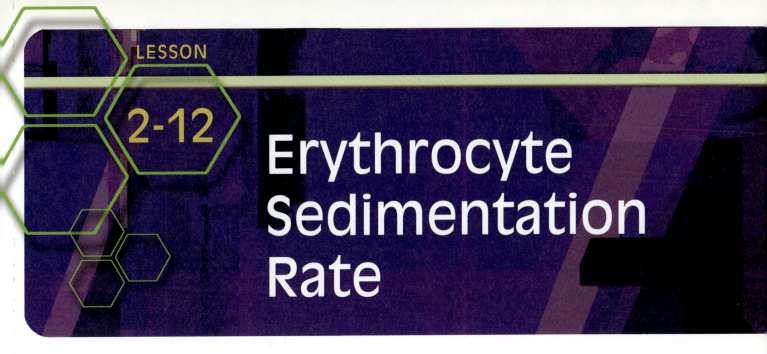

Erythrocyte Sedimentation Rate

LESSON OBJECTIVES

After studying this lesson, the student will:

■ Explain the purpose of performing an erythrocyte sedimentation rate.

■ List four properties of blood that affect the erythrocyte sedimentation rate and explain how the rate is affected by each.

■ List five technical factors that can affect the erythrocyte sedimentation rate and explain how the rate is affected by each.

■ Discuss the relationship of the erythrocyte sedimentation rate to disease.

■ List five pathological conditions that affect the erythrocyte sedimentation rate.

■ State the reference ranges for three erythrocyte sedimentation rate methods.

■ Perform an erythrocyte sedimentation rate.

■ Discuss safety issues specific to the performance of the erythrocyte sedimentation rate.

■ List aspects of quality assessment especially relevant to the erythrocyte sedimentation rate.

■ Define the glossary terms.

GLOSSARY

acute phase proteins / proteins that increase rapidly in serum during acute infection, inflammation, or following tissue injury

aggregate / the total substances making up a mass; a cluster or clump of particles

inflammation / a non-specific protective response to tissue injury

polycythemia / an excess of red blood cells in the peripheral blood

rouleau(x) / group(s) of red blood cells arranged like a roll of coins

sedimentation / the process of solid particles settling to the bottom of a liquid

Westergren tube / a slender pipet marked from 0 to 200 mm, used in the Westergren erythrocyte sedimentation rate method

Wintrobe tube / a slender, thick-walled tube, used in the Wintrobe erythrocyte sedimentation rate

INTRODUCTION

The erythrocyte sedimentation rate (ESR), or *sed rate*, is a commonly performed laboratory test. The ESR test measures the rate at which erythrocytes sediment in blood under standardized conditions. It is a nonspecific indicator of **inflammation** and is elevated in acute and chronic inflammation and also in malignancies. The ESR can also be used to evaluate the treatment and course of certain inflammatory diseases.

The sedimentation of blood was one of the principles of ancient Greek medicine. As early as 1836, in the more modern era of medicine, it was noticed that some factor in plasma increased the sinking rate of erythrocytes in whole blood. A procedure very similar to today's ESR test was first used in laboratory medicine around 1915 as a pregnancy test. Shortly after that, the ESR was used to screen for tuberculosis. Since the mid-1930s, the ESR test has been used as a test to detect inflammation and inflammatory disease.

PRINCIPLE OF THE ERYTHROCYTE SEDIMENTATION RATE TEST

The ESR test is based on the principle of **sedimentation,** the process of solid particles settling to the bottom of a liquid. In a sample of anticoagulated blood left undisturbed, the erythrocytes gradually separate from the plasma and settle to the bottom of the container. The rate at which the erythrocytes settle or fall under controlled laboratory conditions is the ESR.

To perform the manual ESR test, a sample of anticoagulated blood is placed in a calibrated tube of standard dimensions and set in a rack in a vertical position for an exact time. At the end of the time, the distance the erythrocytes have fallen from the plasma meniscus (at the zero mark) is measured in millimeters (mm) and reported as the ESR (Figure 2-72).

In blood samples from most healthy persons, erythrocyte sedimentation occurs slowly. In many diseases, particularly inflammatory diseases, the rate of sedimentation is rapid. In some cases, the rate is proportional to the severity of the disease.

FACTORS AFFECTING THE ERYTHROCYTE SEDIMENTATION RATE

Factors that affect the rate of erythrocyte sedimentation in a blood sample are: (1) properties of the plasma, (2) properties of the erythrocytes, and (3) technical factors.

Properties of Plasma

In normal blood, erythrocytes suspended in the plasma form few, if any, **aggregates** or clusters. Therefore, the mass of the falling (settling) erythrocytes is small and the rate of sedimentation is slow.

In abnormal blood, the erythrocytes sometimes form aggregates called **rouleaux.** This phenomenon is called rouleaux because the cells are arranged like rolls or stacks of coins (Figure

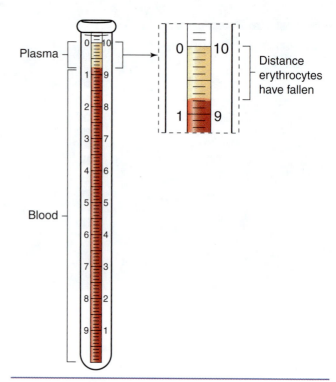

FIGURE 2-72 Illustration of sedimentation of cells in the erythrocyte sedimentation rate (ESR). Example shows a sedimentation of 8 mm

2-73), causing an increase in effective mass and an increased rate of sedimentation. (Clumps or clusters of cells are heavier than single cells and will settle more rapidly.) Rouleaux formation is influenced by the amount and type of plasma proteins present in a blood sample. Increased levels of proteins such as fibrinogen, **acute phase proteins**, or other plasma globulins enhance the tendency of RBCs to form rouleaux and therefore increase the sedimentation rate.

Properties of Erythrocytes

The ESR can be affected by the size, shape and number of RBCs.

Size

Macrocytic cells sediment more rapidly than microcytic cells because of their large size (increased mass).

Shape

The shape of the erythrocytes can also affect the ESR. For example, in sickle cell anemia the irregularly shaped erythrocytes cannot aggregate and the ESR is low or zero. Spherocytic cells also sediment at a slow rate.

Number

The ESR is affected by the red blood cell count. The sedimentation rate can be rapid in some anemias because the blood contains fewer erythrocytes. Therefore, the hematocrit or RBC count should be checked on samples that have elevated ESRs to determine if the elevated rate is due to inflammation or to anemia.

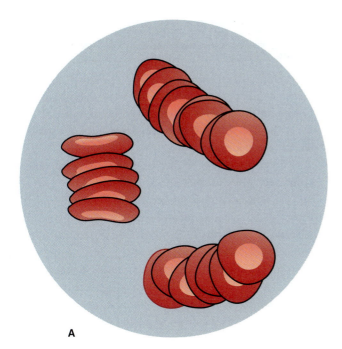

A

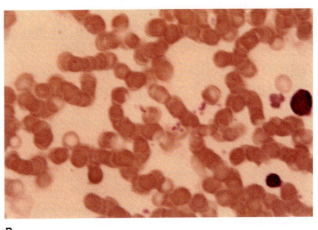

B

FIGURE 2-73 Rouleaux formation: (A) Illustration of red
blood cells forming "stacks of coins" (rouleaux);
(B) rouleaux formation in a peripheral blood smear

When the erythrocyte number is increased, as in **polycythemia**, the erythrocytes settle slowly and the ESR is low.

Technical Factors Affecting the Erythrocyte Sedimentation Rate

Technical factors such as temperature, timing, tube size, pipetting technique, sample mixing, and tube tilting or vibration during incubation will affect the sedimentation rate and can be a source of error in the test (Table 2-17). The precautions listed below must be followed to perform the test correctly.

- The sedimentation tube must be kept exactly vertical during the test; even minor degrees of tilting can greatly increase the ESR.

- The test should be set up on a counter free from vibra-tion. Vibrations, such as those occurring on a counter where a centrifuge is running, will cause a falsely increased ESR.

- The temperature in the testing area should be kept constant (20°C to 25°C) while the test is being performed. Low temperatures cause erythrocytes to settle more slowly.

- The ESR test should be set up within 2 hours after the blood sample is collected. However, blood collected in ethylenedi-aminetetraacetic acid (EDTA) can be stored at 4°C for up to 6 hours for most ESR methods but must be brought to room temperature before the test is performed.

- The length and diameter of the sedimentation tube affect the rate of sedimentation. Therefore, standardized tubes must be used in the test.

- Anticoagulated blood samples must be well-mixed immediately before setting up the ESR test.

- Careful pipetting technique should be used when diluting blood samples and filling the sedimentation tube. Air bubbles in the tube will interfere with test accuracy.

TABLE 2-17. Technical errors that can cause a false increase or decrease in the ESR	
FALSE INCREASED RATE	**FALSE DECREASED RATE**
Tube tilted (not vertical)	Low temperature of blood
Test >1 hour	Air bubbles in tube
Improper blood dilution	Test <1 hour
Improper mixing of blood	Improper blood dilution
Room temp >25°C	Improper mixing of blood
Vibration of tube during test	Room temp <20°C

- The test must be timed accurately. The ESR increases with time.

METHODS OF PERFORMING THE ESR

There are several methods of performing the ESR test, each with advantages, disadvantages, and different levels of sensitivity.

Safety Precautions

  Performing a manual ESR involves handling whole blood; the technician may also perform the venipuncture. Standard Precautions must always be observed. Appropriate personal protective equipment and engineering controls must be used. All sharps must be handled properly and disposed of in sharps containers.

CURRENT TOPICS

RELATIONSHIP OF ERYTHROCYTE SEDIMENTATION RATE TO DISEASE

Because the erythrocyte sedimentation rate is a nonspecific test, it is not diagnostic of any particular condition or disease. However, when the ESR is increased, it can be an indicator of inflammation somewhere in the body. *Inflammation is a response of body tissues to injury or irritation, usually characterized by pain, swelling, redness, and heat (see Lesson 4-1).*

The ESR is elevated in conditions that cause changes in plasma proteins, including inflammatory diseases such as rheumatic fever, rheumatoid arthritis, and lupus erythematosus. The ESR can also be increased in acute and chronic infections, tuberculosis, viral hepatitis, and Hodgkin's disease and other cancers. Multiple myeloma, a malignant condition affecting B lymphocytes, causes an increased ESR because large amounts of immunoglobulins (proteins) are present in plasma.

Changes in red blood cells can also affect the ESR. Patients with microcytic anemia can have an increased ESR when no inflammation is present. By contrast, in sickle cell anemia, the ESR is low or sometimes zero, because the sickled cells cannot form rouleaux.

The ESR can also be increased when there is no disease present. For instance, pregnant females often have an increased ESR because of the increase in plasma fibrinogen which usually accompanies pregnancy. Table 2-18 lists conditions in which the ESR is increased and in which it is decreased.

Although the ESR is not used for a specific diagnosis, the test is often used to follow the course of treatment of inflammatory diseases, such as treatment for rheumatoid arthritis. The ESR would be expected to decrease when treatment is successful. The ESR test can also be used to detect inflammation when white blood cell (WBC) counts are not elevated. For example, elderly patients can have normal WBC counts even in the presence of acute infection.

TABLE 2-18. Conditions in which the erythrocyte sedimentation rate may be increased or decreased

INCREASED SEDIMENTATION RATE	DECREASED SEDIMENTATION RATE
Pregnancy	Presence of sickle cells
Anemia	Polycythemia
Macrocytosis	Spherocytosis
Inflammatory diseases	Microcytosis
Cancer	Increased plasma viscosity
Acute and chronic infections	
Multiple myeloma	
Increased plasma fibrinogen	
Increased plasma globulins	
Tuberculosis	

Quality Assessment

The ESR is affected by environmental and technical factors as well as properties of the sample. The procedure for the ESR method being performed must be followed carefully, with special attention to technical factors that can affect the test, including test setup, proper specimen mixing, temperature, and timing. The procedure must include the use of commercial controls approved for use with the particular ESR method used. Control solutions for the ESR test are available from several suppliers. Some controls can be used with both manual and automated methods; others are made for particular methods. The regular use of controls helps ensure that the ESR values reported by the laboratory are valid.

Manual Methods

Two manual methods described in this lesson are the Wintrobe and the Westergren (Modified). EDTA anticoagulated venous blood is used. The blood must be well-mixed before setting up the test.

Westergren Method

The Westergren ESR method is performed using a **Westergren tube** (or pipet) graduated from 0 to 200 mm and a Westergren rack for holding the tubes. The Westergren test is more sensitive and complex than the Wintrobe method, requiring predilution of the blood with sodium citrate or saline before the pipet is filled. The test has been modified in recent years and most laboratories now perform the Modified Westergren method. It is the Clinical and Laboratory Standards Institute's method of choice.

Sediplast ESR System

Modified Westergren kits are available that have closed systems with self-filling disposable tubes and premeasured diluent (Figure 2-74A). These kits eliminate the biohazard risks present in the original Westergren method and also provide accurate filling of the tube. The use of one of these kits, the Sediplast ESR System, is detailed in the Student Performance Guide at the end of this lesson and in Figure 2-75.

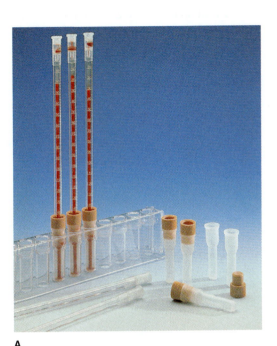

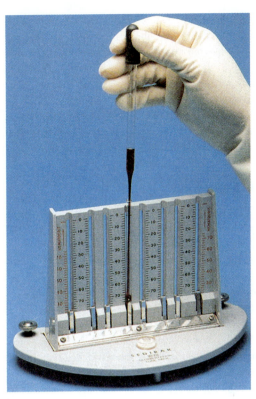

A   **B**

FIGURE 2-74 Erythrocyte sedimentation tubes: (A) Sediplast ESR System (*Photo courtesy of Polymedco, Inc.*); (B) filling Wintrobe tube in a SediRak

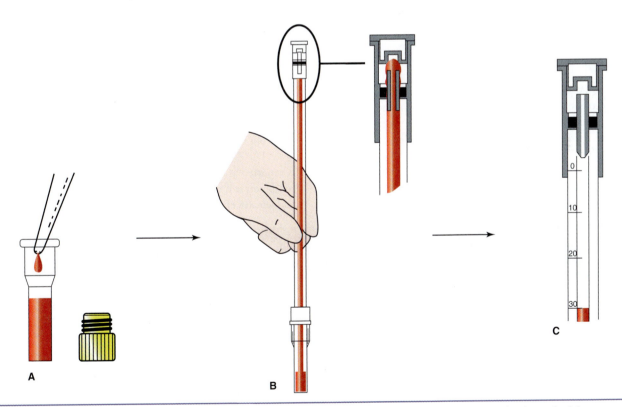

A   **B**   **C**

FIGURE 2-75 Steps for Sediplast ESR test: (A) pipet blood into vial containing diluent; (B) insert tube through vial stopper and allow tube to fill and autozero (inset); (C) read sedimentation distance after 1 hour using marking on tube

In the Sediplast ESR System, anticoagulated blood is mixed with premeasured diluent in the sedivial. After mixing, the Westergren tube is inserted into the vial with a twisting motion until the tube reaches the bottom of the vial. The blood column will automatically zero itself, and any extra blood will overflow into the sealed reservoir. The vial containing the tube is placed in the sedimentation rack for exactly 1 hour. At the end of the hour, the distance the erythrocytes have fallen is measured using the markings on the tube and is reported in millimeters per hour.

Wintrobe Method

The Wintrobe ESR method is performed using a **Wintrobe tube** graduated from 0 to 100 mm (0 to 10 cm) and with a capacity of 1 mL of blood (Figure 2-74B). The use of disposable Wintrobe tubes is recommended because of the biohazard involved in disinfecting and cleaning reusable tubes.

The Wintrobe tube is placed in a special sedimentation rack and is filled to the 0 mark with 1 mL of well-mixed anticoagulated blood using a long-stemmed pipet. The rack holds the tube vertical. At the end of 1 hour, the distance the erythrocytes have fallen in the blood sample is measured using the markings on the tube. The distance is recorded in mm (Figure 2-72).

The advantages of the Wintrobe method are its simplicity and the lack of expensive equipment. However, this method is not as sensitive as the Westergren ESR method.

Automated Methods

The SEDIMAT, Ves-Matic, and Zeta Sedimentation Ratio are three automated methods for performing the ESR.

SEDIMAT

The SEDIMAT system is manufactured by Polymedco and uses the principles, supplies, and procedures of the Sediplast system. The filled Sediplast Westergren tube is placed into the SEDIMAT automated ESR reader. The reader displays the results of each sample on an LCD display. The results are also stored in memory and can be printed out using the attached thermal printer. The system eliminates technician bias and variability in technique among technicians.

Ves-Matic

The Ves-Matic ESR system is an automated walkaway analyzer. A venipuncture is performed using a special vacuum tube that draws 1 mL of blood into a solution of sodium citrate. The tube is placed directly into the analyzer; the ESR is determined by infrared light and the results are available in approximately 22 minutes.

Zeta Sedimentation Ratio

The Zeta Sedimentation Ratio (ZSR) is performed using a special, small-bore capillary tube that is filled with blood and spun for 3 to 4 minutes in a special centrifuge called the Zetafuge (Beckman Coulter). This centrifuge alternately compacts and disperses the red blood cells under standardized centrifugal force. The tube is then read on a special reader to obtain a value called the zetacrit, which represents the percentage of sedimented erythrocytes. The zetacrit value is divided into the patient's hematocrit (also a percentage) and the result is the ZSR, expressed as a percentage.

The ZSR's advantages are that it is rapid, corrects for anemia, and requires only a small blood sample, which is desirable for pediatric patients. However, a special centrifuge and reader are required to perform the test.

REFERENCE RANGES FOR THE ERYTHROCYTE SEDIMENTATION RATE

Each ESR method has its own set of reference values. Specific instructions must be followed for the method used. Results must be compared with the appropriate reference ranges for the method used.

Reference values for the Sediplast ESR (Modified Westergren), Wintrobe ESR, and ZSR are given in Table 2-19. Sediplast and Wintrobe results are reported in millimeters per hour (mm/hr). The reference values for the Wintrobe method are lower than for the Sediplast, because blood is not diluted in the Wintrobe method.

The ZSR is calculated from the hematocrit and zetacrit, and is reported as a percentage. Since the ZSR value is corrected for red blood cell volume, the reference range is the same for males and females of all ages.

TABLE 2-19. One-hour reference ranges for Sediplast ESR (Modified Westergren) and Wintrobe ESR methods and reference ranges for ZSR

		SEDIPLAST ESR (mm)	WINTROBE ESR (mm)	ZSR PERCENTAGE (%) (ALL AGES)
Males:	<50 years	0–15	0–9	40–51 normal
	>50 years	0–20	0–9	51–54 borderline
				≥55 elevated
Females:	<50 years	0–20	0–20	
	>50 years	0–30	0–20	

CASE STUDY

The laboratories at Community Hospital were being remodeled, and some equipment had to be moved temporarily from one laboratory room to another. On Friday the workmen had moved a tabletop centrifuge from the urinalysis station into one of the hematology labs. On Monday, Martha arrived at work in hematology. Her responsibility was to perform erythrocyte sedimentation rates (sed rates) and to run the hematology cell counter. However, when Martha went to the ESR workstation, she noticed that the centrifuge had been moved onto the same counter. The technician from the urinalysis lab said he would be using the centrifuge most of the morning. Martha then told her supervisor that no sed rates could be performed until the centrifuge was removed from that counter.

1. Why did Martha tell the supervisor no sed rates could be performed? Was she simply upset because someone else was working in her lab? Explain your answer.
2. What technical factors can affect the Westergren ESR method?

SAFETY Reminders

- Observe Standard Precautions.
- Wear appropriate personal protective equipment and use appropriate engineering controls.

PROCEDURAL Reminders

- Follow the manufacturer's instructions for the test method being used.
- Be sure the blood has been adequately mixed before performing the the ESR test.
- Read test results at the appropriate time interval after setup.
- Be sure to use reference values specific to the test method used.

SUMMARY

The ESR is a nonspecific test. The results can be used to detect inflammation that may not be detected by other tests. The test can also be used to follow the progress of certain diseases. Since the test is affected by many factors, the technician must follow the instructions for the specific method and take care to eliminate environmental and technical factors that could cause erroneous test results.

REVIEW QUESTIONS

1. Why would an ESR be performed?
2. What four properties of blood affect the ESR? Explain how the ESR is affected by each of these factors.
3. Name five conditions or diseases in which the ESR would be increased.
4. What two conditions usually have a low ESR?
5. What are the reference values for the ESR using the Wintrobe method? Westergren method?
6. Name four technical factors that can affect the sed rate.
7. Name two automated methods for performing an ESR.
8. Define acute phase proteins, aggregate, inflammation, polycythemia, rouleau(x), sedimentation, Westergren tube, and Wintrobe tube.

STUDENT ACTIVITIES

1. Complete the written examination for this lesson.
2. Practice performing the ESR as outlined on the Student Performance Guide.
3. Evaluate the effect of technical factors on the ESR: set up three ESR tests on the same blood sample. Treat one tube according to the test procedure, place one in the refrigerator, and place one at an angle at room temperature. At the end of 1 hour, compare the results from the three tests and explain them.

Student Performance Guide

LESSON 2-12 Erythrocyte Sedimentation Rate

Name _____ Date _____

INSTRUCTIONS

1. Practice performing the ESR test following the step-by-step procedure.
2. Demonstrate the ESR procedure satisfactorily for the instructor using the Student Performance Guide. Your instructor will determine the level of competence you must achieve to obtain a satisfactory (S) grade.

NOTE:
Consult the manufacturer's package insert for specific instructions for the ESR kit being used.

MATERIALS AND EQUIPMENT

- gloves
- antiseptic
- sample of venous blood collected in EDTA
- sediplast kit (or other ESR kit):
  - Sedivial and rack
  - Sediplast autozeroing pipet
  - Micropipetter capable of delivering up to 1.0 mL
- timer
- surface disinfectant
- biohazard container
- acrylic safety shield or face protection
- sharps container

PROCEDURE

Record in the comment section any problems encountered while practicing the procedure (or have a fellow student or the instructor evaluate your performance).

S = Satisfactory
U = Unsatisfactory

You must:	S	U	Comments
1. Wash hands and put on gloves			
2. Assemble equipment and materials for Sediplast ESR. Put on face protection or position acrylic safety shield			
3. Mix blood sample gently for 2 minutes			
4. Remove stopper on sedivial and fill to the indicated mark with 0.8 mL blood. Replace stopper and invert vial several times to mix (or mix using pipet)			
5. Place sedivial in Sediplast rack on a level surface			

You must:	S	U	Comments
6. Insert the disposable Sediplast autozeroing pipet gently through the piercable stopper with a twisting motion and push down until the pipet rests on the bottom of the vial. The pipet will autozero the blood, and any excess will flow into the sealed reservoir compartment			
7. Set timer for 1 hour			
8. Return blood sample to proper storage. (If no laboratory work will be performed during the incubation, remove gloves, discard appropriately, and wash hands. Reglove before handling test materials)			
9. Let the pipet stand undisturbed for exactly 1 hour and then read the results of the ESR: Use the scale on the tube to measure the distance from the top of the plasma to the top of the red blood cells			
10. Record the sedimentation rate: ESR (Mod. Westergren, 1 hr) = _____ mm			
11. Dispose of Sediplast pipet and vial in appropriate biohazard or sharps container			
12. Clean work area with surface disinfectant			
13. Remove gloves and discard in biohazard container			
14. Wash hands with antiseptic			

Evaluator Comments:

Evaluator _____ Date _____

Principles of Automated Hematology

LESSON OBJECTIVES

After studying this lesson, the student will:

- Describe the history of the quantitation of blood cells.
- Compare the accuracy and precision of manual and automated blood cell counting methods.
- Name two automated cell-counting technologies.
- Give an example of an instrument that uses each type of counting technology.
- Explain the principle of electrical impedance.
- Explain the principle of light scatter.
- Explain the principle of flow cytometry.
- Discuss quality control and quality assessment procedures for automated hematology.
- Discuss hazards associated with hematology instrumentation and precautions that should be followed when using hematology analyzers.
- Define the glossary terms.

GLOSSARY

aperture / an opening

electrolyte solution / a solution that conducts an electrical current

fluorescent / having the property of emitting light of one wavelength when exposed to light of another wavelength

histogram / a graph that illustrates the size and frequency of occurrence of articles being studied

impedance / resistance in an electrical circuit

index of refraction / the ratio of the velocity of light in one medium, such as air, to its velocity in another material

laser / a narrow, intense beam of light of only one wavelength going in only one direction

INTRODUCTION

Humans have long been fascinated with blood, associating it with life in themselves and animals. In the 1600s, William Harvey recorded his observations of red blood cells as they passed through the capillaries. However, it was not until the mid-19th century, that a way to quantitate the blood cells was developed.

In 1855, researchers devised the first counting chambers (hemacytometers) for viewing and counting cells using a microscope. Hemacytometers were gradually improved and standardized by changing the background color of the glass and adding some metal to the etched lines to make them brighter. By using special diluting pipets and these hemacytometers, blood cells in a specific volume of blood could be quantitated.

Blood cells were routinely counted manually until the late 1950s. In 1956, W. H. Coulter patented a device that counted blood cells using the method of *electrical impedance*, also known as *aperture impedance*. This invention made performance of blood cell counts faster, easier, and more available.

The first hematology instruments performed only the red blood cell and white blood cell counts. The hemoglobin measurement was added later. Instruments are now available that provide direct or calculated values for 60 or more parameters. In these instruments, only the white and red blood cells, hemoglobin, platelets, and reticulocytes are directly counted or measured. The hematocrit and indices values are calculated from the red blood cell count and hemoglobin results. The automated results are more accurate and precise than manual counts. Manual counts have a coefficient of variation (CV) of approximately ±10%, whereas reliable instrument counts have a CV of about ±1% to 2%. Examples of the information available from various instruments is shown in Table 2-20.

TWO BASIC CELL-COUNTING TECHNOLOGIES

Electrical impedance was the only automated cell-counting method until the 1970s, when light-scatter cell-counting technology was developed. Today's cell counters are based on one of these two technologies.

Principle of Electrical-Impedance Cell Counting

Blood cells to be counted by electrical impedance are diluted in an **electrolyte solution** that conducts electricity. An electrical current flows in the electrolyte solution from one electrode to another across the **aperture** (opening) (Figure 2-76).

Blood cells are poor conductors of electricity. As a cell suspended in the electrolyte solution passes through the aperture, the nonconducting cell causes an **impedance**, or interruption, of the electrical circuit. The impedance causes a pulse in the electrical circuit. These pulses are counted as cells. The size of the impedance is proportional to the size of the cell causing it. Therefore, the instrument records not only how many cells pass through the aperture but also the size of each cell.

All electrical-impedance cell counters are based on Coulter's principles. The instruments using these principles

---

TABLE 2-20. Examples of results available on hematology analyzers

RBC	MCH	Left shift
WBC	MCHC	Atypical lymphs
HGB	RDW*	Hypochromia
HCT	immature granulocytes	RBC fragments
MCV	3-part differential	Nucleated RBCs
PLT count	5-part differential	Reticulocyte
MPV**		count

* *RDW is red cell distribution width, a measure of RBC anisocytosis*

** *MPV is mean platelet volume, a measure of the volume of the average platelet*

Note: Instruments are available that perform other measurements of blood components; many results are only performed for research purposes

---

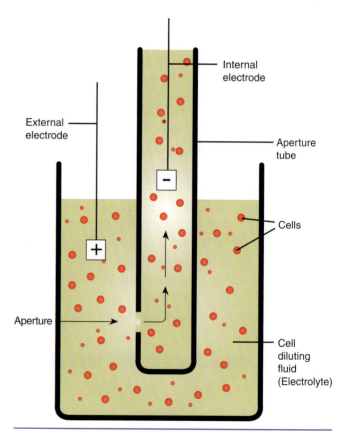

FIGURE 2-76 Illustration of electrical-impedance method of cell counting

have also been adapted for industrial use to count other types of particles in solutions.

Improvements in Electrical-Impedance Counting

Electrical-impedance cell counters had some inherent problems. As cells passed through the aperture, cells not passing through the center of the aperture were measured as being larger than their real size. Also, cells that became trapped in the aperture were counted repeatedly, falsely increasing a count. Accuracy and precision were improved by modifying cell counters so that the flow was channeled to the center of the aperture and the pulses were also electronically edited. The information obtained was then more accurate for the purpose of sizing cells. Most cell counters display this sizing information on a screen in a graph called a **histogram**. The relative numbers of cells are plotted on the Y-axis and the relative cell sizes are plotted on the X-axis (Figure 2-77).

Examples of Electrical-Impedance Instruments

Hematology instruments manufactured by several companies use electrical-impedance technology (Figure 2-78). Beckman Coulter, Inc., markets a variety of such instruments, including the COULTER ONYX for laboratories performing 10 to 100 complete blood counts (CBCs) per day and the COULTER Ac•T diff2 for laboratories such as POLs that perform 1 to 50 CBCs per day. The Serono-Baker 7000, 8000, and 9000 series are all suitable for the workload in a small laboratory or a hematology or oncology practice. The ABBOTT Cell-Dyn 3500 uses electrical impedance and an optical method. Many of these automatic cell counters perform 50 to 110 tests per hour, require small quantities of blood for testing, and have closed-tube sampling capability to reduce risk of exposure to blood.

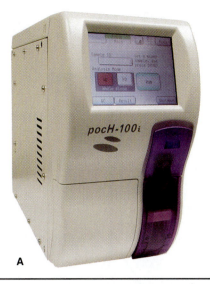

A

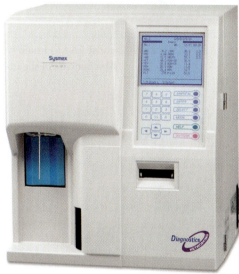

B

FIGURE 2-78 Hematology cell counters: (A) pocH-100i; (B) KX-21 (*Courtesy Sysmex America, Inc. All rights reserved*)

Principle of Light-Scatter Cell Counting

In light-scatter cell counters, a **laser** beam or tungsten-halogen light beam is directed at a stream of blood cells passing through a narrow channel. The channel is narrow to force the cells to pass through in single file. When the light beam strikes a cell, the beam is scattered at an angle. Each type of cell causes a different angle of scatter. This angle depends on the volume, shape, and **index of refraction** of the cell. However, the size of the cell has the most important effect on the scatter. Sensors detect how much light is scattered and how much of the beam is absorbed by the cell (Figure 2-79A).

The laser light is monochromatic, which means it has only one wavelength and travels in only one direction. These two characteristics allow it to be more finely tuned than the tungsten-halogen light beam and enable it to produce scatter patterns more useful in diagnostic hematology. One disadvantage is that laser-

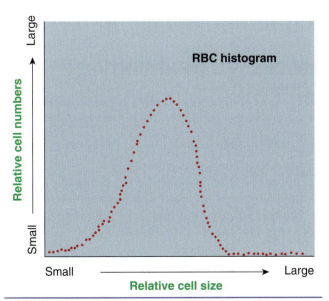

FIGURE 2-77 Example of histogram showing relative red blood cell numbers plotted versus red blood cell size

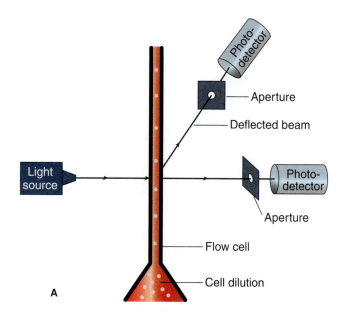

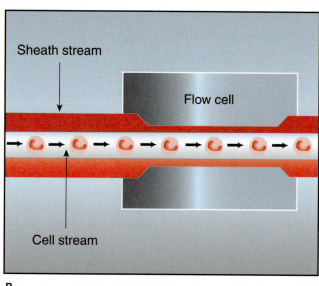

FIGURE 2-79 Light scatter technology: (A) schematic illustrating light-scatter method of cell counting; (B) schematic of sheath-flow, used to focus the cells hydrodynamically

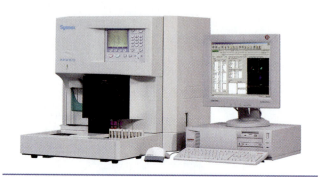

FIGURE 2-80 Sysmex XT 2000i hematology analyzer

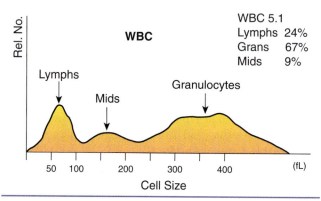

FIGURE 2-81 Histogram of three-part differential illustrating normal white blood cell count and differential

beam instruments cannot be calibrated with the same materials as other cell counters. Only human blood cells can be used for calibrating the laser counters.

An important feature added to light-scattering technology is *sheath-flow*, in which the cells are focused hydrodynamically (Figure 2-79B). This feature improves performance and also helps avoid the cleaning and maintenance problems of electrical impedance models.

Examples of Cell Counters Using Light Scatter Technology

Light scatter is used in the Beckman Coulter GEN-S series, the LH 755, HMX, and MAXM. The GEN-S performs reticulocyte counts, makes a blood smear, and performs a five-part differential for each sample (Table 2-21). The LH 755 and the Abbott SMS also make smears from each blood sample. The Sysmex XT 2000i uses flow technology and performs a reticulocyte count, a five-part differential, and a fluorescent optical platelet count (Figure 2-80). The Abbott Cell-Dyn 4000 combines aperture-impedance with light-scatter technology.

AUTOMATED DIFFERENTIAL COUNTING

Several instruments incorporate a differential count into the cell counter.

Three-Part Differential

As in the cell counters, two major technology types were developed for automated differential counting: electrical-impedance and laser light scatter. Beckman Coulter produces the COULTER Ac•T diff2, a cell-impedance instrument that provides a three-part differential useful as a screening device. The Beckman Coulter Ac•T 8 and Ac•T 10 produce a two-part differential; the "K" series offers a three-part differential. Serono-Baker's "Baker 9000" series also performs a three-part differential count (Table 2-21).

For these instruments to produce an automated differential, the cells must be subjected to a special reagent. This reagent

TABLE 2-21. Examples of hematology analyzers, the technology used, and the type of differential reported

TECHNOLOGY USED	INSTRUMENT	TYPE OF DIFFERENTIAL REPORTED
Electrical-impedance	Beckman COULTER ONYX	5 part
	Beckman COULTER Ac •T diff2	3 part
	Serono-Baker	3 part
Light-scattering	Beckman COULTER VCS, STKS, GEN-S, LH 755	5 part
	Sysmex XT 2000i	5 part
Combination of electrical-impedance and light-scattering	ABBOTT Cell-Dyn 4000	5 part

shrinks the cytoplasm of each type of white blood cell to a different degree, with the lymphocytes shrinking the most. This allows cells to be sorted by size into three distinct classifications: lymphocytes, mononuclear cells, and granulocytes. Cells of 35 to 99 fL (femtoliters) are grouped as lymphocytes, cells of 100 to 200 fL are called mononuclear cells (mids), and cells greater than 200 fL are called granulocytes (Figure 2-81).

The three-part differential is a screening device. It does not separate the granulocytes into neutrophils, eosinophils, and basophils. The instrument flags abnormal results to alert the operator that conditions such as abnormal red or white blood cell counts, atypical lymphocytes, or giant platelets, may be present.

Five-Part Differential Counting

Several hematology analyzers provide five-part differentials (Table 2-21). In the usual five-part differential, the white blood cells are sorted into neutrophils, lymphs, monocytes, eosinophils, and basophils, creating a histogram (Figure 2-81). Any variant lymphs or other immature cells are included in an additional category called LUCs (large unstained cells).

Beckman Coulter's VCS technology uses three cell parameters—volume (V), conductivity (C), and light scatter (S)—to count and classify white blood cells. VCS modules can be incorporated into counters such as the COULTER STKS, GEN-S, and MAXM to produce a CBC with automated five-part differential. The instruments require as little as 100 μL of blood per sample, and can process up to 75 samples per hour. For the laboratory performing 100 to 1000 CBCs per day, the GEN-S system provides 33 parameters, including five-part differential and reticulocyte analysis. A five-part differential and 26 parameters are available on the COULTER MAXM. The COULTER ONYX provides 18 parameters including a five-part differential and is suitable for labs performing 10 to 100 CBCs per day.

ABBOTT Diagnostics markets the Cell-Dyn 3000, 3700, and 4000 instruments that provide a five-part differential by multi-angle polarized light-scatter separation (MAPSS). This method does not alter or shrink the cells. It characterizes each individual cell by the light-scatter pattern from four specific angles.

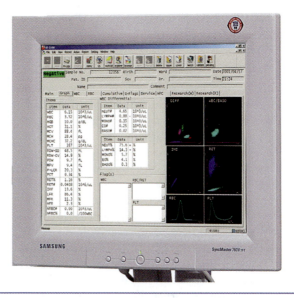

FIGURE 2-82 Five-part differential cytogram shown in right side of monitor (*Courtesy Sysmex America Inc. All rights reserved*)

Cytochemical Staining Differentials

The first instrument that used cytochemical staining to create a differential count was the Hemalog D from the Technicon Corporation in 1975. The instrument performed a CBC and five-part differential. In this instrument, certain chemicals, such as peroxidase and alcian blue, which affect the various white blood cells in specific ways, were added to the blood sample. The sample stream was then subjected to a light beam, and the scatter was measured and recorded. From that information, the total white blood cell (WBC) count and five-part differential were reported. The display of this information is called a *cytogram* or *scattergram* (Figure 2-82). The Sysmex XT2000i and Technicon H series multichannel analyzers incorporate this technology.

Image-Processing Instruments

In the 1980s, automated image-processing of differentials was introduced. This technology was based on storing thousands of images of normal peripheral cells in the memory of the instrument's

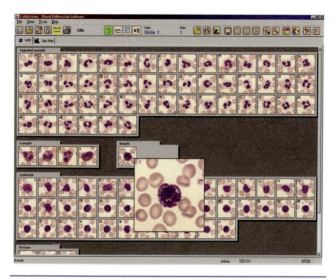

FIGURE 2-83 Sysmex CellaVision DM96 screen showing image-recognition differential counting (*Courtesy Sysmex America, Inc. All rights reserved*)

computer. The instrument scanned the blood smear and compared the cells with the images in its memory. The differential results were affected by some of the same disadvantages of the manual differential counting system—reliance on a well-made smear, good cell distribution, and proper staining technique. The instrument was almost too sensitive. Even though it could match a human technologist in cell recognition, it lacked the reasoning power of humans to think about the abnormality it recognized. Therefore it required that every abnormal cell be reviewed by a technologist.

Neither the LARC, nor the Hematrak, the two initial image-processing instruments, is currently distributed in the United States. However, Sysmex now markets the Cella Vision DM96, which displays on a screen the cells that require reviewing so the technician does not have to find the particular smear and examine it under the microscope (Figure 2-83).

FLOW CYTOMETRY

Flow cytometers (*cyt* means cell, *meter* means measure) are used in both clinical and research applications. These instruments combine the principles of light-scatter with light excitation and emission of **fluorescent** signals. The clinical and research areas that use flow cytometry include:

- Hematology
- Immunology
- Tumor cell analysis
- Genetics
- Microbiology

In the flow cytometer, cells to be analyzed are hydrodynamically focused in a sheath of liquid. As they approach the detector, they are focused into single file. This focused flow intercepts a light source, usually a laser. A series of photodetectors collects the light emissions and converts the data to electrical signals. Flow cytometers can generate multi-parameter data from particles and cells in the

size range of 0.5 to 40 μm in diameter, and can analyze up to 10,000 cells per second. A computer manages the data that is generated.

Cells to be analyzed can be obtained from venipuncture, bone marrow aspirates, body fluids, or solid tissues such as tumors that have been disrupted to release the individual cells. One use of flow cytometry is to distinguish and quantitate subsets of lymphocytes. This is important in leukemias, lymphomas, AIDS or HIV infections and autoimmune diseases. The Beckman Coulter XL is a benchtop instrument used in clinical laboratories. The Beckman-Coulter ELITE-ESP and the Dako Cyomation MoFli are high-speed cell sorters for use in research.

QUALITY ASSESSMENT AND QUALITY CONTROL FOR AUTOMATED HEMATOLOGY

Instrument manufacturers have responded to laboratories' need for better quality assessment by designing instruments that can help the laboratory spot quality control (QC) problems, correct failures, and store and retrieve QC data. Manufacturers provide calibrators, control specimens, and technical service hotlines. Subscription to a proficiency testing (PT) program also allows a laboratory's performance to be compared to the performance of similar laboratories.

Many instruments, especially larger ones, record the patient's I.D. from bar codes on the sample tube, helping to decrease transcription errors. Some instruments store up to 10,000 patient records at a time. A technologist can access a screen and compare a patient's results on one day with those from another day.

Some instruments also prepare Levey-Jennings charts for each run of control samples. In addition, as each control sample is run, any value not within the QC limits of the facility is flagged. The Levey-Jennings screen can be accessed to see if a trend or shift might be developing. At the end of the month, the complete QC record can be printed out.

An inexpensive method of quality control involves choosing five to 10 patient samples within reference ranges from a day's workload and reanalyzing them the next day on the same instrument. Statistical methods can then be used to calculate whether there is a significant change between the two sets of values.

SAFETY IN AUTOMATED HEMATOLOGY

 Automation substantially increases accuracy and reduces the time required to complete hematology testing. However, the use of instruments poses physical, chemical, and biological hazards. Standard Precautions must be followed and personal protective equipment (PPE) worn when using these instruments and performing maintenance and repairs, because the internal parts of the instrument can become contaminated with blood. Safety rules to guard against physical and chemical hazards must be followed.

Routine maintenance or repair of an instrument can present several hazards. Some instruments automatically perform

CASE STUDY

Cheryl works the evening shift in an urgent care clinic. The first patient of the evening is a patient with a fever. Dr. McCloud ordered a WBC count and differential. The hematology analyzer in the clinic is one that performs cell counts and three-part differentials. Cheryl collected the blood, but when she tried to use the analyzer, it malfunctioned, displaying "Error 9!" message. When Cheryl consulted the instrument's operating manual to find the corrective action, she found that the error 9 message indicated that the services of a certified repair technician were required.

1. Cheryl should:
   a. Tell the physician that it is impossible to perform the test
   b. Perform a manual WBC count and differential
   c. Tell the physician the test will be done after the instrument is repaired
   d. Send the test to a reference laboratory the next day
   e. Attempt to repair the analyzer since the test results are needed
2. Explain your answer.

routine maintenance procedures, but if the technician must do the procedures, the manufacturer's instructions must be closely followed. Repairs should be performed only by trained personnel. Removal of the outside instrument case should be attempted only by authorized personnel because of the hazard of electrical shock.

Chemical hazards are present in the reagents used by the instruments when performing analyses. The material safety data sheets (MSDSs) accompanying the chemicals must be read and understood by everyone using them. If differential slides must be stained, all chemical precautions must be observed.

Preparation of the blood sample for analysis and use of hematology controls and calibrators potentially expose technicians to bloodborne pathogens. Instruments with a through-the-cap sampler and that produce an automated differential greatly reduce this risk.

SUMMARY

The advent of the Coulter electrical-impedance counting technology revolutionized cell counting. Automated counts have a CV of $\pm 1\%$ to 2% compared with $\pm 10\%$ for manual counts. One improvement in cell-counting technology was to channel the flow through the aperture and edit the signals. Another improvement was sheath-flow, which reduced the need for frequent cleaning and maintenance of the aperture. Light-scatter technology was also introduced for cell counting. Today's instruments can perform cell counts, white blood cell differentials, reticulocyte counts, red cell indices, and several other parameters. Flow cytometry has increased the ability of the laboratory to classify and sort cells into categories.

Hematology analyzers have simplified and somewhat reduced the hematology workload. At the same time, they have increased the laboratory's capacity and ability to perform a variety of hematology tests. It is the responsibility of every laboratory professional to ensure that correct controls and calibration materials are used for all procedures. When a laboratory maintains a good QC and quality assessment program and participates in a certified PT program, the physician can have confidence in the results used to guide patient treatment.

REVIEW QUESTIONS

1. Describe the history of blood cell counting after Harvey's observations.

2. How does the coefficient of variation for manual blood cell counts compare with that for automated counts?

3. Name two types of technology used to count blood cells and give an example of each type.

4. Discuss the importance of quality assessment and QC for automated instruments.

5. What is the difference between the technologies used for three-part differential counters and five-part differential counters?

6. Explain what information is illustrated by a histogram.

7. Explain the principle of flow cytometry.

8. List three uses of flow cytometers.

9. Define aperture, electrolyte solution, fluorescent, histogram, impedance, index of refraction, and laser.

STUDENT ACTIVITIES

1. Complete the written examination for this lesson.

2. Investigate the use of automation in large hematology laboratories and in small practices. How do their needs differ?

3. Interview someone who works in a hematology laboratory and find out what type of hematology testing is performed there.

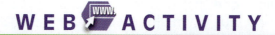

WEB ACTIVITY

Use the Internet to find operating manuals or brochures for hematology analyzers. Find out the instruments' test capacities. Calculate the time required to manually perform 50 CBCs with differential counts and compare with the time required using a hematology analyzer that performs a five-part differential count.

UNIT 3

Basic Hemostasis

UNIT OBJECTIVES

After studying this unit, the student will:

- Explain the processes involved in hemostasis.
- Discuss the use of instrumentation in coagulation testing.
- Discuss two principles of clot detection used in hemostasis instruments.
- Discuss disorders of hemostasis.
- Explain the bleeding time test.
- Perform a prothrombin time test.
- Perform an activated partial thromboplastin time test (APTT).
- Perform a rapid coagulation test.

UNIT OVERVIEW

Unit 3 is an introduction to the complex topic of hemostasis—the processes of stopping bleeding and the subsequent dissolution of clots. Lesson 3-1, Principles of Hemostasis, outlines the basic mechanisms of hemostasis. The lesson also provides a foundation for understanding the principles of routine coagulation testing and basic instrumentation. Disorders of hemostasis, including inherited and acquired conditions of platelets and coagulation factors, are discussed in Lesson 3-2.

The bleeding time test, a screening procedure that is abnormal in some blood-clotting disorders, is discussed in Lesson 3-3. The bleeding time test is not specific for a particular deficiency, but it is presented in this unit as an introduction to the principles involved in hemostasis.

The prothrombin time and the activated partial thromboplastin time, frequently ordered coagulation screening tests, are covered in Lessons 3-4 and 3-5. These tests illustrate the ability of plasma proteins to form a fibrin clot. Lesson 3-6 includes the principles of some rapid tests for hemostatic function, such as the D-dimer and ACT tests. Both manual and automated methods are presented.

Unit 3 covers some basic coagulation procedures performed in clinical laboratories. However, these procedures represent only a few of the large number of tests performed in the coagulation laboratory and are included to illustrate some basic principles of hematology and coagulation.

READINGS, REFERENCES, AND RESOURCES

Goodnight, S. & Hathaway, W. E. (2001). *Disorders of hemostasis & thrombosis: a clinical guide.* (2nd ed.). Lancaster, PA: McGraw Hill.

Greer, J. P., et al. (Eds.). (2003). *Wintrobe's clinical hematology.* (11th ed.). Baltimore: Lippincott Williams & Wilkins.

Harmening, D. M. (Ed.). (2001). *Clinical hematology and fundamentals of hemostasis.* (4th ed.). Philadelphia: F. A. Davis.

Henry, J. B. (Ed.). (2006). *Clinical diagnosis and management by laboratory methods.* (21st ed.). Philadelphia: W.B. Saunders.

Jacobs, D. S., et al. (2001). *The laboratory test handbook.* (5th ed.). Cleveland: Lexi-comp.

McClatchey, K. D. (Ed.). (2002). *Clinical laboratory medicine.* (2nd ed.) Baltimore: Lippincott Williams & Wilkins.

O'Shaughnessy, D., et al. (Eds.). (2005). *Practical hemostasis and thrombosis.* Ames, IA: Blackwell Publishers.

Rogers, G. M. (2001). *Case studies in hemostasis: Laboratory diagnosis and management.* Chicago: American Society of Clinical Pathology.

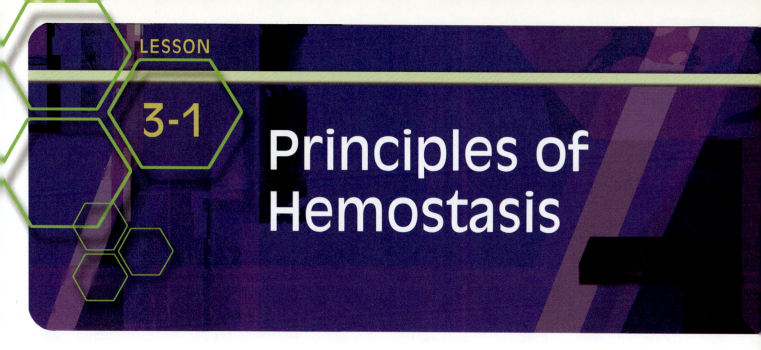

Principles of Hemostasis

LESSON OBJECTIVES

After studying this lesson, the student will:

- Explain the interaction of the blood vessels, platelets, and coagulation factors in hemostasis.
- Explain the mechanisms of platelet adhesion and aggregation.
- List the coagulation factors.
- List the coagulation factors produced in the liver.
- Diagram the intrinsic pathway of hemostasis.
- Diagram the extrinsic pathway of hemostasis.
- Diagram the common pathway of hemostasis.
- Explain regulatory mechanisms in hemostasis.
- Explain dissolution of the fibrin clot.
- Define the glossary terms.

GLOSSARY

adhesion / the act of two parts or surfaces sticking together

aggregation / the collecting of separate objects into one mass

arteriosclerosis / abnormal thickening and hardening of the arterial walls, causing loss of elasticity and impaired blood circulation

atherosclerosis / a form of arteriosclerosis in which lipids, calcium, cholesterol, and other substances deposit on the inner walls of the arteries

coagulation / the process of forming a fibrin clot

coagulation factors / a group of plasma proteins (and the mineral calcium) involved in blood clotting

collagen / a protein connective tissue found in skin, bone, ligaments, and cartilage

D-dimer / one of the products formed from the breakdown of fibrin by plasmin

embolus (pl. emboli) / a mass (clot) of blood or foreign matter carried in the circulation

endothelium / the layer of epithelial cells that lines blood vessels and the serous cavities of the body

fibrin / a protein formed from fibrinogen by the action of thrombin

fibrin degradation products / degradation products formed when plasmin cleaves fibrin or fibrinogen; formerly fibrin split products

fibrinogen / a plasma protein produced in the liver and converted to fibrin through the action of thrombin

fibrinolysis / enzymatic breakdown of a blood clot

hemorrhage / uncontrolled bleeding

hemostasis / the process of stopping bleeding, which includes clot formation and dissolution

intravascular / within the blood vessels

ionized calcium / in the body, a mineral that plays an important role in hemostasis

plasmin / an enzyme that binds to fibrin and initiates breakdown of the fibrin clot (fibrinolysis)

plasminogen / the inactive precursor of plasmin

prothrombin / the precursor of thrombin; factor II

thrombin / a protein formed from prothrombin by the action of thromboplastin and other factors in the presence of calcium ions; factor II_a

thromboplastin / a lipoprotein found in endothelium and other tissue; coagulation factor III; also called tissue factor

thrombus (pl. thrombi) / a blood clot that obstructs a blood vessel

vasoconstriction / narrowing of the diameter of a blood vessel

INTRODUCTION

Blood normally circulates through the body in a liquid form via the arteries, veins, and capillaries. Problems arise when blood is lost from the vessels by bleeding, or when an **intravascular** clot obstructs a blood vessel.

Hemostasis is the process of stopping the loss of blood from blood vessels. This process involves four interrelated and interdependent systems, as shown in Figure 3-1. These are the blood vessels, platelets, blood coagulation factors, and components of the clot dissolution system (fibrinolysis).

PRINCIPLES OF HEMOSTASIS

In the majority of patients, hemostasis functions normally; bleeding is stopped by clot formation, and unwanted clot formation is prevented by the body's circulating inhibitors. However, con-

genital and acquired abnormalities can affect hemostasis. An abnormality can be minor and result only in easy bruising, or it can cause a life-threatening incident, such as a **hemorrhage**, or uncontrolled bleeding.

The Role of Blood Vessels

The vascular phase of hemostasis includes a variety of responses that occur when a blood vessel is damaged. One reaction is **vasoconstriction**, the narrowing of the vessel to reduce blood flow to the damaged area. When a vessel is completely severed, the cut ends retract and are compressed by the contraction of skeletal muscle. Small capillary vessels seal themselves together if the damaged edges touch. **Collagen**, a protein connective tissue exposed when the **endothelium** lining the blood vessels is damaged, plays an important role in platelet activation.

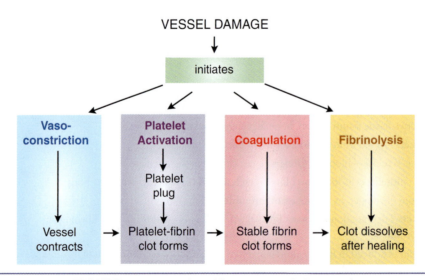

FIGURE 3-1 Interaction of four processes in hemostasis

The Role of Platelets

Platelets have a rounded disk-like shape while circulating in the bloodstream. However, platelets undergo a shape change when they come in contact with the exposed collagen in the wall of a damaged blood vessel. This contact with collagen initiates platelet **adhesion**, the act of the individual platelets sticking to the damaged edge of the vessel. Normal adhesion also requires a plasma protein, von Willebrand's factor (VIII:vWF), and a platelet glycoprotein.

As platelets adhere to the exposed endothelium, they become activated and react by releasing substances from their granules. The platelets then change from the normal discoid shape into a spherical one, with pseudopods forming over their surfaces. This shape change is initiated by the release of ADP from the platelets and the exposed endothelium. These spiny platelets react with each other to form an aggregate. The **aggregation** reaction also requires sufficient calcium and fibrinogen. Because of the large number of platelets present in circulating blood, a platelet plug forms in seconds to stop bleeding in a small wound, such as a capillary puncture (Figure 3-2).

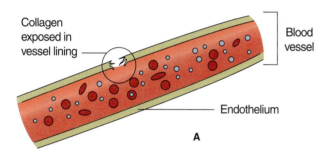

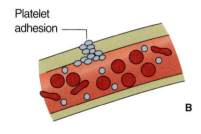

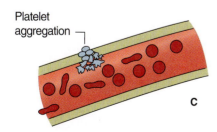

FIGURE 3-2 Illustration of platelet action in a small wound: (A) collagen exposed in vessel lining; (B) platelet adhesion; (C) platelet aggregation

Although platelets are not complete cells, they are quite active chemically. Over 40 substances are secreted from platelets during the release reaction that accompanies aggregation.

The Role of Coagulation Factors

The **coagulation factors** are plasma proteins, except for **ionized calcium** (Ca^{++}), a mineral, formerly called Factor IV. The protein coagulation factors are produced in the liver and circulate in the blood in an inactive form. When a vessel becomes damaged, a series of complex reactions leads to the activation of coagulation factors, resulting in formation of a fibrin clot.

The coagulation factors are numbered I through XIII, in the order in which they were discovered, not in the order of their action. (The numbers IV and VI are no longer used.) Factors II, VII, IX, and X are vitamin K–dependent—this means that vitamin K is required for these factors to be synthesized. In addition, two of the factors are named but have no number. The active forms of the factors are designated by the subscript letter a after the number. For example, activated factor XII is XII_a. The coagulation factor numbers and names are listed in Table 3-1.

Coagulation factor interaction involves very complex reactions. However, the entire process can be summarized in two general reactions: 1) the conversion of prothrombin to thrombin in the presence of thrombokinase and calcium, and 2) the conversion of fibrinogen to fibrin due to the action of thrombin (Figure 3-3).

TABLE 3-1. The coagulation factors

FACTOR NUMBER	NAME
Factor I	Fibrinogen
Factor II	Prothrombin
Factor III	Thromboplastin, tissue factor (TF)
	Ionized Calcium (Ca^{++})
Factor V	Prothrombin accelerator
Factor VII	Proconvertin
Factor VIII:C	Antihemophilic factor (AHF)
Factor IX	Christmas factor
Factor X	Stuart-Prower factor
Factor XI	Plasma thromboplastin antecedent (PTA)
Factor XII	Hageman factor (contact factor)
Factor XIII	Fibrin-stabilizing factor
[*no number assigned*]	Fitzgerald factor (high-molecular-weight kininogen)
[*no number assigned*]	Fletcher factor (prekallikrein)

Note: *Some references may use different names for the numbered factors.*

These two basic concepts developed in 1905 are still valid today. The only changes are the additions of the intermediate plasma-coagulation factors and calcium. The result is the production of a stable fibrin clot to stop bleeding and then dissolution of the clot when it is no longer needed.

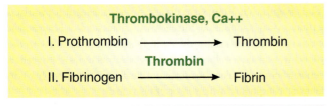

FIGURE 3-3 Simplified diagram showing conversion of prothrombin to fibrin

Fibrinolysis

The fibrin clot serves as a temporary structure until the damaged area heals. The clot is then digested by the action of enzymes. This complex process is called **fibrinolysis**. Two important components of the fibrinolytic system are **plasminogen** and **plasmin**. Plasminogen is present in circulating blood and must be activated to become plasmin. On activation, plasmin binds to fibrin in the clot, initiating its breakdown.

This process breaks fibrinogen and fibrin into **fibrin degradation products (FDPs)** consisting of intermediate fragments X and Y and fragments D and E. This has led to the development of rapid tests, such as those for **D-dimer**, to detect these fragments that can interfere with both polymerization of fibrin and platelet aggregation (Lesson 3-6).

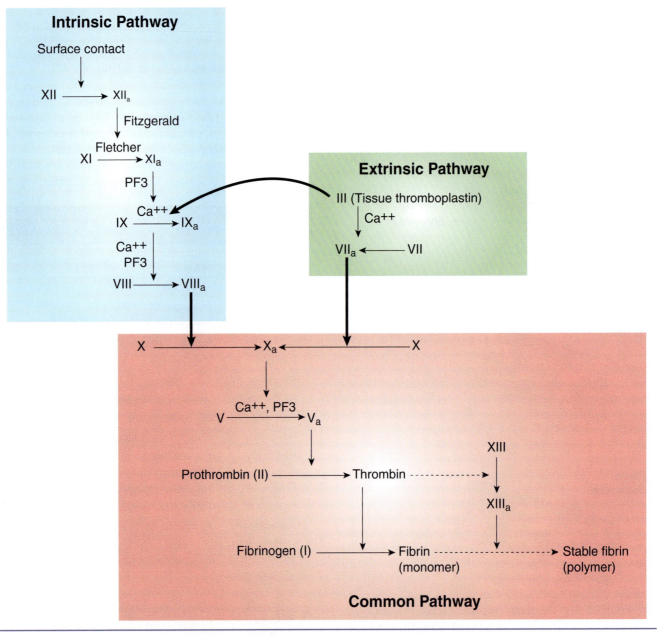

FIGURE 3-4 A modification of the cascade or waterfall hypothesis of hemostasis of MacFarlane (1964) and Davie and Ratnoff (1964)

THE COAGULATION PATHWAYS

The three coagulation pathways are the common, intrinsic, and extrinsic pathways. The **coagulation** process involves activation of the common pathway by either the extrinsic or the intrinsic pathway. There is also some interaction between the extrinsic and the intrinsic pathways. Figure 3-4 illustrates the three pathways.

The Extrinsic Pathway

The extrinsic pathway is so named because one of the coagulation factors involved, factor III, is not present in circulating blood. Factor III, also called tissue factor or **thromboplastin**, is released when blood vessel endothelium is damaged. Factor III is a lipoprotein composed of protein and phospholipid and acts as a cofactor in the activation of factor VII to VII$_a$. Calcium is required for the reaction. Activated factor VII then participates in the reaction converting X to X$_a$ (Figure 3-4).

The Intrinsic Pathway

All of the factors required to activate the intrinsic pathway are present in the circulating blood. This pathway is initiated when factor XII, contact factor, is activated by contact with certain surfaces to form XII$_a$. The final reaction in the intrinsic pathway is the conversion of factor VIII to VIII$_a$. Platelet factor 3 (PF3), a phospholipid released from the platelet membranes, is also required in the activation of factor VIII to factor VIII$_a$ by IX$_a$. Factor IX can also be activated by factor III (tissue factor). Factor VIII$_a$ converts factor X to X$_a$ (Figure 3-4). The intrinsic pathway is also activated when blood contacts a glass syringe or tube during blood collection.

The Common Pathway

Whether the activation occurs by the intrinsic or the extrinsic pathway, the result is the conversion of factor X to X$_a$. The remainder of the activation sequences follow a common pathway (Figure 3-4). A complex reaction involving X$_a$, V, phospholipid, and calcium results in the activation of **prothrombin** to **thrombin**. Thrombin then acts as a catalyst in the conversion of **fibrinogen** to **fibrin** to form a fibrin clot. The fibrin clot is stabilized by factor XIII$_a$.

CONTROL MECHANISMS IN HEMOSTASIS

In normal circumstances, a clot forms only at the site of injury. Regulating systems prevent an isolated injury from initiating the clotting mechanism throughout the body. Normal endothelium lining the blood vessels can also act as a regulator, preventing platelets from adhering and aggregating. In addition, some plasma proteins act as circulating coagulation inhibitors to prevent the formation of unwanted clots.

Intravascular Clotting

Sometimes the hemostasis mechanism goes amiss and intravascular blood clots become a problem. In **atherosclerosis**, a form of **arteriosclerosis,** blood vessel walls become rough and irregular. This can cause platelets to become activated and initiate the formation of clots within the blood vessels (intravascular clotting). A blood clot attached to a vessel wall is called a **thrombus,** but when it breaks off and travels through the circulatory system, it is called an **embolus**. Emboli are very dangerous because they become lodged in small vessels in the brain, lungs, and other organs. They can cause serious damage and sometimes death unless they are dissolved.

Anticoagulant Therapy

The two types of anticoagulants used for prevention and treatment of thrombosis are heparin and Coumadin (sodium warfarin). Heparin administered intravenously is effective immediately but is usually used only short-term. Both Coumadin and heparin can be administered orally and used long-term. Patients who have undergone major surgical procedures or joint replacement (hip or knee) are at risk for blood clot formation. The oral anticoagulants allow them to return home and be treated as outpatients. Patients with certain conditions such as atherosclerosis or phlebitis may have oral anticoagulants (blood thinners) prescribed long-term to prevent the formation of thrombi. These patients must be monitored by having their coagulation times checked at regular intervals.

HEMOSTASIS TESTS

Coagulation analyzers range from relatively simple ones to more complex, fully automated ones. The technology that has been used the longest is based on the detection of a fibrin clot using a moving wire probe. Now, most instruments use electromechanical methods or photo-optical density to detect clot formation. In the former, the clot formation is detected by laser; in the latter, the change in transmitted light is measured as the clot forms. Some coagulation analyzers use only plasma for testing; others use whole blood.

Plasma Tests

Tests for function of the coagulation factors have traditionally been performed on patient plasma samples. The FibroSystem by Becton Dickinson has been used for many years (Figure 3-5). It

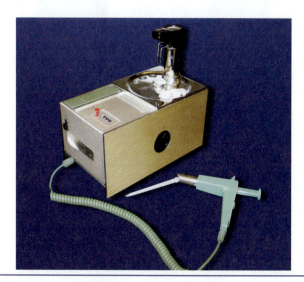

FIGURE 3-5 The FibroSystem

works on the principle of fibrin clot detection with a moving wire probe. This instrument can be used for prothrombin time (PT), activated partial thromboplastin time (APTT), and fibrin assays. The technologist must insert the samples into the fibrometer, add the reagents, and start the timer. When a clot is detected the probe stops moving and the time elapsed is displayed.

Other more automated hemostasis instruments are now in common use. They range from semiautomated to fully automated. With the fully automated models, a tray or rack of plasma tubes can be placed into the machine with identification, such as bar coding. The technologist is then free to perform other duties in the laboratory. The CA-7000 from Sysmex Corp. can generate up to 500 results per hour. This instrument uses clot detection, as well as chromogenic and immunological methods (Figure 3-6).

Helena Laboratories markets the Cascade 480, which automatically aspirates plasma samples directly from blood-collection tubes. The ELECTRA 1000C, manufactured by Medical Laboratory Automation, Inc. (MLA), has an automated specimen-processing and identification system. The COAG-A-MATE series of instruments, marketed by bioMérieux, has been popular in both small and large laboratories.

An additional line of coagulation analyzers known as the ACL series is marketed by Beckman Coulter. The smallest and simplest of them is the ACL. Its test menu includes prothrombin time, fibrinogen, APTT, thrombin time, protein C, protein S, and factor assays. Other analyzers in the series, ACL 1000 through 7000, can sample directly from the blood-collecting tube, reducing technicians' exposure risk.

Whole Blood Tests

Systems have been developed to meet the need for rapid testing. The HEMOCHRON Signature Plus Coagulation Analyzers from International Technidyne Corporation perform several rapid coagulation tests using whole blood. The results of some tests are available in less than 2 minutes and can be performed at point of care.

Three additional point-of-care coagulation analyzers are the GEM PCL, the ACT PLUS, and the CoaguChek S. The GEM PCL's test menu includes APTT, prothrombin time, and activated clotting time test (ACT). The sample size required is just 50 µL of whole blood available from capillary puncture. The APTT and prothrombin time test can also be performed on a blood sample drawn into a citrate tube. The ACT PLUS gives results for prothrombin time and aPTT on whole blood, citrated blood, or plasma samples. The prothrombin time test using the CoaguChek S from Roche Diagnostics is CLIA-waived (Figure 3-7).

Platelet Aggregation Tests

Platelet aggregation can be tested using instruments specially made for the purpose (Figure 3-6B). A tube containing a suspension of the patient's platelets is inserted into the instrument.

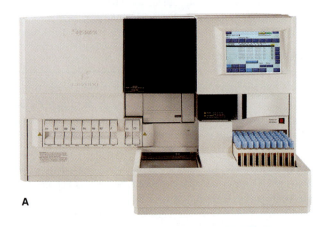

A

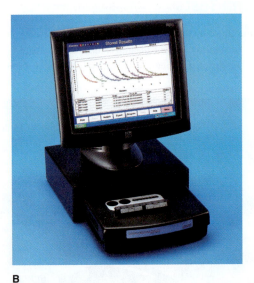

B

FIGURE 3-6 Two types of analyzers used in the coagulation laboratory: (A) Sysmex CA-7000 (*Courtesy of Sysmex America, Mundelein, IL, all rights reserved*); (B) Platelet Aggregation Profiler, Model PAP 8E (*Courtesy of Bio/Data Corporation, Horsham, PA*)

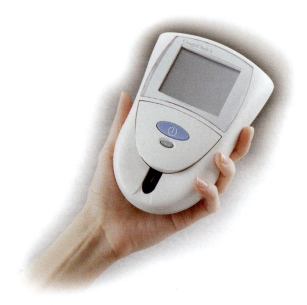

FIGURE 3-7 An example of a handheld coagulation analyzer (*Photo courtesy of Roche Diagnostics Corp., Indianapolis, IN*)

Reagents that induce platelet aggregation, such as collagen, epinephrine, or ristocetin, are added to the suspension. The amount of light transmitted as the platelets aggregate into clumps is proportional to the degree of aggregation; as more platelets aggregate, the suspension clears. The instrument displays a graph illustrating the response.

SAFETY PRECAUTIONS

Instruments substantially increase accuracy and reduce the time required to complete coagulation testing. However, these instruments do pose physical, chemical, and biological hazards. Routine maintenance or repair of an instrument can present several hazards, including shock hazard. Standard Precautions must be followed and personal protective equipment (PPE) worn when performing maintenance and repairs, because the instrument can be contaminated with blood and/or toxic reagents.

Some instruments automatically perform routine maintenance procedures, but if the technician must do them, the manufacturer's instructions must be closely followed. Repairs should be performed only by trained personnel. Removal of the outside case should be attempted only by authorized personnel because of the hazard of electrical shock.

Chemical hazards are present in the reagents used by the instruments when performing analyses. The material safety data sheets (MSDS) accompanying the chemicals must be read and understood by everyone using them.

Preparation of the blood sample for analysis and use of controls and calibrators potentially exposes the worker to bloodborne pathogens (BBPs). Instruments that have a through-the-cap sampler greatly reduce the risk.

QUALITY ASSESSMENT

Every laboratory professional must ensure that correct controls and calibration materials are used and the results verified for each procedure. Standards and controls are available for all coagulation tests whether performed on an instrument or manually. Some instruments, such as the HEMOCHRON line, have both an electronic quality control check and a liquid quality control check at defined intervals as set by the supervisor.

Specimen collection is an important part of laboratory quality. The venipuncture must be performed with minimal trauma to the vein to avoid contaminating the sample with tissue factor. The blood must have 3.2% sodium citrate added in the proportion of one part anticoagulant to nine parts blood. When a laboratory maintains a good QA program and participates in a certified proficiency testing program, the physician can have confidence in the results used to guide patient treatment.

SUMMARY

Hemostasis, the process of stopping the loss of blood, is a delicate balance between coagulation and fibrinolysis. This balance is maintained by the interaction of the blood vessels, platelets, coagulation factors, and components of the fibrinolytic system. Abnormalities in any part of the system can cause conditions ranging from mild to life-threatening.

Tests for hemostatic function can be as simple as the platelet count and prothrombin time or as complex as assays for factor deficiencies and platelet aggregation tests. Automated and semiautomated instruments are available to perform coagulation tests and have simplified and somewhat reduced the workload in the laboratory. Small, simple-to-operate instruments have made it possible to perform more testing in physician office laboratories and at point of care. In some cases, patients can now perform testing at home with small, handheld meters.

Patients receiving oral anticoagulant therapy must be tested at regular intervals. Through good quality assessment programs, the physician and patient can have confidence that test results are accurate and can be relied on for diagnosis, treatment, and management of hemostatic disorders.

REVIEW QUESTIONS

1. List the four interrelated systems that have a role in hemostasis.
2. Describe the blood vessels' role in hemostasis.
3. Outline the role of platelets in clot formation.
4. Describe the role of the coagulation factors in hemostasis.
5. List the coagulation factors that are vitamin K dependent.
6. Explain how atherosclerosis can cause thrombus formation.
7. Name the two important components of the fibrinolytic system.
8. Name the three pathways in the coagulation cascade and the factors involved in each.
9. What types of blood specimens can be used for coagulation testing?
10. Explain the advantages of using the new whole blood coagulation testing instruments.
11. Name two instruments that use plasma for coagulation tests.
12. Explain how platelet aggregation testing is performed.
13. How could vitamin K deficiency affect hemostasis?
14. Define adhesion, aggregation, arteriosclerosis, atherosclerosis, coagulation, coagulation factors, collagen, D-dimer, embolus, endothelium, fibrin, fibrin degradation products, fibrinogen, fibrinolysis, hemorrhage, hemostasis, intravascular, ionized calcium, plasmin, plasminogen, prothrombin, thrombin, thromboplastin, thrombus, and vasoconstriction.

STUDENT ACTIVITIES

1. Complete the written examination for this lesson.

2. Research the use of instruments for coagulation testing. How do the requirements of physician office laboratories differ from those of hospital laboratories?

3. Interview an employee of a hematology or coagulation laboratory and ask about the types of coagulation testing performed.

4. Research and report on laboratory tests of platelet function.

5. Interview a cardiac rehabilitation educator about causes and complications of atherosclerosis.

WEB ACTIVITIES

1. Use the Internet to find information about correlating coagulation results from point-of-care testing instruments with results from the main or reference laboratory.

2. Use the Internet to find conditions that can cause vitamin K deficiency.

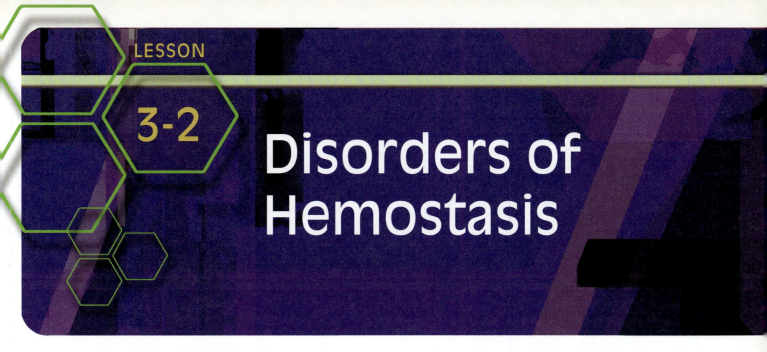

Disorders of Hemostasis

LESSON OBJECTIVES

After studying this lesson, the student will:

- List and discuss two inherited and two acquired abnormalities of platelets.
- List and discuss two inherited and two acquired abnormalities of coagulation factors.
- List the coagulation factors that are vitamin K dependent.
- Name three tests for evaluating hemostatic function.
- Explain how disseminated intravascular coagulation (DIC) occurs.
- Define the glossary terms.

GLOSSARY

disseminated intravascular coagulation (DIC) / a bleeding disorder characterized by widespread thrombotic and secondary fibrinolytic reactions

hemophilia / a bleeding disorder resulting from a hereditary coagulation factor deficiency or dysfunction

petechiae / small, purplish hemorrhagic spots on the skin

INTRODUCTION

Hemostasis disorders have a variety of causes. A disorder can be inherited, such as classic hemophilia, or acquired, such as abnormalities resulting from a vitamin K deficiency. Acquired abnormalities can also arise because of medications, such as the effect of aspirin on platelet aggregation. Other drugs or treatments can accelerate clot formation. These inherited and acquired disorders of hemostasis affect patients' lives and require a combination of clinical examination, laboratory tests, and investigation into family medical history for diagnosis.

HEREDITARY DISORDERS OF HEMOSTASIS

Inherited Factor Disorders

The **hemophilias** are inherited diseases in which there is a deficiency or functional disorder in one or more of the coagulation factors (Table 3-2). Classic hemophilia, called *hemophilia A*, is caused by a functional deficiency of coagulation factor VIII, the VIII:C protein.

319

Hemophilia B, also called Christmas disease, is named after the first patient in which it was studied. The defect in Christmas disease is a functional deficiency of coagulation factor IX.

Hemophilias A and B are inherited as sex-linked recessive genes carried on the X chromosome. Since males inherit one X and one Y, if the inherited X chromosome carries the recessive hemophilia gene, the disease will be expressed. Since females have two X chromosomes, those who carry the recessive hemophilia gene on one X chromosome will not manifest the disease because the normal X chromosome will be dominant. These females are called *carriers* and can pass the recessive gene to their offspring. Therefore, the diseases are limited almost exclusively to males, although there have been rare cases documented in females.

The clinical symptoms of hemophilias A and B are identical. Affected infants do not have symptoms unless they undergo circumcision or other surgery. However, as the child grows and is subject to bumps and falls, large bruises appear. Abnormal bleeding occurs into the joints, causing swelling and pain. In addition, bleeding occurs in the mouth, muscles, renal tract, and gut and after dental extractions.

The most common inherited factor deficiency is *von Willebrand's disease* (vWD). It is not really a disease, but is a condition caused by a deficiency or functional abnormality of von Willebrand factor (vWF). The vWF is a portion of the factor VIII molecule, the VIII:vWF segment. Although the deficiency is in a coagulation factor, it results in alteration of platelet adhesion. Most cases of von Willebrand's disease are mild, and display symptoms such as nose bleeds, bleeding of the gums, and easy bruising. Unlike the classic hemophilias, von Willebrand's disease is inherited as an autosomal trait, and so can occur in both males and females.

Although rare in occurrence, coagulation problems can be caused by either quantitative or functional deficiencies of other coagulation factors.

Inherited Platelet Disorders

Several inherited disorders of platelets cause prolonged bleeding in the patient (Table 3-2). *Bernard-Soulier syndrome* is a disorder in which the platelets are larger than normal and are present in normal or decreased numbers. The platelets' ability to adhere is decreased because of a defect in the surface membrane. Affected patients develop small, purplish spots on the skin called **petechiae**. They also suffer gastrointestinal bleeding, nosebleeds, abnormal menstrual bleeding, or intracranial bleeding. The disease can be severe and even fatal.

In *Glanzmann's thrombasthenia*, the platelet count and platelet morphology are usually normal. The platelets have the ability to adhere to collagen but do not have normal aggregation. If a smear is made from the patient's capillary blood or venous blood without an anticoagulant, the platelets do not form the characteristic clumps. The defect has been found to be in the surface membrane of the platelets. The patient's bleeding problems are similar to those of the Bernard-Soulier patient.

As discussed in the previous section, von Willebrand's disease (vWD) is caused by an abnormality or deficiency in part of the Factor VIII molecule. However, the condition is often grouped with platelet disorders because the major effect is on the platelets. In the condition, the platelet count is normal but the adhesion function of platelets is diminished, resulting in bleeding from slight injuries.

ACQUIRED DISORDERS OF HEMOSTASIS

Acquired disorders of hemostasis can cause either abnormal bleeding or thrombus formation. The disorders can affect one or more of the coagulation factors or the platelets (Table 3-2).

Acquired Factor Disorders

Acquired factor disorders can be due to:

- Vitamin K deficiency
- Disseminated intravascular coagulation
- Circulating inhibitors to coagulation factors

Severe deficiency of vitamin K causes decreased production of the vitamin K-dependent coagulation factors, factors II, VII, IX, and X. The oral anticoagulant Coumadin, often prescribed to reduce unwanted clotting, acts as a vitamin K antagonist, causing a decrease in the vitamin K-dependent factors. Other causes of vitamin K deficiency include insufficient vitamin K in diet (rare), malabsorption of vitamin K from the intestine, and prolonged treatment with antibiotics.

Disseminated intravascular coagulation (DIC) is a serious condition in which a pathological process initiates coagulation

TABLE 3-2. Acquired and inherited disorders of hemostasis

COAGULATION FACTOR DISORDERS

ACQUIRED	INHERITED
Vitamin K deficiency	Hemophilia A
Anticoagulant therapy	Hemophilia B
Disseminated intravascular coagulation (DIC)	von Willebrand's disease
	Deficiencies or dysfunction of coagulation factors

PLATELET DISORDERS

ACQUIRED	INHERITED
Aspirin ingestion	von Willebrand's disease
Decreased mega-karyocyte production	Bernard-Soulier syndrome
Idiopathic thrombo-cytopenic purpura (ITP)	Glanzmann's thrombasthenia

This table lists only a few disorders and is not meant to be a comprehensive list.

and secondary fibrinolysis. Depending on the balance between the two systems, there may be thrombosis or bleeding, or a combination of the two. Some conditions that contribute to DIC are crushing injuries; certain bacterial, viral, or rickettsial infections; and drug reactions.

DIC occurs when intravascular coagulation is triggered. This causes fibrin deposition in blood vessels, which in turn uses up the available supply of coagulation factors. Microthrombi form in vital organs, including the kidneys, lungs, heart, and brain. The fibrinolytic system is then activated, releasing fibrin fragments that can act as coagulation inhibitors.

Another cause of bleeding disorders is the development of circulating inhibitors to coagulation factors. These inhibitors, also called circulating anticoagulants, usually are autoantibodies directed at one or more of the clotting factors, causing the factor(s) to be removed from the blood, creating a factor deficiency.

Acquired Platelet Disorders

Acquired platelet disorders can arise from several sources (Table 3-2). *Idiopathic thrombocytopenic purpura (ITP)* occurs when the immune system makes antibodies against the patient's own platelets. Acquired thrombocytopenia can occur when the spleen enlarges from disease. The enlarged spleen traps many platelets inside the spleen (sequestration), reducing the number of circulating platelets. Infection by certain viruses can decrease the bone marrow production of megakaryocytes. Ingestion of aspirin affects the aggregation of platelets for up to 8 to 10 days by inhibiting the platelet-release reaction (Table 3-2).

TESTS OF HEMOSTATIC FUNCTION

Examination of hemostatic function can involve testing the platelets, the blood vessels, or the coagulation factors. The tests can include the prothrombin time, activated partial thromboplastin time (APTT), bleeding time, and platelet count. Expected laboratory results for some disorders of hemostasis are shown in Table 3-3.

The platelet count, discussed and performed in Lesson 2-6, is a quantitative test for platelets. However, even if the platelet count is in the normal reference range, a bleeding problem can still exist if the platelets do not function normally.

Bleeding time is a screening test for quantitative or qualitative abnormalities in the platelets, and also for vascular integrity of the capillaries (Lesson 3-3). When bleeding time is prolonged, more definitive tests, such as platelet adhesion and platelet aggregation, must be performed.

Prothrombin time is a measure of the extrinsic pathway and is discussed at length in Lesson 3-4. The APTT, discussed in Lesson 3-5, is a test of intrinsic pathway function. Instruments used in coagulation testing are discussed in Lesson 3-1 and Lesson 3-6, Rapid Hemostasis Tests.

Safety Precautions

 For hemostasis tests that are performed on plasma samples, anticoagulated blood must be centrifuged to separate the cells from the plasma. The worker can potentially be exposed to pathogens if the collection tube stopper must be removed and the plasma transferred by pipet. To avoid exposure, Standard Precautions must always be followed. Appropriate personal protective equipment (PPE) such as gloves and face protection must be worn. With newer instruments that use whole blood or pierce the tube stopper to obtain the plasma, the risk of exposure is somewhat reduced. However, the worker must always observe the safety policies and procedures of the workplace.

Quality Assessment

Specimen collection for hemostasis tests must be performed carefully. Venipuncture must be performed with minimum trauma to the vein and surrounding tissues. Tests of the coagulation pathways, such as prothrombin time, are designed to artificially activate the coagulation factors in a plasma sample to measure the clotting time. Tissue or vessel damage during venipuncture releases thromboplastin into the sample, activating the extrinsic pathway prematurely, causing erroneous test results. In addition, the blood-collecting tube must contain the correct type and amount of anticoagulant.

TABLE 3-3. Expected coagulation test results for some disorders of hemostasis

CONDITION	BLEEDING TIME	PROTHROMBIN TIME	ACTIVATED PARTIAL THROMBOPLASTIN TIME
Hemophilia A	Normal	Normal	Abnormal
Hemophilia B	Normal	Normal	Abnormal
von Willebrand's disease	Prolonged	Abnormal	Abnormal
Anticoagulant therapy	Normal	Abnormal	Abnormal
Glanzmann's thrombasthenia	Prolonged	Normal	Normal

CURRENT TOPICS

HEMOPHILIA

Hemophilia, the oldest known inherited blood disorder, is caused by low levels or complete lack of a blood protein essential for clotting. Hemophilia A is caused by a deficiency in Factor VIII; hemophilia B is caused by a lack of Factor IX.

There are about 20,000 hemophiliacs in the United States; approximately 85% have hemophilia A, and the rest have hemophilia B. Each year about 400 babies are born with the disorder. The severity of the disease is related to the levels of functional coagulation factors in the blood. Approximately 70% of patients have less than 1% of the normal factor level and therefore have severe disease. However, when factor level is increased to just 5% of normal, the patient usually has only a mild form of disease and bleeding events are rare except after injuries or surgery.

Treatment—Treatment of hemophilia has historically involved transfusion of plasma containing the needed factor. This traditionally has been *on-demand* therapy given only when bleeding symptoms appear. Usually by that time bleeding into the joints has already occurred. This repeated internal bleeding causes joint damage. In some European countries, treatments are given periodically to keep the factor level high enough to prevent bleeding, joint destruction, and hemorrhage. However, because these patients must have a venous catheter to have frequent access to the veins, there is an increased risk of infection.

The most serious challenges to successful treatment are:

■ Maintaining safety of blood products

■ Managing inhibitor formation

■ Preventing irreversible joint damage

■ Preventing life-threatening hemorrhage

■ Making progress toward a cure

The Hemophilia Treatment Centers and National Institutes of Health (NIH) sponsor over 100 hemophilia treatment centers around the United States. These organizations also coordinate treatment and offer grants for scientific research into improved treatment. For example, after hurricanes Katrina and Rita in 2005, they organized efforts to ensure that patients could receive treatments in Houston, Texas.

In the past, safety of blood products used for treatment of hemophilias has been a major concern. With improved testing methods and techniques to inactivate viruses, the risk of becoming infected with HIV or one of the hepatitis viruses is now mostly a thing of the past. However, there is still concern over the potential of these products to transmit emerging diseases such as variant Creutzfeldt-Jakob disease (vCJD)—the human form of mad cow disease.

Research—Factor VIII can now be produced by biotechnology. This recombinant Factor VIII is entirely free of blood components. Although the cost is higher for this form, it is clearly the choice for infants because it is free of viruses and plasma proteins that can cause allergic reactions and immunosuppression. Clinical trials are now in progress using recombinant Factor IX. In early 2005, the NIH announced research grants to be awarded for development of:

■ Modified Factor VIII or IX proteins with improved biological activity and/or increased functional half-life

■ Drugs to improve the activity or biological availability of factors

■ Novel hemostatic agents such as small molecules to promote hemostasis

■ Ways to use immunosuppressive agents to prevent immune response to factor therapies

Although hemophilia remains a potentially life-threatening condition, progress is being made. Gene therapy has been done experimentally in mice and dogs, but a clinical trial with human subjects has not been approved. The prognosis should improve as more scientific research is applied to patient care.

SUMMARY

Hemostasis disorders can result from abnormalities or deficiencies in platelets, coagulation factors, or both. Disorders can be inherited or acquired and can cause conditions ranging from mild to life-threatening. Hemophilias A and B are examples of inherited disorders of hemostasis. Certain drugs and cancer treatments can cause an acquired thrombocytopenia. Vitamin K deficiency can cause decreased production of coagulation factors, an acquired condition that can be reversed by increasing vitamin K in the body. Development of rapid, portable test systems for detection of hemostasis disorders, as well as treatments such as recombinant Factor VIII, contribute to better diagnosis and treatment of these disorders.

REVIEW QUESTIONS

1. Name two acquired and two inherited disorders of platelets.

2. What is the effect of aspirin on platelets?

3. List the vitamin K–dependent coagulation factors.

4. Name two hereditary disorders of coagulation factors.

5. Explain the differences between hemophilia A and hemophilia B.

6. Explain why hemophilia A and hemophilia B are almost exclusively limited to males.

7. What percent of hemophilia patients have hemophilia B?

8. Discuss conditions that contribute to DIC.

9. How does the defect in von Willebrand's disease affect platelets?

10. Define disseminated intravascular coagulation, hemophilia, and petechiae.

STUDENT ACTIVITIES

1. Complete the written examination for this lesson.

2. Research and report on a hemostasis disorder.

WEB ACTIVITIES

1. Find information about treatment(s) of hemophilias using the Internet and report on them.

2. Use the Internet to find information on the genetics governing the inheritance of hemophilia B.

3. Find information about DIC using the Internet. Report on the clinical signs, treatments, and laboratory tests used to identify and evaluate the condition.

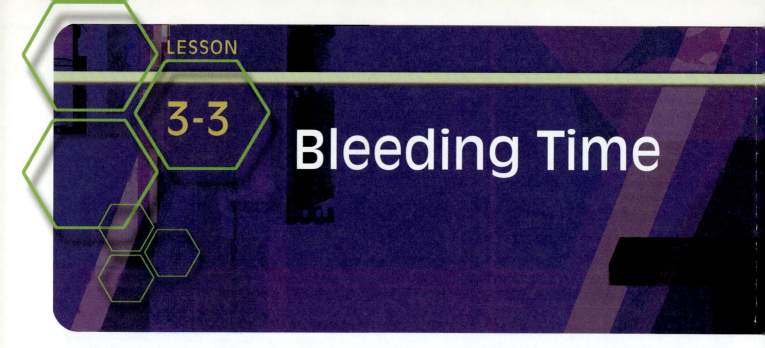

Bleeding Time

LESSON OBJECTIVES

After studying this lesson, the student will:

- State the purpose of the bleeding-time test.
- Name and describe two methods used to determine bleeding time and list the reference values of each.
- List three conditions in which bleeding time will be prolonged.
- Interpret the results of a bleeding time test.
- List the safety precautions to be observed in performing a bleeding time.
- Discuss quality assessment procedures to be followed when performing a bleeding time test.
- Define the glossary terms.

GLOSSARY

dysfunction / impaired or abnormal function

INTRODUCTION

The bleeding-time test is a screening procedure used to evaluate the function of platelets and small blood vessels. The test is performed by making a small standardized incision of capillaries. The length of time required for the bleeding to stop is noted and recorded.

Hemostasis, the cessation of bleeding, involves a series of complex interactions. The components that must interact are:

- Blood vessels
- Blood platelets
- Plasma proteins known as coagulation factors

The blood vessels must be able to constrict and slow blood flow after an injury. This property is known as vasoconstriction.

The platelets react within seconds after an injury to form a plug and release certain chemical activators. The coagulation factors are activated by the platelets and the tissue factor released from the injured tissue.

When all the hemostasis components interact and function properly, a clot is formed and bleeding stops. Failure of the clotting mechanism can be due to the absence, deficiency, or improper function of any of the components. Failure of the hemostatic or clotting mechanism can result in hemorrhage, uncontrolled bleeding.

Decreased numbers of platelets (thrombocytopenia), platelet **dysfunction**, and ingestion of aspirin or other drugs can prolong bleeding time. Aspirin can affect platelet function for up to 8 to 10 days. Except for von Willebrand's disease, abnormality or deficiency of one of the coagulation factors does not usually affect the bleeding time.

PRINCIPLE OF THE BLEEDING TIME TEST

The bleeding time tests the functions of the platelets and the capillary blood vessels by measuring the time required for a small standardized skin incision to stop bleeding. The test indirectly evaluates platelet numbers and function. When a vessel is injured, platelet adhesion and aggregation must occur to form a platelet plug at the site of injury. The bleeding time test also measures the ability of the capillaries to contract and slow blood flow to the area.

METHODS OF MEASURING BLEEDING TIME

Two ways of measuring bleeding time are the Ivy method and the Duke method. The Ivy method, although the more difficult to perform correctly, is preferred because it can be somewhat standardized. The Duke method is rarely performed. Both methods present difficulties in obtaining reproducible results. All coagulation tests must be performed carefully and accurately by well-trained technicians.

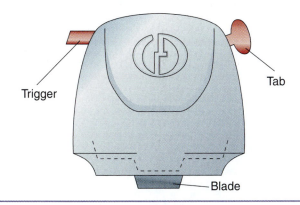

FIGURE 3-8 Illustration of a device used in the bleeding-time test

Safety Precautions

  Standard Precautions must be observed while performing the bleeding-time test. Appropriate personal protective equipment, including gloves and a fluid-resistant laboratory coat, must be worn by the technician. In addition, the blades of the bleeding-time device or lancet are potentially dangerous. All sharps must be handled carefully and discarded in a sharps container. The filter paper should be disposed of in the biohazard waste container.

Quality Assessment

  The bleeding time procedure must be carefully followed so that the test results are reliable.

- The proper area of the arm must be used.
- The alcohol-cleansed site must be allowed to dry completely before the test is performed.
- Pediatric-sized bleeding-time devices should be used when performing the test on infants and children.
- The filter paper should touch only the drop of blood, not the incision.
- Timers must be checked for accuracy on a regular basis.

Ivy Bleeding Time

The Ivy bleeding-time test is performed by making an incision in the forearm and measuring the time required for bleeding to stop.

This method is usually performed using devices such as Simplate or Surgicutt, which make a standardized incision (Figures 3-8 and 3-9). Proper incision depth and length differs for infants and children and for adults. Bleeding-time devices are available in sizes appropriate for these groups. Patients must be informed that this procedure can cause scarring.

A blood-pressure cuff is placed around the patient's arm above the elbow, and the pressure is increased to 40 mm of mer-

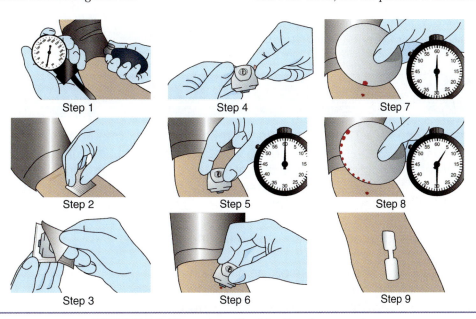

Step 1 Step 4 Step 7
Step 2 Step 5 Step 8
Step 3 Step 6 Step 9

FIGURE 3-9 Illustration of Ivy bleeding-time procedure

TABLE 3-4. Reference ranges for bleeding-time tests*

METHOD	REFERENCE RANGE
Ivy	2–9 minutes
Duke	1–3 minutes

* Each laboratory should establish its own reference ranges for bleeding time.

SAFETY Reminders

- Observe Standard Precautions.
- Discard the used puncture device in the biohazard sharps container.
- Discard the used filter paper in the appropriate biohazard waste container.

cury to standardize the pressure in the capillaries. This pressure is held constant for the entire procedure.

The forearm is cleansed with 70% alcohol. A standardized incision is made on the inner surface of the forearm in an area free of large superficial blood vessels (Figure 3-9). A timer is started when the first drop of blood appears. At 30-second intervals, the blood is blotted with filter paper without touching the puncture site. When bleeding ceases, the time is noted and the pressure cuff removed. The technician should stop the test if bleeding continues more than 15 minutes. The time between the first appearance of blood and the stopping of blood flow is the bleeding time.

Normal bleeding time by the Ivy method is 2 to 9 minutes (Table 3-4).

Duke Bleeding Time

The Duke bleeding-time test was used for many years but is rarely performed today. The Duke bleeding-time test is performed by making an incision in the earlobe and measuring the time required for bleeding to cease.

To perform the test, the earlobe is cleansed with alcohol and allowed to dry. A puncture is made with a sterile lancet, and timing is begun when the first drop of blood appears. The blood is blotted every 30 seconds with filter paper without touching the actual puncture site. The timer is stopped when bleeding ceases. The time elapsed is reported as the bleeding time. Normal bleeding time by the Duke method is 1 to 3 minutes (Table 3-4).

PROCEDURAL Reminders

- Do not perform the bleeding-time test if the patient has taken aspirin products within the last 8 to 10 days.
- Ensure that the incision site is warm before performing the test.
- Choose an incision site free of superficial veins.
- Allow the alcohol-cleansed puncture site to dry completely before making the incision.
- Do not wipe away the first drop of blood that appears after the incision is made.
- Touch only the drop of blood, not the incision, with the filter paper.
- Stop the test if bleeding continues more than 15 minutes in the Ivy test and notify the supervisor.

CASE STUDY

Ms. Clark, a 63-year-old patient, had been taking an aspirin-containing over-the-counter medication daily for mild arthritic pain. She was scheduled for minor surgery, and her surgeon ordered an Ivy bleeding-time test after Ms. Clark reported that she had several bruises but did not remember injuring herself. The bleeding-time was 11 minutes; the surgeon postponed the surgery and told Ms. Clark to stop taking the medication.

1. When should the surgeon order another bleeding-time test?
    a. When the bruises are gone
    b. 8 to 10 days after the last dose of the pain reliever
    c. After results from other coagulation tests are received
    d. About 3 to 5 days after pain reliever is discontinued
2. Explain your answer.

SUMMARY

The bleeding time has often been used as a presurgery screening test. It is not specific for any one condition, but an abnormally long bleeding time can indicate problems with either capillary or platelet function. A prolonged bleeding time can signal the need to do further coagulation testing. The physician can order a platelet count, a blood smear for platelet morphology, and other tests such as platelet aggregation. All Standard Precautions must be observed while performing the bleeding-time test. The laboratory's quality assessment policies must be followed to ensure valid test results.

REVIEW QUESTIONS

1. What functions are measured by the bleeding-time test?
2. What three components interact to produce hemostasis?
3. How do the number and function of platelets affect the bleeding time?
4. Explain the procedure for the Ivy bleeding-time test.
5. Describe the quality assessment procedures that must be observed when performing the bleeding-time test.
6. State the reference range for bleeding time by the Ivy method.
7. List safety precautions that should be observed when performing a bleeding-time test.
8. What incision site is used for the Ivy method? For the Duke method?
9. Define dysfunction.

STUDENT ACTIVITIES

1. Complete the written examination for this lesson.
2. Practice explaining the bleeding-time procedure to a patient.
3. Practice applying a blood pressure cuff, inflating to 40 mm Hg, and maintaining the pressure for 5 minutes.
4. Practice performing a bleeding-time test as outlined in the Student Performance Guide.
5. Find out which bleeding-time test is performed in a local laboratory.

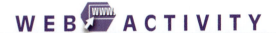

W E B   ACTIVITY

Use the Internet to research the mechanisms by which nonsteroidal anti-inflammatory drugs (NSAIDs) such as aspirin and ibuprofen affect bleeding time. Find out if acetaminophen affects the bleeding time.

Student Performance Guide

Name _____ Date _____

INSTRUCTIONS

1. Practice performing a bleeding-time test (Ivy method) following the step-by-step procedure.
2. Demonstrate the bleeding-time procedure satisfactorily for the instructor using the Student Performance Guide. Your instructor will determine the level of competency you must achieve to obtain a satisfactory (S) grade.

NOTE: *Always follow manufacturer's directions for the type of bleeding-time device used.*

MATERIALS AND EQUIPMENT

- gloves
- face shield
- antiseptic
- sterile cotton balls or gauze
- 70% alcohol or alcohol swabs
- blood-pressure cuff
- filter paper
- timer
- surface disinfectant
- biohazard container
- sharps container
- butterfly bandage
- commercial bleeding-time device such as Simplate or Surgicutt, including instructions

PROCEDURE

Record in the comment section any problems encountered while practicing the procedure (or have a fellow student or the instructor evaluate your performance).

S = Satisfactory
U = Unsatisfactory

You must:	S	U	Comments
1. Assemble equipment and materials. Put on face protection			
2. Wash hands and put on gloves			
3. Explain the procedure to the patient			
4. Seat the patient and explain that the test can cause a small scar; have the patient rest the arm palm side up			
5. Choose a site containing no visible blood vessels on the inner surface of the forearm approximately 5 cm below the cubital crease			
6. Cleanse the site with 70% alcohol. Wait for the alcohol to dry completely			

You must:	S	U	Comments
7. Place the blood-pressure cuff on the arm above the elbow and inflate to 40 mm Hg pressure (for adults). Maintain that pressure during the test			
8. Set a sharps container within reach			
9. Prepare the bleeding time device following manufacturer's instructions			
10. Make the incision following the instructions included with the bleeding-time device. Start the timer when the incision is made			
11. Discard the device into the sharps container			
12. Touch the filter paper to the drop of blood after 30 seconds; do not touch the incision			
13. Repeat step 12 every 30 seconds until no blood appears on the filter paper			
14. Stop the timer			
15. *Remove the blood pressure cuff*			
16. Cleanse the site gently with sterile gauze or a cotton ball; apply a butterfly bandage to minimize the chance of scarring. Advise the patient to leave the bandage in place for 24 hours			
17. Discard filter paper in biohazard container			
18. Wipe the work area with surface disinfectant			
19. Remove and discard gloves in biohazard container. Wash hands with antiseptic			
20. Report result as the time on the timer			

Evaluator Comments:

Evaluator _____ Date _____

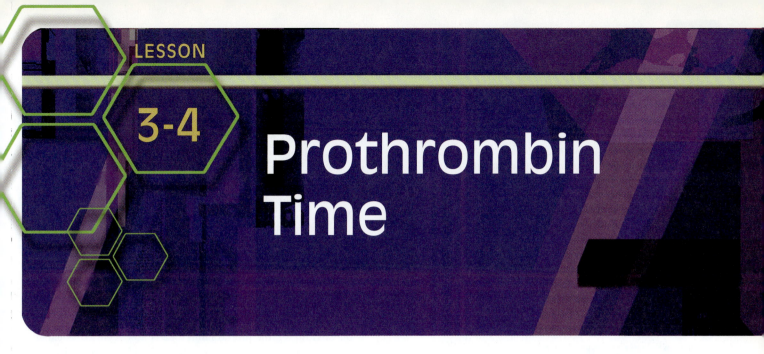

Prothrombin Time

LESSON OBJECTIVES

After studying this lesson, the student will:

- Discuss the role of prothrombin in blood coagulation.
- Explain the major use of the prothrombin time test.
- Perform a prothrombin time test.
- State the reference values for the prothrombin time test.
- Name three point-of-care testing instruments for prothrombin time.
- Explain the importance and use of the international normalized ratio (INR).
- Calculate the INR value.
- List two instruments that use whole blood samples for the prothrombin time test.
- Discuss safety procedures that must be followed when performing the prothrombin time.
- Discuss quality assessment procedures for the prothrombin time test.
- Define the glossary terms.

GLOSSARY

Coumadin / an anticoagulant derived from coumarin that is administered orally to prevent or slow clotting

enzyme / a protein that causes or accelerates changes in other substances without being changed itself

international normalized ratio (INR) / a way of reporting a prothrombin time that takes into consideration the sensitivity of the thromboplastin used and the mean of the normal prothrombin time in the facility's population

international sensitivity index (ISI) / a value assigned to each lot of thromboplastin to compensate for variations in sensitivities of thromboplastin from different sources

prothrombin time / a coagulation screening test used to monitor oral anticoagulant therapy

vitamin K / a vitamin essential for production of coagulation Factors II, VII, IX, and X

INTRODUCTION

The **prothrombin time (PT)** or *pro time*, one of the most frequently performed coagulation tests, evaluates the function of the extrinsic and common pathways of hemostasis. It is used not only as a pre-surgery coagulation screening test, but also to monitor **Coumadin** (warfarin) anticoagulant therapy. Patients may have the prothrombin time performed in a physician office laboratory (POL), a hospital outpatient laboratory, or a reference laboratory. Prothrombin time results can be used to guide the physician in regulating the patient's anticoagulant dosage. The test was developed by Dr. A. J. Quick, who named it prothrombin time because he thought it measured only prothrombin. Even though it was later discovered that the test actually measures prothrombin plus additional factors, it is still called the prothrombin time.

PRINCIPLE OF THE PROTHROMBIN TIME TEST

The hemostasis pathway is normally activated when damage occurs to blood vessel endothelium or to body tissue. The extrinsic pathway converts Factor X, a proenzyme, to the enzyme X_a which in turn converts prothrombin to the enzyme thrombin (Figure 3-10). An **enzyme** is a protein that is able to cause or accelerate changes in other substances without being changed.

Thrombin acts on fibrinogen to form fibrin monomers that make up the initial unstable clot.

Prothrombin (Factor II) is produced in the liver and is **vitamin K** dependent. A deficiency of vitamin K causes reduced amounts of the factor to be produced and can result in bleeding. The prothrombin time is used as a coagulation screening test to measure the extrinsic pathway (Figure 3-10). Its major use is to monitor oral anticoagulant therapy since these anticoagulants decrease the production of prothrombin and factors VII, IX, and X in the liver. The prothrombin time results in factor deficiencies and other conditions are compared in Table 3-5.

Reference Values for Prothrombin Time

The accepted prothrombin time reference value is 10 to 13 seconds. However, the prothrombin time is now reported as either the prothrombin ratio or the **international normalized ratio (INR)**. The prothrombin ratio compares the patient's result with the mean of the normal population of the facility. The INR is used to standardize prothrombin time reporting among different laboratories. Because each lot of thromboplastin can have a different sensitivity in the prothrombin test, an **international sensitivity index (ISI)** is assigned to each reagent lot by the manufacturer. The ISI is used in the INR formula to compensate for varying sensitivities of thromboplastin reagent. Before the INR was used,

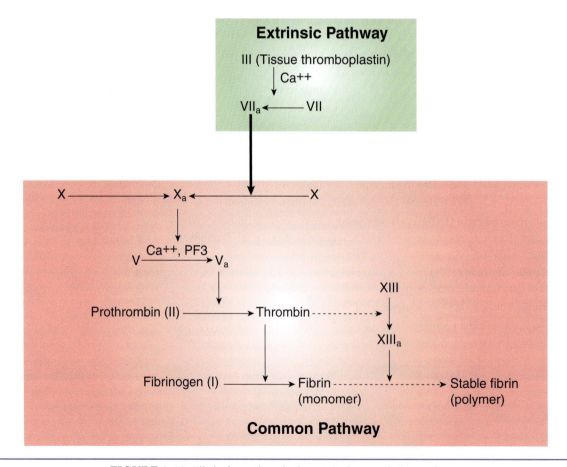

FIGURE 3-10 Fibrin formation via the extrinsic coagulation pathway

Calculate the International Normalized Ratio (INR) where:
patient prothrombin time = 23 seconds
mean normal protime of the facility = 10.5 seconds
ISI = 1.2

$$INR = \left(\frac{Patient\ result\ in\ seconds}{Mean\ normal\ of\ the\ facility\ in\ seconds} \right)^{ISI}$$

$$INR = \left(\frac{23\ sec}{10.5\ sec} \right)^{1.2}$$

$$INR = (2.1)^{1.2}$$

$$INR = 2.52$$

FIGURE 3-11 One example of calculating the international normalized ratio (INR)

a patient could have a prothrombin time test performed on the same day at different laboratories and have different results. The reference value for the INR is 1.0 to 1.4. See Figure 3-11 for an example of calculating the INR.

PERFORMING THE PROTHROMBIN TIME TEST

The prothrombin time can be performed manually, using the FibroSystem, using a multitest instrument that runs several hemostasis tests on the same sample, or using small, handheld instruments. The manual method is rarely used except for research, but it has the advantage of being able to see the clot as it forms. The FibroSystem has been used for decades; moving wires detect the formation of the clot in the sample cup and stop the timer. In higher volume laboratories, the test is performed on instruments that are capable of performing several hemostasis tests on the same plasma sample. Most of these detect clot formation by photo-optical means. The newest instruments are small, handheld devices that perform several different tests, one at a time or the same sample in duplicate.

Safety Precautions

Performing the prothrombin time involves handling patient blood and control plasmas. In addition, the technician may also perform the venipuncture and process the specimen before testing it. Standard Precautions must be observed to protect the worker from bloodborne pathogens.

Quality Assessment

Quality assessment for the prothrombin-time test includes collecting and processing the specimen, analyzing control plasmas, and performing the test procedure.

- The venipuncture must be clean, since trauma to the vein or surrounding tissues releases tissue factor into the specimen.

TABLE 3-5. Prothrombin time results in various conditions

CONDITION	PROTHROMBIN TIME RESULTS
Factor Deficiencies	
VIII	Normal
XI	Normal
XII	Normal
II	Prolonged
V	Prolonged
VII	Prolonged
X	Prolonged
Other Conditions	
Coumadin therapy	Prolonged
Heparin therapy	Prolonged
Liver disease	Prolonged
Vitamin K deficiency	Prolonged

- The ratio of anticoagulant to blood is critical: one (1) part anticoagulant to nine (9) parts blood.

- The filled tube should be immediately inverted to gently mix the blood and anticoagulant.

- While separating the plasma from the blood cells by centrifugation, the tube of blood must be stoppered to prevent exposure to the air.

- All specimens, controls, and instruments must be at the proper temperature before the test is performed.

Collecting the Specimen

The specimen for the prothrombin time must be collected with minimal trauma to the vein and surrounding tissue to prevent the release of tissue thromboplastin into the sample. The blood is drawn into a tube that contains a 3.2% solution of sodium citrate. The vacuum tube contains 0.5 ml of the anticoagulant and is manufactured to draw 4.5 mL of blood. It is essential that the proportion of anticoagulant to blood be one (1) part anticoagulant to nine (9) parts blood in order for the test results to be valid. The tube of blood must be centrifuged as soon as possible and the plasma transferred to a clean tube for use in the assay. The plasma is usually assayed within 4 hours of collection; however, the operating procedures of the facility or reference laboratory must be followed. If a procedure calls for prewarming the sample, it should not stand at 37° C for more than 5 minutes before being tested. The expiration date of collection tubes must be checked and be valid because the anticoagulant can evaporate over time.

Manual Method

In the manual method, the plasma and reagents are warmed in separate tubes in a heat block or waterbath. After warming,

0.1 mL of patient plasma is forcefully added to 0.2 mL of reagent while the tube is in the waterbath. A timer is started, and at the end of 10 seconds the tube is picked up, held horizontally in good light, and gently tilted back and forth until a thickening appears (Figure 3-12). This is the fibrin clot, and the timer is stopped when it appears. The time for the clot to form is recorded in seconds. It is recommended that the test be run in triplicate. Timing of the first test will be approximate, and the remaining two should agree with each other. Abnormal and normal control plasmas are analyzed with the patient samples.

FibroSystem

In the FibroSystem method, the plasma and reagents are warmed as in the manual method. When the warming time is up, the reagent cup is placed into the center well of the instrument. The automatic pipetter on the instrument is used to draw up and then expel the patient sample into the reagent cup. This action simultaneously starts the timer and lowers the detector into the cup. (See Lesson 3-1, Figure 3-5.) Two wire probes detect the formation of the clot and stop the timer. The tests are performed in duplicate and the results averaged. Abnormal and normal plasma controls are analyzed with the patient samples.

Coagulation Analyzers

Several types of coagulation instruments are available for the higher-volume laboratory. The plasma samples are prepared and placed into the instrument sample tray. The operator enters patient information and the test information into the instrument, indicating which tests to run on each sample. Most instruments detect clot formation by photo-optical density and print out a report or send the results directly to the laboratory computer system.

Point-of-Care Instruments

Many instruments are available for point-of-care (POC) or near-patient coagulation testing (Figure 3-13). Clot formation is detected by either electromechanical means or by photo-optics. Examples of these analyzers are the HEMOCHRON Jr. Signature Plus and the ProTime, both from International Technidyne (ITC), and the CoaguChek S from Roche Diagnostics. Another small instrument, the ACT PLUS by Medtronic, can analyze whole blood, citrated blood, or plasma for the prothrombin time test or the activated partial thromboplastin time (APTT). The ProTime is marketed as a tool to monitor Coumadin therapy. Prothrombin times performed on both the CoaguChek S and the ProTime are CLIA–waived, which makes them suitable for use in POLs and at POC.

The HEMOCHRON microcoagulation instruments use electromechanical means to detect clot formation. Each individual test cuvette is contained in a foil packet that must be at room temperature before the test can be run. The test cuvette is inserted into the instrument to begin warm-up, which takes approximately 30 seconds. The blood sample is whole blood obtained by capillary puncture (or venipuncture without anticoagulant). When the instrument is ready, a tone alerts the operator and the screen displays *add sample*. The operator then has 5 minutes to obtain the blood sample from the patient. Two hundred microliters (0.2 mL) of blood are added to the cuvette sample well in the instrument and the *start* key is depressed. Inside the instrument, the cuvette is tilted, moving the blood back and forth between two laser detectors. The instrument signals test completion when cessation of blood movement in the cuvette is detected. The patient results are displayed as the plasma equivalent and as the INR. Electronic controls and liquid controls can be run at set intervals on the instrument, scheduled by the supervisor.

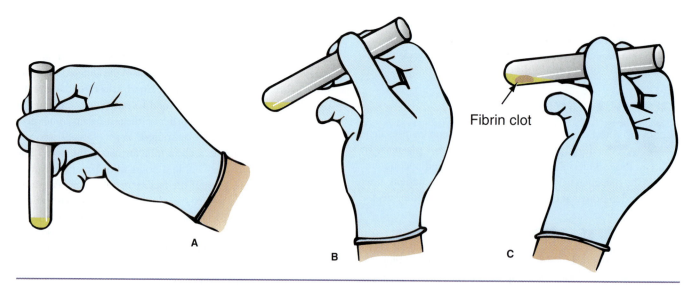

Fibrin clot

A   B   C

FIGURE 3-12 Illustration of the manual tilt-tube prothrombin time method: (A) lift tube out of waterbath; (B) tilt tube horizontally; (C) observe formation of fibrin clot

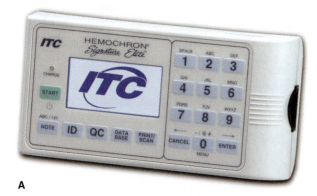

A

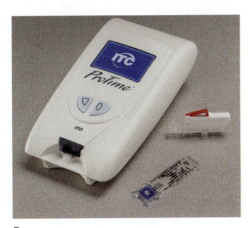

B

FIGURE 3-13 Small point-of-care coagulation analyzers:
(A) HEMOCHRON Signature Elite; (B) ProTime
(*Photos courtesy of ITC, Edison, NJ*)

REPORTING PROTHROMBIN TIME RESULTS

The most common use of the prothrombin time test is monitoring the effectiveness of Coumadin or coumarin-derived anticoagulant drugs. These drugs are prescribed for patients who are in danger of forming clots, such as those with artificial heart valves, phlebitis, other circulatory problems, or those undergoing joint replacement. The test is performed at regular intervals, such as weekly or every 2 weeks. The physician uses the results to regulate the dose.

Prothrombin times can be reported (1) in seconds, (2) as the prothrombin ratio, or (3) as the INR. The prothrombin ratio is obtained by dividing the patient's prothrombin time by the time of the normal control. The INR is calculated by using the patient's prothrombin time, the prothrombin time of the normal control plasma, and an index supplied by the manufacturer for each lot of prothrombin time reagent (thromboplastin) (Figure 3-11).

The goal for patients who are on anticoagulant therapy because of unwanted clot formation, artificial heart valve, or other conditions is to keep the anticoagulant dosage sufficient to maintain the INR between 1.5 and 2.5. When results are reported in seconds, the usual goal is to keep the patient's prothrombin time at about 16 to 18 seconds, or 1.3 to 1.5 times the normal control value.

SAFETY Reminders

- Observe Standard Precautions.
- Treat all control solutions as if potentially infectious.

PROCEDURAL Reminders

- Avoid trauma to vein and surrounding tissues when performing a venipuncture for prothrombin time.
- Be sure that venous blood is collected using one (1) part anticoagulant to nine (9) parts blood.
- Ensure that the correct type of sample is used for the instrument.
- Keep waterbath or heat block temperature at 37° C.
- Warm test sample and reagents for the times specified in the package inserts and manufacturer's instructions.
- Follow an established quality-control program, testing both normal and abnormal plasmas.

SUMMARY

The prothrombin time (or protime) remains one of the most frequently requested coagulation tests. It is used to evaluate the function of the extrinsic and common pathways. It not only is used as a coagulation screening test, but also is widely used to monitor patients receiving Coumadin therapy. These patients are tested at regular intervals, sometimes as often as weekly. The prothrombin time was formerly reported only in seconds. However, it was discovered that there could be disagreement among values obtained on the same sample at different facilities because of variations in the sensitivities of thromboplastin. A sensitivity index, the ISI, is now assigned to each lot of thromboplastin. This index is used to calculate the INR, a value that should represent a patient's prothrombin time result without regard to where the test was performed.

Historically, the FibroSystem was used to perform the prothrombin time test, but now optical technologies are used for coagulation testing. Instruments that use whole blood and require very small samples, obtainable by fingerstick, have simplified prothrombin testing. Tests performed on some of these instruments are CLIA-waived. Although the prothrombin time test has been greatly

C A S E   S T U D Y

A 54-year-old man had been injured in an industrial accident 10 years earlier. He had received two blood transfusions at the time of the accident, and in the intervening years, it was discovered that he had severe liver damage from a hepatitis C infection. He had a prothrombin time (PT) test performed along with other screening tests in preparation for him to have minor surgery.

1. What is a likely result?
   a. The PT was within the reference (normal) range.
   b. The PT result was shorter than the reference range.
   c. The PT was longer than the reference (normal) range.
2. Explain your answer.

simplified, the institution's safety and quality assessment procedures must be followed to assure worker safety and reliable test results.

REVIEW QUESTIONS

1. What is the role of prothrombin in blood coagulation?

2. How does the physician use results from the prothrombin time?

3. Explain how a manual prothrombin time is performed.

4. Explain how to perform a prothrombin time using the FibroSystem.

5. What is the reference value for the prothrombin time test? For the INR?

6. List three ways of reporting prothrombin times.

7. What is the desired range for the prothrombin time of a patient receiving oral anticoagulant therapy?

8. What anticoagulant is used to collect blood for a prothrombin time? What concentration?

9. List four conditions in which the prothrombin time is prolonged.

10. List two instruments that use whole blood samples for the prothrombin time test.

11. Calculate the prothrombin ratio of a patient's sample that gave a prothrombin time result of 21 seconds, while the normal control was 12 seconds.

12. Calculate the INR if the ISI is 1.15, the prothrombin time is 20 seconds, and the mean of normal is 10 seconds. Is it within therapeutic range?

13. Explain why Factor VIII deficiency doesn't affect prothrombin time results.

14. Define Coumadin, enzyme, international normalized ratio, international sensitivity index, prothrombin time, and vitamin K.

STUDENT ACTIVITIES

1. Complete the written examination for this lesson.

2. Practice pipetting with a FibroSystem pipet.

3. Practice performing the prothrombin time as outlined in the Student Performance Guide.

4. If another analyzer is available, perform the prothrombin time on the same sample tested with the FibroSystem. Compare the results.

W E B 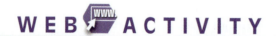 A C T I V I T Y

Use the Internet to find information about a handheld POC analyzer used for performing the prothrombin time. Write a paragraph describing the instrument, procedure, sample size, etc.

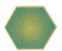 # Student Performance Guide

LESSON 3-4 Prothrombin Time

Name _____ Date _____

INSTRUCTIONS

1. Practice performing the prothrombin time test following the step-by-step procedure.

2. Demonstrate the prothrombin time test satisfactorily for the instructor, using the Student Performance Guide. Your instructor will determine the level of competency you must achieve to obtain a Satisfactory (S) grade.

NOTE: Follow manufacturer's directions for instrument and reagents used

MATERIALS AND EQUIPMENT

- gloves
- centrifuge
- face protection
- commercial source of thromboplastin-$CaCl_2$
- citrated human plasma, recently collected
- normal controls
- abnormal controls
- distilled water for reconstituting controls
- biohazard container
- surface disinfectant
- laboratory tissue
- antiseptic
- test tube rack
- calculator with exponential function

For Manual Method

- test tubes (13 × 75 mm)
- waterbath at 37° C
- pipets to transfer 0.1 and 0.2 mL
- timer

For Automated Method

- coagulation instrument, such as FibroSystem or HEMOCHRON Jr.
- supplies for instrument
- capillary puncture supplies

PROCEDURE

Record in the comment section any problems encountered while practicing the procedure (or have a fellow student or the instructor evaluate your performance).

S = Satisfactory
U = Unsatisfactory

You must:	S	U	Comments
1. Wash hands, put on face protection, and put on gloves			
2. Obtain citrated blood sample (if not provided)			
3. Centrifuge the specimen as specified in reagent package insert			
4. Remove the plasma and transfer to a clean test tube. Label with patient identification			

You must:	S	U	Comments

5. Perform a manual prothrombin time:
   a. Check that waterbath temperature is 37° C
   b. Pipet 0.2 mL of thromboplastin-CaCl$_2$ reagent into seven labeled tubes (three for the patient, two for each normal and abnormal control)
   c. Place tubes in rack in waterbath
   d. Pipet sufficient patient plasma and control plasmas (0.4 to 0.5 mL each) to perform the test in triplicate in another set of appropriately labeled tubes
   e. Place tubes in rack in waterbath
   f. Allow patient sample, controls, and reagent to warm for the prescribed amount of time
   g. Draw up 0.1 mL patient plasma and forcibly expel into tube containing reagent, starting timer simultaneously
   h. Allow tube to remain in waterbath about 10 seconds
   i. *Work quickly*—pick up the tube, wipe the outside with tissue, start tilting tube slowly back and forth in front of good light source
   j. Stop the timer at the first sign of thickening (clot) in the moving liquid and record the time
   k. Repeat steps 5g–5j using another tube of warmed reagent. Remember that the first time is approximate, and the second and third should agree with each other
   l. Perform steps 5g–5j in duplicate for each control sample
   m. Report results: Report average of patient's second and third times; record the times for the controls

6. Perform an automated prothrombin time using the FibroSystem (If instrument is not available, proceed to step 7)
   a. Turn on instrument. If using the instrument's pipetter, be certain it is turned "OFF"
   b. Label desired number of sample cups and place in heat block (patient samples should be run in duplicate)
   c. Pipet 0.2 mL of thromboplastin-CaCl$_2$ into cups, following manufacturer's instructions
   d. Pipet sufficient patient plasma and controls (0.4 to 0.5 mL) into separate cups to allow for duplicate testing of patient and controls
   e. Allow all components to warm the prescribed amount of time. Place one sample cup with measured thromboplastin CaCl$_2$ into center well of instrument
   f. Draw up 0.1 mL of patient plasma
   g. Turn pipetter "ON"

You must:	S	U	Comments
h. Expel plasma into center cup containing 0.2 mL of thromboplastin-CaCl$_2$. The timer will start automatically when the plunger is depressed, if using instrument's pipet i. Wait for timer to stop, signaling the formation of a clot j. Record the time in seconds k. Gently wipe probe wires with laboratory tissue between determinations l. Repeat steps 6e–6k using patient plasma m. Average the two times and report the results n. Repeat steps 6e–6k for each control o. Record the times for the controls p. Turn off instrument			
7. Perform a prothrombin time using a small handheld instrument. These instructions are for a HEMOCHRON type instrument using a whole blood sample. Follow the instructions for the instrument that is being used. a. Allow test pack to come to room temperature. Assemble all other supplies b. Perform quality control checks if necessary c. Insert the cuvette into the instrument to initiate the prewarm/self-check mode (approximately 30 seconds) d. Observe the display screen for any error messages e. Wait for the audible signal that sounds when the instrument is ready. The screen will display "Add Sample" and "Press Start" NOTE: If the test is not run the instrument will go into timeout at the end of 5 minutes indicating that the test cuvette must be discarded and a new one obtained f. Obtain the fresh whole blood sample and immediately dispense one drop (0.2 mL) into the sample well of the cuvette in the instrument. Fill the well flush to the top. If a large drop forms a dome, push it over into the outer sample well NOTE: Bubbles make the sample invalid. Do not force blood into the pin in the center of the sample well g. Depress the START key h. Wait for the single beep that signals the completion of the test i. Record the results; they will be displayed as the plasma equivalent value and the INR. The results will remain displayed for an additional 120 seconds			
8. Return all equipment to proper storage			
9. Dispose of all contaminated articles in biohazard container and contaminated sharps in sharps container			

You must:	S	U	Comments
10. Wipe counter with surface disinfectant			
11. Remove and discard gloves in biohazard container			
12. Wash hands with antiseptic			

Evaluator Comments:

Evaluator _____ Date _____

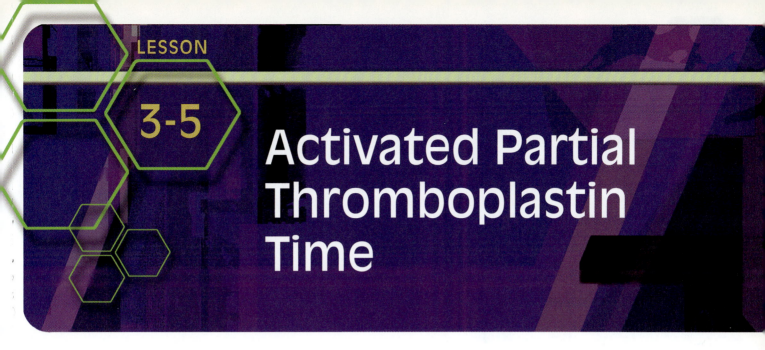

Activated Partial Thromboplastin Time

LESSON OBJECTIVES

After studying this lesson, the student will:

- Explain the principle of the activated partial thromboplastin time (APTT).
- Explain the reasons for performing an APTT.
- Explain which parts of the coagulation pathway are checked in the APTT.
- List the coagulation factor deficiencies detected by the APTT.
- Give the reference values for the APTT.
- List safety precautions to be observed when performing the APTT.
- Discuss why quality assessment policies and procedures are important in the performance of the APTT.
- Define the glossary term.

GLOSSARY

partial thromboplastin / the lipid portion of thromboplastin, available as a commercial preparation; formerly cephaloplastin

INTRODUCTION

The activated partial thromboplastin time (APTT) is used to monitor heparin therapy and screen for function of the intrinsic and common pathways of hemostasis (Figure 3-14). The APTT is named because the test reagent contains activators such as kaolin or silica to activate the contact factors in the intrinsic pathway. Calcium chloride ($CaCl_2$) is also added to supply the ionized calcium required for fibrin formation by the intrinsic pathway.

The APTT test is sensitive to mild deficiencies of factors XII, XI, IX, and VIII and Fletcher and Fitzgerald factors. It is also useful for detecting deficiencies of factors X, V, II, and fibrinogen (I), although these factor deficiencies must be

slightly more severe to cause a prolonged APTT. Factors VII, XIII, and platelet factor 3 (PF3) are not assayed in the APTT (Figure 3-14).

Partial thromboplastin is the reagent used in performing the APTT. Partial thromboplastin, the lipid portion of tissue thromboplastin, is manufactured from human or bovine brain tissue or derived from soybeans. Since partial thromboplastin performs the function of PF3 in the APTT test, platelet abnormalities will have no effect on the APTT.

The formation of a fibrin clot in the APTT can occur only if factors in the intrinsic pathway—XII, XI, IX, and VIII—and those in the common pathway—I, II, V, and X—are present in sufficient amounts and are functional (Table 3-6).

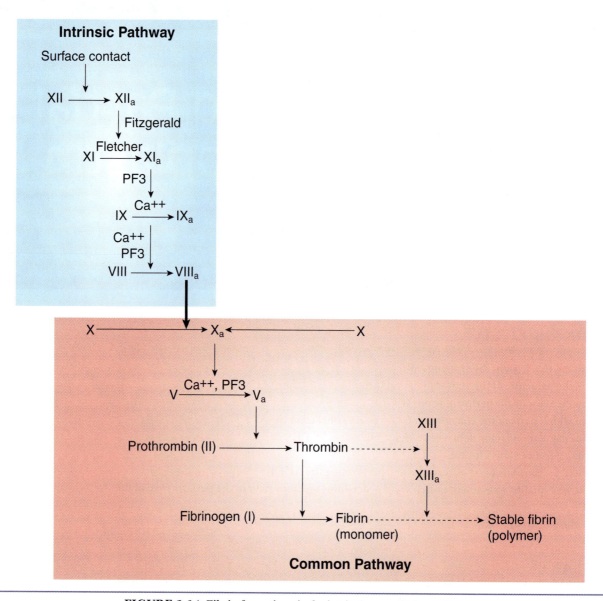

FIGURE 3-14 Fibrin formation via the intrinsic coagulation pathway

TABLE 3-6. Hemostasis pathways and coagulation factors tested by the activated partial thromboplastin time (APTT)	
FACTORS OF INTRINSIC PATHWAY	**FACTORS OF COMMON PATHWAY**
XII	I
XI	II
IX	V
VIII	X
Fitzgerald	
Fletcher	

REFERENCE VALUES FOR THE APTT

The mean reference value for the normal APTT is usually about 35 seconds. Some laboratories use a range of 31 to 39 seconds. It is best if each laboratory establishes its own normal range by periodically testing several plasmas from normal patients. Table 3-7 gives examples of conditions that affect the APTT. When the APTT is used to monitor heparin therapy, the usual goal is to keep the patient's APTT 1.5 to 2.0 times the APTT of the normal plasma control.

PERFORMING THE ACTIVATED PARTIAL THROMBOPLASTIN TIME

The APTT can be performed on a FibroSystem, a multi-sample coagulation analyzer, or using small POC-type analyzers. Semi-automated multi-sample analyzers have been in use many years

TABLE 3-7. Various conditions that affect the activated partial thromboplastin time (APTT)

CONDITION	EFFECT ON APTT
Factor Deficiencies	
I, II, V, VIII, IX, X, XI, XII	Prolonged
VII, XIII	No effect
Other Conditions	
Heparin therapy	Prolonged
Vitamin K deficiency	Prolonged

in larger facilities but are now also designed for small laboratories. The small handheld analyzers can be used for near-patient or POC testing, in physician office laboratories (POLs), and for home testing by patients.

Safety Precautions

 Standard Precautions must be observed to protect the worker from exposure to bloodborne pathogens. Appropriate personal protective equipment must be used. Performing the APTT can expose the worker to the patient's blood specimen unless the coagulation instrument can sample through the stopper.

Quality Assessment

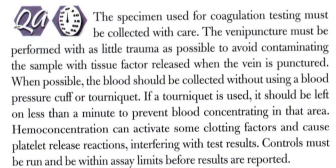 The specimen used for coagulation testing must be collected with care. The venipuncture must be performed with as little trauma as possible to avoid contaminating the sample with tissue factor released when the vein is punctured. When possible, the blood should be collected without using a blood pressure cuff or tourniquet. If a tourniquet is used, it should be left on less than a minute to prevent blood concentrating in that area. Hemoconcentration can activate some clotting factors and cause platelet release reactions, interfering with test results. Controls must be run and be within assay limits before results are reported.

Collecting the Specimen

Blood is collected using 3.2% sodium citrate anticoagulant. The proportions are one (1) part sodium citrate (0.5 mL) to nine (9) parts (4.5 mL) blood. Vacuum tubes are available containing this volume and also in a smaller size for pediatric use. After collection, the whole blood sample is centrifuged, and the plasma is removed and placed in another tube. The plasma should be stored covered at 4° C until used for the test. The test should be run within 4 hours of collection.

FibroSystem Method

The procedure for the APTT using the FibroSystem is similar to that of the prothrombin time. The patient plasma, the activated partial thromboplastin, and CaCl₂ are prewarmed in the heat-

block for at least 3 minutes but no more than 10 minutes. The patient samples are prepared by adding 0.1 mL of patient plasma and 0.1 mL of thromboplastin reagent into the patient sample cups. These are allowed to warm and activate for 3 minutes. To initiate the clotting reaction, the warmed CaCl₂ is added using the FibroSystem automatic pipet, which simultaneously starts the timer and lowers the probes into the reaction cup. The two wire probes stir the sample until a clot is detected, which stops the timer. Normal and abnormal controls must be run with the patient samples.

Point-of-Care Instruments

The APTT can be performed quickly and easily using an instrument such as the International Technidyne (ITC) HEMOCHRON Jr. or HEMOCHRON Signature Elite. The individual test cuvettes contain all the needed reagents and are enclosed in foil packets. The packet must be brought to room temperature before the cuvette is removed. The test cuvette is inserted into the instrument to begin the 30 second warm-up cycle. The instrument assays whole blood from either capillary puncture or venipuncture (without anticoagulant). When the instrument is ready, an audible tone alerts the operator, and *add sample* is displayed on the screen. The technician then has 5 minutes to obtain the blood specimen from the patient. A large drop of blood (0.2 mL) is added to the sample well in the center of the cuvette, and the *Start* key is depressed to begin the assay. Inside the instrument, the blood is mixed with the cuvette reagents and the mixture is moved back and forth within the cuvette. When the clot forms, laser detectors sense that movement has ceased and the timer is stopped. The instrument reports the result as a plasma equivalent in seconds.

Other small, handheld instruments are available to perform the APTT. These require only a small blood sample and can use whole blood for the assay. In these instruments the formation of a clot is detected either by photo-optical density or laser detectors. Photo-optical density is used for clot detection in the

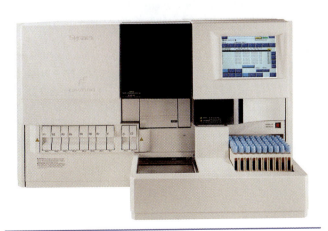

FIGURE 3-15 Sysmex CA-7000 automated coagulation analyzer (*Courtesy of Sysmex America, Mundelein IL, all rights reserved*)

COATRON and COATRON M-1 from TECO. The ACT PLUS from Medtronic also uses laser technology.

Coagulation Analyzers

The APTT can be run on the automated and semi-automated analyzers that are capable of performing several different assays on a sample (Figure 3-15). The technician loads the samples into the sample tray, enters the patient ID, and enters the tests that are to be run on each specimen. The analyzer performs the requested assays and then prints a report or sends the results directly to the computer system.

SUMMARY

The APTT is useful to monitor patients who are on heparin therapy. In addition, it is used as a screening test for abnormalities in the intrinsic and common pathways. A fibrin clot can form only if factors XII, XI, IX, and VIII in the intrinsic pathway and I, II, V, and X in the common pathway are functional and present in sufficient amounts. The APTT does not test platelet function since the partial thromboplastin added in the test procedure performs the function of platelet factor 3.

The APTT can be performed on multi-function coagulation instruments in the laboratory or on one of many handheld POCT instruments. The instructions for each instrument must be followed carefully because some of the instruments can use only plasma samples and others can use plasma, whole blood, or

SAFETY Reminders

- Observe Standard Precautions.
- Handle control plasma as if potentially infectious.
- Discard used sharps in biohazard sharps container.

PROCEDURAL Reminders

- Read and follow the manufacturer's instructions for the reagents and instruments used.
- Review quality assessment section before performing procedure.
- Perform venipuncture with care.
- Use the proper ratio of blood to anticoagulant.
- Remove plasma from red blood cells promptly and perform test within 4 hours of collection.

CASE STUDY

Alice Morrow came to the outpatient laboratory to have blood drawn for coagulation testing. Usually Ms. Morrow did not have problems getting blood drawn. On that particular morning, the phlebotomist had difficulty, but he did finally obtain about 3 mL of blood in the vacuum collection tube which contained 0.5 mL of sodium citrate. When Ms. Morrow's results were received the next day, her physician was surprised at the test results. Ms. Morrow told the physician about the circumstances of the blood being drawn.

1. Why did her physician order the test to be repeated?
   a. The physician knew there was a problem with the laboratory's instrument.
   b. The laboratory waited too long to centrifuge the blood specimen.
   c. The ratio of anticoagulant to blood was incorrect.
   d. The physician thought Ms. Morrow had a serious disease.
2. Explain your answer.

citrated blood. Standard Precautions must be observed while performing the test. In addition, all quality assessment procedures of the facility and the instrument manufacturer must be followed for test results to be valid.

6. Why is CaCl₂ added in the APTT?

7. Why are activators added to the plasma during the APTT?

8. Define partial thromboplastin.

REVIEW QUESTIONS

1. Which hemostasis pathway is measured by the APTT?

2. What conditions could cause a prolonged APTT?

3. What is one use of the APTT?

4. List two coagulation factors not measured by the APTT.

5. Why is the extrinsic pathway not measured by the APTT?

STUDENT ACTIVITIES

1. Complete the written examination for this lesson.

2. Practice performing the APTT as outlined in the Student Performance Guide.

3. If available, use a coagulation analyzer to perform the APTT on the same sample tested using the FibroSystem. Compare the results obtained with the two instruments.

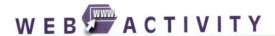

WEB ACTIVITY

Using the Internet, find examples of two APTT instruments that use whole blood. Explain the advantages of using a whole blood sample.

Student Performance Guide

LESSON 3-5 Activated Partial Thromboplastin Time

Name _____ Date _____

INSTRUCTIONS

1. Practice performing the APTT following the step-by-step procedure.

2. Demonstrate the APTT procedure satisfactorily for the instructor, using the Student Performance Guide. Your instructor will determine the level of competency you must achieve to receive a satisfactory (S) grade.

NOTE: Follow manufacturers' instructions for instrument and reagents used.

MATERIALS AND EQUIPMENT

- face protection
- gloves
- citrated blood sample or venipuncture materials required for obtaining citrated blood
- clinical centrifuge
- commercial control plasmas
- biohazard container
- sharps container
- antiseptic
- surface disinfectant
- FibroSystem and pipetter (or other coagulation analyzer)
- FibroSystem tips and cups
- 37° C heat block
- commercial partial thromboplastin
- CaCl₂, 0.02 M
- capillary puncture supplies
- HEMOCHRON or other POCT-type coagulation analyzer and test packets

PROCEDURE

Record in the comment section any problems encountered while practicing the procedure (or have a fellow student or the instructor evaluate your performance).

S = Satisfactory
U = Unsatisfactory

You must:	S	U	Comments
1. Assemble materials and equipment and turn on instrument to warm up. Wash hands and put on face protection			
2. Put on gloves			
3. Obtain citrated blood sample by venipuncture and label with patient's name (or use commercial plasma controls)			
4. Centrifuge the blood sample for 5 minutes at 1,500 rpm to obtain the plasma			
5. Follow instructions for the instrument being used. Check to see that heat block is at 37° C			

You must:	S	U	Comments
6. Reconstitute the partial thromboplastin according to manufacturer's instructions			
7. Label sample cups: normal control, abnormal control, patient name, partial thromboplastin, and $CaCl_2$			
8. Pipet enough partial thromboplastin into reagent cup(s) to have 0.1 mL for each test (which should be run in duplicate)			
9. Pipet enough control plasma into labeled cups to have 0.1 mL for each test			
10. Pipet into the reagent cups enough $CaCl_2$ to have 0.1 mL for each test			
11. Allow reagents and plasmas to prewarm for at least 3 minutes and not more than 10 minutes			
12. Place a clean cup in the reaction well of the instrument and pipet 0.1 mL partial thromboplastin into it			
13. Perform the APTT on a normal control plasma by pipetting 0.1 mL of normal control into the cup containing the 0.1 mL of prewarmed partial thromboplastin (in the reaction well)			
14. Let the mixture warm and activate for 3 minutes			
15. Draw up 0.1 mL prewarmed $CaCl_2$, turn on pipetter, and dispense $CaCl_2$ into the cup in the reaction well. The probe will lower into the cup and the timer will start automatically and stop when a fibrin clot is detected			
16. Record the time from the instrument's timer			
17. Repeat the test (steps 9–16) on the normal control plasma			
18. Average the results and report the APTT in seconds			
19. Perform the APTT in duplicate using the abnormal control plasma, following steps 9–18			
20. If all control values are within acceptable limits, repeat steps 9–18, using patient plasma			

21. If POCT instrument is not available, go to step 22. If POCT instrument is available follow general steps 21a–21j and the manufacturer's guidelines for the exact procedure. (Procedure given is for HEMOCHRON)
  a. Allow test packet to reach room temperature (refrigerated packets require almost an hour). Assemble capillary puncture supplies
  b. Perform quality control checks if needed
  c. Insert the room temperature cuvette into the instrument to initiate the pre-warm/self-check mode (approximately 30 seconds)			

You must:	S	U	Comments
d. Observe the display for any error messages e. Listen for the audible tone that signals the instrument is ready f. Wait for the screen to display "add sample" g. Perform the capillary puncture and immediately dispense one drop of blood directly into the center of the cuvette sample well. Fill the well flush to the top. (*Air bubbles make the test invalid.*) If a large drop of blood extends above the top simply push it over into the outer sample well. Do not force the blood sample into the pin in the center of the well h. Depress the START key i. Wait for the audible tone to signal completion of the test j. Record the results: the APTT will be displayed as the plasma equivalent result in seconds **NOTE:** The result will be displayed for an additional 120 seconds after the test cuvette is removed			
22. Dispose of all biohazard waste in biohazard container			
23. Dispose of contaminated sharps in sharps container			
24. Turn instrument off and return all equipment to proper storage			
25. Wipe counter with surface disinfectant			
26. Remove and discard gloves in biohazard container; wash hands with antiseptic			

Evaluator Comments:

Evaluator _____ Date _____

Rapid Hemostasis Tests

LESSON OBJECTIVES

After studying this lesson, the student will:

■ List two conditions that could require rapid hemostasis testing.

■ Discuss the role of heparin in anticoagulant therapy.

■ Discuss the reasons for close monitoring of heparin levels.

■ Explain the breakdown of fibrinogen and fibrin into smaller molecules.

■ Perform a test for D-dimers.

■ Perform a test for activated clotting time.

■ Discuss safety precautions that must be observed when performing rapid hemostasis tests.

■ Explain why it is important to follow quality assessment procedures when performing coagulation testing.

■ Define the glossary terms.

GLOSSARY

angioplasty / surgical repair of a vessel

D-dimer / one of the products formed from the breakdown of fibrin by plasmin

deep vein thrombosis (DVT) / occurrence of a thrombus within a deep vein, usually of the leg or pelvis

disseminated intravascular coagulation (DIC) / a bleeding disorder characterized by widespread thrombotic and secondary fibrinolytic reactions

fibrin degradation products (FDP) / degradation products formed when plasmin cleaves fibrin or fibrinogen; formerly fibrin split products

pulmonary embolism / occlusion of a pulmonary artery or one of its branches, usually produced by an embolus that originated in a deep vein of the leg or pelvis

XDP / fibrin-degradation products that contain the D-dimer cross-linked region

INTRODUCTION

Some medical situations require rapid hemostasis test results. These include circumstances in which the patients are receiving heparin therapy or when conditions such as disseminated intravascular coagulation (DIC), deep vein thrombosis (DVT) or pulmonary embolism are suspected. Hemostasis tests used to help in diagnosis or in prescribing treatment for these conditions include the activated clotting time (ACT) and APTT for monitoring heparin therapy. Tests for fibrinogen/fibrin degradation products (FDP), such as the D-dimer test, are used for suspected cases of DIC, DVT, or pulmonary embolism. Several small portable coagulation analyzers are available that can be used at point of care to perform these tests in just a few minutes.

HEPARIN THERAPY

Heparin is an anticoagulant that inhibits the activated forms of Factors IX, X, XI, and XII as well as platelet release factor. It is prescribed to prevent thrombosis in patients undergoing cardiac **angioplasty**, joint replacement and other procedures with risk of clot formation. Heparin can also be prescribed in patients who have thrombosis or emboli. Because patients vary in their response to heparin, and heparin from different sources has varying activity, the blood levels of the anticoagulant must be closely monitored during therapy.

ACT and APTT Tests

Several small handheld instruments can perform the ACT and APTT tests used to evaluate the effectiveness of heparin therapy. Some instruments require plasma samples but others can use whole blood, citrated blood, or citrated plasma. The sample size is small, ranging between 10 and 200 μL. When whole blood is used, the total time to obtain test results is reduced.

Instrumentation

Examples of these instruments are the ACT PLUS from Medtronic and the HEMOCHRON analyzers from ITC. The Bayer Rapidpoint measures prothrombin time, APTT, and HMT (Heparin Management Test), a version of the ACT. The HMT test is especially useful for monitoring patients recovering from a thrombus or embolus and who are receiving moderate to high doses of heparin.

DISSEMINATED INTRAVASCULAR COAGULATION, DEEP VEIN THROMBOSIS, AND PULMONARY EMBOLISM

Disseminated intravascular coagulation (DIC) is a life-threatening condition in which widespread thrombosis and secondary hemorrhaging occur due to a malfunction in the mechanisms that maintain the balance between clotting and dissolution of the clot (fibrinolysis). The result is pathological clotting and/or excessive clot dissolution. Patients can develop DIC from injuries that cause widespread damage to the vascular system, such as crushing injuries received in construction or automobile accidents. Certain bacterial and viral infections can also cause DIC. The hemorrhaging is caused by fibrinolysis combined with depletion of platelets and coagulation factors.

Deep vein thrombosis (DVT) and **pulmonary embolism** are conditions that can be difficult to diagnose by clinical symptoms alone. DVT is the formation of a thrombus or thrombi caused by slow blood flow or stasis in the large veins, usually of the legs, due to long periods of inactivity. Pulmonary embolism can be a complication of DVT. Pulmonary embolism is a potentially lethal condition caused when a clot dislodges, is carried to the lungs, and blocks a pulmonary vessel. Rapid diagnosis and treatment are essential to recovery.

Formation of FDP and XDP

During fibrinolysis, both fibrinogen and fibrin are cleaved by plasmin to yield various degradation products called **fibrin degradation products (FDP)** as shown in Figure 3-16. Lysis of stable fibrin clots also results in the formation of cross-linked fibrin degradation products, called **XDPs**. The derivatives of XDPs are proteins called **D-dimers**. It is important to distinguish between FDPs and XDPs since the presence of XDPs indicates a more serious condition.

Tests for FDP and XDP (D-dimer)

FDP and XDP can be measured using either latex agglutination assays or one of the small handheld analyzers made for near-patient testing. Available tests can distinguish between FDPs and XDPs or D-dimers. The latex agglutination tests consist of latex beads coated with a monoclonal antibody specific for the D-dimer. When the patient sample is mixed with the test kit reagents on a special slide, any D-dimer present is bound to the antibody on the beads and visible agglutination forms.

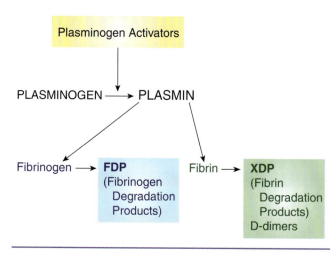

FIGURE 3-16 Illustration of the fibrinolytic pathway showing formation of D-dimers

PERFORMING RAPID HEMOSTASIS TESTS

Rapid hemostasis tests can be performed in a variety of situations. Near-patient testing can be performed to monitor heparin therapy using one of the small handheld analyzers that performs ACT, HMT, or APTT tests. The presence of D-dimers can be detected within minutes using latex agglutination tests or instrumentation if DIC, pulmonary embolism, or deep vein thrombosis is suspected.

Safety Precautions

Standard Precautions must be observed when handling patient specimens and control reagents. Appropriate personal protective equipment (PPE) must be worn when collecting the blood specimen and performing the test. The controls for rapid hemostasis tests are made from human blood and should be considered potentially infectious. Safety needle devices must be used when venipuncture is performed. All used materials should be discarded into appropriate biohazard and sharps containers.

Quality Assessment

Some instruments can analyze only one type of blood specimen; other instruments can use whole blood, citrated blood, or citrated plasma. The technician must know the type of sample the particular instrument can analyze, since an instrument can be damaged if the wrong specimen is used, such as using whole blood when only plasma should have been used. All quality assessment procedures of the facility must be followed when using the instruments.

Specimen collection must be performed following manufacturers' instructions. Venipuncture must be performed without trauma to avoid release of tissue thromboplastin into the specimen. Blood should be collected in sodium citrate when citrated plasma is required for tests such as the D-dimer and APTT plasma tests. Heparin or EDTA anticoagulants cannot be used.

All reagents must be brought to room temperature before the tests are performed. The policies of the facility and manufacturers' package inserts must be followed concerning the number of controls to be run. For D-dimer latex agglutination tests, pipetting must be precise; the tests must be read immediately at the specified time to avoid false-positive reactions caused by drying of the latex.

Tests for D-dimer

Tests for D-dimer are useful in diagnosing DIC, DVT, and pulmonary embolism. The reference values for FDP are: any value less than 0.20 μg/mL is considered negative; any value greater than 0.20 μg/mL is considered positive.

Manual Latex Agglutination Tests

The DADE Dimertest Latex Assay is specific for the D-dimers formed from the degradation of stable fibrin. A highly specific

monoclonal antibody (anti-D-dimer) binds to any D-dimer present in the specimen. The quantity of D-dimer in the patient's plasma is proportional to the quantity of fibrin being cleaved.

Latex agglutination assays are available from Remel to detect D-dimer in serum or plasma and FDPs in serum and urine (Figure 3-17). The Wellcotest D-dimer assay can be used for qualitative and semi-quantitative assays. It is more specific than the FDP test because the monoclonal antibody coated on the latex beads is specific for D-dimer. Results are available in 3 minutes. The Thrombo-Wellcotest, considered by some to be the gold standard for FDP assays, can be used for urine or blood. It has high sensitivity, and can detect low levels of FDPs. Results are available in only 2 minutes making it valuable for emergency situations.

To perform the latex tests, the patient sample is mixed with the test kit reagents on a special slide provided with the test kit. The sample and reagent are stirred together and a timer is set for the appropriate incubation period. Immediately at the end of the time period, the slide is inspected for agglutination. The presence of agglutination is a positive result; absence of agglutination is a negative result.

Automated D-dimer Analysis

Instrumentation such as the Di-Stat D-dimer (Fisher Diagnostics) and the DIMEX (Teco) can assay for D-dimer in just minutes. These systems report qualitative and quantitative results for the D fragment in a plasma specimen. Latex particles coated with monoclonal antibody react with any D fragment present in the patient plasma sample. The amount of aggregation that develops is proportional to the amount of D fragment present in the plasma. Results from this test have a negative predictive value of 100% for

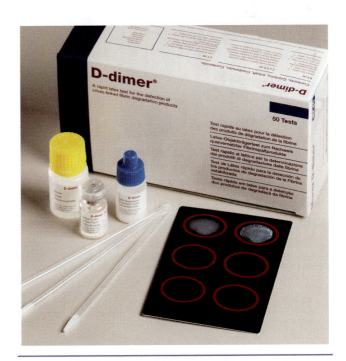

FIGURE 3-17 Rapid latex agglutination test for D-dimers showing positive (right) and negative (left) reactions (*Photo courtesy of Remel, Inc., Lenexa, KS*)

pulmonary embolism and 94% for DVT; in other words, a negative result predicts with 100% certainty that pulmonary embolism is not present and predicts with 94% certainty that DVT is not not present. The Cardiac Reader (Roche Diagnostics) assays D-dimer as well as several cardiac markers (Figure 3-18).

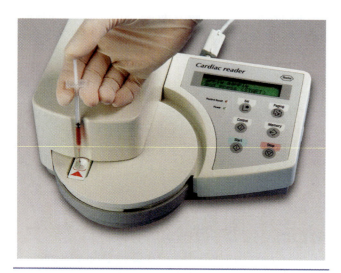

FIGURE 3-18 The Cardiac Reader, a small coagulation analyzer that can measure D-dimers (*Courtesy of Roche Diagnostics Corp., Indianapolis, IN*)

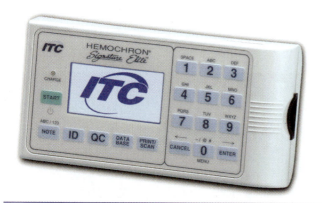

FIGURE 3-19 HEMOCHRON Signature Elite (*Photo courtesy of ITC, Edison, NJ*)

Activated Clotting Time Test

HEMOCHRON Analyzer

HEMOCHRON analyzers such as the HEMOCHRON Jr. and Signature Elite are handheld analyzers that can perform tests such as prothrombin time, APTT, and ACT (Figure 3-19 and Table 3-8). Each test system has specific cuvettes containing the reagents for the test to be performed. For each test, 200 μL of whole blood is collected. A 90-second warmup period and instrument self-check are initiated by inserting a test cuvette into the instrument. The blood sample is added to a collection cup in the prewarmed cuvette. After the sample is added, the START key is pressed.

Inside the analyzer, the blood is mixed with the cuvette reagents and the sample is moved back and forth in test channels and monitored for clot formation. As the clot begins to form, a photometer with two optical detectors registers the endpoint when movement of the blood has slowed. A single beep indicates completion of the test and the test result is displayed on the instrument screen.

The ACT is a diagnostic test in which whole blood is added to a test tube containing a clotting activator such as kaolin, celite, silica, or glass particles and the blood is monitored for clot formation. The ACT+ performed by the HEMOCHRON uses a cuvette containing a mixture of silica, kaolin, and phospholipids as the activator. The reactions take place in the cuvette inside the analyzer. Detection of a clot by the photometer determines the test endpoint. The ACT+ test result is automatically converted to a reference celite-ACT value reported in seconds (Table 3-8).

Bayer Rapidpoint

The Bayer Rapidpoint is a small POCT instrument that performs prothrombin time, APTT, and the heparin management test (HMT), a version of the ACT. The HMT is especially valuable for monitoring patients receiving heparin therapy to prevent blood clots or to treat clotting disorders.

GEM PCL

The GEM PCL (Instrumentation Laboratory) requires 50 μL of whole blood each for the ACT, prothrombin time test, and APTT. Plasma samples from citrated blood can also be used for the prothrombin time test and the APTT. Results are available in less than 5 minutes.

TABLE 3-8. Reference values for prothrombin time, activated partial thromboplastin time (APTT), and activated clotting time (ACT) using the HEMOCHRON

| TEST | WHOLE BLOOD | | PLASMA EQUIVALENT | |
	MEAN	RANGE	MEAN	RANGE
PT	19 sec	17–22 sec	12.5 sec	11.3–13.6 sec
APTT	110 sec	93–127 sec	24 sec	24–30 sec
ACT+	121 sec	89–153 sec	None	None

SAFETY Reminders

- Observe Standard Precautions when handling patient and control samples.
- Discard all used materials in appropriate biohazard containers.

PROCEDURAL Reminders

- Follow manufacturer's directions for specimen collection.
- Collect specimens for the D-dimer rapid slide test and HEMOCHRON plasma tests in citrate anticoagulant only.
- Equilibrate all specimens and reagents to room temperature before using.
- Run two levels of controls with each batch of patient samples.

SUMMARY

The development of portable coagulation analyzers and rapid coagulation tests has made possible rapid diagnosis of some hemostasis problems, resulting in improved patient care. With this new technology has also come the introduction of new types of tests such as ACT, HMT, and D-dimer, which provide the physician valuable information quickly in life-threatening situations. These technologies ensure improved on-site monitoring of patient status during procedures such as open-heart surgery. They also enable coagulation testing to be performed at point of care and in physician office laboratories, which is more efficient than patients having to go to larger off-site laboratories for testing.

REVIEW QUESTIONS

1. List two conditions that could require rapid hemostasis testing.
2. What anticoagulant is administered to patients undergoing cardiac angioplasty?
3. How does heparin inhibit clotting?
4. Why is it important to monitor heparin levels?
5. List two tests used to monitor heparin therapy.
6. What mechanisms occur in DIC that make it life-threatening?

CASE STUDY

Jason Moore had returned from Europe on a long transatlantic flight the previous day. During the flight, he had gotten chilled and developed a cough and some chest pain. Jason had been especially tired and spent a lot of time sleeping during the flight. Although the cough was uncomfortable, he was more concerned about the pain in his right calf. He called his physician who instructed him to go to the emergency department. After hearing about his trip, the emergency department physician suspected DVT and ordered a D-dimer test that could be performed quickly using an instrument. The test result was negative. The physician told Jason he did not have a pulmonary embolism but did possibly have DVT, requiring immediate treatment and hospitalization.

DVT is a threat to people who experience long periods of sitting and inactivity. The slowing of blood flow from prolonged inactivity plus possible vessel constriction due to pressure from the edge of the seat or tight trouser material can cause platelets to adhere and aggregate. Thrombi can form if travelers do not get up and walk around at regular intervals. It is also important for travelers to keep hydrated by drinking lots of juices and water during long flights.

1. Why did the physician order a D-dimer test?
2. Why was it important to use a test system that had a high negative predictive value?
3. What over-the-counter medication could possibly help prevent DVT? Why might this help?

7. The D-dimer test detects degradation products from the breakdown of which clotting proteins?

8. Name three conditions the D-dimer test can help to diagnose.

9. Name three small handheld analyzers that perform the ACT.

10. Define angioplasty, D-dimer, deep vein thrombosis, disseminated intravascular coagulation, fibrin degradation products, pulmonary embolism, and XDP.

STUDENT ACTIVITIES

1. Complete the written examination for this lesson.

2. Practice performing a rapid test for D-dimer as outlined in the Student Performance Guide.

3. Practice performing an ACT as outlined in the Student Performance Guide.

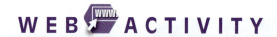

WEB ACTIVITY

Use the Internet to gather information on DIC, DVT, or pulmonary embolism. For one of these conditions, report on the cause(s), symptoms, factors considered in diagnosis, laboratory tests that aid in diagnosis, and treatment.

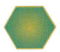

Student Performance Guide

LESSON 3-6 Rapid Hemostasis Tests

Name _____ Date _____

INSTRUCTIONS

1. Practice performing a rapid test for fibrin-degradation products or ACT following the step-by-step procedure.

2. Demonstrate the procedure for either fibrin-degradation products or the ACT satisfactorily for the instructor, using the Student Performance Guide. Your instructor will determine the level of competency you must achieve to receive a satisfactory (S) grade.

NOTE: The following is a general procedure for detecting D-dimer fragments using the DADE Dimertest and a general procedure for the performance of an ACT using the HEMOCHRON system. The manufacturers' instructions for the specific methods or instruments being used must be followed.

MATERIALS AND EQUIPMENT

- face protection
- gloves
- marking pencil
- blood-collection equipment:
  - syringe venipuncture equipment (ACT test)
  - vacuum tube blood collection equipment (D-dimer test), including citrate collection tube
  - capillary puncture materials
- commercial kit for detecting D-dimer fragments
- pipets and tips to deliver 20 and 100 μL
- disposable plastic test tubes and test tube rack (optional, for semi-quantitative D-dimer test)
- mechanical slide rotator (optional)
- HEMOCHRON or other handheld instrument for determining ACT, including cuvettes and whole blood controls
- surface disinfectant
- antiseptic
- biohazard container
- sharps container

PROCEDURE

Record in the comment section any problems encountered while practicing the procedure (or have a fellow student or the instructor evaluate your performance).

S = Satisfactory
U = Unsatisfactory

You must:	S	U	Comments
1. Assemble equipment and materials			
2. Wash hands and put on face protection and gloves			
3. Perform the manual test for D-dimers (DADE Dimertest Latex Assay). If manual test is not available skip to step 4 a. Obtain plasma from a citrated specimen b. Allow the reagents and specimen to equilibrate to room temperature			

357

You must:	S	U	Comments
c. Mark patient identifications and control in white areas of the slide			
d. Mix the contents of the latex beads reagent bottle; hold the bottle vertically and add one drop of latex beads to each test area			
e. Dispense 20 μL of undiluted patient plasma or control solution adjacent to the latex beads in each test area			
f. Promptly mix the latex beads and plasma together until the test area is covered; *use a new stirrer for each test area and discard each after use*			
g. Rotate the slide gently for 3 minutes, manually or using a rotator			
h. Exactly 3 minutes after mixing, check for agglutination (clumping); make observations before the mixtures begin to dry out to avoid false-positive reactions. A positive result is white agglutination on a black background; a negative result is a homogeneous white mixture on a black background			
i. Record the results for the patient and the positive and negative controls			
j. Optional: if test is positive, perform the semi-quantitative test following the manufacturer's instructions			
k. If controls are within acceptable limits, report the patient results			
4. Perform activated clotting time (ACT+) using HEMOCHRON or other POC-type instrument (The whole blood controls must be prepared 15 minutes before use; follow the manufacturer's instructions for rehydration and use)			
a. Insert the cuvette into the slot to start the instrument			
b. Perform capillary puncture or obtain a fresh whole blood specimen (1 to 2 mL)			
c. Wait for message "ADD SAMPLE" to appear and add the blood sample to the center well of the cuvette			
d. Fill the well to the top; avoid bubble formation. Allow excess sample to spill over into the outer well			
e. Depress the START button			
f. Wait for the result to be displayed			
g. Repeat steps 4a through 4f for both levels of controls or as directed by the instructor. Refer to the acceptable range provided with each quality control kit			
h. If the controls are within the acceptable range, report the patient results			
5. Dispose of sharps in sharps container			

You must:	S	U	Comments
6. Discard all contaminated sharps into sharps container and other contaminated materials into biohazard container			
7. Disinfect the work area with surface disinfectant			
8. Remove and discard gloves in biohazard container and wash hands with antiseptic			
9. Return other equipment to storage			

Evaluator Comments:

Evaluator _____ Date _____

Basic Immunology and Immunohematology

UNIT OBJECTIVES

After studying this unit, the student will:

- Describe how principles of immunology are used in the clinical laboratory.
- Explain the mechanisms of humoral and cell-mediated immunity.
- Explain the principles of four types of immunological tests.
- Discuss the function of the immunohematology department.
- Perform ABO grouping.
- Perform Rh typing.
- Perform a rapid immunoassay for infectious mononucleosis.
- Perform a latex agglutination assay for rheumatoid factors.

UNIT OVERVIEW

Immunology is the study of the body's immune system and includes a variety of subdisciplines such as the study of immune diseases, tissue typing, blood banking, and organ transplantation. Even though most laboratories have a separate immunology department, every department in the laboratory uses immunological principles and procedures in some way. Therefore, a basic knowledge of immunology is necessary to understand the principles of many laboratory tests.

Serology was the term first used for laboratory immunology because early immunological tests used serum for testing, and tests were designed around the *antigen-antibody* reaction. Today, *serological* procedures are more properly called immunological procedures because they use serum, whole blood, urine, and other body fluids, as well as cells or tissues in a variety of test methods. A general name used for these tests is *immunoassay*. A brief introduction to principles of immunology and basic techniques used in the immunology laboratory are described in Lesson 4-1.

Immunohematology, or blood banking, is the branch of immunology that uses immunological principles to identify and study the blood groups. While some blood banking procedures are relatively simple, such as routine ABO grouping and Rh typing, complex procedures such as compatibility testing for blood transfusion, antibody identification, and tissue typing are also performed in that department. Lesson 4-2 provides an introduction to immunohematology. Information and procedures for ABO grouping are discussed in Lesson 4-3. The Rh system and Rh typing procedures are discussed in Lesson 4-4.

Immunology laboratories perform a variety of tests to detect, identify, and quantitate antibodies and to aid in diagnosing infectious diseases such as hepatitis, AIDS, influenza, and infectious mononucleosis. Lesson 4-5 explains the principle of a chromatographic immunoassay, a rapid immunological test, and how it is used in diagnosing infectious mononucleosis. Lesson 4-6 explains qualitative and semi-quantitative rapid agglutination assays, using as an example the test for rheumatoid arthritis, an autoimmune disease. Principles of the immunoassays presented in Lessons 4-5 and 4-6 can be applied to many other immunoassays.

Immunological tests are used in chemistry, hematology, microbiology, and toxicology to detect and quantitate hormones (as in Lesson 5-6, Urine hCG Tests), identify subsets of blood cells, identify pathogenic microorganisms, and monitor drug levels. Workers in all laboratory departments should have a good foundation and understanding of immunological principles.

READINGS, REFERENCES, AND RESOURCES

American Association of Blood Banks. (2005). *Technical manual of the American Association of Blood Banks* (15th ed.). Bethesda, MD.

Flynn, J. C., Jr. & Kaszczuk, S. (Eds.). (1998). *Essentials of immunohematology*. Philadelphia: W. B. Saunders Co.

Forbes, B. A., et al. (2002). *Bailey & Scott's diagnostic microbiology* (11th ed.). St. Louis: Mosby Year Book.

Harmening, D. (Ed.). (2005). *Modern blood banking and transfusion practices* (5th ed.). Philadelphia: F. A. Davis Company.

Henry, J. B. (Ed.). (2006). *Clinical diagnosis & management by laboratory methods.* (21st ed.). Philadelphia: W. B. Saunders Company.

Paul, W. E. (Ed.). (2003). *Fundamental immunology* (5th ed.). Philadelphia: Lippincott Williams & Wilkins.

Peakman, M. & Vergani, D. (1997). *Basic and clinical immunology*. London: Churchill Livingstone.

Roitt, I. M. (2001). *Roitt's essential immunology* (10th ed.). Malden, MA: Blackwell Publishers.

Rose, N. R., et al. (2002). *Manual of clinical laboratory immunology* (6th ed.). Washington, D.C.: American Society for Microbiology.

Sacher, R. A. & McPherson, R. A. (2000). *Widmann's clinical interpretation of laboratory tests* (11th ed.). Philadelphia: F. A. Davis Company.

Turgeon, M. L. (1995). *Fundamentals of immunohematology: Theory and technique* (2nd ed.). Baltimore: Williams & Wilkins.

Widmann, F. K. & Itatani, C. A. (1998). *An introduction to clinical immunology and serology* (2nd ed.). Philadelphia: F. A. Davis Company.

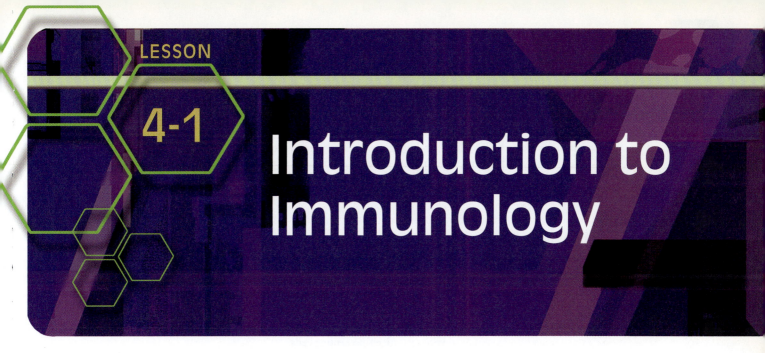

4-1

Introduction to Immunology

LESSON OBJECTIVES

After studying this lesson, the student will:

- Explain the differences between natural resistance and acquired immunity.
- Describe the process of inflammation.
- State three characteristics of specific immunity.
- Explain the differences between humoral and cell-mediated immunity.
- Name the major cells that bring about specific immunity and describe their functions.
- Explain what is meant by primary and secondary lymphoid tissue.
- Diagram the structure of an immunoglobulin molecule.
- Name the five immunoglobulin classes and give characteristics of each.
- Explain the principle of agglutination and give an example of how it is used in the laboratory.
- Explain the principle of precipitation and describe three types of agar precipitation techniques.
- Explain the principles of labeled antibody tests and name three types of labels used.
- Define the glossary terms.

GLOSSARY

agglutination / the clumping or aggregation of particulate antigens due to reaction with a specific antibody

allergy / a condition resulting from an exaggerated immune response; hypersensitivity

anamnestic response / rapid increase in blood immunoglobulins following a second exposure to an antigen; booster response or secondary response

antibody (Ab) / serum protein that is induced by, and reacts specifically with, a foreign substance (antigen); immunoglobulin

antigen (Ag) / foreign substance that induces an immune response by causing production of antibodies and/or sensitized lymphocytes that react specifically with that substance; immunogen

autoimmune disease / disease caused when the immune response is directed at one's own tissues (self-antigens)

B lymphocyte (B cell) / the type of lymphocyte primarily responsible for the humoral immune response

cell-mediated immunity / immunity provided by T lymphocytes and cytokines

complement / a group of plasma proteins that can be activated in immune reactions, can cause cell lysis, and can help initiate the inflammatory response

cytokine / any of various non-antibody proteins secreted by cells of the immune system and that help regulate the immune response; lymphokine

dendritic cells / cells in lymphoid tissues that form a network to trap foreign antigens

enzyme immunoassay (EIA) / an assay that uses an enzyme-labeled antibody as a reactant

epitope / the portion of an antigen that reacts specifically with an antibody; antigenic determinant

humoral immunity / immunity provided by B lymphocytes and antibodies

immunocompetent / capable of producing a normal immune response

immunocompromised / having reduced ability or inability to produce a normal immune response

immunoglobulins (Ig) / antibodies; serum proteins that are induced by and react specifically with antigens (immunogens)

immunology / the branch of medicine encompassing the study of the immune processes and immunity

immunosuppression / suppression of the immune response by physical, chemical, or biological means

inflammation / a nonspecific protective response to tissue injury brought about primarily by release of chemicals such as histamine and serotonin and action of phagocytic cells

lymphokines / non-antibody proteins produced by lymphocytes in response to antigen stimulation and that play a role in regulating the immune response; cytokines

macrophages / long-lived phagocytic tissue cells derived from blood monocytes and that function in destruction of foreign antigens and serve as an antigen-presenting cells

monoclonal antibody / antibody derived from a single cell line or clone

plasma cell / a differentiated B lymphocyte that produces antibodies

polyclonal antibodies / antibodies derived from more than one cell line

precipitation / formation of an insoluble antigen-antibody complex

primary lymphoid organs / organs in which B and T lymphocytes acquire their special characteristics; in humans, the bone marrow and thymus

radioimmunoassay (RIA) / an assay using a test component labeled with a radioisotope

secondary lymphoid tissue / tissues in which lymphocytes are concentrated, such as the spleen, lymph nodes, and tonsils

seroconversion / the appearance of antibody in the serum of an individual following exposure to an antigen

serology / the study of antibodies and antigens in serum using immunological methods

T lymphocyte (T cell) / the type of lymphocyte responsible for the cell-mediated immune response

thymus / a gland, located near the thyroid, that is a primary lymphoid tissue

titer / in serology, the reciprocal of the highest dilution that gives the desired reaction; the concentration of a substance determined by titration

INTRODUCTION

Immunology, the study of the immune system, developed from the study of immunity. Early immunologists were physicians who worked to develop ways of providing immunity to infectious disease. They produced vaccines for bacterial and viral diseases such as smallpox, diphtheria, and tetanus.

As knowledge advanced, it became evident that the immune system had much broader functions than just providing protection from invading microorganisms. It was recognized that a healthy immune system is fundamental to overall good health. The immune system is involved not only in preventing or fighting infectious disease but also in providing protection from toxins and tumors (cancers).

The immune system can also be involved in the initiation of disease. For example, **allergies** such as hay fever or a poison ivy rash are brought on by an exaggerated immune response. **Autoimmune diseases** such as rheumatoid arthritis and lupus erythematosus result when components of the immune system react against one's own tissues. Deficiencies or malfunctions of the immune system can allow cancer cells to grow or allow the development of life-threatening infections by normally nonpathogenic (opportunistic) organisms.

This lesson presents an overview of immunology and an introduction to principles of common immunological tests. A basic understanding of immunology is required to be able to generate or use much of the data in today's clinical laboratory.

IMMUNOLOGY IN THE CLINICAL LABORATORY

Assays based on immunological principles are used in essentially all departments in the clinical laboratory where analytical tests are performed. These assays vary widely in design and purpose. Immunological assays are used to:

- Aid in the diagnosis of infectious diseases by detecting serum antibodies to bacteria, viruses, and parasites
- Detect or identify microorganisms using commercial antibodies
- Detect substances unrelated to the immune system, such as drugs or hormones, using antigen-antibody reactions
- Type blood and tissue
- Identify cell markers
- Evaluate patient immune function in cases of recurring infections, poor wound healing, or other symptoms indicating a possible problem with the immune response

THE IMMUNE SYSTEM

The immune system is a remarkably complex organization of tissues, cells, cell products, and biologically active chemicals, all of which interact to produce the *immune response*. The immune system provides specific defense mechanisms against a variety of foreign substances called **antigens (Ag)**. These antigens can be molecules, viruses, blood cells, tumor cells, bacteria, or fungi. For a substance to be strongly antigenic (capable of stimulating the immune response), the molecule must contain protein or carbohydrate. However, only small sections of these molecules, called **epitopes**, are antigenic.

Natural Resistance Versus Specific Immunity

All of us have an innate *natural resistance* to harmful substances as a result of physical barriers, such as the skin and mucous membranes, and protective secretions, such as mucus, stomach acid, and enzymes in tears. Also participating in this natural resistance are the phagocytic action of cells such as neutrophils and **macrophages**, and natural biochemicals and proteins that work together to initiate protective reactions such as **inflammation** (Figure 4-1). These responses are nonspecific. Previous exposure to an antigen is not required for initiation of the inflammatory response, and the response is the same to a variety of substances and organisms.

The inflammatory response also contributes to the initiation of the specific immune response through interaction of macrophages and lymphocytes. The *specific immune response* (specific immunity) is the type of immune response that recognizes and remembers different antigens. It is this response that most people refer to as immunity or the immune response.

Specific immunity is characterized by three properties:

- Recognition
- Specificity
- Memory

Recognition refers to the immune system's ability to recognize differences in vast numbers of antigens in the environment and to distinguish them from self (one's own tissues).

Specificity refers to the ability to direct a response toward a specific antigen without reacting with other similar antigens.

Memory refers to the immune system's ability to remember an antigen long after initial exposure. This ability, also called the **anamnestic response**, is the basis for immunizations. For example, a childhood immunization against the mumps virus

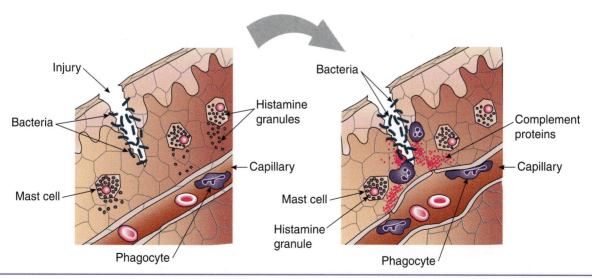

FIGURE 4-1 Inflammation: (left) tissue injury initiates a non-specific inflammatory response near the injured site and mast cells release histamine into tissue; (right) histamine causes capillary dilation (redness) and plasma leaks into tissue (swelling). Complement proteins and cytokines attract phagocytic cells which engulf and digest bacteria and tissue debris. On healing, histamine and complement signals cease, and tissue returns to normal

will provide years of protection because the body's immune cells remember the viral antigens in the vaccine and will respond if they come in contact with the virus again, even years after the immunization. After a child has a disease such as chickenpox, the child usually develops lifelong immunity to the disease because of the memory response.

Cells, Tissues, and Organs of the Immune System

Lymphocytes are important cells that help bring about the specific immune response. The two major types of lymphocytes are **T lymphocytes (T cells)** and **B lymphocytes (B cells)**, each having different functions in immunity. Lymphocytes circulate in the blood and in the lymph fluid and are also concentrated in lymphoid tissues throughout the body.

Lymphocytes are produced in the bone marrow and mature in the primary lymphoid organs. The bone marrow and the **thymus** are the **primary lymphoid organs** in mammals. In humans, B cells mature in the bone marrow and T cells mature in the thymus. The spleen, lymph nodes, and tonsils are examples of **secondary lymphoid tissues** where lymphocytes can be found (Table 4-1).

Two Types of Specific Immunity: Humoral and Cell-Mediated

The two types of specific immunity are **humoral immunity** and **cell-mediated** (cellular) **immunity** (Table 4-2). Both of these responses display recognition, specificity, and memory. The response that predominates is determined by the type of lym-

phocyte that provides the major response to the antigen. Many other cells contribute to and participate in immune responses and overall immunity through complex interactions, including granulocytes, monocytes, tissue macrophages, and **dendritic cells**.

Humoral Immunity

B lymphocytes, or B cells, are responsible for humoral immunity and provide primary protection against bacteria, toxins, and circulating antigens. B lymphocytes produce **antibodies (Ab)**, serum proteins that react specifically with antigens. **Plasma cells**

TABLE 4-1. Primary and secondary lymphoid organs and tissues

PRIMARY LYMPHOID ORGANS

Thymus

Bone marrow (bursa equivalent)

SECONDARY LYMPHOID ORGANS AND TISSUES

Lymph nodes

Spleen

Gut-associated lymphoid tissue (GALT)

    Peyer's patches

    Appendix

    Tonsils

Bronchus-associated lymphoid tissue (BALT)

CURRENT TOPICS

INFLAMMATION

The inflammatory response is initiated by tissue injury from any trauma, mild or severe. The trauma can be internal or external and can be caused by burns, puncture wounds, toxins, bacteria, and other foreign substances, as well as by autoimmune disease. The outward signs of inflammation are *redness, swelling, heat,* and *pain.* For example, when a superficial scratch becomes red, swollen, and tender, it is because of the inflammatory response, a nonspecific response that promotes healing.

The typical inflammatory response is initiated when damaged tissue releases several different chemicals such as histamine, serotonin, and bradykinin. The immediate result of this chemical release is that capillary vessels become *leaky,* allowing fluid to move into the tissue (causing swelling) and isolate any foreign substances from the rest of the body (Figure 4-1). The chemicals are also chemotactic, which means they attract phagocytic white blood cells to the site. These cells engulf microorganisms that might have

been introduced at the trauma site as well as dead or damaged cells. The phagocytes eventually die and accumulate at the site, forming what is commonly called *pus,* a combination of dead tissue cells and live and dead phagocytes. When the body senses that the foreign substance has been eliminated, the chemical releases cease and tissue returns to normal.

The inflammatory response just described is a simplified version of the complex interactions that occur during inflammation. Also involved are the actions of **complement** proteins and many types of cytokines released by cells such as lymphocytes and macrophages. Cytokines have far-reaching functions, which include recruiting cells such as neutrophils and *natural killer cells* to the site, causing fever by influencing the hypothalamus, and stimulating hematopoietic stem cells to produce more immune cells.

Acute inflammation is a natural part of the immune response. However, inflammation can occur inappropriately and lead to tissue destruction, such as occurs in autoimmune disorders, cardiovascular disease, and some degenerative disorders.

are differentiated B lymphocytes and are the most efficient antibody-producing cells (Table 4-2).

Most vaccines work by stimulating humoral immunity. For instance, the DPT vaccine contains three antigens—tetanus toxoid (an inactive toxin), killed *Bordetella pertussis* (the bacterium that causes whooping cough), and killed *Corynebacterium diptheriae,* (the bacterium that causes diphtheria). After injection with these antigens, specific antibody is produced against each antigen. When a child who has received DPT vaccine is subsequently exposed to *B. pertussis,* the specific anti-*B. pertussis* antibodies stimulated by the vaccine will provide protection.

Cell-Mediated Immunity

T lymphocytes, or T cells, help bring about **cell-mediated immunity**, providing protection against viruses, fungi, tumor cells, and intracellular organisms. Cell-mediated immunity is initiated by the interaction of T cells with *foreign cells* and with antigens presented by macrophages and dendritic cells in secondary lymphoid tissue. T cells secrete **lymphokines**, also called **cytokines**, small molecules that communicate with other cells to help regulate the immune response (Table 4-2).

IMMUNOGLOBULINS

Immunoglobulins (Ig), or antibodies, are proteins produced by plasma cells and secreted into body fluids in response to antigen exposure. Immunoglobulins circulate in the blood and make up approximately 10% to 15% of serum protein.

Antibodies are named by placing the prefix *anti* before the antigen with which the antibody reacts. For example, one type of test for AIDS detects the presence of antibodies to HIV (anti-HIV). The antibody specific for the A blood group antigen on group A red blood cells is called *anti-A.*

TABLE 4-2. Comparison of humoral and cell-mediated immunity

IMMUNITY	CELLS RESPONSIBLE	MEDIATED BY	PROTECTION PROVIDED
Humoral	B cells (plasma cells)	Antibodies	Bacteria, toxins
Cell-mediated	T cells	Cells and lymphokines	Viruses, fungi, tumors

Structure and Function of Immunoglobulins

A typical immunoglobulin or antibody molecule consists of four polypeptide chains, two heavy (large) chains, and two light (smaller) chains. These are bound together to form a shape similar to the letter *Y* (Figure 4-2). The majority of antibodies are bivalent, that is, each antibody molecule contains two epitope-combining sites, one located at the end of each arm of the Y.

An antigen entering the body triggers the production of immunoglobulins that react specifically with epitopes found in that antigen. This specific reaction is a physical binding and can be compared to a lock-and-key, with the immunoglobulin being the lock and the epitope the key (Figure 4-3). This physical binding inactivates antigens and targets them for destruction, providing an important defense mechanism. Epitopes are very small, only about five to six amino acids in a protein and four to five sugar residues in a carbohydrate. Since a particular epitope may only occur once or twice on a molecule, a specific antibody may be able to bind to only one or two sites.

CURRENT TOPICS

T LYMPHOCYTE SUBSETS

The designations T lymphocytes or T cells refer to several subsets of lymphocytic cells, each with different functions. T cells are the major players in cell-mediated immunity, which is initiated when T cells encounter antigen processed and presented by cells such as macrophages and dendritic cells in the secondary lymphoid tissues.

The pool of T cells consists of subsets of cells, each with specific responsibilities in the immune response. One way these subsets are identified is by the presence of *markers,* called CD markers, on the T-cell membrane. Two T-cell categories that are often measured in the immunology laboratory are *CD4 cells,* also called helper T cells, and *CD8 cells,* called cytotoxic cells. (A CD4 cell has the CD4 marker on its membrane; a CD8 cell has the CD8 marker on its cell membrane.)

CD4 cells cooperate with B cells to optimize antibody production and also contribute to regulation of the immune response by secreting cytokines, which influence the action of other cells of the immune system. CD8 cells are responsible for destroying tumor cells and virus-infected cells.

The human immunodeficiency virus (HIV) infects and destroys CD4 cells. To monitor treatment or estimate immune suppression in HIV-infected patients, CD4 and CD8 cells are counted using flow cytometry (discussed later in this lesson). The results can be reported as the CD4/CD8 ratio, CD4 and CD8 percentages, or absolute CD4 and CD8 counts. The normal CD4/CD8 ratio ranges from approximately 0.8 to 3.0, and is usually ≥ 1.0. For example, a ratio of 2 would indicate two CD4 cells for each CD8 cell. In HIV infection the ratio can fall to 0.1, meaning only one CD4 cell for each ten CD8 cells. Because CD4 cells are important to immune regulation and antibody production through their effects on B cells, the loss of CD4 cells due to HIV infection produces a profound immunodeficiency.

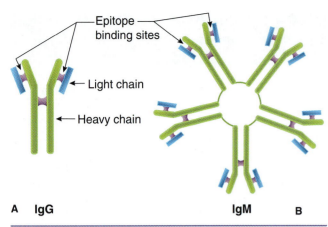

A IgG   IgM   B

FIGURE 4-2 Structure of (A) IgG monomer and (B) IgM pentamer. IgG monomer is composed of four polypeptide chains, two heavy (H) chains and two light (L) chains, all connected by disulfide bonds. IgM is composed of five monomers bound together by disulfide bridges. The heavy chains in each class differ slightly, IgG having gamma (γ) chains, and IgM having mu (μ) chains. Each monomer has two epitope-binding sites

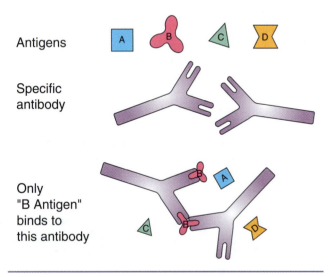

FIGURE 4-3 Illustration of the lock-and-key specificity of the antigen-antibody reaction

Classes of Immunoglobulins

The five classes of Ig in humans are:

- Immunoglobulin G (IgG)
- Immunoglobulin M (IgM)
- Immunoglobulin A (IgA)
- Immunoglobulin D (IgD)
- Immunoglobulin E (IgE)

Although the antibody classes are structurally similar, each has particular characteristics and functions (Table 4-3).

IgG

IgG is the antibody class in highest concentration in serum. It is also called gamma globulin or immune globulin. IgG, once pro-

TABLE 4-3. Characteristics and functions of immunoglobulin classes

CLASS	CHARACTERISTICS/ FUNCTIONS
IgG	Long-lasting immunity, crosses placenta
IgM	First response antibody
IgA	Present in secretions
IgD	Function unknown
IgE	Allergic reactions

duced, remains in serum for a long time and provides long-lasting immunity. It is also the only immunoglobulin class that crosses the placenta.

A newborn is born with humoral immunity that mirrors its mother's humoral immunity. This is called *passive immunity,* because the infant did not produce the antibodies. These maternal IgGs cross the placenta and provide newborns with important immunity that lasts for several months. However, as the infant's level of maternal antibody decreases, the infant becomes susceptible to diseases. The infant's own immune system will be stimulated to produce antibodies when she is exposed to infectious agents or given vaccines. This is called *active immunity.*

IgM

IgM, the second most abundant antibody, is approximately five times larger than IgG. IgM is a pentamer, five immunoglobulin molecules bound together in a manner that leaves 10 epitope-binding sites free (Figure 4-2). Because of its large size and many binding sites, IgM is useful in agglutination reactions. IgM is the first antibody produced in response to an antigen but does not provide long-lasting immunity. It is also the first class of antibody to be produced by newborns after birth. Immunological tests based on detection of antibody in patient serum or plasma are usually measuring IgG or IgM.

IgA

IgA is called the secretory antibody because it is the predominant immunoglobulin in tears, saliva, breast milk, and secretions of the respiratory and intestinal tract. IgA provides protection against organisms that invade through these sites. IgA in breast milk provides passive immunity to newborns in addition to the passive immunity supplied by maternal IgG.

IgD

IgD is present in very small amounts in serum. Little is known of the biological function of IgD.

IgE

IgE is present in very small amounts in serum. IgE is involved in some allergic reactions, such as hay fever and food allergies. IgE production also increases in parasitic infections. Allergy skin tests can be used to detect IgE sensitization to allergens. More specific immunoassays, combining patient serum with specific allergens to detect antigen-specific IgE, enable diagnosis of allergies to foods, pollens, chemicals, drugs, and various other substances.

Primary Versus Secondary Antibody Response: Anamnestic Response

The *primary antibody response* is the immune response occurring after the first exposure to an antigen. The first antibody detectable in plasma following initial antigen exposure is IgM, which usually appears in serum 3 to 4 days after exposure. The IgM concentration quickly peaks and then drops rapidly over a few weeks.

IgG is detectable 1 to 2 weeks after antigen exposure. The IgG level peaks within a few weeks and gradually decreases over a period of months (Figure 4-4).

Measurement or detection of IgM can provide information estimating when an individual was exposed to an organism or antigen. Since IgM is produced early and declines quickly, detection of IgM indicates acute disease (recent exposure). A rise in IgG concentration in serum samples collected 2 to 3 weeks apart also indicates recent exposure. **Seroconversion** is the term used when an antibody becomes detectable in the serum of a patient who has previously tested negative.

The anamnestic response, or *secondary antibody response,* is seen after reexposure to an antigen. Because immune cells remember the antigen, antibody production increases rapidly and IgM and IgG levels rise quickly (within 2 to 3 days) following antigen reexposure. In the secondary response, IgG reaches higher levels than in the primary response, and remains detectable in the serum for months to years (Figure 4-4). Booster vaccinations are based on the principle of the anamnestic response.

DISEASES INVOLVING THE IMMUNE SYSTEM

The immune system provides important protection from disease in **immunocompetent** individuals, that is, individuals who have intact functioning immune responses. Any deficiency or damage to the immune system makes an individual more susceptible to disease, or **immunocompromised**.

Immune deficiencies can be mild or severe and can be acquired or congenital. Most abnormalities of the immune system are acquired. Many drugs, especially corticosteroids and cancer chemotherapy agents, cause **immunosuppression** as an unwanted side effect. Infection with HIV results in interference with immune function, causing infected persons to become susceptible to opportunistic organisms such as *Pneumocystis,* an organism that causes no problems for healthy individuals.

Malignancies of the immune system such as leukemias and lymphomas can occur. Disease or abnormalities can also occur when the immune system is overactive, as in allergies (hypersensitivities), or is misdirected, as in autoimmune diseases.

Immune deficiencies can be a result of inherited genes or of a developmental abnormality in the fetus. While these conditions are uncommon, the effect is usually severe, causing a shortened life expectancy. Table 4-4 lists some diseases and conditions involving the immune system.

IMMUNOLOGICAL TESTS

In the clinical laboratory, tests based on principles of immunology are diverse and in wide use.

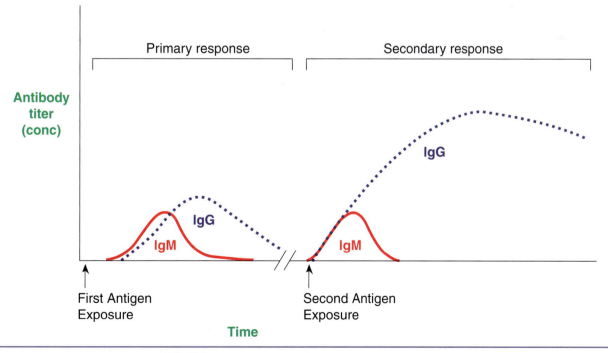

FIGURE 4-4 Comparison of immunoglobin M (IgM) and immunoglobin G (IgG) levels in the primary and secondary antibody responses

TABLE 4-4. Diseases or conditions associated with immune system abnormalities

DISEASE CATEGORY	EXAMPLES
Autoimmune diseases	Rheumatoid arthritis, lupus erythematosus, Type 1 diabetes, myasthenia gravis
Hypersensitivities	Rhinitis, asthma, dermatitis
Malignancies	Lymphomas, leukemias, multiple myeloma
Acquired immuno-deficiencies	Infections, systemic disease, malignancies, reactions to drugs, irradiation
Congenital immuno-deficiencies	DiGeorge syndrome, agammaglobulinemia, SCID (severe combined immune deficiency)

TABLE 4-5. Immunological-based diagnostic methods in order of increasing sensitivity

Precipitation

Agglutination

Complement fixation

Labeled antibody techniques (radio immunoassay, enzyme immunoassay, fluorescent antibody)

Flow cytometry

Tests of Immune Function

Many tests are designed to measure immune function or to detect immune deficiencies or irregularities. These include quantitation of lymphocyte subsets such as CD4 and CD8 cells, quantitation of immunoglobulin subgroups, tests of leukocyte function, allergy tests, and tests for complement components. Most tests of immune function are performed in special immunology laboratories, usually located only in larger hospitals or reference laboratories.

Tests Based on Antigen-Antibody Reactions

Because of the unique properties of antibodies in recognizing and distinguishing among closely related antigens, antibodies are incorporated into many clinical laboratory tests. Some tests use the patient's immune response to help diagnose infections by detecting antibodies to infectious agents in patient specimens, as in HIV, influenza, hepatitis, or rubella tests. These have commonly been called **serology** tests because serum is the usual patient specimen tested. The presence of microbial antigens can be detected in patient specimens using commercial microbe-specific antibodies, as in hepatitis and HIV viral antigen tests on serum. Other laboratory tests use the antigen-antibody reaction to measure or detect a substance not a part of the immune system, such as using antibodies to measure drug or hormone levels, or to identify bacterial species in the microbiology laboratory.

Monoclonal and Polyclonal Antibodies

Antibodies used in immunological tests can be monoclonal or polyclonal. **Monoclonal antibodies** are antibodies of one class and one specificity (react with only one epitope) and are derived from one (mono) clone, or cell line. Monoclonal antibodies are produced in laboratories and used as reagents in many immuno-diagnostic kits. **Polyclonal antibodies** are mixtures of antibodies

produced by more than one (poly) cell line and having more than one epitope specificity. Serum or plasma antibodies are polyclonal. For instance, a bacterial infection would stimulate many plasma cells to produce protective anti-bacterial antibodies, with antibodies from each plasma cell possibly recognizing a different epitope of the bacterium.

Test Sensitivity and Specificity

Laboratories choose test methods based on the sensitivity and specificity of the method. *Specificity* refers to the ability to detect only the substance for which the test is designed. Reaction with other substances (cross-reactivity) decreases the specificity of the test and causes false positive reactions.

Sensitivity refers to the lower limit of detection, or the lowest concentration capable of being detected by a test method (Table 4-5). Failure to detect small amounts of a substance in a test will result in false-negative reactions.

Semi-quantitative and Quantitative Tests

Many immunological procedures are qualitative and are reported only as negative or positive. Others are semi-quantitative or quantitative. Semi-quantitative procedures usually require testing serial dilutions to estimate antibody (or sometimes antigen) concentrations. The relative concentration of the antibody is estimated by making serial dilutions and determining the maximum dilution still capable of causing a visible reaction. Immunoglobulin concentration is expressed as the **titer**, or the reciprocal of the highest dilution showing a reaction. (The procedure for serial dilutions is given in Lesson 1-11.) Quantitative immunological tests are infrequent in everyday practice but include tests such as absolute T-cell counts, measuring concentration of Ig subclasses, and drug assays.

PRINCIPLES OF ANTIGEN-ANTIBODY TESTS

Examples of tests that incorporate the antigen-antibody reaction include:

- Agglutination tests
- Agar precipitation tests
- Nephelometric assays

- Complement fixation tests
- Fluorescent antibody (FA) tests
- Enzyme immunoassays (EIAs)
- Chromatographic immunoassays
- Radioimmunoassays (RIAs)
- Flow cytometry techniques

Assays based on agglutination, precipitation, and nephelometric techniques are sometimes called *indirect* assays because they depend on the formation of a visible reaction, which can only happen when substances are in relatively large amounts. Labeling techniques, including enzyme immunoassays, radioimmunoassays, fluorescent antibody tests, and flow cytometry, are called *direct* assays. This means they are sensitive tests that can be designed to detect individual particles, cells, or antigens.

Agglutination

Agglutination is the visible clumping or aggregation of cells or particles due to reaction with specific antibody (Figure 4-5). IgM is the antibody class that reacts best in agglutination reactions because of its large size and multivalent binding capacity. Antigen-coated cells or particles, such as red blood cells or latex beads, will be linked together and form visible clumps when reacted with sufficient antibody. The presence of agglutination indicates a positive test. Blood typing (Lessons 4-3 and 4-4) and bacterial identification are based on the agglutination reaction. The classic test for rheumatoid arthritis (described in Lesson 4-6) is also based on this principle. Slide agglutination tests can give a qualitative or semi-quantitative result.

Semi-quantitative tests can also be performed in special microtiter plates, using red blood cells as the agglutinating particles. Serial dilutions of serum are made and tested to determine the maximum dilution capable of causing agglutination, which is reported as a titer. In these plates, nonagglutinated particles concentrate in a small dot in the bottom of the well, and agglutinated particles create a diffuse pattern spread over the bottom of the round well.

Precipitation

Agar Precipitation

Precipitation is the formation of an insoluble complex when a specific antibody is reacted with a soluble antigen (Figure 4-6). IgG is the antibody class that reacts best in precipitation reactions. Agar or agarose, gelatin-like substances, provide a matrix for the reactions. The formation of a visible white precipitate in the agar is a positive reaction. However, precipitation can only occur when antigen and antibody are in the correct proportions. Excess of either will inhibit formation of a visible precipitate. Radial immunodiffusion, rocket electrophoresis, and immunoelectrophoresis are examples of agar precipitation tests.

Radial Immunodiffusion (RID)

An example of a *radial immunodiffusion* (RID) test used in clinical laboratories is the test to estimate the concentration of IgG, IgM, or IgA in a patient's serum. Agar plates, about the size of a microscope slide, can be purchased that contain anti-human IgG (or anti-human IgA or IgM) diffused through the agar. The agar contains small wells. Each well is filled with serum, a serum dilution, or a standard (known amount of IgG), and the plate is incubated several hours. As

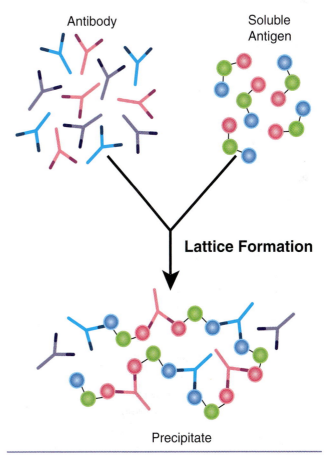

Antibody   Soluble Antigen

Lattice Formation

Precipitate

FIGURE 4-6 Precipitation reaction. Soluble antigen reacts only with specific antibody to form a lattice. When the size of the lattice complexes becomes large enough, a visible white precipitate forms

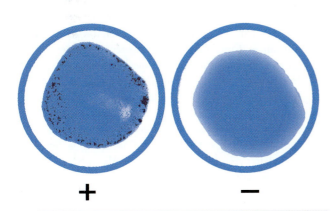

$+$ $-$

FIGURE 4-5 Agglutination reaction: reaction on left is positive ($+$); reaction on right is negative ($-$) (*Courtesy of Remel, Inc., Lenexa, KS*)

the IgG in the serum or standard diffuses out of the well and into the agar, it reacts with the anti-IgG in the agar and forms a white ring of precipitation around the well (Figure 4-7A). The diameter of the ring is proportional to the concentration of IgG in the sample. A standard curve is constructed using the diameters of the rings produced by the IgG standards and the concentrations of the IgG standards. The concentration of the unknown is determined by comparing its precipitation diameter with the standard curve.

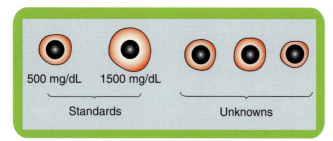

A   **Radial Immunodiffusion**

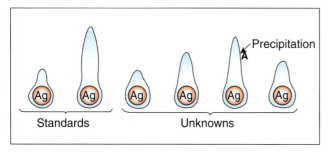

B   **Rocket Electrophoresis**

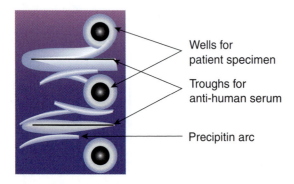

Wells for patient specimen

Troughs for anti-human serum

Precipitin arc

C   **Immunoelectrophoresis**

FIGURE 4-7 Examples of agar precipitation techniques. (A) radial immunodiffusion: rings of precipitation form when serum diffuses out of wells and reacts with specific antibody in agar; (B) rocket electrophoresis: under the influence of electric current, serum proteins move out of wells and react with antibody in agar to form rocket-shaped precipitation patterns; (C) immunoelectrophoresis: arcs of precipitation form in agar indicating reaction of serum proteins with anti-human serum antibody

Rocket Electrophoresis

Rocket electrophoresis is similar to radial immunodiffusion. A slide of antibody-containing agar is used. Standard-sized wells along one side of the slide are filled with standards or the serum that is being tested. An electric current is then applied to the agar to accelerate movement of the substances in the wells into the agar. Movement of charged molecules in response to an electric current is called *electrophoresis*. At the point where the antibody concentration in the agar is in the correct proportion to the substance applied to the wells, precipitation occurs (Figure 4-7B), forming a cone or *rocket*-shaped precipitation pattern. The rocket height is proportional to the concentration of the sample. A standard curve is constructed using the measurements of the standards, and the concentration of the unknown is determined by referring to the standard curve.

Immunoelectrophoresis

Immunoelectrophoresis is used primarily to examine serum globulins for abnormalities. Two wells and a trough are cut into an agar slide. The trough runs lengthwise in the agar between the two wells. A patient serum is inoculated to one well and a standard normal serum to the other. Electric current is applied to the slide, which causes migration of substances in the well toward the positive or negative poles, depending on the particular characteristics of the molecules. (Most proteins have a negative charge and migrate to the positive pole.) The second stage of the test is to inoculate anti-human serum into the trough. This serum diffuses into the agar from the trough, contacting the proteins from the wells. After incubation, precipitin lines will be visible as arcs in the agar (Figure 4-7C). The precipitin lines formed by the unknown serum are compared to the standard to look for abnormalities or missing proteins.

Nephelometry

The use of nephelometric techniques allows immunological tests based on precipitation methods to be automated. When specific antibody is reacted with soluble antigen, a suspension of very small particles forms which can be measured using an instrument called a nephelometer. Nephelometry is based on the principle that a suspension of small particles will scatter light when a beam is passed through it (Figure 4-8). The scattered light is collected electronically and quantitated. The greater the amount of light scatter, the more concentrated the suspension of particles.

In practice, antigen and antibody are combined in proportions to cause formation of small antigen-antibody complexes that remain suspended during measurement. A beam of light is passed through the suspension, and the light scatter is compared to scatter from standard mixtures. The amount of unknown is determined from a standard curve. Many tests that formerly were performed by agar precipitation techniques have been adapted to nephelometry, and many automated immunology analyzers are available that operate on the principle of nephelometry. Tests for immunoglobulin subclasses and specific plasma proteins such as haptoglobin, α-1 antitrypsin, rheumatoid factor, complement proteins, or C-reactive protein, can be performed quickly by nephelometry.

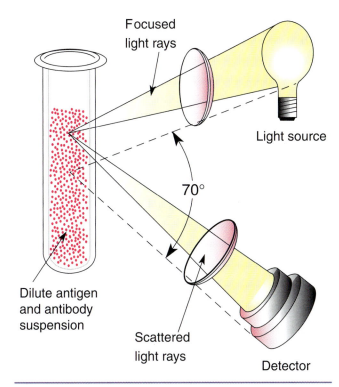

Focused
light rays

Light source

70°

Dilute antigen
and antibody
suspension

Scattered
light rays

Detector

FIGURE 4-8 Illustration of principle of nephelometry. Light is passed through a solution of antigen-antibody (Ag-Ab) complexes. The amount of light scattered as it interacts with Ag-Ab is measured and is proportional to the concentration of Ag-Ab complexes

Complement Fixation

Complement fixation (CF) is a sensitive method for detecting an antigen-antibody reaction and is used to detect specific antibody in patient serum. CF assays are less sensitive than labeled antibody techniques, such as enzyme immunoassays. CF procedures are lengthy, complicated to perform, and require many controls. These tests are performed primarily in research and reference laboratories to detect unusual viral or fungal infections for which test kits are not available.

Labeled Antibody Techniques

Several types of immunological tests use *labeled* antibodies. Molecules (labels) such as dyes, enzymes, or radioisotopes are conjugated (attached) to the antibodies (Figure 4-9). Attaching labels to the immunoglobulins does not interfere with the immunoglobulins' ability to bind to antigens. Labeled antibody techniques are among the most sensitive immunoassays available. Examples of labeled antibody techniques include **enzyme immunoassays (EIAs)**, **radioimmunoassays (RIAs)**, membrane or immunochromatographic assays, fluorescent antibody techniques, Western blotting, and flow cytometry.

Enzyme Immunoassay

EIAs use enzyme-labeled antibodies to cause a visible reaction (Figure 4-9). The tests can be designed to detect either antibody in patient serum, or antigen, such as viral antigen, in a patient specimen. Early EIAs were complex procedures, but many of today's tests, although sophisticated in internal design, require little expertise to perform.

The following description of a test for serum rubella antibodies to determine immunity to rubella can be used as an example of how an EIA works.

1. Patient serum is added to a reaction vessel, such as a well in a microtiter plate, that is coated with rubella viral antigen.

2. After an incubation period to allow any specific antibody in the patient serum to bind to the viral antigen, the patient serum is gently washed away to remove nonspecific unbound antibody.

3. A second antibody directed against human IgG (anti-human IgG), and having an enzyme label attached, is dispensed into the well and allowed to incubate. If anti-rubella was present in the serum and became bound to the viral antigen, the second labeled antibody will bind to the anti-rubella. If no anti-rubella was present in the serum, the second labeled antibody will not bind.

4. The well is again washed to remove unbound, enzyme-labeled antibody, and a colorless substrate specific for the enzyme is added to the well. If the substrate is converted to a colored form, indicating that enzyme-labeled secondary antibody was present, the test is positive. The color intensity can be estimated visually or measured using a special spectrophotometer capable of reading microtiter plates. The amount of color produced is proportional to the amount of bound enzyme-linked antibody. Absence of color is a negative test.

Membrane or Chromatographic Immunoassays

Numerous tests are based on variations of the EIA. These are sometimes called membrane immunoassays, chromatographic immunoassays, or immunochromatographic assays. In membrane EIAs, most or all of the reagents are incorporated in an absorbent membrane enclosed in a plastic cassette. When a sample (serum or urine) is added, it migrates through the membrane reacting with the antibody and reagents and forming a color (Figure 4-10). Most of these tests are simple to perform and interpret, even though the technology is complex. Examples of membrane EIAs include over-the-counter pregnancy test kits, tests for Group A *Streptococcus,* influenza, and *Helicobacter pylori.* Many EIA kits are CLIA-waived.

Protein Immunoblotting Techniques

Protein *immunoblotting* techniques, sometimes called Western blots, combine electrophoresis with principles of labeled antibody tests. The secondary antibodies used in immunoblotting can be labeled with enzymes, fluorescent dyes, or radioisotopes. These techniques are primarily performed in special chemistry, reference, or research laboratories. Immunoblotting is used to confirm positive results in HIV rapid screening tests. The immunoblotting procedure detects

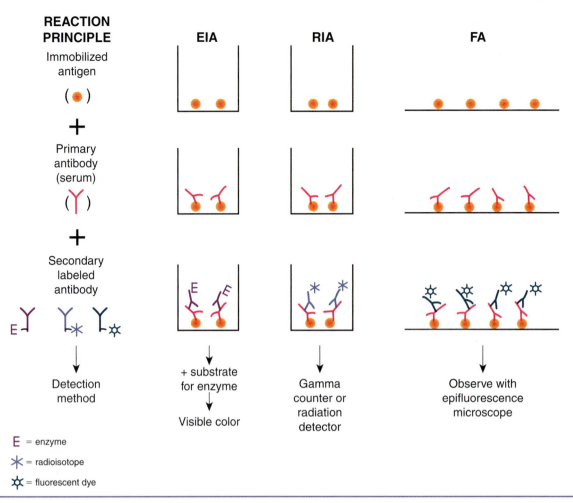

FIGURE 4-9 Comparison of antibody labeling techniques: (left) enzyme immunoassay (EIA); (center) radioimmunoassay (RIA); (right) fluorescent antibody (FA) assay

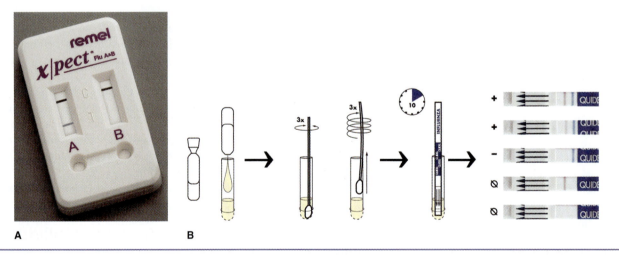

FIGURE 4-10 Examples of membrane immunoassays for influenza. (A) Test for influenza A and B showing results for a patient that has influenza. A patient serum was applied to wells A and B; the upper black "C" lines indicate internal controls are working properly; blue "T" line in window A is a positive result for influenza A; absence of blue "T" line in window B is a negative result for influenza B (*Courtesy of Remel, Inc., Lenexa, KS*). (B) Antigens in nasal swab are extracted, test strip is immersed in reagent, and colored lines indicate control results and test results (⊘ indicates invalid test) (*Courtesy of Quidel, Inc., San Diego, CA*)

patient antibodies to the p24 antigen of the human immuno-deficiency virus.

Radioimmunoassay

RIAs were some of the earliest of the modern generation of immunoassays. The first sensitive and reliable drug and hormone assays were RIAs. They are similar in principle to enzyme immunoassays and can be used to detect antigen or specific serum antibody. However, instead of an enzyme, a radioisotope is used as the label (Figure 4-9), and results are measured by using a radiation detector to quantitate radiation in the reaction vessel. EIAs have replaced many RIAs because the EIA reagents are more stable and the hazards of using radioactive materials are eliminated.

Fluorescent Antibody Techniques

In fluorescent antibody (FA) tests, a fluorescent dye is conjugated to the antibody. These dyes fluoresce when excited by a beam of ultraviolet (uv) light, and epifluorescence microscopes must be used to read and interpret the reactions (Figure 4-9 and Lesson 1-10). Fluorescent antibody tests can be direct or indirect and can be used to detect antibody in patient serum or antigen in a patient specimen. Fluorescent antibody tests are used in microbiology and parasitology and in detecting autoantibodies present in autoimmune diseases such as lupus.

Treponema pallidum infection (syphilis) can be diagnosed by incubating patient serum with a prepared slide containing a laboratory strain of *Treponema*. The slide is gently washed to remove unbound, nonspecific antibody, and the specimen is then incubated with fluorescent labeled anti-human globulin. The slide is washed again and then examined microscopically. Presence of fluorescent-stained spirochetes indicates that the patient serum was positive for antitreponemal antibodies. *Mycobacteria* and *Cryptosporidium* are also identified using fluorescent antibod-ies. For these tests, a slide preparation prepared from the patient specimen is reacted with commercial microorganism-specific antibody. This first antibody can be fluorescently labeled (direct test) or, if not, is followed with a second labeled antibody (indirect test). Presence of fluorescing microorganisms of the correct morphology indicates that the patient is infected with the suspect microorganism. Indirect techniques are more sensitive than direct because more than one molecule of fluorescent-labeled second antibody can bind to the first antibody, increasing the amount of fluorescence.

Flow Cytometry or Cell Sorting

In clinical medicine, flow cytometry is used primarily in immunology and hematology laboratories; instruments are also available for use in urinalysis. This technique is useful when cells in suspension need to be identified, categorized, or separated into groups.

The term *flow cytometer* comes from cell (*cyto*) measurement (*meter*) as cells *flow* through a special narrow channel in single file. Usually, cell suspensions are treated with a fluorescent label. The suspensions are then directed through a narrow channel and pass by a laser beam in single file. Cells passing through the beam are counted, cell or nuclear size is measured, or fluorescence pattern detected, and this information is stored in a database. A screen displays the information graphically showing cell percentages for each cell category, or size distribution. Some instruments can measure three different fluorescent colors, so three types of cells can be analyzed and sorted into groups simultaneously. Instruments capable of cell sorting can separate cells by category and keep them alive for later use. Flow cytometry has many applications and is useful in separating blood cells or subpopulations of lymphocytes. Applications of flow cytometry to hematology and urinalysis are discussed in Lessons 2-13 and 5-5.

CASE STUDY

Ahmed came to see his physician because he had fever, headache, and fatigue for over a week and still was not feeling well. His physician ordered several tests for infectious diseases, including tests for influenza, toxoplasmosis, West Nile virus, and Epstein-Barr virus. These tests were performed by testing Ahmed's serum for both IgG and IgM antibody to the various infectious agents. The following results were reported:

	IgG	IgM
Influenza A	negative	negative
Toxoplasma	positive	negative
West Nile virus	negative	positive
Epstein-Barr virus	positive	negative

What agents can be ruled out as the cause of Ahmed's illness? Why? What is a possible cause of his illness? Explain your answer.

SUMMARY

This lesson is a brief introduction to the basic principles of immunology needed to understand procedures in the remaining lessons in this unit. Knowledge of the cells and organs of the immune system and the mechanisms of immune responses aids in comprehending how laboratory tests work, not only immunology tests but tests performed in all laboratory departments. Because many tests are based on the antigen-antibody reaction, knowledge of the structure and functions of antibody subclasses is important. A variety of tests use immunological principles. Many immunological tests, such as membrane EIAs, have been designed to be very easy to perform despite being based on complex principles. These tests give rapid results and many are CLIA-waived.

Tests using antigen-antibody reactions can be indirect or direct. Indirect tests include agglutination, agar precipitation techniques, and nephelometric assays and are not as sensitive as direct tests. Direct assays include several types of labeled antibody assays, using enzymes, fluorescent dyes, radioisotopes, or other labels. It is impossible to cover the complex topic of immunology in a single lesson, but it is hoped that the student will be stimulated to seek more information on this topic.

REVIEW QUESTIONS

1. What are the differences between specific immunity and natural resistance?

2. What are the differences between humoral and cell-mediated immunity?

3. What are the three characteristics of specific immunity?

4. What type of immunity most commonly develops from vaccinations?

5. Draw an IgG molecule. Show where the epitope binding sites are.

6. Name the five classes of immunoglobulins. Which is the most abundant?

7. Which immunoglobulin class gives long-lasting immunity?

8. Which immunoglobulin class participates in allergic reactions?

9. Explain the principle of agglutination.

10. What tests are based on the principle of precipitation?

11. What is meant by labeled antibody? What types of labels are used in immunological tests?

12. How does the sensitivity of labeled antibody tests compare to that of precipitation and agglutination tests?

13. Explain the principle of flow cytometry and discuss how it is used in the clinical laboratory.

14. How do qualitative tests differ from quantitative tests?

15. Discuss how the inflammatory response stimulates healing.

16. How are lymphocyte markers used in tests for HIV?

17. Why is newborn immunity called passive immunity?

18. How do monoclonal antibodies differ from polyclonal antibodies?

19. Define agglutination, allergy, anamnestic response, antibody, antigen, autoimmune disease, B lymphocyte, cell-mediated immunity, complement, cytokine, dendritic cells, enzyme immunoassay, epitope, humoral immunity, immunocompetent, immunocompromised, immunoglobulins, immunology, immunosuppression, inflammation, lymphokines, macrophages, monoclonal antibody, plasma cell, polyclonal antibodies, precipitation, primary lymphoid organs, radioimmunoassay, secondary lymphoid tissue, seroconversion, serology, T lymphocyte, thymus, and titer.

STUDENT ACTIVITIES

1. Complete the written examination for this lesson.

2. Look in magazines, newspapers, or other sources for information on the role of the immune system in allergies.

W E B   ACTIVITIES

1. Use the Internet to find information on two brands of analyzers used for immunology testing. Compare the principle of operation of each and list tests that are included in the test menus.

2. Research an autoimmune disease, immune deficiency disease, or infectious disease diagnosed by immunological methods using reliable Internet sources. Report on the cause of the disease, symptoms, methods of diagnosis, and appropriate clinical laboratory tests.

Introduction to Immunohematology

LESSON OBJECTIVES

After studying this lesson, the student will:

- Discuss the functions of the immunohematology, or blood banking, department.
- Explain the process of blood donation.
- Discuss requirements that must be met by blood donors.
- Name eight tests that must be performed on donated blood before it can be used.
- Name blood components that can be obtained from a unit of donated blood.
- Name five procedures performed in the blood bank department.
- Discuss the safety procedures that must be followed in the blood bank.
- Explain the importance of quality assessment policies to the operation of the blood bank.
- Define the glossary terms.

GLOSSARY

American Association of Blood Banks (AABB) / international association that sets blood bank standards, accredits blood banks, and promotes high standards of performance in the practice of transfusion medicine

apheresis / the process of removing a specific component, such as platelets, from donor blood, and returning the blood to donor circulation

blood bank / clinical laboratory department where blood components are tested and stored until needed for transfusion; immunohematology department; transfusion services; also the refrigerated unit used for storing blood components

immunohematology / the study of the human blood groups; in the clinical laboratory, often called blood banking or transfusion services

transplant / living tissue placed into the body; the placing of living tissue into the body

INTRODUCTION

Immunohematology is the study of the human blood groups. In the clinical laboratory, the field of immunohematology can include:

- Evaluation of blood donors
- Collection and processing of donor blood
- Testing patient blood for blood group antigens
- Matching patient with compatible blood before transfusion
- Tissue typing
- Forensic studies
- Paternity tests
- Genetic studies

This lesson presents an introduction to the clinical practice of immunohematology, and includes information about the routine functions of the immunohematology or **blood bank** department. Also included is information about blood donation and the collection and processing of donor blood. A discussion of the ABO blood group and procedures for ABO grouping are described in Lesson 4-3. The importance of the Rh blood group and procedures for Rh typing are given in Lesson 4-4.

HISTORY OF TRANSFUSION MEDICINE

The earliest recorded blood transfusion was attempted shortly after William Harvey discovered blood circulation in 1628. For several decades following, crude blood transfusions were tried numerous times, sometimes transfusing blood from animals to humans, mostly with disastrous results. This eventually led to the prohibition of transfusion in the late 1600s.

In 1818, Dr. James Blundell, an English obstetrician, successfully transfused a woman suffering from post-partum hemorrhage using her husband's blood. He continued to experiment with transfusion, with some success, and also devised instruments for use in transfusion. In 1867, Joseph Lister proposed using antiseptic techniques during transfusions. In the late 1800s, U.S. physicians experimented with transfusing milk into patients, but because of adverse reactions, the physicians switched to saline. Throughout all of this time, some patients did well, some developed infections, and some suffered immediate severe reactions and died. Physicians had no way to anticipate which transfusions would be successful and which would fail.

In 1900, Karl Landsteiner discovered the ABO blood group and, in 1930, received the Nobel Prize for this discovery. Following this landmark discovery, other physicians began developing ways to improve transfusion success. Patient blood was mixed with donor blood to look for reactions before transfusion; the inheritance of blood groups was worked out; anticoagulants were developed that could preserve blood for longer periods; the Rh blood group, as well as other minor blood groups, was discovered; the first blood *depot* for storing donated blood was established during World War I; the first hospital blood bank in the United States was established in 1937 in Chicago; and in 1940 the U.S. government established a nationwide blood collection program which was instrumental in saving lives during World War II.

Beginning around 1950, and for the next three decades, improvements in blood banking were rapid and dramatic: sterile plastic blood bags were manufactured, improved blood preservation methods extended shelf life of blood to 35 days, donor units were screened for hepatitis B, and hospital blood banks were established all over the country, even in small hospitals. Blood use increased dramatically as its value in trauma and major surgeries such as open heart surgery was recognized. Specialized treatments using components such as platelet concentrates, fresh frozen plasma, and anti-hemophilic factor (AHF) were used to treat bleeding disorders.

In the early 1980s, the discipline of transfusion medicine became a medical specialty. About this time the first cases of AIDS began to appear. In 1984 the cause of AIDs was proven to be the human immunodeficiency virus (HIV), and the virus was shown to be transmissible by blood. This immediately caused drastic changes in donor blood screening and intensified research into developing sensitive, reliable tests for HIV, to avoid transmitting HIV from an infected donor to a patient. The need to guarantee a safe blood supply led not only to the development of sensitive tests to detect HIV but also to improved tests for other infectious agents. As new infectious diseases emerge, blood bank specialists act quickly to develop screening tests for the infectious agent and to tighten donation requirements so that potentially infected individuals are excluded from donating blood.

IMMUNOHEMATOLOGY OR BLOOD BANK DEPARTMENT

The application of immunohematology principles in the clinical laboratory is usually carried out in the **blood bank**, or *transfusion services*, department. The commonly used designation blood bank comes from the fact that blood units have traditionally been stored or *banked* in one location.

On a daily basis, technicians working in the blood bank are responsible for typing patient blood, testing blood for usual antibodies related to the blood groups, matching compatible blood units to patients for transfusion, and providing special components such as platelets for transfusion. Depending on the size of the hospital, the blood bank department may also perform blood group studies in paternity questions and work with transplant teams and tissue typing laboratories to ensure safe organ and tissue transplants (Table 4-6). Because the blood bank department is responsible for preparing and testing components that will be administered intravenously, or transplanted, to patients, its operation is regulated by the Food and Drug Administration (FDA). Standards for blood banking practice are issued by the **American Association of Blood Banks (AABB)**, an agency that also accredits blood banks.

DONOR BLOOD

The AABB estimates that approximately 15 million units of blood are donated each year, from about half as many donors. Donations are made at community blood donation centers as well as mobile blood donation centers that go to malls, schools, churches, and

TABLE 4-6. Tests performed in immunohematology laboratories

Routine blood typing

Evaluation of blood donors

Providing compatible components for transfusion

Testing blood for unusual blood group antibodies

Collection and processing of donor blood

Tissue typing

Forensic studies

Paternity tests

Genetic studies

TABLE 4-7. Diseases and infectious agents capable of being transmitted by blood transfusion

VIRUSES	PARASITIC DISEASES	BACTERIAL DISEASES
Hepatitis A virus (rare)	Babesiosis	Syphilis*
Hepatitis B virus*	Chagas	
Hepatitis C virus*	Malaria	
Cytomegalovirus		
Human immuno-deficiency virus (HIV)*		
HTLV-I*		
HTLV-II*		
West Nile virus*		

*Denotes donor blood is tested for this disease/agent

TABLE 4-8. General health requirements for blood donors

PARAMETER	CRITERIA
Age	>16 and conforming to state law
Weight	110 pounds
Temperature	≤99.5°F (≤ 37.5° C)
Blood pressure	<180/<100 mm Hg
Hemoglobin	>11 g/dL (or >33% Hct)

Requirements can differ slightly among blood collection agencies and according to state laws.

other areas participating in blood drives. Each year, these donations provide blood components for over 4 million patients, including trauma victims, surgical patients, and patients with bleeding disorders or diminished blood cell production.

Most hospitals acquire donor blood from blood donor processing centers, such as those operated by the American Red Cross (ARC) or other independent, nonprofit blood donation agencies. Blood donation centers work to provide safe blood for transfusion, and this begins with accepting blood donation only from healthy donors. Potential blood donors can be volunteer donors, paid or professional donors, or replacement donors. Volunteer donors provide the majority of donated blood in the United States and are highly recruited because the quality of volunteer donated blood is considered to be high. Several methods are used to eliminate unsafe blood from entering the blood supply—strictly enforced donor eligibility standards, verification of donor I.D., donor medical screening, laboratory testing of donor blood, confidential exclusion of donors, and checks of donor records.

Blood Donor Requirements

Although donated blood is tested for several infectious agents, it is impossible to test every unit for all possible agents (Table 4-7). Before donating, prospective donors are provided educational materials explaining the requirements that must be met to be accepted as a donor, as well as diseases, conditions, or medical history that would cause a donor to be excluded from donating. Potential donors who elect to continue with the process after reading the materials are given a brief physical examination and asked to answer extensive questions about their medical history. The questions are designed both to ensure that donation will not present a health risk to the donor and also to exclude donors whose blood might present a hazard if transfused. The safety of the blood supply depends on the education of donors and honesty of donors in answering these questions. The privacy of prospective donors must be respected while obtaining medical history so that donors are not reluctant to provide honest answers.

The physical examination includes weight, temperature, blood pressure, pulse rate, blood hemoglobin level, and evaluation of general health and demeanor of donor (Table 4-8). The health questionnaire may contain as many as 100 questions, asking about date of last donation, current medications, recent immunizations, previous and existing diseases or medical conditions, and travel or residency outside of the United States. Behavioral history is also questioned, including questions about sexual behavior, illegal drug use, recent tattoos, body piercing, acupuncture, and electrolysis among others. Ultimately the physician in charge of the donation center makes the final decision on whether to accept, defer, or exclude a donor.

Donor Blood Collection

All materials used to collect donor blood are sterile, so there is no danger of transmitting disease to the donor. Blood is collected by venipuncture from a large vein in the arm, usually the cephalic vein, after sterilizing the puncture site. Approximately one pint (0.5 L) of whole blood is collected into a sterile closed bag con-

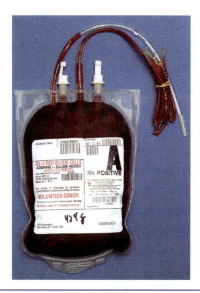

FIGURE 4-11 Donor blood bag with attached segmented tubing

TABLE 4-9. Tests for infectious diseases performed on donated blood (as of June 2006)

ANTIBODY TESTS	ANTIGEN TESTS
Hepatitis B core antibody (anti-HBc)	Hepatitis B surface antigen (HBsAg)
Hepatitis C virus antibody (anti-HCV)	Nucleic acid amplification testing (NAT):
HIV-1 (anti-HIV-1)	HIV-1
HIV-2 (anti-HIV-2)	Hepatitis C virus
HTLV-I antibody (anti-HTLV-I)	West Nile virus (WNV)
HTLV-II antibody (anti-HTLV-II)	
Serologic test for syphilis	

taining a citrated anticoagulant and dextrose. This process takes approximately 10 to 20 minutes. A small portion of the blood remains in sealed, segmented tubing external to the sterile unit (Figure 4-11). Each tubing segment is coded to match the code on the blood bag. The blood in these tubing segments is used for various tests so that unit sterility is maintained until it is transfused. At the time of donation, blood is also collected into vacuum tubes to be used for typing donor blood and other screening tests.

Adults average about 10 pints of blood in their circulation. The fluid lost from donation is replenished by the body in about 24 hours; the red blood cells are replaced in a few weeks. Blood donors must wait a minimum of 56 days (8 weeks) between donations of whole blood.

Another type of donation is called **apheresis**, the process of removing one blood component and returning the remaining blood components to the donor's circulatory system. Apheresis can take 1 to 2 hours to complete and requires special cell-separating machines. This process can be used to donate red blood cells, plasma, platelets, and granulocytes. *Plateletpheresis* is the process of removing only platelets from donor blood. One plateletpheresis session provides up to five times more platelets than are present in one platelet component prepared from whole blood.

Processing and Testing Donor Blood

Technologists in donor processing centers determine the ABO group and Rh type of donor blood, screen the blood for unusual antibodies to blood group antigens, and perform several other tests before releasing it to hospitals. Most of these tests are designed to eliminate potentially infectious units from being transfused. Blood is tested for syphilis and for antibodies to hepatitis B and C viruses, HIV (HIV-1 and HIV-2), and human T-cell lymphotropic virus types I and II (HTLV-I, HTLV-II). Units are also tested for HIV, hepatitis, and West Nile viral antigens using very sensitive nucleic acid amplification tests (NATs) which

detect viral genetic material. Any unit that is confirmed positive for any of these tests must be discarded, and the donor must be notified and placed on a list prohibiting them from giving blood. Table 4-9 lists the tests for infectious agents performed on donor blood in the United States in 2006. The list has expanded, and will continue to expand, as new infectious diseases emerge.

Blood Components

Blood is normally collected as whole blood, which contains red and white blood cells and platelets suspended in plasma. Donated blood can be left as whole blood or separated into several components, depending on the needs of the medical community in the region. In this way more than one patient can benefit from the donation of one unit of blood. Three components easily obtained from a donor unit are:

- Red blood cells
- Platelets
- Plasma (fresh frozen plasma, FFP)

After testing and processing, the blood components are distributed to hospitals for use. Blood components must be kept within a very narrow temperature range until used. Temperature controlled units, such as blood bank refrigerators and freezers, are used for storing some components (Figure 4-12). These units are fitted with temperature alarms and backup power sources, and temperature is monitored and recorded daily (minimum).

Red blood cells are used for patients with low hemoglobin or hematocrit who need improved oxygen-carrying capacity of blood. With improvements in anticoagulants in the last several years, units of red blood cells can now be stored for up to 42 days. Plasma is a source of proteins such as albumin, globulins, fibrinogen, and other clotting proteins, as well as electrolytes. If the plasma is frozen within hours after collection, it is designated as FFP and is useful in treating bleeding disorders due to deficiency of clotting factors. Platelet units (platelet concentrates) are prepared by centrifuging plasma to obtain platelet-rich plasma. Platelets are used to treat thrombocytopenia and other platelet disorders.

Many other components can be prepared from donor blood but are used less frequently than red blood cells, platelets, and FFP. These components are usually prepared in a facility other than the blood donation center and include cryoprecipitated anti-hemophilic factor (AHF), Factor VIII concentrate, Factor IX concentrate, and immune globulins, including Rh immune globulin.

PROCEDURES PERFORMED IN THE HOSPITAL BLOOD BANK

Blood banking is the term commonly used to refer to the tests routinely performed in this department. Most routine blood banking procedures are based on the agglutination reaction. These procedures include:

- ABO grouping
- Rh typing
- Compatibility testing before blood transfusion
- Typing of donor blood
- Screening for and identification of unusual blood group antibodies
- Tests for hemolytic disease of the newborn

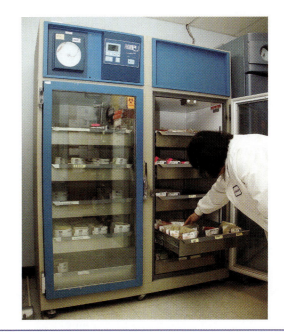

FIGURE 4-12 Refrigerated blood bank for storing blood components

CURRENT TOPICS

ARTIFICIAL BLOOD AND BLOOD SUBSTITUTES

It is estimated that someone in the United States needs a blood transfusion every 2 to 3 seconds. During holidays or extreme winter weather, through the news media we often hear about blood shortages and pleas for people to donate blood. Emergencies and natural disasters create immediate needs for increased donor units. Trauma victims needing blood must wait for a transfusion until they can reach a medical facility and laboratory testing can identify compatible blood.

What can be done to address these problems? For decades researchers have been searching for a blood substitute, or way to make artificial blood. Research funded by the military began decades ago, searching for a portable, stable product to transfuse into wounded personnel suffering oxygen deprivation from blood loss in the battlefield.

Research for blood substitutes continues today, using two main approaches: (1) use of liquid *perfluorochemicals*, synthetic chemicals related to Teflon, administered intravenously under high oxygen pressure and (2) use of *cell-free stable hemoglobin* molecules derived from blood cells or genetically engineered. (The term *oxygen therapeutics* is often used in place of artificial blood as it more closely approaches the function of the products.) The ideal blood substitute would provide rapid oxygen delivery to the patient's tissues while eliminating risk of transmission of infectious agents from a donor to patient. It would also (1) eliminate blood shortages, (2) have a long shelf life, (3) require no special storage conditions, and (4) be universally compatible. Each research approach has advantages and disadvantages, but neither has been able to overcome a major disadvantage which is the short half-life of the product in plasma, making it useful for only a few hours.

Clinical trials of several products have been conducted in animals and some in humans. Some hemoglobin products are already in limited use. Oxyglobin, a chemically stabilized hemoglobin, has been used successfully since 1998 to treat canine anemia. A stabilized bovine hemoglobin product is used in South Africa to treat severely anemic human adult patients. In the United States, blood substitutes have been tested in healthy volunteers and found to be safe in small amounts. As these products come into wider use, they will be useful at trauma sites to provide a means to stabilize oxygen-deprived patients until they can receive donor blood.

ABO is the major blood group. The Rh group is the second in importance. All donor blood and patients who might receive donor blood must have the ABO group and Rh type determined. These procedures are described in Lessons 4-3 and 4-4. Although donor units are labeled with ABO and Rh type before they are released to hospitals, the hospital blood banks repeat typing on all donor components.

The blood of patients requiring a transfusion must be matched to a compatible component. This test is called a *cross-match*, or *compatibility testing*. It involves combining patient serum with donor red blood cells and examining for an agglutination reaction. This is to be sure the patient has no antibody that could react with donor blood and cause an adverse reaction in the patient.

Safety in the Blood Bank

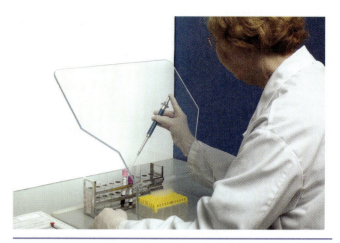

Standard Precautions must be followed when performing all blood bank procedures, whether at donor processing centers or hospital blood banks. Gloves and appropriate personal protective equipment (PPE) must be worn. Exposure control methods, such as working behind an acrylic safety shield (Figure 4-13), must be used to protect against exposure to blood and blood products. Because most reagents used in blood banking originate from human blood products, all reagents must be handled as if potentially infectious. Disposable supplies should be used, and surfaces should be disinfected frequently. Safety rules must be followed when using electrical equipment and instruments with moving parts, such as centrifuges.

Quality Assessment

It is crucial to patient well-being that testing performed in the immunohematology department is of the highest quality and performed with the utmost attention to accuracy. Blood is a living tissue; a blood transfusion is a tissue **transplant**. The same precautions must be used with blood transfusions as with organ transplants. The donor blood must be collected and stored in a

FIGURE 4-13 Exposure control method: acrylic safety shield used to prevent exposure to blood and reagents made from blood

manner that maintains the sterility of the blood and the viability of the cells. Test results are used to match donor blood to the patient. Transfusion of the wrong blood into a patient can cause severe adverse reactions, such as kidney shutdown, or even death.

Strict quality assessment and assurance procedures must be followed in the blood bank department. Mandatory quality assessment guidelines include:

- Documenting proper working condition of refrigerators, freezers, water baths, centrifuges, and any other equipment used in preparing, testing, and storing blood components
- Monitoring temperatures at all times to ensure that components are constantly stored within acceptable temperature ranges
- Visual inspection and testing of reagents at designated intervals and recording results
- Observing reagent expiration dates
- Running appropriate controls

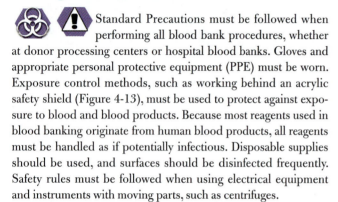

CASE STUDY

Suri, a 31-year-old woman, heard about a need for blood donors in her area on the local television news broadcast. She went to the local blood donation center to volunteer to donate. Results of her physical examination and medical history included these findings:

		Medications:		Travel in past year:	
Temperature	98.5°F				
Weight	115	Aspirin (last 8 days)	no	Europe	no
Hematocrit	31%	Birth control pills	yes	Canada	yes
Blood pressure	110/70	Antidepressant	yes	Africa	no

(If necessary, use information from the ARC or AABB Web sites in addition to Table 4-8 to answer the following questions.)

1. Are any of the findings above reasons for deferring donation? If so, which one(s)?
2. Name three medications that can cause a donor to be permanently or indefinitely excluded from donating blood.

Special attention must be paid to patient and donor blood identification. Tests must be performed following standard operating procedure. Observation and interpretation of results must be carefully recorded. Manufacturer's instructions must be followed for the particular reagents used.

SUMMARY

Immunohematology covers several areas of study. These areas include research to ensure a safe blood supply, increase shelf life of donor blood, and develop artificial blood. Clinical practices are also continually evaluated to determine the best transfusion therapies for patients.

In the clinical laboratory, immunohematology procedures are performed in the blood bank or transfusion services department. Here personnel type patient and donor blood and provide compatible blood components for transfusion. The utmost care must be taken in all blood bank procedures to ensure that the patient ultimately receives a transfusion which is life-saving, not life-threatening, or otherwise detrimental to his or her health.

Blood donor collection and processing agencies work to provide a safe blood supply by screening donors through physical examinations and medical questionnaires. Donor blood is also screened for several infectious agents before it is released into the donor pool. Immunohematology is a challenging field, and requires dedicated, capable technologists working to provide the best possible patient care.

REVIEW QUESTIONS

1. What viral tests are performed on donated blood before it can be released to hospital blood banks?

2. Name three components that can be obtained from a unit of donor blood.

3. Which governmental agency regulates blood banks?

4. What are the two major blood groups?

5. What is meant by artificial blood? Why would it be beneficial?

6. What benefit could be gained by giving FFP to a patient?

7. What benefit is derived from transfusing red blood cells into a patient?

8. What important contribution was made to immunohematology by Karl Landsteiner? How did this change the practice of immunohematology?

9. Name five procedures performed in blood banks.

10. Explain the safety precautions that must be used when performing blood bank procedures.

11. Why is it essential to have a comprehensive quality assessment program in place in blood banks?

12. Define American Association of Blood Banks, apheresis, blood bank, immunohematology, and transplant.

STUDENT ACTIVITIES

1. Complete the written examination for this lesson.

2. Visit a blood donor center and find out how donated blood is collected, tested, and processed for distribution. Ask for information about how apheresis is performed. Ask for a copy of the donor education information and donor questionnaire.

W E B   A C T I V I T I E S

1. Use the Internet to find specific blood donor requirements. From Web sites such as those of the ARC or AABB, find and print or download a donor medical questionnaire. Name 10 conditions or criteria that would cause a potential donor to be deferred or excluded.

2. From reliable Web sites such as those of the Centers for Disease Control and Prevention (CDC), ARC, or AABB, find out if the following diseases present risk of transmission by blood transfusion: SARS, vCJD, Lyme disease, and smallpox.

3. Search the Internet for information on *autologous* blood donation. Write a paragraph about it, including a definition and explanation of how it differs from regular blood donation.

4. Search the Internet for information about freezing blood cells for long-term storage. Describe how this process is performed and discuss advantages and disadvantages.

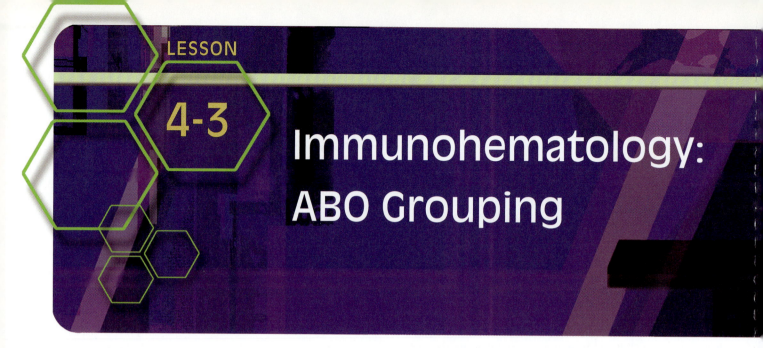

Immunohematology: ABO Grouping

LESSON OBJECTIVES

After studying this lesson, the student will:

- Name the four blood groups in the ABO system and state their frequencies in the United States.
- Explain the inheritance of the ABO blood groups.
- Name the blood group antigens and antibodies in the ABO system.
- Explain forward and reverse grouping.
- Perform ABO slide grouping and interpret the results.
- Perform ABO tube grouping and interpret the results.
- Describe grading of agglutination in tube grouping.
- Explain the use of gel typing in the blood bank.
- Discuss safety precautions that must be observed when performing ABO grouping.
- Discuss the importance of using controls and following quality assessment policies in the blood bank.
- Define the glossary terms.

GLOSSARY

allele / one of two (or more) alternate forms of a gene responsible for hereditary variation

antiserum / serum that contains antibodies

blood bank / department in the clinical laboratory where blood components are tested and stored until needed for transfusion; refrigerated unit used for storing blood components

blood group antibody / a serum protein (immunoglobulin) that reacts specifically with a blood group antigen

blood group antigen / a substance or structure on the red blood cell membrane that stimulates antibody formation and reacts with that antibody

codominant / in genetics, a gene that is expressed in the heterozygous state, that is, in the presence of a different allelic gene

forward grouping / the use of known antisera (antibodies) to identify unknown antigens on a patient's cells; forward typing; direct grouping

genes / segments of DNA that code for specific proteins or enzymes and that are the structural units of heredity

histocompatibility testing / performance of assays to determine if donor and recipient tissue are compatible

human leukocyte antigen (HLA) / one of several antigens present on leukocytes and other body cells that are important in transplant rejection

major histocompatibility complex (MHC) / the group of genes responsible for producing antigens such as HLA that contribute to the failure of organ and tissue transplants

reverse grouping / the use of known cells (antigens) to identify unknown antibodies in the patient's serum or plasma

serological centrifuge / a centrifuge that spins small tubes such as those used in blood banking; serofuge

INTRODUCTION

The major blood group system is the ABO system, where individuals are grouped as one of four major types: A, B, AB, or O. ABO grouping tests are based on the principle of agglutination. The grouping tests can be performed by slide, tube, or gel methods. The slide method is quick and easy and requires no special equipment. However, the tube and gel methods are both more sensitive than the slide test and are used in clinical laboratories.

The ABO group of patient and donor blood must be determined before a blood transfusion can be given. Blood group determination must also be performed before organ transplantation and in questions of paternity, forensic investigations, and genetic studies. This lesson presents information about the ABO blood group system and procedures for slide, tube, and gel methods of ABO grouping.

THE ABO SYSTEM

The ABO blood group system was discovered by Karl Landsteiner around 1900. All individuals can be placed into one of four major groups: A, B, AB, or O. In the United States, approximately 45% of the population is group O and 40% is group A. Only 11% of the population is B, and 4% is AB (Table 4-10). Distribution differs greatly according to specific racial and ethnic groups. Approximately 63% of the world's population is group O.

Blood Group Antigens

ABO grouping is based on the presence or absence of two **blood group antigens** designated A and B. These antigens are found on the cell membranes of red blood cells, as well as platelets and leukocytes. The blood group antigens are products of inherited allelic **genes**. Each individual inherits one blood group **allele** from each parent—the *A*, *B*, or *O* allele. *A* and *B* are **codominant** with respect to each other. Therefore, persons who inherit both an *A* and *B* allele will express both A and B antigens. A person who inherits one *O* allele and an *A* (or *B*) allele will express only A (or B) antigen. Individuals who inherit two *O* alleles have neither A nor B antigens expressed.

Individuals are grouped according to the antigens present on their blood cells: a person who is group A has A antigen; a person who is group B has B antigen; a person who is group AB has A and B antigens; and a person who is group O has neither A nor B antigen (Table 4-11). The ABO grouping procedures are agglutination tests. A and B antigens on patient or donor red blood cells are detected by reacting the cells with known (commercial) antibodies in a procedure called **forward grouping**, or direct grouping.

Blood Group Antibodies

The discovery of the A and B antigens was accompanied by the discovery of the corresponding ABO **blood group antibodies** in human blood.

Blood group antibodies are named according to the antigen with which they react: an antibody that reacts with A antigen (A red blood cells) is called anti-A; an antibody that reacts with B antigen (B red blood cells) is called anti-B. The blood group O was so named because the red blood cells have neither A nor B antigen; therefore, there is no anti-O antibody.

TABLE 4-10. ABO blood group frequencies in the United States*

GROUP	PERCENTAGE OF POPULATION
A	40%
B	11%
O	45%
AB	4%

* From AABB Website, 2007

TABLE 4-11. Antigens and antibodies of the ABO system

ABO GROUP	ANTIGEN ON RED BLOOD CELLS	ANTIBODY IN SERUM
A	A	Anti-B
B	B	Anti-A
AB	A and B	Neither anti-A nor anti-B
O	Neither A nor B	Both anti-A and anti-B

ABO blood group antibodies occur naturally in serum and are of the immunoglobin M (IgM) class. If an antigen is missing from an individual's cells, the antibody specific for the missing antigen will be present. For example, group A individuals have anti-B antibody in their serum. An individual who is group O has both anti-A and anti-B since O cells have neither A nor B antigen (Table 4-11). Testing patient blood for the presence of the blood group antibodies is called **reverse grouping**, confirmatory grouping, or indirect grouping. It is performed by reacting serum or plasma with (commercial) red blood cells whose A and B antigens are known.

Although the blood group antigens are present on red blood cells of newborns, the blood group antibodies are not well developed at birth. The ABO antibodies may not be easily detectable until the age of about 6 months. For this reason, only forward grouping is reliable in newborns and young infants.

Importance of ABO Grouping

The ABO group must be determined before procedures such as blood transfusion can be performed. An individual should be transfused with blood of the same ABO blood group. Because of the presence of the naturally occurring antibodies to A and B antigens, severe transfusion reactions can occur if blood is not matched properly.

The rule to follow in transfusing blood is to *avoid giving the patient an antigen he does not already have*. In an emergency, O blood can be used because it contains neither A nor B antigen. For this reason, people of blood group O are called *universal donors*.

SAFETY PRECAUTIONS

 Standard Precautions must be followed when performing all **blood bank** procedures. Gloves and appropriate personal protective equipment (PPE) must be worn to protect against exposure to blood and blood products. Exposure control methods should be used to protect against accidental exposure to blood and blood typing reagents. Since most blood grouping reagents originate from human blood, all reagents must be handled as if potentially infectious. Disposable labware and supplies should be used and discarded into appropriate biohazard or sharps containers. Counter surfaces should be disinfected frequently with surface disinfectant. Safety rules must be followed to protect from physical and electrical hazards when using electrical equipment and instruments with moving parts, such as centrifuges.

QUALITY ASSESSMENT

 Quality assessment procedures will be outlined in the blood bank standard operating procedure (SOP) manual. This manual will incorporate standards for good blood banking practice developed by the American Association of Blood Banks (AABB), an agency that also accredits blood banks. The blood bank department must also follow Food and Drug Administration (FDA) guidelines and is subject to FDA inspections.

Mandatory quality assessment guidelines include:

- Documenting proper working condition of refrigerators, freezers, water baths, centrifuges, and any other equipment used in preparing, testing, and storing blood components and reagents
- Monitoring temperatures at all times to ensure that components are constantly stored within acceptable temperature ranges
- Inspecting visually and testing reagents at designated intervals and recording results
- Observing reagent expiration dates
- Running appropriate controls and verifying reagent performance

Special attention must be paid to patient and specimen identification. Patients having tests performed by the blood bank department are issued special armbands that are coded to the patient's blood specimen to help avoid a chance of misidentification.

Observations of reactions must be carefully interpreted and recorded. Manufacturers' instructions must be followed for the particular reagents used.

In immunohematology, the quality of laboratory testing can have a direct, immediate impact on the patient. A blood transfusion is a potentially lifesaving event. Errors or mistakes in identifying specimens, performing grouping tests, or interpreting grouping results can lead to serious consequences. Technologists who work in the blood bank must be highly trained, conscientious, and vigilant.

PRINCIPLE OF ABO SLIDE GROUPING

The slide test detects A or B antigens on red blood cells by combining the patient's blood cells with a known **antiserum** on a slide and observing for agglutination. If the antigen present on the cells corresponds to the antibody in the antiserum, the antibody will bind to the antigen and cause clumping of the cells, or agglutination. If the antigen is not present on the cells, no agglutination will be observed.

Performing ABO Slide Grouping

ABO slide grouping is performed using commercial typing slides or microscope slides. One drop of commercial anti-A serum is added to one labeled slide, and one drop of anti-B serum is added to a separate labeled slide. A drop of well-mixed capillary or venous blood is placed adjacent to each drop of antiserum (Figure 4-14). The anti-A is mixed with the drop of blood using a disposable applicator stick, stirrer, or spreader. The procedure is repeated with the anti-B and the other drop of blood using a clean stirrer.

The slides are then rocked gently for 2 minutes and observed for agglutination using good lighting. Agglutination, a positive reaction, will appear as a clumping together of the red blood cells (Figure 4-15). Absence of agglutination is a negative reaction. The reactions with each antiserum should be recorded as positive (+) or negative (0).

CURRENT TOPICS

ABO GROUPS AND ORGAN AND TISSUE TRANSPLANTS

Tissues or organs that are typically transplanted include kidney, liver, cornea, skin, pancreas, bone marrow, heart, lung, intestine, and bone. Transplants that occur from one body site to another in the same individual are called *autologous* or *allogeneic transplants*, or *autografts*. An example of this would be skin grafts that are taken from one part of the body and transferred to a burned area. Since autografts are of one's own tissue, the problem of possible tissue rejection is eliminated.

Transplants from a donor of the same species are called *homologous transplants, homografts,* or *allografts*. Examples of these would be a sister donating a kidney to her brother, or a person receiving a heart transplant. According to the U.S. Department of Health and Human Services, approximately 27,000 people received organ transplants in the United States in 2004, or about 74 people each day. Over 90,000 are waiting to receive organ donation.

Before a transplant can take place, the donor tissue or organ must be matched to the recipient (see Figure 4-16). In the case of blood transfusions, which are tissue transplants, the ABO group and Rh type of the recipient is matched to the ABO group and Rh type of the donor blood. The ABO group must also be considered in other tissue and organ transplants because A and B antigens are present not only on red blood cells, platelets, and leukocytes but also on many other cells in the body, particularly endothelial and epithelial cells.

The second level of tissue matching involves **histocompatibility testing**, assays to determine if donor and recipient share some tissue antigens. The **major histocompatibility complex (MHC)** is a complex of closely associated genes that code for highly variable antigens expressed on most cells of the body. The antigens of the MHC distinguish one individual from another and are the principle barrier to the ability to transplant tissues and organs from one individual to another. Several antigens produced by the MHC genes are required for the immune response. Some of the most important are called **human leukocyte antigens (HLA)**, named because they were first discovered on leukocytes. However, these antigens are on many body cells, and many different forms can be expressed by the MHC based on our inheritance. Therefore, family members are more likely to have some of the same antigens and be a compatible donor. It is usually impossible to find a perfect HLA match because only identical twins have identical HLA antigens. However, when more HLA antigens are shared by donor and recipient, the chances of transplant rejection are lessened.

Transplant Rejection—The body's normal response to the introduction of foreign material is to mount an immune response and reject the foreign body. This reaction occurs when homologous transplants are performed. Matching donor histocompatibility antigens to the recipient minimizes the chances of rejection. However, it is also necessary to use immunosuppressive drugs to further minimize the chances of rejection. Rejection can be acute, chronic, or a graduated phenomenon, but often rejection can be treated successfully with increased drug therapy. Individuals who receive homologous transplants usually must remain on immunosuppressive drugs for the remainder of their lives.

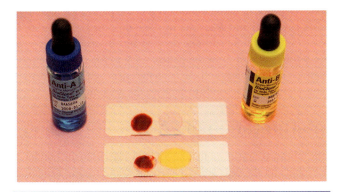

FIGURE 4-14 ABO slide grouping procedure: Top slide contains blood plus anti-A; bottom slide contains blood plus anti-B

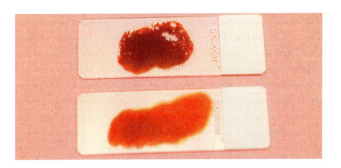

FIGURE 4-15 Illustration of agglutination of blood cells by anti-A in ABO slide grouping. Agglutination of cells with anti-A in the top slide and absence of agglutination with anti-B in the bottom slide indicates the patient is group A

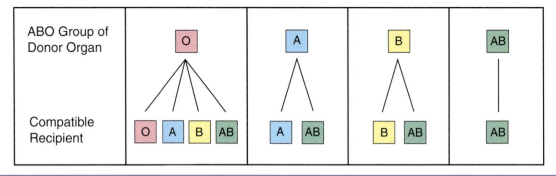

FIGURE 4-16 ABO compatibility chart for tissue and organ transplant

TABLE 4-12. Reactions of ABO groups with anti-A and anti-B sera

BLOOD GROUP	REACTIONS OF CELLS WITH: ANTI-A	ANTI-B
A	+	0
B	0	+
AB	+	+
O	0	0

+ = agglutination
0 = no agglutination

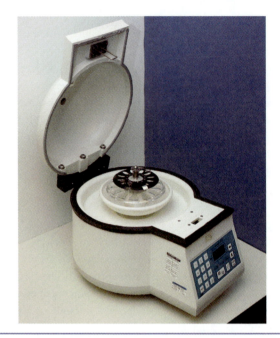

FIGURE 4-17 Serological centrifuge

Interpretation of Slide Grouping Results

If only the A antigen is present on the red blood cells, the blood cells will agglutinate with anti-A but not with anti-B. If only B antigen is present, the blood cells will agglutinate with anti-B but not with anti-A. Group O blood cells will not agglutinate with either anti-A or anti-B. Group AB blood will agglutinate with both anti-A and anti-B (Table 4-12).

PRINCIPLE OF ABO TUBE GROUPING

Tube testing is a more sensitive and reliable method of determining a patient's blood group than is slide testing. Tube testing is used in blood banks and in clinical laboratories; slide testing is more likely to be used in classrooms. Tube grouping requires dilution of the blood with saline to make a 2% to 5% suspension of cells.

ABO tube grouping consists of (1) direct or forward grouping, which identifies the antigens on the cells, and (2) reverse or confirmatory grouping, which identifies the blood group antibodies in the serum. A serological centrifuge can be used to speed up the reaction (Figure 4-17). A **serological centrifuge** is a specialized centrifuge that spins small test tubes.

Performing Forward Grouping

Forward or direct grouping identifies the antigens present on red blood cells by reacting a suspension of cells with commercial anti-

A and anti-B sera and observing for agglutination after centrifugation. If a centrifuge is not available, the reactions can be observed after allowing the tubes to sit undisturbed at room temperature for 15 to 30 minutes.

A 2% to 5% red blood cell suspension is made by adding 18 to 19 drops of saline to one drop of the patient's blood. Two tubes labeled *A* and *B* are set up: one drop of anti-A serum is placed in the *A* tube and one drop of anti-B serum is placed in the *B* tube. One drop of the patient's 2% to 5% cell suspension is added to each tube, and the contents are mixed. The tubes are centrifuged for 30 seconds to enhance the reaction.

Interpretation of Forward Grouping

The tubes are tapped gently to loosen the cells from the bottom of the tube, and the cells are observed for agglutination. Clumping of the cells is a positive reaction indicating the antigen present on the cells corresponds to the antibody placed in the test tube (Tables 4-12 and 4-13). Reactions should be graded using a plus system: neg (no agglutination); w+ (weak reaction); and 1+, 2+, 3+, and 4+ (strongest agglutination). Figure 4-18 gives an illustration and description of each grade of reaction.

TABLE 4-13. ABO forward and reverse grouping results

ABO GROUP	FORWARD GROUPING		REVERSE GROUPING		
	Reactions of Cells with:		Reactions of Plasma with:		
	Anti-A	Anti-B	A Cells	B Cells	O Cells
O	0	0	+	+	0
A	+	0	0	+	0
B	0	+	+	0	0
AB	+	+	0	0	0

0 = no agglutination
+ = agglutination

Performing Reverse Grouping

Reverse (indirect or confirmatory) grouping identifies the antibodies present in a patient's serum or plasma by reacting the plasma with a commercial 2% to 5% suspension of group A cells and a commercial 2% to 5% suspension of group B cells and observing for agglutination.

Two drops of the patient's plasma are added to each of three tubes marked *a*, *b*, and *control*. One drop of the group A cell suspension is added to tube *a*, one drop of group B cell suspension is added to tube *b*, and one drop of a 2% to 5% suspension of patient cells is added to the *control* tube. The contents of the tubes are mixed, and the tubes are centrifuged for 30 seconds.

Interpretation of Reverse Grouping

The tubes are tapped gently, and the cells are observed for agglutination and the reactions graded (Figure 4-18). A positive test, agglutination, indicates that the antibody present in the patient's plasma corresponds to the antigen on cells added to the tube. The control tube should always be negative for agglutination since it contains only the patient's plasma and cells. Reverse grouping results should confirm the results of forward grouping (Table 4-13).

PRINCIPLES OF GEL TYPING

Improvements are constantly being made in the technology of blood bank testing. Automated and semi-automated systems are available for blood grouping and crossmatching. Solid-phase and gel or column typing methods can be automated allowing some walk-away testing. This is particularly helpful when staffing is low and technologists must work in more than one department on their shift.

Gel typing is sensitive and specific, and the procedure can be standardized, verified, and validated. Testing is performed in a card prefilled with gels mixed with the appropriate reagent (Figure 4-19). A dilution of patient cells is pipetted onto the gel column and the card is incubated. The card is centrifuged and read. Agglutinated cells will not travel through the gel but remain at the top of the column, a positive reaction. Nonagglutinated

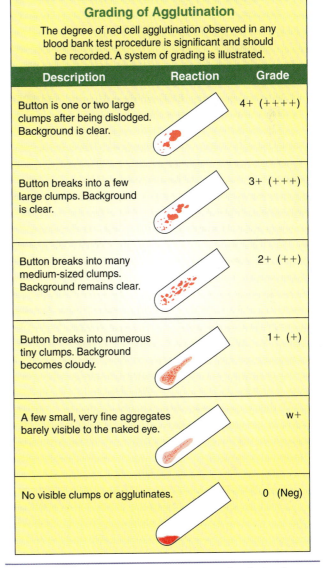

Grading of Agglutination

The degree of red cell agglutination observed in any blood bank test procedure is significant and should be recorded. A system of grading is illustrated.

Description	Reaction	Grade
Button is one or two large clumps after being dislodged. Background is clear.		4+ (++++)
Button breaks into a few large clumps. Background is clear.		3+ (+++)
Button breaks into many medium-sized clumps. Background remains clear.		2+ (++)
Button breaks into numerous tiny clumps. Background becomes cloudy.		1+ (+)
A few small, very fine aggregates barely visible to the naked eye.		w+
No visible clumps or agglutinates.		0 (Neg)

FIGURE 4-18 Illustration of grading of agglutination reactions in ABO tube typing

cells travel through the gel to the bottom of the column, a negative reaction (Figures 4-19 and 4-20). Since some gel typing reactions are stable for several hours, tests can be retained and reread if necessary.

Minimal handling of reagents and specimens increases biosafety. Use of gel tests eliminates variables due to worker technique. Clear, stable, well-defined endpoints mean objective and reproducible interpretation of test results, as well as reduced need to repeat tests. Although cost containment is an important issue in health care today, the blood bank must continue to maintain strict standards and use the best available methods, even if it means that the cost of services must rise.

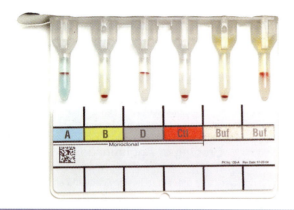

FIGURE 4-19 Gel typing card with columns (from left) for ABO forward grouping, Rh D typing and control, and ABO reverse grouping. Patient specimen shown is "A positive."

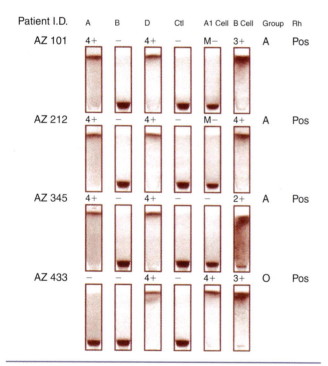

Patient I.D.	A	B	D	Ctl	A1 Cell	B Cell	Group	Rh
AZ 101	4+	−	4+	−	M−	3+	A	Pos
AZ 212	4+	−	4+	−	M−	4+	A	Pos
AZ 345	4+	−	4+	−	−	2+	A	Pos
AZ 433	−	−	4+	−	4+	3+	O	Pos

FIGURE 4-20 Gel typing report form. Shown are reports of ABO and Rh D typing on four patient specimens using the Ortho ProVue automated immunohematology testing system. Tests from left are forward grouping (patient cells and anti-A and anti-B), Rh D and control, and reverse grouping (A and B cells and patient plasma). Cells at bottom of column indicate absence of agglutination, a negative reaction. Agglutinated cells form a layer at top of column and indicate a positive reaction

SAFETY Reminders

- Review safety precautions before performing procedures.
- Observe Standard Precautions when performing blood-grouping procedures.
- Wear buttoned fluid-resistant laboratory coat and other appropriate PPE.
- Discard all used glassware in sharps container.
- Observe equipment safety rules when operating the serofuge.

PROCEDURAL Reminders

- Review quality assessment section before performing procedures.
- Follow manufacturer's directions regarding the storage and use of all commercial reagents.
- Do not use reagents beyond expiration dates.
- Perform quality control procedures at specified intervals and record results.
- Observe timing carefully when performing slide tests.
- Use a 2% to 5% cell suspension for tube grouping.
- Use good lighting to observe reactions.
- Do not shake tubes too vigorously; weak agglutination reactions can be dispersed and misinterpreted.
- Record results as soon as they are observed.

CRITICAL THINKING 1

Type O blood is considered the *universal* donor group. If a patient other than one in blood group O must receive a transfusion of group O blood, it is best to transfuse that patient with O packed or washed red cells rather than O whole blood. Explain why this is so.

CRITICAL THINKING 2

A couple expecting their first child had ABO grouping performed. The husband was group AB and the wife was group O. What are the possible ABO groups of the fetus?

SUMMARY

The antigens and antibodies of the major blood group system, the ABO system, can be detected by simple agglutination tests performed by slide, tube, or gel methods. The gel methods have many advantages, such as conservation of reagents and possibility of automation and walk-away technology. In addition, gel tests can be retained and reinterpreted if questions arise.

Determination of ABO blood group is performed in hospital blood banks, blood donor centers, and other settings such as forensic laboratories. Blood bank or immunohematology tests can often have life-changing consequences. These tests can lead to such outcomes as patients receiving transfusions of blood components, determination or ruling out of parentage, or evidence provided in forensic cases.

Blood banks, whether in hospitals or donor centers, are the only clinical laboratory service regulated by the FDA. Technologists who work in this department must be of the highest caliber and must adhere to strict quality assessment policies and procedures to ensure that a safe product is available for transfusion and that the patient receives the proper components.

REVIEW QUESTIONS

1. Name the four groups in the ABO system.
2. State the frequency of each ABO group in the U.S.
3. What antigens present on red blood cells determine the ABO groups?
4. What antibody is present in the serum of a person who is group B? Group O?
5. What is forward grouping?
6. What is reverse grouping?
7. What agglutination results would be observed when testing group A blood with anti-A and anti-B? When testing group AB blood?
8. How does ABO tube testing differ from ABO slide testing?
9. How are the results of tube grouping tests interpreted? Explain the system of grading agglutination.
10. What safety precautions should be observed in ABO grouping?
11. Explain why adherence to quality assessment policies and procedures is important in the blood bank department.
12. Explain the principle of gel typing and list some of its advantages.
13. What is the MHC? How is it involved in tissue and organ transplants?
14. Define allele, antiserum, blood bank, blood group antibody, blood group antigen, codominant, forward grouping, genes, histocompatibility testing, human leukocyte antigen, major histocompatibility complex, reverse grouping, and serological centrifuge.

STUDENT ACTIVITIES

1. Complete the written examination for this lesson.

2. If possible, visit a hospital blood bank and find out how ABO testing is performed.

3. Practice performing ABO groupings as outlined in the Student Performance Guides, using the worksheets.

4. Survey blood groups in your classroom. Make a chart showing the percentages of each ABO group. Do your percentages agree with published percentages?

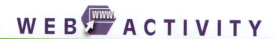

WEB ACTIVITY

Use the Internet to find two types of gel or solid-phase blood typing materials. Download or request package inserts. Read about instruments used to process and read the gel typing cards. Write a short report about one of the instruments, including information about how the gel card results are read, how many samples can be processed each hour, etc.

Student Performance Guide

LESSON 4-3 Immunohematology: ABO Grouping—I. Slide Method

Name _____ Date _____

INSTRUCTIONS

1. Practice performing the slide method of ABO grouping following the step-by-step procedure.

2. Demonstrate the slide method of ABO grouping satisfactorily for the instructor, using the Student Performance Guide. Your instructor will determine the level of competency you must achieve to receive a satisfactory (S) grade.

NOTE: Reagent package inserts should be consulted for specific instructions before test is performed.

MATERIALS AND EQUIPMENT

- gloves
- antiseptic
- face protection and/or acrylic safety shield
- EDTA (ethylenediaminetetraacetic acid) anticoagulated blood specimens
- optional—capillary puncture materials: alcohol swabs, lancets, cotton balls or gauze, and capillary collection vials or tubes
- timer
- pen or pencil for labeling slides
- applicator sticks or stirrers
- disposable transfer pipets
- commercial anti-A
- commercial anti-B
- microscope slides or cell typing slides
- ABO Worksheet I
- surface disinfectant
- biohazard container
- sharps container

PROCEDURES

Record in the comment section any problems encountered while practicing the procedure (or have a fellow student or the instructor evaluate your performance).

S = Satisfactory
U = Unsatisfactory

You must:	S	U	Comments
1. Assemble equipment and materials and wash hands			
2. Put on face shield or position acrylic safety shield on work area and put on gloves			
3. Perform slide grouping following steps 3a through 3g a. Obtain two slides, label one *A* and one *B* b. Place one drop of anti-A serum on the *A* slide and one drop of anti-B serum on the *B* slide. Do not allow dropper to touch the slide c. Dispense one drop of well-mixed venous blood or freshly collected capillary blood adjacent to the antiserum on each slide using a disposable pipet. Do not allow pipet to touch slide			

395

You must:	S	U	Comments
d. Use a disposable stirrer to mix the blood and anti-serum on slide *A* into an area about the size of a quarter. Repeat the procedure on the *B* slide, using a clean stirrer e. Rock the slides gently for 2 minutes and observe for agglutination using strong lighting f. Record agglutination results on ABO Worksheet I: agglutination = +; no agglutination = 0 g. Determine the blood group and record			
4. Repeat steps 3a through 3g using additional blood samples			
5. Discard all specimens appropriately or return them to storage as directed by instructor			
6. Discard disposable labware into appropriate biohazard and sharps containers			
7. Return reagents and equipment to proper storage			
8. Clean work area with surface disinfectant			
9. Remove gloves and discard into biohazard container			
10. Wash hands with antiseptic			

Evaluator Comments:

Evaluator _____ Date _____

◆ ABO Worksheet I

LESSON 4-3 Immunohematology: ABO Grouping—Slide Method

Name _____   Date _____

Specimen I.D.	AGGLUTINATION RESULTS*		INTERPRETATION
	Anti-A	Anti-B	ABO Group
_____	_____	_____	_____
_____	_____	_____	_____
_____	_____	_____	_____
_____	_____	_____	_____
_____	_____	_____	_____

* Record results as:

0 = no agglutination

+ = agglutination

Student Performance Guide

LESSON 4-3 Immunohematology: ABO Grouping—II. Tube Method

Name _____ Date _____

INSTRUCTIONS

1. Practice performing ABO grouping by the tube method following the step-by-step procedure.
2. Demonstrate the tube method for ABO grouping satisfactorily for the instructor, using the Student Performance Guide. Your instructor will determine the level of competency you must achieve to receive a satisfactory (S) grade.

NOTE: Reagent package inserts should be consulted for specific instructions before test is performed.

MATERIALS AND EQUIPMENT

- gloves
- antiseptic
- face protection and/or acrylic safety shield
- EDTA anticoagulated blood specimens
- wax pencil or Sharpie for labeling tubes
- blood bank saline (physiological saline)
- plastic, disposable transfer pipets
- commercial anti-A
- commercial anti-B
- commercial A cells (2% to 5% suspension)
- commercial B cells (2% to 5% suspension)
- disposable test tubes, 13 × 75 mm
- test tube rack
- timer
- optional: serological centrifuge capable of spinning 13 × 75 mm tubes at 2000 to 2500 rpm
- ABO Worksheet II
- surface disinfectant
- biohazard container
- sharps container

PROCEDURE

Record in the comment section any problems encountered while practicing the procedure (or have a fellow student or the instructor evaluate your performance).

S = Satisfactory
U = Unsatisfactory

You must:	S	U	Comments
1. Assemble equipment and materials. Put on face shield or position acrylic safety shield on work area			
2. Wash hands and put on gloves			

3. Perform ABO forward tube grouping following steps 3a through 3i
  a. Prepare a 2% to 5% suspension of patient cells by placing one drop of a well-mixed blood specimen into a test tube and adding 18 to 19 drops of saline. Label the tube *patient cells*
  b. Label two test tubes *A* and *B*			

You must:	S	U	Comments
c. Place one drop of anti-A in tube *A* and one drop of anti-B in tube *B* d. Place one drop of the 2% to 5% patient cell suspension in each tube and mix gently e. Place tubes in serological centrifuge and spin 30 seconds **NOTE:** Balance the centrifuge by placing tubes opposite each other. (If no centrifuge is available, allow tubes to stand at room temperature for 15 to 30 minutes and go to step 3g) f. Allow the centrifuge to come to a complete stop and remove the tubes g. Tap each tube gently to loosen cells from the bottom of the tube and observe cells for agglutination using good lighting. Grade agglutination using the guide in Figure 4-18 h. Record results from each tube on Worksheet II i. Determine the blood group of the sample and record			
4. Perform ABO reverse grouping on the blood sample following steps 4a through 4k a. Centrifuge the blood specimen, remove 0.5 to 1.0 mL of plasma from the sample, and place it in a clean test tube b. Label three test tubes *a, b,* and *control* c. Place two drops of plasma into each of these tubes d. Place one drop of a 2% to 5% commercial suspension of A cells into tube *a* and mix e. Place one drop of a 2% to 5% commercial suspension of B cells into tube *b* and mix f. Place one drop of the patient's 2% to 5% cell suspension into *control* tube and mix g. Place tubes in serological centrifuge (be sure to balance tubes in rotor) and spin 30 seconds (or allow tubes to sit at room temperature 15 to 30 minutes and go to step 4i) h. Remove the tubes from the centrifuge after it stops completely i. Tap each tube gently and observe cells for agglutination. Grade agglutination using guide in Figure 4-18 j. Record the results from each tube on ABO Worksheet II k. Determine the blood group of the sample and record			
5. Compare results of forward grouping with results of reverse grouping of the same sample. Reverse grouping should agree with results of forward grouping			
6. Repeat forward and reverse grouping (steps 3 and 4) on additional blood specimens if available			

You must:	S	U	Comments
7. Discard all specimens appropriately or store specimens as directed by instructor			
8. Discard disposable labware into appropriate biohazard or sharps container			
9. Return all equipment and reagents to proper storage			
10. Clean work area with surface disinfectant			
11. Remove gloves and discard in biohazard container			
12. Wash hands with antiseptic			

Evaluator Comments:

Evaluator _____ Date _____

ABO Worksheet II

Name _____ Date _____

Specimen I.D.	DIRECT (FORWARD) GROUPING*		INTERPRETATION	INDIRECT (REVERSE) GROUPING*			INTERPRETATION
	Anti-A	Anti-B	ABO Group	A Cells	B Cells	Control	ABO Group
_____	_____	_____	_____	_____	_____	_____	_____
_____	_____	_____	_____	_____	_____	_____	_____
_____	_____	_____	_____	_____	_____	_____	_____
_____	_____	_____	_____	_____	_____	_____	_____
_____	_____	_____	_____	_____	_____	_____	_____

* Record results as:

0 = no agglutination

w+ = fine agglutinates, most cells not agglutinated

1+ = numerous tiny clumps, cloudy background

2+ = several small to medium clumps, clear background

3+ = a few large clumps, clear background

4+ = two to three large clumps, clear background

Immunohematology: Rh Typing

LESSON OBJECTIVES

After studying this lesson, the student will:

- Explain the importance of the Rh blood group system.
- Discuss the antigens of the Rh system and explain how they are inherited.
- Name two ways in which immunization to the Rh D antigen may occur.
- Name two problems that can occur as a result of immunization to the D antigen.
- Explain why Rh D immune globulin (RhIG) is used.
- Perform Rh D slide typing.
- Interpret the results of Rh D typing.
- Explain the significance of the weak D antigen.
- Describe safety precautions that should be observed while performing Rh D typing.
- Discuss quality assessment policies and procedures that must be followed to ensure reliable typing results.
- Define the glossary terms.

GLOSSARY

antihuman globulin test / a sensitive test that uses a commercial antihuman globulin reagent to detect human globulin coated on red blood cells; antiglobulin test; Coombs' test

genotype / the allelic genes that are responsible for a trait

hemolytic disease of the newborn (HDN) / a condition in which maternal antibody targets fetal red blood cells for destruction

phenotype / in blood banking, the blood type as determined by blood typing tests

Rh D immune globulin (RhIG) / a concentrated, purified solution of human anti-D antibody used for injection; RhoGam

INTRODUCTION

The Rh blood group, discovered in the 1940s, is the second most important human blood group system. The system got its name from the rhesus monkeys being used in the experiments when the system was discovered.

Rh typing can be performed by slide, tube, or gel methods. Tube and gel methods are used in blood banks. Rh typing must be performed on all donor blood and on patient blood before a blood transfusion can be given. Rh typing is also a routine part of the prenatal workup.

THE Rh BLOOD GROUP SYSTEM

The Rh blood group system is composed of many antigens. The first antigen of the Rh system recognized was the D antigen. It remains the most important antigen in the system because it is the most antigenic and the only one for which blood is routinely tested. Like the antigens of the ABO system, Rh antigens are products of inherited genes and are present on the surface of red blood cells. Unlike the ABO system, other blood and tissue cells do not express the Rh antigens. Also unlike the ABO system, antibodies to Rh antigens do not occur naturally in serum.

Rh D Antigen

The major antigen in the Rh system is the D antigen. Red blood cells that possess the D antigen are called Rh D positive. Cells that lack the D antigen are called Rh D negative. It has become common to refer to the Rh D antigen simply as D antigen, and Rh D-positive blood as D-positive blood or Rh-positive blood.

The D antigen occurs in the majority of the population, but the incidence differs according to ethnic group (Table 4-14). Donor blood, in addition to being labeled with the ABO group, must be labeled as Rh positive or Rh negative (Figure 4-21), referring to presence or absence of the Rh D antigen.

Weak D Antigen

Some individuals have a form of the D antigen that reacts weakly in the typing procedure. Blood giving a weak reaction with anti-D is called weak D, or D^U, and is considered D positive.

Blood cells expressing the weak D antigen can also give a negative reaction in routine Rh D typing. In these cases, the *weak D test* must be performed before the Rh D type can be reported. Donor blood can only be labeled D negative after the weak D test confirms that no D antigen is detectable. Laboratories permit only specially qualified workers to perform the weak D test.

The test for detection of weak D uses the principles of the **antihuman globulin test**, a sensitive method of detecting antibody bound to red blood cells by using a commercial antihuman immunoglobulin G (IgG) reagent (AHG). Red blood cells incubated with commercial anti-D of the IgG class and initially showing no reaction are tested further by the weak D test. The red blood cells are washed several times to remove any unbound anti-D and are then incubated with antihuman IgG. This anti-IgG will react with any anti-D IgG that became bound to the red blood cells during the initial typing test. The cells are centrifuged and are observed for agglutination macroscopically. If no agglutination is seen, the cells are observed microscopically for agglutinates. Only blood that is negative macroscopically and microscopically in the weak D test is labeled D negative.

Rh Antigens Other than D

Over three dozen antigens have been identified in the Rh system. Many of these antigens are rare. However, four Rh antigens rank next in importance behind D. The most common name for these antigens are C (big C), c (little c), E (big E), and e (little e). In certain cases, blood is typed for these Rh antigens in addition to typing for D. Infrequently, an individual negative for one of these antigens (C, c, E, e), if exposed to blood containing the antigen, will produce antibodies against it. Three ways of naming Rh antigens are listed in Table 4-15 and explained in Current Topics (page 407).

TABLE 4-14. Frequency of Rh D-positive and D-negative blood in different populations		
ETHNIC GROUP	**D POSITIVE (%)**	**D NEGATIVE (%)**
Caucasian	84	16
African-American	93	7
African	99	1
Asian	99	1
Western European (Basque)	65	35
Native American Indian	99	1

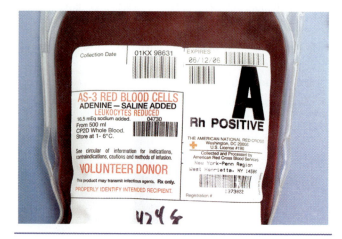

FIGURE 4-21 Donor bag containing A positive blood

TABLE 4-15. Comparison of Fisher-Race, Wiener, and Rosenfield methods of naming Rh antigens

FISHER-RACE METHOD	WIENER METHOD	ROSENFIELD (ET AL.) SYSTEM
D	Rh_o	Rh 1
C	rh'	Rh 2
E	rh"	Rh 3
d*	Hr_o	—
c	hr'	Rh 4
e	hr"	Rh 5

* no d antigen has been found. d denotes absence of D antigen

Rh Antibodies

Although antibodies to Rh antigens do not occur naturally in the blood, antibody to D antigen (anti-D) can be produced by a D-negative individual who becomes sensitized or immunized to the D antigen. This can occur during pregnancy (see information on hemolytic disease of the newborn) or following blood transfusion with D-positive blood. Anti-D, when produced, is of the immunoglobin G (IgG) class.

Importance of Rh Typing

It is important to test for the D antigen in all patients who are to receive transfusions so that the correct type of blood will be given. Rh D-negative patients should only be transfused with Rh D-negative blood. Testing for the D antigen is also used to identify females at risk of giving birth to an infant with hemolytic disease of the newborn (HDN), in family genetic studies, and in legal cases to establish parentage.

Rh TYPING PROCEDURES

The Rh D antigen is identified using agglutination techniques. Venous anticoagulated blood is the preferred specimen, but capillary blood can also be used.

Safety Precautions

 Standard Precautions must be followed when collecting blood specimens and when performing typing. Gloves and other appropriate personal protective equipment (PPE) must be worn when performing the procedures. Used slides or tubes must be discarded in a biohazard container for sharps. All reagents must be treated as if potentially infectious since many are derived from human blood. Centrifuge safety rules must be followed, including always balancing tubes in the rotor and allowing the centrifuge to come to a complete stop before opening the lid.

CURRENT TOPICS

NOMENCLATURE AND INHERITANCE OF THE Rh SYSTEM

Three nomenclatures (naming systems) have been suggested for the Rh system. These nomenclatures were suggested by different researchers to correlate the antigen names with the proposed method of inheritance. The three naming systems are those of Fisher and Race, Weiner, and Rosenfield et al. Manufacturers of blood bank reagents use one or more of these naming systems on their products (Table 4-15). The Fisher-Race nomenclature is used most frequently, because of its simplicity. However, the method of inheritance of Rh genes suggested by Fisher and Race has been shown to be incorrect.

Three sets of genes code for the Rh antigens, D, C, E, c, and e. The genes are positioned very close to each other on one chromosome, causing the three genes on each chromosome to be inherited as a group. The genes coding for C and c antigens are alleles of the same gene and are codominant.

This means that if a person inherited one allele for C and one allele for c, both antigens (Cc) would be expressed. The genes coding for E and e antigens are alleles of another gene, are also codominant, and are located near the C/c alleles. The alleles D and d are located at the third closely linked site. The D allele codes for the D antigen, but no antigen has been discovered to be expressed by the d allele. The D allele is said to be dominant over the d allele.

Each individual inherits three alleles from one parent and three from the other. For example, if an individual inherits CDe alleles from one parent and cDe from the other, the individual's **genotype** for these three genes would be CDe/cDe. Their red cell **phenotype**, the detectable expression of the inherited genes, would be C+, c+, D+, and e+. The most common allelic combination found in Rh D-negative individuals is cde/cde, meaning that the only Rh antigens detectable on their red cells would be c and e (a phenotype of c+, e+). A person of genotype CDe/cde would express C, D, and e antigens (remember there is no d antigen).

CURRENT TOPICS

HEMOLYTIC DISEASE OF THE NEWBORN DUE TO Rh

Hemolytic disease of the newborn (HDN) is a condition in which antibody from the mother enters the fetal circulation and destroys the fetal red blood cells. In the past, HDN was caused primarily by maternal anti-D reacting with D antigen on the fetal red cells. However, through prenatal testing and aggressive use of methods to prevent HDN caused by D antigen, non-D Rh antigens (such as C, c, E, or e) are now responsible for the largest proportion of HDN.

HDN can occur when a D-negative mother becomes pregnant with a D-positive fetus. During pregnancy or at birth, some of the fetus's D-positive blood cells can leak into the mother's circulatory system, stimulating her immune defenses to produce antibodies—essentially she becomes immunized to D cells. This antibody (anti-D) is of the IgG class, which can cross the placenta and enter fetal circulation. Bleeding of fetal blood into the mother is called *feto-maternal hemorrhage* (FMH). Situations that can cause the mother's exposure to fetal cells include:

- Amniocentesis or other invasive procedure
- Miscarriage or abortion
- Ectopic pregnancy
- Heavy bleeding during pregnancy
- The birth process

In most cases women are not exposed to fetal blood until the time of birth, which means that the first baby usually will not have HDN. However, large amounts of newborn blood often leak into the mother's circulation during delivery. If a D-negative woman is exposed to D-positive blood and produces anti-D antibodies, these can cross the placenta in subsequent pregnancies. If a subsequent fetus also has D-positive red cells, the anti-D will cause destruction of the fetus's red blood cells—thus the name *hemolytic* disease of the newborn.

Symptoms and Consequences of HDN

The mother of a fetus with HDN usually experiences no symptoms during pregnancy unless the HDN is very severe.

For this reason it is very important that at-risk expectant mothers have prenatal screenings in their first trimester to determine their Rh D type and to test for any anti-D antibodies that may already be present. These mothers will also usually have frequent fetal monitoring so that any signs of fetal stress will be detected early. The father can also be typed—there is no risk of Rh D HDN when both parents are D negative.

HDN can be mild to severe; the degree of severity is usually related to the mother's antibody level and the length of time during the pregnancy that she produced antibodies. In mild cases, signs of HDN may not be detected until birth and can include anemia, jaundice, or breathing problems. In very severe cases, heart failure or brain damage can occur or even stillbirth or miscarriage.

Prevention of Rh D HDN

Since 1968 it has been possible to prevent almost all cases of HDN due to the D antigen by administering injectable **Rh (D) immune globulin (RhIG)** to the D-negative mother. Development of this treatment was a significant breakthrough in obstetrics and is estimated to have saved the lives of approximately 10,000 babies each year. RhIG is a concentrated solution of anti-D purified from human plasma. When RhIG is administered at the appropriate time, it will prevent the mother from producing her own antibody to D cells. The injected anti-D will bind to any red blood cells from the fetus that have entered her blood, causing them to be eliminated from circulation, and preventing her immune system from being stimulated. Current treatment regimen is to give Rh-immune globulin at 28 weeks of pregnancy and within 72 hours after birth of a D-positive baby. RhIG is also given after events such as miscarriage, abortion, or amniocentesis. By receiving the injection at 28 weeks and after delivery, sensitization will be prevented and Rh D incompatibility should not be a problem during the next pregnancy. This treatment must be repeated with every pregnancy unless it is positively known that the fetus/baby is D negative. This treatment is only successful with D antigen incompatibilities.

Quality Assessment

Accuracy in Rh typing and reporting results is critical to a patient's well-being. To prevent errors, quality assessment policies must be followed. These will be outlined in the institution's standard operating procedure manual and will include practices such as:

- Identifying patient, patient specimen, reagents, and test vessels with accuracy
- Visually inspecting typing antisera for contamination
- Testing commercial cells and antisera at designated intervals with controls
- Using and storing reagents according to manufacturer's directions and observing expiration dates
- Observing strict timing limits for slide typing tests so that cell drying will not be mistaken for cell agglutination
- Carefully interpreting and recording results

Rh Slide Typing

To perform Rh D slide typing, a drop of commercial anti-D antiserum is added to a labeled microscope slide. A large drop of whole blood is added to the slide. The blood and antiserum are mixed with a stirrer and spread over at least one-half of the slide. The slide is placed on a heated, lighted viewbox to heat it to 37°C. The box is rocked back and forth for 2 minutes while the mixture is observed for agglutination (Figure 4-22). The presence or absence of agglutination is recorded.

Several types of commercial anti-D are available for Rh typing, including high protein anti-D, chemically modified anti-D, monoclonal anti-D, and saline anti-D. Quality control procedures and instructions for use can differ for each type of antiserum. Recommendations in package insert(s) for the reagents being used must be followed.

A negative control is usually prepared and tested along with the patient sample when using high protein anti-D. This is prepared by mixing a nonantibody protein control solution with patient blood.

Rh Tube Typing

Rh tube typing is more sensitive than slide typing. Rh D tube typing is performed as for ABO grouping. A 2% to 5% suspension is made from the patient's cells. One drop of this suspension is mixed with one drop of anti-D and the tube is centrifuged. The cell pellet is gently dislodged and observed for agglutination, and the reaction is graded. Since the patient serum contains no natural anti-D antibody, reverse or confirmatory typing is not performed.

Commercial anti-D is available as monoclonal antisera, polyclonal antisera, purified IgG antisera, purified IgM antisera, combinations of IgG and IgM, and chemically modified antisera. Many laboratories routinely type each specimen with two different types of anti-D to increase the chances of detecting weak D antigen. It is important to carefully follow the manufacturer's directions for each type of antisera.

Laboratories must have a clear written procedure regarding D typing and interpretation. It is particularly vital that weak D-positive donor blood not be misidentified as D-negative blood. If that were to happen, a D-negative person could be given blood containing D antigen. Some laboratories have a policy of transfusing a weak D patient with D-negative blood. However, blood from weak D donors is labeled D positive and is only transfused into D-positive patients.

Interpreting Results of Rh Typing

If a patient is Rh D positive, the patient's cells will agglutinate when reacted with anti-D. If the patient is Rh D negative, no agglutination will be present (Table 4-16). Depending on laboratory policy, negative Rh D typing results must be confirmed with a weak D (D^U) test before being reported.

The control slide or tube should always be negative for agglutination. If the control is positive, the test is invalid and must be repeated using a different method or different reagents. Positive control results can be due to contaminated control serum or abnormalities in the patient blood sample.

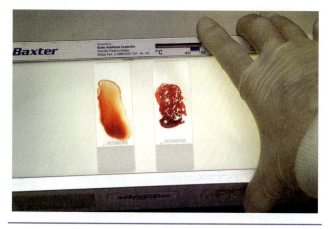

FIGURE 4-22 A heated, lighted viewbox is used for Rh slide typing. Specimen on right is D positive

TABLE 4-16. Interpretation of results of Rh D typing

REACTIONS OF CELLS WITH:

Anti-D	Control Serum	Interpretation
+	0	Rh (D) positive
0	0	Presumptive Rh D negative; confirm with weak D (D^U) test before reporting
+	+	Unable to interpret; repeat test using another method

+ = agglutination
0 = no agglutination

Gel Typing for Rh D

Gel cards used for ABO typing also contain columns for D typing (see Lesson 4-3). The tests are performed and interpreted as for the ABO forward and reverse grouping. Dilute red cell suspensions are added to the columns that contain a gel matrix and antiserum or control reagent. Under controlled centrifugation, the cells are forced into the gel matrix, where they contact anti-D or control reagent. If D antigen is not present on the red cells, the cells will fall to the bottom of the column without reacting with the antisera. Anti-D in the gel will bind to D-positive cells, causing agglutination and preventing the cells from traveling through the gel. A cell layer remaining at the top of the column is a positive result.

PROCEDURAL Reminders

- Review quality assessment section before performing procedure.
- Always follow manufacturers' instructions for the use of reagents.
- Identify patient and patient specimens correctly.
- Label slides and tubes accurately.
- Perform Rh D slide typing at 37°C, using a lighted, heated viewbox.
- Observe Rh slide typing reactions within 2 minutes
- Confirm negative Rh D slide typing with a tube test or a test for weak D (D^U).

SAFETY Reminders

- Review Safety Precautions section before beginning procedure.
- Observe Standard Precautions when performing typing tests.
- Wear fluid-resistant, buttoned laboratory coat and other appropriate PPE.
- Discard all used supplies appropriately.
- Wipe work area with surface disinfectant frequently.

SUMMARY

The Rh blood group system is composed of red blood cell antigens that are products of inherited genes. The D antigen is the major antigen in the system, but other lesser antigens, including C, c, E, and e, are also important in blood banking. Donor blood units and potential transfusion recipients are routinely typed for D antigen. Rh typing can be performed by slide, tube, or gel methods. D-negative typing results must be confirmed by a test for weak D.

CASE STUDY 1

Mr. Morris came into the blood donation center to donate blood. When the processing center performed initial ABO and Rh D typing of his blood, the results indicated that Mr. Morris was A negative. The ABO grouping was done by tube typing, and the Rh D typing was done by the slide method.

The next step for the processing center should be:
a. Label the blood A negative
b. Repeat the ABO grouping by the slide test that is more reliable
c. Perform further typing to test for weak D before labeling unit

CASE STUDY 2

Mrs. Rodriguez, who had been typed as B negative, needed a transfusion. The only blood available was B positive and O negative. Which should she receive? Explain your answer.

CASE STUDY 3

Mr. Gupta, whose genotype was *CDe/CDe*, was transfused with D-negative blood.

Which of the following could occur?
a. He could produce anti-d
b. He could produce anti-c
c. He could produce anti-E
d. He could produce anti-e

Determining the Rh D type is especially important in transfusion medicine and in obstetrics. Persons who are typed as D negative should only be transfused with blood that is also D negative. Rh D-negative expectant mothers must be monitored and treated with Rh immune globulin to prevent the possibility of the fetus developing HDN. Testing for the Rh D antigen must be performed, interpreted, and reported only by qualified personnel.

REVIEW QUESTIONS

1. What is the major antigen in the Rh system?
2. What circumstances must exist before anti-D antibody is produced by an individual?
3. What is the weak D antigen?
4. Explain how HDN occurs.
5. Why is Rh D typing performed?

6. Why must D-positive blood not be transfused into a D-negative patient?
7. Which is more sensitive, slide or tube typing?
8. Why is reverse typing not done for the Rh system?
9. Explain how the major Rh antigens are inherited.
10. Define antihuman globulin test, genotype, hemolytic disease of the newborn, phenotype, and Rh D immune globulin.

STUDENT ACTIVITIES

1. Complete the written examination for this lesson.
2. Practice performing Rh D typing on several blood samples as outlined in the Student Performance Guide, using the worksheet.
3. Survey the Rh D types in your class. Compare your findings with the distribution of D antigen in the United States.

WEB 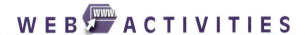 ACTIVITIES

1. Use the Internet to find information about transfusion reactions.
2. Use the Internet to find information about different types of Rh typing sera.

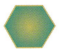

Student Performance Guide

LESSON 4-4 Immunohematology: Rh Typing

Name _____ Date _____

INSTRUCTIONS

1. Practice performing Rh D typing following the step-by-step procedure.

2. Demonstrate Rh D typing satisfactorily for the instructor, using the Student Performance Guide. Your instructor will determine the level of competency you must achieve to obtain a satisfactory (S) grade.

NOTE: Package inserts should be consulted for specific instructions before test is performed.

MATERIALS AND EQUIPMENT

- gloves
- antiseptic
- face protection and/or acrylic safety shield
- serological centrifuge
- test tube rack
- serological tubes, 13 × 75 mm
- blood bank saline (physiological saline)
- disposable transfer pipets
- microscope slides
- applicator sticks or stirrers
- anti-D serum (anti-Rh$_o$)
- Rh protein control
- EDTA blood specimens
- lighted viewbox
- Rh typing worksheet
- wax pencil or sharpie
- timer
- surface disinfectant
- biohazard container
- sharps container

PROCEDURE

Record in the comment section any problems encountered while practicing the procedure (or have a fellow student or the instructor evaluate your performance).

S = Satisfactory
U = Unsatisfactory

You must:	S	U	Comments
1. Assemble equipment and materials. Put on face protection or position acrylic safety shield in work area			
2. Wash hands and put on gloves			
3. Perform Rh D slide typing following steps 4 through 14			
4. Turn on viewbox. Label two microscope slides *D* and *C* (control)			
5. Place one drop of anti-D serum on the *D* slide			
6. Place one drop of Rh protein control on the *C* slide			
7. Place one large drop of patient's well-mixed whole blood on each slide			

You must:	S	U	Comments
8. Mix blood and anti-D with an applicator stick, spreading the mixture over at least one-half of the slide			
9. Repeat procedure for the control slide using a clean applicator stick			
10. Place slides on the lighted viewbox and start timer			
11. Tilt the viewbox slowly back and forth for 2 minutes			
12. Observe the slides for agglutination at the end of 2 minutes			
13. Record results on worksheet: agglutination = +; no agglutination = 0			
14. Determine the Rh type and record on worksheet			
15. Repeat steps 4 through 14 on other blood samples, as directed by instructor			
16. Perform tube typing on a specimen (or go to step 24)			
17. Prepare a 2% to 5% suspension of the blood specimen by adding 18-19 drops of saline to 1 drop of well-mixed blood			
18. Label one tube *patient* and one tube *control*			
19. Add 1 drop of patient cell suspension to each labeled tube			
20. Add 1 drop of anti-D to *patient* tube and 1 drop of Rh protein control to *control* tube			
21. Mix contents of tubes and centrifuge for 30 seconds			
22. Gently tap tubes to loosen cell pellets and observe for agglutination			
23. Grade reactions and record results on worksheet. NOTE: Absence of agglutination in patient tube requires a test for weak D before the patient can be definitively typed as D negative			
24. Discard specimens, tubes, and slides in appropriate biohazard or sharps container			
25. Clean equipment and return to proper storage			
26. Clean work area with surface disinfectant			
27. Remove gloves and discard in biohazard container			
28. Wash hands with antiseptic			

Evaluator Comments:

Evaluator _____ Date _____

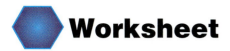

Worksheet

LESSON 4-4 Immunohematology: Rh Typing

Name _____ Date _____

| | AGGLUTINATION RESULTS* | | INTERPRETATION** |
Specimen I.D.	Anti-D	Protein Control	Rh Type
_____	_____	_____	_____
_____	_____	_____	_____
_____	_____	_____	_____
_____	_____	_____	_____
_____	_____	_____	_____

*Record tube typing results as:

0 = no agglutination

w+ = fine agglutinates, most cells not agglutinated

1+ = numerous tiny clumps, cloudy background

2+ = several small to medium clumps, clear background

3+ = few large clumps, clear background

4+ = two to three large clumps, clear background

**Record interpretation as:

Rh D positive or

presumptive Rh D negative

4-5

Immunology: Rapid Test for Infectious Mononucleosis

LESSON OBJECTIVES

After studying this lesson, the student will:

- Explain the cause of infectious mononucleosis (IM).
- List five clinical symptoms of IM.
- Explain how hematological and immunological findings are used in diagnosing IM.
- Name two types of tests used to diagnose IM.
- Perform a rapid test for IM and interpret the results.
- Explain the safety precautions that must be observed when performing the test for IM.
- Discuss procedures that must be followed to ensure the quality of results for the IM test.
- Define the glossary terms.

GLOSSARY

chronic fatigue syndrome (CFS) / a syndrome characterized by prolonged fatigue and other nonspecific symptoms, and for which the cause remains unknown

Epstein-Barr virus (EBV) / a virus that infects lymphocytes and is the cause of IM

hepatosplenomegaly / enlargement of the liver and spleen

heterophile antibodies/ antibodies that are increased in IM

incubation period / the time elapsed between exposure to an infectious agent and the appearance of symptoms

infectious mononucleosis / a contagious viral disease caused by Epstein-Barr virus

latent / dormant; in an inactive or hidden phase

lymphadenopathy / a condition in which the lymph glands are enlarged or swollen

lymphocytosis / an increase above the normal number of lymphocytes in the blood

INTRODUCTION

Infectious mononucleosis (IM), commonly called *mono* or *kissing disease,* is a contagious viral disease that affects mostly the 15- to 25-year-old age group. The disease is caused by infection of B lymphocytes with the **Epstein-Barr virus (EBV)**, a member of the herpes group of viruses and one of the most common human viruses.

Infectious mononucleosis (IM) is accompanied by a variety of nonspecific symptoms that are also present in other diseases. Early diagnosis of IM is usually based on laboratory test results combined with clinical symptoms.

The most common immunologic test for IM is a rapid test that gives reliable results and is simple to perform. Some test kits for IM are included in the list of CLIA-waived tests.

DIAGNOSIS OF INFECTIOUS MONONUCLEOSIS

Diagnosis of infectious mononucleosis is based on clinical symptoms, hematological findings, and immunological test results.

Clinical Symptoms

Clinical symptoms of IM are nonspecific and include fatigue, fever, sore throat, weakness, headache, and **lymphadenopathy**, or swollen lymph nodes. Patients can have some or all of these symptoms. During the acute phase, patients can also have **hepatosplenomegaly**, enlargement of the liver and spleen.

The **incubation period**, or the time between exposure to the virus and the appearance of symptoms, ranges from 4 to 6 weeks. Symptoms generally last for 1 to 4 weeks and seldom last for more than 4 months. When the illness lasts more than 6 months, it is frequently called chronic EBV infection and should be investigated further to determine if it meets the criteria for **chronic fatigue syndrome (CFS)**.

Hematological Findings

Infectious Mononucleosis causes changes in the circulating lymphocytes that can be detected by a white blood cell differential count and evaluation of white blood cell morphology from a stained blood smear. Usually **lymphocytosis**, an increase in lymphocytes, occurs and large numbers (from 10% to >20%) of the lymphocytes are *atypical* or *reactive* (Figure 2-61, Lesson 2-9).

Immunological Findings

Immunological tests for infectious mononucleosis are based on the detection of **heterophile antibodies** in the patient's serum or blood. Heterophile antibodies react with similar antigens in more than one species and are usually of the IgM class. Individuals with infectious mononucleosis begin producing heterophile antibodies early in the infection.

Detection of heterophile antibodies combined with hematological and clinical findings provide the basis for diagnosing IM. The immunological test for IM is usually positive after the first week of illness. The level of heterophile antibodies peaks at 2 to 4 weeks after onset of symptoms and declines to low levels by 12 weeks. The reason these antibodies are produced is unclear, but the antibodies are associated specifically with IM. If the first immunological test is negative and clinical symptoms remain after a week, the patient should be retested.

IMMUNOLOGICAL TESTS FOR INFECTIOUS MONONUCLEOSIS

Several commercial kits are available to test for IM. The specimen used can be plasma, serum, or whole blood. Many of the kits are CLIA-waived when used with whole blood. If either serum or plasma is used, the tests are usually categorized as moderately complex. Test kits provide all the necessary reagents, materials, and controls needed to perform the test.

Two Types of Rapid Tests

Rapid tests for IM detect heterophile antibodies present in the blood of IM patients. Some kits are based on agglutination principles, with the end reaction being the presence or absence of agglutination. Other kits are immunochromatographic assays, which produce a color reaction. Both types are adaptations of the Davidsohn differential test for heterophile antibodies, a time-consuming, cumbersome test that was developed in the mid 1900s. Some rapid tests treat the patient sample to remove non-heterophile antibodies and then react it with an antigen that binds only to heterophile antibodies. Because heterophile antibodies react with antigens found in several species, including bovine, sheep, and horse red blood cells, one or more of these are used as a source antigen in test kits.

Immunochromatographic Assays

In the past, many laboratory tests were lengthy procedures, requiring special equipment and glassware, preparation and pipetting of several reagents, large sample volumes, and several complicated steps and incubations. Today, however, through the use of analyte-specific antibodies, complex test procedures have been miniaturized and simplified. Solid-phase immunochromatographic assays are now available for a multitude of analytes. In these assays, reagents and reactants are immobilized on membranes that are enclosed in individual test units. In most cases, these assays require only that the technician add a few drops of patient sample and perhaps one or two more reagents to a test cartridge. The test results are usually available in minutes.

By substituting the appropriate analyte-specific antibody into the test unit during manufacture, the same solid-phase technology can be used to detect several analytes. For this reason, many test cartridges made by a single company appear identical except for the label indicating which analyte can be detected using the test unit.

Principle of Immunochromatographic Assay for Infectious Mononucleosis

The procedure for detecting the heterophile antibodies of IM described in this lesson is the QuickVue+ Infectious Mononucleosis test (Quidel Corp.), an immunochromatographic assay (Figures 4-23 and 4-24). The technology of this test is described in detail as an example of the basis of design of many such assays.

In the QuickVue+ Infectious Mononucleosis test, a membrane strip that provides solid support for the assay is housed in a plastic unit. One end of the membrane lies under the sample well, which contains an absorbent pad that promotes an even flow of sample through the membrane (Figure 4-23). Adjacent to the sample area, the membrane is coated with blue latex beads conjugated to goat antihuman IgM antibodies.

In the next membrane zone, which is exposed in the *read result* window, two reagents are immobilized (bound to the membrane). The first is blue latex beads immobilized in a pattern to provide a preprinted horizontal line. This line is visible when the test unit package is opened. The second reagent in this area is a bovine erythrocyte extract, which is immobilized in a vertical configuration (but not visible). The third zone of the membrane is exposed in the *test complete* window and contains an immobilized reagent in a vertical configuration. This reagent is capable of binding the antibody-blue latex conjugate to produce a visible vertical blue line. An absorbent pad is situated at the opposite end of the membrane from the sample end to retain fluid after the reaction is completed. A drying agent in the membrane keeps the reactive agents stabilized until the test is used.

Patient sample is added to the sample well followed by developer, which is simply an inert solution that provides enough volume to promote capillary movement of the sample through the membrane. As the sample moves through the membrane, it mobilizes the first anti-IgM-blue latex conjugate, which binds to IgM antibodies in the sample. This mixture is carried (with the sample) across the membrane to the bovine erythrocyte zone.

If heterophile antibodies of IM are in the sample, they will bind to the immobilized bovine erythrocyte extract and be held in place. Because these IgM antibodies also have the goat-anti-IgM-blue latex bound to them, a visible blue vertical line forming a + sign will appear in the *read result* window (Figure 4-24). If no heterophile antibody is present in the sample, this line will not form, leaving only the preprinted horizontal (−) blue line visible. The fluid sample will continue to move across the membrane carrying the antibody-blue latex conjugate until it contacts the binding agent in the *test complete* window. As the antibody-latex conjugate is bound, a blue line will appear, indicating the test is complete.

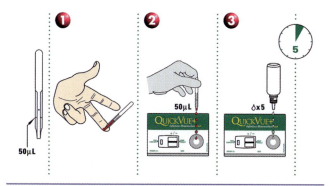

FIGURE 4-23 QuickVue+ Infectious Mononucleosis test. (1) collect blood sample, (2) add sample to well, (3) add reagent, and observe result after 5 minutes (*Courtesy of Quidel Inc., San Diego, CA*)

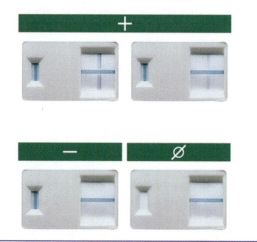

FIGURE 4-24 Reaction windows showing positive (top), negative (bottom left), and invalid (Ø, bottom right) results with QuickVue+ IM test (*Courtesy of Quidel Inc., San Diego, CA*)

PERFORMING THE RAPID TEST FOR INFECTIOUS MONONUCLEOSIS

The manufacturer's instructions and the package insert provided with each kit must be strictly followed when performing and interpreting the test.

Safety Precautions

Standard Precautions must be observed when performing immunological tests. Gloves and other appropriate personal protective equipment (PPE) must be worn. Patient samples and control sera made from human blood products must be treated as if potentially infectious. Used test components must be discarded into appropriate biohazard containers.

Quality Assessment

Manufacturer's instructions and package insert for the kit being used must be followed. Reagents must be stored and used according to package inserts and should not be used beyond the expiration dates. Positive and negative serum controls provided with kits should be tested along with the patient sample to ensure that all reagents or kits are reacting correctly. Reagents from different kit manufacturers must not be interchanged. Reactions must be recorded and interpreted carefully, following the instructions in the package insert and the laboratory's procedure manual.

Specimen Collection

The test can be performed using whole blood from capillary puncture or venous whole blood that is either heparinized or has had ethylenediaminetetraacetic acid (EDTA) anticoagulant added. The test can also be performed using serum, heparinized plasma, or EDTA-anticoagulated plasma.

Test Procedure

The reaction unit should be removed from its sealed pouch just before the test is to be run. A separate reaction unit is used for each patient sample and each control. A positive control and a negative control provided with the kit should be run as outlined in the laboratory's standard operating procedure (SOP) manual. The reaction unit contains three areas: *add* well, to which reagents and specimen are added; *read result* window for reading and interpreting reaction; and *test complete* window, which indicates if the test is working properly (Figure 4-24). The *read result* window should be observed before the unit is used to be sure a blue horizontal line is visible.

One drop (50 μL) of whole blood, serum, or plasma is introduced into the *add* well, using the pipette provided in the kit. If capillary blood is used, it should be drawn up to the line of the capillary tube included in the kit and the entire contents of the tube dispensed into the *add* well. Five drops of developer are dispensed into the *add* well while the dropper bottle is held vertically. The unit is allowed to remain undisturbed for 5 minutes and the reaction is read.

CURRENT TOPICS

CLINICAL SIGNIFICANCE OF EPSTEIN-BARR VIRUS INFECTION

Occurrence—The Epstein Barr Virus (EBV) occurs worldwide, and most people become infected with EBV sometime during their lives. In the United States, an estimated 95% of the population has been infected by the time they reach age 40. There are no known associations between active EBV infection and problems during pregnancy, such as miscarriages or birth defects. Infants become susceptible to infection with EBV as soon as maternal antibody protection (present at birth) disappears. Many become infected with EBV during childhood, but these infections usually either cause no symptoms or are indistinguishable from the other mild, brief illnesses of childhood. When infection with EBV occurs during adolescence or young adulthood, it causes infectious mononucleosis up to 50% of the time.

Virus Persistence—Although the symptoms of infectious mononucleosis usually resolve in 1 or 2 months, the virus remains latent, or dormant, in a few cells in the throat and blood for the rest of the person's life. Periodically, the virus can reactivate and be found in the saliva of infected persons even in the absence of symptoms. EBV also establishes a lifelong latent infection in some cells of the body's immune system.

Transmission—Most people who are exposed to an individual with infectious mononucleosis have already been infected with EBV and so are not at risk for developing infection. Transmission of this virus does not normally occur through the air or blood but requires intimate contact with the saliva of an infected person. In fact, healthy individuals can carry and spread the virus intermittently their whole life. These people are usually the primary source for person-to-person transmission. For this reason, transmission of EBV is almost impossible to prevent.

Protective measures—Persons with active infectious mononucleosis can spread the infection to others for a period of weeks. However, no special precautions or isolation procedures are recommended, since the virus is also found frequently in the saliva of healthy people. There is no specific treatment for infectious mononucleosis, other than treating the symptoms. No antiviral drugs or vaccines are available. Some physicians prescribe a short course of steroids to control the swelling of the throat and tonsils; steroids are also believed by some to decrease the overall length and severity of illness.

Rapid Immunological Test for IM—Routine testing for the heterophile antibody, the basis of the rapid tests for IM, is the method of choice for diagnosing infectious mononucleosis. In patients with symptoms compatible with infectious mononucleosis, a positive rapid test for heterophile antibodies is diagnostic, and no further testing is necessary.

False-positive results can occur in a small number of patients, and false-negative results can occur in as many as 10% to 15% of patients, primarily in children younger than 10 years of age. When rapid IM tests or heterophile test results are negative, additional laboratory testing may be needed to differentiate EBV infections from a mononucleosis-like illness induced by agents such as cytomegalovirus (CMV), adenovirus, or the parasite *Toxoplasma gondii*. This can be done by testing a patient's serum for antibodies to various EBV-associated antigens, tests that are expensive and more difficult and time-consuming than are the rapid slide tests. Direct detection of EBV in blood or lymphoid tissues is a research tool and is not available for routine diagnosis.

TABLE 4-17. Interpretation of results with QuickVue+ Infectious Mononucleosis test

Positive test	Any shade of blue vertical line forming a plus (+) sign in the *read result* window along with a blue line in the *test complete* window
Negative test	No blue vertical line in *read result* window along with a blue line in the *test complete* window
Invalid test	1. No line in *test complete* window after 10 minutes, or 2. Blue color fills *read result* window after 10 minutes

Reading and Interpreting Results

Reactions that must be interpreted include the internal controls and patient results, as well as the reactions obtained with the positive and negative serum controls (external controls).

Internal Controls

Internal procedural controls are incorporated into immunochromatographic assays as one way of ensuring that the tests are set up correctly and the test unit is working properly. The Quidel IM test includes both negative and positive internal controls. Failure of an internal control indicates either that the test was not performed properly or the reagents were not working properly. The internal controls should be read and interpreted before reading patient results (Table 4-17 and Figure 4-24).

A clear *background* (other than the blue reaction lines) in the *read result* window at the end of the timed test is an internal negative control. If a blue color fills the *read result* window, the results are invalid.

A blue line appearing in the *test complete* area is an internal positive control, indicating that the unit is performing correctly. If no blue line forms in the *test complete* window after 10 minutes, the results are invalid and patient results from the test cannot be reported.

External Controls

Positive and negative controls included with the test kit should be tested in the same manner as patient samples, using a separate test unit for each control. A vertical line forming a (+) should appear in the *read result* window with the positive control serum. No vertical line should form when the negative control is used in the test. A blue line must form in the *test complete* window for the external control tests to be valid.

Patient Results

The *read result* window is observed for the test reaction. The presence of heterophile antibodies of IM (a positive result) is indicated by the formation of any shade of a blue vertical line forming a (+) in the *read result* window. The test is interpreted as negative if no vertical blue line appears in the *read result* window (Table 4-17 and Figure 4-24).

SAFETY Reminders

- Review safety precautions before performing procedure.
- Follow Standard Precautions when performing immunological tests.
- Discard all contaminated items in appropriate biohazard containers.

CASE STUDY

Michaela, a college student, developed fever and sore throat a few days before spring break. She went to her university's health center, where the staff physician ordered a rapid immunological test for IM, but the results were negative. Michaela went home for spring break, and her symptoms continued. After staying in bed for about a week, she went to see her hometown physician, who ordered another rapid immunological test for IM. The results were positive. However, Michaela began to improve within a few days.

Michaela's mother called the university health center and complained that its testing was not reliable and she was unhappy with the level of health care her daughter was receiving.

Was her complaint valid?
Give your explanation for this scenario.

PROCEDURAL Reminders

- Review quality assessment section before beginning procedure.
- Follow manufacturer's directions for the kit being used.
- Use positive and negative controls along with patient samples.
- Observe and interpret results carefully.

SUMMARY

Infectious mononucleosis is a contagious viral disease occurring primarily in teens and young adults. It is caused by infection with EBV, which is common worldwide. By the age of 40, most individuals have had an EBV infection, often subclinical (without noticeable symptoms). Although there is no specific treatment for IM, in most cases the disease runs its course without complications.

Diagnosis of IM is made based on a combination of clinical symptoms, hematological findings, and immunological tests. Typical symptoms of IM include fever, sore throat, and lymphadenopathy. Atypical lymphocytes are usually present in peripheral blood. Immunological tests for infectious mononucleosis detect the presence of heterophile antibodies in the patient's blood or serum, a characteristic finding in IM. Simple, rapid tests for IM can be performed at point of care. Some of these rapid IM tests are CLIA-waived.

REVIEW QUESTIONS

1. What is the cause of IM?
2. What are the clinical symptoms of IM?
3. What information can be gained from the hematological test?
4. What is detected in the immunological test for IM?
5. What safety precautions should be followed in performing a rapid test for IM?
6. How soon after IM begins will the immunological test usually be positive?
7. Describe the general principle of a rapid immunologic test for IM.
8. Explain how internal and external controls are used with rapid tests for IM.
9. Define chronic fatigue syndrome, Epstein-Barr virus, hepatosplenomegaly, heterophile antibodies, incubation period, infectious mononucleosis, latent, lymphadenopathy, and lymphocytosis.

STUDENT ACTIVITIES

1. Complete the written examination for this lesson.
2. Practice performing the rapid test for IM as outlined in the Student Performance Guide.

W E B A C T I V I T I E S

1. Using the Internet, find information about a test kit for infectious mononucleosis. Obtain the package insert or manufacturer's information and explain the test design.
2. Using the Internet, look for information about chronic fatigue syndrome. Find out how it can be distinguished from infectious mononucleosis.
3. Use the Internet to find information about the Epstein-Barr virus. Write a one-page report on the virus, including the family of viruses it belongs to and the types of infections it causes.

Student Performance Guide

LESSON 4-5 Immunology: Rapid Test for Infectious Mononucleosis

Name _____ Date _____

INSTRUCTIONS

1. Practice performing the rapid test for IM following the step-by-step procedure.
2. Demonstrate the rapid test for IM satisfactorily for the instructor, using the Student Performance Guide. Your instructor will determine the level of competency you must achieve to obtain a satisfactory (S) grade.

NOTE: Procedure given is for QuickVue+ Infectious Mononucleosis test by Quidel Corp. Package insert for the kit should be followed. If another kit is used, the manufacturer's instructions for that kit must be followed.

MATERIALS AND EQUIPMENT

- capillary puncture supplies
- gloves
- face shield or acrylic safety shield
- antiseptic
- test serum, plasma, or whole blood
- timer
- surface disinfectant
- test kit for IM including instructions, test units, dispensers, reagents, and controls
- biohazard container
- sharps container

PROCEDURE

Record in the comment section any problems encountered while practicing the procedure (or have a fellow student or the instructor evaluate your performance).

S = Satisfactory
U = Unsatisfactory

You must:	S	U	Comments
1. Assemble equipment and materials. Put on face protection or set up acrylic safety shield			
2. Wash hands and put on gloves			
3. Remove test cartridge from its sealed pouch and place it on a level well-lit surface. Check to see that *read result* window has a blue horizontal line showing			

4. Dispense patient sample into the cartridge using method a, b, or c below:
a. For venous whole blood samples:
  1) Mix tube of blood well by inverting several times
  2) Draw blood into the sample pipet provided with the kit and dispense one drop into the *add* well			

You must:	S	U	Comments
b. For plasma or serum samples: 1) Draw plasma or serum into the sample pipet provided with the kit 2) Dispense one drop into the *add* well c. For capillary blood: 1) Perform a capillary puncture using the routine procedure 2) Fill the capillary tube provided with the kit to the line (50 µL) 3) Dispense entire contents of tube into *add* well			
5. Immediately add 5 drops of developer to the *add* well while holding the bottle vertically			
6. Start timer. Do not pick up or move test cartridge			
7. Read results at 5 minutes. The *test complete* line must be visible by 10 minutes			
8. Interpret the results (see guide in Table 4-17 and Figure 4-24): a. Positive result—formation of a blue vertical line forming a (+) sign in the *read result* window along with a blue line in the *test complete* window b. Negative result—A blue line in the *test complete* window but no blue vertical line in the *read result* window c. Invalid result—one or more of the following reactions: 1) No line in the test complete window after 10 minutes 2) A blue color filling the *read result* window after 10 minutes			
9. Record results as positive or negative			
10. Repeat test procedure (steps 3 through 9) using positive and negative controls			
11. Discard used materials in appropriate biohazard or sharps container			
12. Store or dispose of specimen appropriately			
13. Clean work area with surface disinfectant			
14. Remove gloves and discard in biohazard container			
15. Wash hands with antiseptic			

Evaluator Comments:

Evaluator _____ Date _____

4-6

Immunology: Slide Test for Rheumatoid Factors

LESSON OBJECTIVES

After studying this lesson, the student will:

- Explain the significance of rheumatoid factors.
- Explain the reasons for performing the test for rheumatoid factors.
- Explain the principle of latex agglutination tests.
- Perform a qualitative latex agglutination test for rheumatoid factors and interpret the results.
- Perform a semi-quantitative latex agglutination test for rheumatoid factors and interpret the results.
- Discuss safety precautions that must be followed when performing the test for rheumatoid factors.
- Discuss quality assessment practices used in performing the test for rheumatoid factors.
- Define the glossary terms

GLOSSARY

arthritis / inflammation of the joints

autoantibody / an antibody directed against the self (one's own tissues)

reciprocal / inverse; one of a pair of numbers (as 2/3 and 3/2) that has a product of one

rheumatoid arthritis (RA) / an autoimmune disease characterized by pain, inflammation, and deformity of the joints

rheumatoid factors (RF) / autoantibodies that are directed against human immunoglobin G (IgG) and are often present in the serum of rheumatoid arthritis patients

synovial / of, or relating to, the lubricating fluid of the joints

INTRODUCTION

Arthritis, an inflammation of the joints, can occur in several diseases. Among these are gout, rheumatic fever, lupus, osteoarthritis, and **rheumatoid arthritis (RA)**. Between 75% and 85% of people with rheumatoid arthritis have elevated levels of **rheumatoid factors (RFs)** in their serum. Rheumatoid factors are **autoantibodies**, usually of the immunoglobin (Ig) M class, directed against human IgG. Rheumatoid factors are not usually elevated in other forms of arthritis. Because of this, the RF test is useful in diagnosing rheumatoid arthritis.

Immunological tests can be used to aid in distinguishing rheumatoid arthritis from arthritis of other causes. Several of these tests are based on the detection of rheumatoid factors in the patient's serum using a latex agglutination method. This lesson describes a rapid slide test for the detection of rheumatoid factors.

PRINCIPLE OF SLIDE AGGLUTINATION TESTS FOR RHEUMATOID FACTORS

Several types of test kits are available for rheumatoid factors. Kits are designed using principles of enzyme immunoassay (EIA), nephelometry, or agglutination. Kits are also available for use with automated immunology instruments.

Most RF slide tests are modifications of a latex agglutination test developed by Singer and Plotz in 1956. In the RF test, small latex particles are coated with specially treated human immunoglobulin (IgG). When serum containing RF is mixed with the IgG-coated latex particles, the rheumatoid factors (which are autoantibodies) bind to the IgG and cause agglutination of the particles (Figure 4-25).

Commercial latex RF kits include the coated latex particles, positive and negative control sera, buffer, and other materials necessary to perform the tests (Figure 4-26). Another type of slide agglutination test is a hemagglutination test that uses specially treated red blood cells to detect RF.

PERFORMING A QUALITATIVE TEST FOR RHEUMATOID FACTORS

The procedure described in this lesson provides general directions for performing a slide latex agglutination test to detect RF.

When performing the test, the instructions in the current package insert for the particular brand of kit in use must be followed.

Safety Precautions

Standard Precautions must be followed and appropriate personal protective equipment (PPE) worn when performing all immunological tests. Control sera produced from human blood must be treated as if potentially infectious. All used materials must be discarded into appropriate biohazard containers.

Quality Assessment

The manufacturer's instructions for the particular kit being used must be followed. Reagents from different manufacturers must not be interchanged. Storage recommendations must be followed, and reagents should not be used beyond the expiration dates.

Positive and negative control sera provided with the kits must be run at the specified intervals and the results recorded. If controls do not give the expected reactions, patient specimens must not be tested until the problem has been identified and corrected.

Specimen Collection and Preparation

Serum is the usual specimen for latex agglutination tests. This is obtained by collecting a red top tube by venipuncture, and separating the serum from the cells by centrifugation. Most RF tests require that, before testing, the serum be diluted 1:20 with a buffer included in the kit. This dilution is necessary because the sera of normal individuals can have low levels of RF. Testing diluted serum assures that only significant levels of RF will be detected in the test.

Test Procedure

To perform the test, one drop of positive control serum, negative control serum, and diluted patient serum are each placed in a separate test area on a slide included in the test kit. One drop of well-mixed latex reagent is dispensed into each test area. Latex reagent is then mixed with each serum using a clean stirrer or

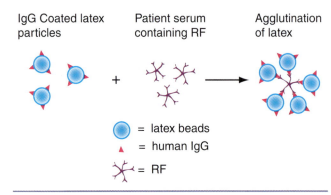

FIGURE 4-25 Principle of latex agglutination test for rheumatoid factors. Rheumatoid factors in serum react with IgG-coated particles to cause agglutination

IgG Coated latex particles   Patient serum containing RF   Agglutination of latex

= latex beads
= human IgG
= RF

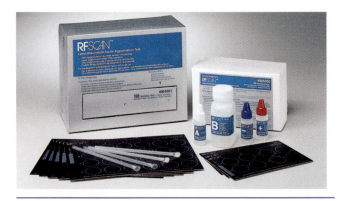

FIGURE 4-26 Rheumatoid factor latex agglutination kit (*Courtesy of Becton Dickinson and Co., Franklin Lakes, NJ*)

CURRENT TOPICS

ARTHRITIS

Arthritis is a general term that means inflammation of the joints. Arthritis is usually a chronic condition involving pain, redness, and swelling of the joints. Arthritis has many causes and can affect any joint in the body. The three most common types of arthritis in older adults are osteoarthritis, gout, and RA.

Osteoarthritis is the type of arthritis commonly seen as people age. It is sometimes called *wear and tear* arthritis. It usually affects joints of the hands, back, neck, hip, knee, or ankle. Cartilage, which cushions the ends of the bones in the joints, wears away, allowing bones to rub against each other. Osteoarthritis can begin in younger individuals, such as in athletes who receive joint injury. Most of us will have evidence of osteoarthritis in at least one joint by the time we become seniors. Although severe osteoarthritis can be debilitating and can severely affect mobility, it does not cause organ damage. There is currently no cure for osteoarthritis, but treatment includes exercise, joint care, treatment of pain, and sometimes joint replacement surgery.

Another type of arthritis is caused by *gout*, a condition seen more commonly in middle-aged men. In this condition, sudden attacks of pain, redness, and swelling occur in the joints of the lower extremities such as the knees, ankles, heels, or toes. These attacks can be precipitated by stress, diet, or the presence of infection and often occur in persons who have a family history of gout. The pain of gout is caused by a buildup of uric acid in the joint. Uric acid is a breakdown product of purines, which are found in many foods. The uric acid crystallizes in the joints, causing pain that usually subsides within a few days. Diagnosis of gout can be confirmed by finding uric acid crystals in a microscopic examination of synovial (joint) fluid. Pain relief is often obtained with over-the-counter anti-inflammatory medications. Lifestyle changes usually can significantly reduce attacks.

RA is an autoimmune disease that usually begins in young adulthood and is more common in women than men. When it begins in childhood, it is called juvenile RA. In RA, the symptoms are usually symmetrical; for example, both hands are usually affected rather than just one. RA affects not only the joints but also other parts of the body, such as skin, lungs, vascular system, and eyes. Much is still unknown about RA, but it is thought that a combination of genetic factors, environmental factors, and hormones play a part in the disease. Some investigators have evidence that infections with certain viruses or bacteria can trigger onset of the disease in individuals with an inherited tendency to RA. There is no specific test for rheumatoid arthritis, but the test for RF is positive in the majority of cases. Other tests for inflammatory disease, such as the erythrocyte sedimentation rate, are also used. Anti-nuclear antibody (ANA) tests can also be positive in rheumatoid arthritis. Treatment for RA includes rest, medications to provide pain relief and reduce inflammation, and powerful medications such as corticosteroids and drugs called biological response modifiers that modify or reduce the immune response.

Diagnosis of the type of arthritis is made using a combination of family and personal medical history, physical examination, X-rays, and laboratory findings. Human leukocyte antigen (HLA) testing can be performed to identify cell markers associated with diseases that display arthritis-like symptoms. Several autoimmune diseases have arthritis-associated symptoms, including ankylosing spondylitis, lupus erythematosus, Sjögren's syndrome, and scleroderma.

---

spreader for each. Each mixture is spread over the entire individual test area. The slide is then rocked or rotated for the specified time (usually 1 to 3 minutes) and observed for agglutination under a bright light.

Interpreting the Results of an RF Test

The area containing the positive control serum should show agglutination. Agglutination appears as small clumps against the background of the slide (Figure 4-27). The negative control serum should have no agglutination. A negative reaction will appear as a smooth solution with no clumping in the test area (Figure 4-27).

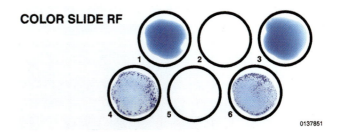

COLOR SLIDE RF

0137851

FIGURE 4-27 Illustration of agglutination in the rheumatoid factor latex test. Wells 1 and 3 have no agglutination and are negative; wells 4 and 6 show agglutination and are positive. (*Courtesy Remel, Inc., Lenexa, KS*)

Absence of agglutination with the patient serum indicates the level of RFs is within normal range and is reported as *negative, no agglutination seen*, or, if diluted serum was used, *titer less than 20*.

Presence of agglutination with the patient serum is considered a positive test and indicates a significantly elevated level of RFs. A semi-quantitative RF test should be performed on positive samples to determine the RF titer.

If undiluted serum is tested and shows agglutination, the serum must be diluted 1:20 or serially diluted and reassayed. Test kits differ in sensitivity. For most test kits, only serum that is positive at a 1:20 (or higher) dilution can be considered positive for RF.

Significance of Results

Diagnosis of RA should not be based on the RF test alone, since other conditions, particularly inflammatory diseases, can also cause a positive RF test. Conversely, since only 75% to 85% of those with RA have increased levels of RF, *a diagnosis of RA cannot be ruled out solely on the basis of a negative test.*

Knowledge of the amount of RF present can be useful in monitoring the course of RA, since RF levels tend to parallel the patient's condition. Patients with active RA usually have higher RF levels than do patients with inactive disease.

PERFORMING A SEMI-QUANTITATIVE TEST FOR RHEUMATOID FACTOR

A semi-quantitative test for RF is performed by testing a series of dilutions of the patient's serum to determine the RF titer. The highest serum dilution showing agglutination (positive reaction) is recorded. The titer, which is the **reciprocal**, or inverse, of the highest dilution giving a positive result, is reported. For example, dilutions of 1:40, 1:80, and 1:160 were made from a serum that was positive in the qualitative test. When the dilutions were tested for RF, the 1:40 dilution showed agglutination and the 1:80 and 1:160 dilutions were negative. This serum would be reported to have an RF titer of 40 (the reciprocal of the 1:40 or 1/40 serum dilution).

SAFETY Reminders

- Review safety precautions before beginning procedure.
- Observe Standard Precautions when performing assays.
- Discard used materials in appropriate biohazard containers.
- Handle controls and reagents produced from human products as if potentially infectious.

PROCEDURAL Reminders

- Review quality assessment section before beginning procedure.
- Follow manufacturer's instructions for the kit used.
- Perform semi-quantitative test if initial test for RF is positive.
- Use good lighting to observe latex agglutination.
- Run positive and negative controls each time a patient sample is tested.

CASE STUDY 1

Christy Jenkins, a 23-year-old woman, visited her physician and complained of joint pain and swelling. An RF test was ordered. The technician tested Ms. Jenkins' undiluted serum using a latex agglutination test for RF and observed agglutination. RF-positive and RF-negative serum controls performed as expected.

The technician should:
a. Report the test as negative
b. Report the test as positive
c. Report a titer of 20
d. Repeat the test using diluted serum

CASE STUDY 2

The following reactions were observed after performing a semi-quantitative RF latex agglutination test.

Serum Dilution	Agglutination Reaction
1:20	(+)
1:40	(+)
1:80	(+)
1:160	(−)
1:320	(−)

The RF titer is:

a. 1:80

b. 1:160

c. 80

d. 160

SUMMARY

Arthritis is a condition common in old age. However, different forms of arthritis occur, each with its distinct causes, symptoms, and laboratory findings. Three types of arthritis are osteoarthritis, gout, and RA. Of these, RA is the most severe.

RFs are autoantibodies that are increased in the serum of 75% to 85% of patients with rheumatoid arthritis. The RF test is used in the differential diagnosis of RA. Many tests for RF are based on the principle of latex agglutination. Results of RF tests must be interpreted carefully. Since elevated levels of rheumatoid factors are not detectable in all patients with RA, a negative RF test does not rule out RA. In addition, certain other inflammatory conditions can cause a positive RF test.

REVIEW QUESTIONS

1. What are RFs?

2. An elevated level of RF is often associated with what disease?

3. Explain the principle of the latex agglutination test for RF.

4. Describe the appearance of a positive latex test and a negative latex test.

5. What is the difference between a qualitative and semi-quantitative agglutination test?

6. What is the significance of a positive RF slide agglutination test? Of a negative RF slide agglutination test?

7. Why is serum diluted before performing the RF test?

8. What is a titer?

9. Define arthritis, autoantibody, reciprocal, rheumatoid arthritis, rheumatoid factors, and synovial.

STUDENT ACTIVITIES

1. Complete the written examination for this lesson.

2. Practice performing qualitative and semi-quantitative slide agglutination tests for RF as outlined in the Student Performance Guide.

WEB ACTIVITY

Use the Internet to search for information on RA. Report on the pathology of the disease. Find information about other conditions that have symptoms similar to RA and laboratory tests that are useful in diagnosis.

Student Performance Guide

LESSON 4-6 IMMUNOLOGY: SLIDE TEST FOR RHEUMATOID FACTORS

Name _____ Date _____

INSTRUCTIONS

1. Practice performing the slide test for RF following the step-by-step procedure.

2. Demonstrate the latex slide test for RF satisfactorily for the instructor, using the Student Performance Guide. Your instructor will determine the level of competency you must achieve to obtain a satisfactory (S) grade.

NOTE: Instructions given are general. The procedure should be modified to conform to the manufacturer's instructions provided with the kit being used.

MATERIALS AND EQUIPMENT

- antiseptic
- gloves
- face protection and/or acrylic safety shield
- timer
- test tubes (13 × 75 mm)
- test tube rack
- serum samples
- pipets for delivering 0.05 mL (50 μL), 0.5 mL, 0.95 mL
- RF slide test kit that includes:
  - RF latex reagent
  - RF positive control serum
  - RF negative control serum
  - diluent
  - ringed slides
  - dispensers
- surface disinfectant
- biohazard container
- applicator sticks (if spreaders are not in kit)

PROCEDURE

Record in the comment section any problems encountered while practicing the procedure (or have a fellow student or the instructor evaluate your performance).

S = Satisfactory
U = Unsatisfactory

You must:	S	U	Comments
1. Assemble equipment and materials. Allow all reagents to reach room temperature before performing test			
2. Wash hands and put on gloves			
3. Put on face protection or position acrylic shield			

4. Prepare a 1:20 dilution of the test serum:
  a. Pipet 0.05 mL (50 μL) of serum into a 13 × 75 tube
  b. Pipet 0.95 mL of diluent into the tube and mix well			

5. Label test areas +, −, and *patient*			

You must:	S	U	Comments
6. a. Dispense one drop of positive control serum into (+) ring on slide using dispenser provided with kit b. Dispense one drop of negative control serum into (−) ring on slide using a clean dispenser			
7. Dispense one drop of diluted patient serum (from step 4) into (patient) ring on slide using a clean dispenser			
8. Mix the RF latex reagent well by inverting several times.			
9. Dispense one drop of well-mixed RF latex reagent into each ring containing a control or test serum			
10. Use a spreader to thoroughly mix serum with latex reagent, spreading the mixture over the entire surface of the ring **NOTE:** Be sure to use a separate spreader for each serum or control sample. An applicator stick can be used if no spreaders are included in the kit			
11. Start timer and rock the slide in a figure-eight motion for the appropriate time (usually 1 to 3 minutes)			
12. Observe the ringed areas for agglutination immediately at the end of the appropriate time period			
13. Record the results of the controls and patient serum (agglutination = positive; no agglutination = negative, or titer less than 20)			
14. Perform the semi-quantitative test (steps 15 through 18) if the patient sample is positive for agglutination; if it is negative, go to step 19			
15. Prepare a two-fold serial dilution of patient serum: a. Label five test tubes: 1 (1:40), 2 (1:80), 3 (1:160), 4 (1:320), and 5 (1:640) b. Pipet 0.5 mL of diluent into each tube c. Pipet 0.5 mL of 1:20 dilution of patient serum (from qualitative test, step 4) into tube 1 (1:40) and mix contents of tube well d. Transfer 0.5 mL from tube 1 to tube 2 and mix well e. Transfer 0.5 mL from tube 2 to tube 3 and mix well f. Transfer 0.5 mL from tube 3 to tube 4 and mix well g. Transfer 0.5 mL from tube 4 to tube 5 and mix well			
16. Use each dilution (tubes 1 through 5) as a separate test specimen and perform the latex agglutination test as in steps 5 to 13			
17. Record the agglutination results for each tube			
18. Record the serum RF titer (the reciprocal of the highest dilution that shows agglutination)			
19. Discard specimens and used materials appropriately			

You must:	S	U	Comments
20. Return all reagents and materials to proper storage and clean and disinfect work area			
21. Remove gloves and discard in biohazard container			
22. Wash hands with antiseptic			

Evaluator Comments:

Evaluator _____ Date _____

UNIT 5

Urinalysis

UNIT OBJECTIVE

After studying this unit, the student will:

- Identify the organs of the urinary system.
- Identify the parts of the kidney and state the function of each part.
- Explain how urine is formed.
- Discuss diseases that affect kidney function and urinalysis results.
- Describe proper urine collection and preservation methods.
- Perform a physical examination of urine.
- Perform a chemical examination of urine.
- Perform a microscopic examination of urine sediment.
- Explain how urinalysis results can give important information about the status of a patient's health.
- Perform a urine hCG test and interpret the results.

UNIT OVERVIEW

Urine has long been used as an indicator of a person's health. Analysis of urine is the earliest recorded medical laboratory test. References to testing urine date back to ancient Egyptian hieroglyphics and are found in the writings of Hippocrates. By the middle ages, early physicians often examined urine, sometimes without ever seeing the patient. Although these physicians did not have the sophisticated tests that we have now, they did examine the color, odor, volume, viscosity, and even sweetness of urine. With the invention of the microscope, urine sediment could be examined and identified microscopically.

In the first half of the 1900s, when laboratory medicine was in its infancy, many chemical tests were developed for urine. For the most part, however, these tests were complex and time-consuming, causing urine testing to be rather impractical and infrequently done. With the development of the rapid reagent strip test, urinalysis became an important part of the routine physical examination.

Modern urinalysis has two major advantages: (1) urine is an easily obtained specimen and (2) much information can be obtained about the body's metabolism through rapid, simple, reliable, and inexpensive tests. Most physical examinations include a routine urinalysis, in which several tests are performed on one urine sample. The routine urinalysis is one of the most frequently performed laboratory procedures.

Changes occur in urine when kidney disease or certain other diseases are present. Urinalysis can be performed to detect physical, chemical, and microscopic characteristics that indicate disease of, or damage to, the urinary system. Urine tests can also detect metabolic end products that indicate particular diseases unrelated to the urinary system. Urinalysis results can give the physician valuable information about a patient's health and information useful in diagnosing disease or following the course of treatment.

This unit presents basic information about the urinary system, proper collection of urine specimens, procedures for performing a routine urinalysis, and the urine test for human chorionic gonadotropin (hCG). Lesson 5-1 contains fundamental information about the anatomy of the urinary system, kidney structure and function, urine formation and composition, and diseases that affect the urinary system. This information provides a foundation for understanding the importance of urine testing and test results.

Lesson 5-2 describes routine and special urine collection procedures. Lessons 5-3, 5-4, and 5-5 describe the tests that make up the three parts of the routine urinalysis—the physical, chemical, and microscopic examinations of urine. Lesson 5-6, Urine hCG Tests, is included in this unit because hCG tests, commonly used to detect pregnancy, are often performed in the urinalysis section of the laboratory.

READINGS, REFERENCES, AND RESOURCES

General/Immunology

Baker, F. J., et al. (2000). *Baker & Silverton's introduction to medical laboratory technology.* (7th ed.). London: Arnold.

Barrett, J. T. (1998). *Microbiology and immunology concepts.* Philadelphia: Lippincott Williams & Wilkins.

Henry, J. B. (Ed.) (2006). *Clinical diagnosis and management by laboratory methods.* (21st ed.). Philadelphia: W. B. Saunders Company.

Paul, W. E. (Ed.) (2003). *Fundamental immunology.* Philadelphia: Lippincott Williams & Wilkins.

Turgeon, M. L. (2003). *Immunology and serology in laboratory medicine.* (3rd ed.). St. Louis: C. V. Mosby.

Urinalysis and Body Fluids

Bayer encyclopedia of urinalysis. CD-ROM. Tarrytown, NY: Bayer Corp., Diagnostics Division.

Bayer HealthCare, Diagnostics Division. (2004). *Modern urine chemistry.* Tarrytown, NY.

Brunzel, N. A. (2004). *Fundamentals of urine and body fluid analysis.* (2nd ed.) Philadelphia: W. B. Saunders Company.

McBride, L. J. (1998). *Textbook of urinalysis and body fluids: a clinical approach.* Philadelphia: Lippincott-Raven.

Ringsrud, K. M. & Linne, J. J. (1995). *Urinalysis and body fluids: a colortext and atlas.* St. Louis: Mosby Yearbook.

Strasinger, S. K. & Di Lorenzo, M. S. (2001). *Urinalysis and body fluids.* (4th ed.) Philadelphia: F. A. Davis Company.

Package Inserts

ICON II hCG. Package insert. Fullerton, CA: Beckman Coulter, Inc.

ICON 25 hCG. Package insert. Fullerton, CA: Beckman Coulter, Inc.

KOVA System for Standardized Urinalysis. Package insert. Garden Grove, CA: HYCOR Biomedical Corporation.

QuickVue One-Step hCG Urine. Package insert. San Diego, CA: Quidel Corporation.

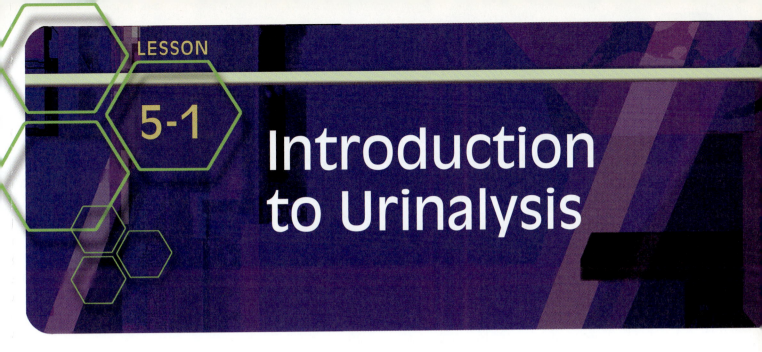

Introduction to Urinalysis

LESSON OBJECTIVES

After studying this lesson, the student will:

- Identify the organs of the urinary system.
- List four major functions of the kidney.
- Identify the parts of the kidney.
- Explain how urine is formed.
- Describe the composition of urine.
- List the three parts of a routine urinalysis.
- Explain the value of performing a routine urinalysis.
- Name three hormones that are produced in the kidneys.
- Name three hormones that influence kidney function.
- Explain the differences between hemodialysis and peritoneal dialysis.
- List three kidney diseases that can cause abnormal urinalysis results.
- List three systemic diseases that can cause abnormal urinalysis results.
- Define the glossary terms.

GLOSSARY

Bowman's capsule / the portion of the nephron that receives the glomerular filtrate

cortex / the outer layer or portion of an organ

cystitis / inflammation of the urinary bladder

dialysate / in kidney dialysis, a solution used to draw waste products and excess fluid from the body

distal convoluted tubule / the portion of a renal tubule that empties into the collecting tubule

glomerular filtrate / the fluid that passes from the blood into the nephron and from which urine is formed

glomerulonephritis / inflammation of the glomeruli

glomerulus (pl. glomeruli) / a small bundle of capillaries that is the filtering portion of the nephron

kidney / the organ in which urine is formed

loop of Henle / the U-shaped portion of a renal tubule between its proximal and distal portions

medulla / the inner or central portion of an organ

nephron / the structural and functional unit of the kidney composed of a glomerulus and its associated renal tubule

439

nephrotoxic / toxic or destructive to kidney cells

peritoneum / a membrane lining the abdominal cavity and containing a fluid that keeps abdominal organs from adhering to the abdominal wall; parietal peritoneum

proximal convoluted tubule / the portion of a renal tubule that collects the filtrate from Bowman's capsule

pyelitis / inflammation of the renal pelvis

pyelonephritis / inflammation of the kidney and the renal pelvis

renal hilus / the concavity in the kidney where nerves and vessels enter or exit

renal pelvis / the funnel-shaped expansion of the upper portion of the ureter that receives urine from the renal tubules

renal threshold / the blood concentration above which a substance not normally excreted by the kidneys appears in urine

renal tubule / a small tube of the nephron that collects and concentrates urine

tubular necrosis / death of the tissue comprising the renal tubules

ureter / the tube carrying urine from the kidney to the urinary bladder

urethra / the canal through which urine is discharged from the urinary bladder

urinary bladder / an organ for the temporary storage of urine

urine / excretory fluid produced by the kidneys

UTI / urinary tract infection

INTRODUCTION

The urinary system has a vital role in regulating many bodily processes. The kidneys are the primary functional organs of the urinary system. The major functions of the kidneys include:

- Elimination of metabolic and toxic waste products from the body
- Regulation of acid-base balance (pH)
- Regulation of the composition and volume of body fluids
- Production of hormones necessary for proper function of body tissues and organs

Through the formation and excretion of urine, a variety of waste products are eliminated from the body. These products, if not removed, can rapidly reach toxic levels and cause death within a few days. The kidneys function as biological purification factories, filtering and cleansing the blood of harmful toxins, metabolic wastes, and excess ions. These wastes then leave the body in the urine. Through a complex process of excretion and reabsorption, the urinary system also regulates blood volume, blood chemistry, pH, electrolyte concentrations, and blood pressure. Hormones produced in organs of the urinary system are integral to proper red blood cell production, blood pressure regulation, and bone calcium absorption.

This lesson presents introductory material about the structure and functions of the urinary system, basic knowledge that is necessary to understand the relationship between the urinary

system and health. Later lessons in this unit explain how routine urinalysis test results can give important information about the state of a patient's health.

THE URINARY SYSTEM

The urinary system is an excretory system consisting of two kidneys, two ureters, the urinary bladder, and the urethra. The **kidneys** are the organs in which urine is formed. Humans have two kidneys, bean-shaped organs that lie on either side of the vertebral column. Connected to each kidney is a **ureter**, a funnel-shaped tube that carries urine from the kidney to the **urinary bladder**, where it is stored. The **urethra** is the canal through which urine is carried from the urinary bladder to the outside. Figure 5-1 is a diagram of the urinary system, showing the kidneys, ureters, urinary bladder, and urethra.

Anatomy of the Kidneys

Each kidney is surrounded by a fibrous protective capsule. The **renal hilus** is the concave region of the kidney where blood vessels, lymphatic vessels, nerves, and the ureter enter or exit the kidney (Figure 5-2). Internally, the kidney has three major regions: the cortex, the medulla, and the renal pelvis (Figures 5-1 and 5-2). The **cortex** is the outermost layer of tissue, lying beneath the capsule. The **medulla** lies beneath the cortex and contains the renal pyramids, cone-shaped tissue masses. The renal columns are extensions of the renal cortex that separate the renal pyramids. Each pyramid and its associated cortical region make

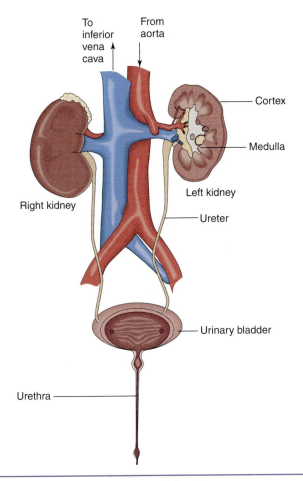

FIGURE 5-1 Organs of the urinary system

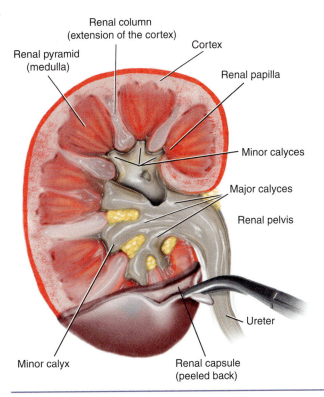

FIGURE 5-2 Cut-away view of the internal anatomy of the kidney

up a kidney lobe. The **renal pelvis** is the funnel-shaped expansion of the upper (proximal) portion of the ureter.

The Nephron

The functional unit in the kidneys is the **nephron** (Figure 5-3). Each kidney has approximately 1 million nephrons, which are located in the kidney cortex. Each nephron is composed of a glomerulus and its associated renal tubule.

The Glomerulus

The **glomerulus**, the filtering unit of the kidney, is composed of a bundle of blood capillaries (Figure 5-3). Surrounding each glomerulus is a layer of cells called **Bowman's capsule**. In the glomerulus, water and other small molecules such as glucose, salt, and urea are filtered from the blood (leave the circulatory system) and pass into Bowman's capsule, while blood cells and larger molecules such as proteins remain in the blood. This filtered glomerular fluid is called the **glomerular filtrate** and is funneled by Bowman's capsule into the renal tubule (Figures 5-3 and 5-4).

The Renal Tubule

A **renal tubule** is associated with each glomerulus. The glomerular filtrate is concentrated as it passes through the renal tubule. The three parts of a renal tubule are (1) the **proximal convoluted**

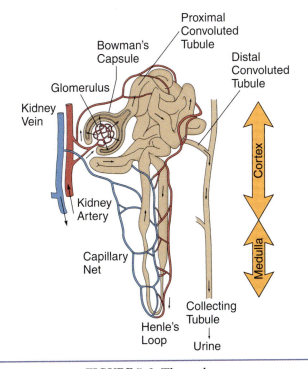

FIGURE 5-3 The nephron

tubule, (2) the **loop of Henle**, and (3) the **distal convoluted tubule**, which empties into a collecting tubule (Figure 5-3). The renal tubule is surrounded by blood capillaries (peritubular capillaries), and portions of the tubule may extend into the medulla of the kidney (Figure 5-3).

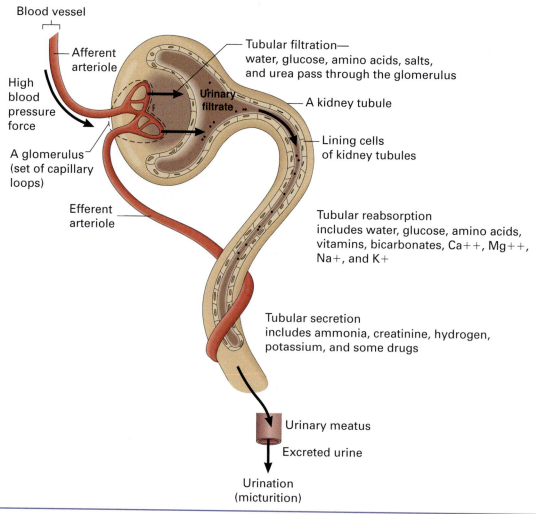

Blood vessel

Afferent arteriole

High blood pressure force

A glomerulus (set of capillary loops)

Efferent arteriole

Tubular filtration—water, glucose, amino acids, salts, and urea pass through the glomerulus

Urinary filtrate

A kidney tubule

Lining cells of kidney tubules

Tubular reabsorption includes water, glucose, amino acids, vitamins, bicarbonates, Ca++, Mg++, Na+, and K+

Tubular secretion includes ammonia, creatinine, hydrogen, potassium, and some drugs

Urinary meatus

Excreted urine

Urination (micturition)

FIGURE 5-4 Diagram of glomerular filtration and tubular reabsorption and secretion (loop of Henle and convoluted and distal tubules not shown)

Urine Formation

Urine is formed by concentration of the glomerular filtrate as it passes through the renal tubules. Substances such as vitamins, electrolytes, amino acids, and glucose are selectively reabsorbed from the filtrate by renal tubular cells. Most of the water in the filtrate is also reabsorbed, producing a concentrated fluid (Figure 5-4). In addition, some molecules, such as potassium and hydrogen ions, are secreted into the filtrate by tubular cells. The resulting concentrated fluid is **urine**, which passes into the collecting tubules, collects in the renal pelvis, and flows through the ureters into the urinary bladder.

The rate of blood flow through the kidneys is extremely high—approximately 1,200 mL of blood are cleansed of waste products each minute. As a result, the glomeruli form approximately 180 L (about 45 gallons!) of filtrate each day. After concentration in the tubules, this volume is reduced to approximately 1 to 2 L of urine produced daily in a healthy adult.

Urine Composition

Approximately 95% of urine is water and the other 5% is solutes (dissolved substances). Urea, a breakdown product of amino acids, is the solute in highest concentration, followed by sodium. Other solutes include potassium, chloride, phosphate and sulfate ions, creatinine, and uric acid, as well as small amounts of bile pigments and calcium, magnesium, and bicarbonate ions (Table 5-1).

Urine composition changes depending on factors such as the time of day (diurnal changes) and the physical state, diet, and health of the individual. In some diseases, substances such as glucose, blood cells, protein, or bile pigments can be present in the urine. Abnormalities in urine composition alert physicians to possible disease.

Hormones and the Urinary System

Kidney function is under the influence of several hormones. In addition, some hormones are produced by the kidneys (Table 5-2).

Hormones That Affect Kidney Function

Hormones that influence kidney function include:

- Parathyroid hormone (PTH)
- Calcitonin
- Aldosterone
- Antidiuretic hormone (ADH)
- Atrial natriuretic peptide (ANP)

TABLE 5-1. Some solutes found in normal urine

Sodium	Magnesium	Urea	Creatinine
Potassium	Vitamins	Uric acid	Phosphate ions
Chloride	Amino acids	Bile pigments	
Bicarbonate ions	Sulfate ions		Calcium ions

TABLE 5-2. Hormones that influence or are produced by the kidneys

HORMONE	FUNCTION
Hormones that influence kidney function	
Aldosterone	Regulates electrolytes, especially potassium
Antidiuretic hormone	Regulates water reabsorption
Atrial natriuretic peptide	Influences sodium excretion
Parathyroid hormone	Regulates calcium reabsorption
Calcitonin	Inhibits calcium reabsorption
Hormones produced by the kidneys	
Erythropoietin	Stimulates red blood cell synthesis
Renin	Influences blood pressure
Active vitamin D_3	Influences bone calcium levels

Parathyroid hormone influences calcium reabsorption in the kidney tubules and works with vitamin D_3 to regulate bone calcium. *Calcitonin* inhibits reabsorption of calcium by kidney tubules, leading to increased calcium loss in urine. *Aldosterone* is a mineralocorticoid that helps regulate electrolytes and promotes urinary potassium excretion. *Antidiuretic hormone,* also called *vasopressin,* regulates water reabsorption by the kidneys. *Atrial natriuretic peptide* is produced by heart cells. It helps reduce plasma volume by increasing sodium excretion in the kidneys.

Hormones Produced by the Kidneys

While kidney function is influenced by hormones such as ADH that are produced in other organs, the kidneys also produce hormones that influence physiologic processes in other parts of the body (Table 5-2). Three hormones produced by the kidneys are:

- Erythropoietin
- Renin
- Active vitamin D_3

Erythropoietin stimulates red blood cell production in the bone marrow. *Renin* indirectly influences blood pressure. *Vitamin D_3*, which is actually a hormone rather than a vitamin, helps regulate bone calcium and phosphorus by increasing absorption of dietary calcium and phosphorus.

Urine Volume

The amount of urine formed daily depends on age, fluid intake, metabolism, blood pressure, diet, hormone balance, and many other factors. Healthy adults excrete between 1 and 2 L of urine per day. *Diuretics* increase urinary output and therefore dilute the urine. Caffeine and some hypertension medications act as diuretics. *Antidiuretic hormone* stimulates water reabsorption by the kidneys, thus creating a concentrated urine and decreasing urine output.

Renal Threshold

Most components present in urine are also present in blood, but in different amounts and proportions. Many small molecules that enter the glomerular filtrate become reabsorbed into the blood as the filtrate passes through the tubules of the nephron. When the blood level of a substance becomes high enough to exceed the tubular reabsorption capacity, then the substance will be excreted in the urine. In those cases, the blood concentration is said to have exceeded the **renal threshold**. For example, the renal threshold of glucose ranges from 160 to 180 mg/dL. At blood glucose levels below this range, glucose is reabsorbed from the filtrate by the tubules. When blood glucose levels exceed this threshold, glucose will be excreted in the urine.

TESTS OF RENAL FUNCTION

Several tests can be performed on urine. Some are simple and rapid, such as the tests included in the routine urinalysis. The routine urinalysis procedure has three parts: the physical and chemical examinations of urine and the microscopic examination of urine sediment. These are described in Lessons 5-3, 5-4, and 5-5.

Abnormalities discovered during a routine urinalysis can lead the physician to request more specific tests of renal function. Serum tests for metabolites such as creatinine and blood urea nitrogen (BUN) are important in monitoring kidney function. Other tests used to assess renal function such as the creatinine clearance test can be performed on 24-hour urine specimens. These tests are often complex and time-consuming. Although the performance of clearance tests are beyond the scope of this text, the procedure for collecting 24-hour urine specimens is covered in Lesson 5-2.

CONDITIONS AND DISEASES AFFECTING URINALYSIS RESULTS

Abnormal urinalysis results can be seen (1) in disorders or diseases of the urinary tract or (2) in situations when disease in other

CURRENT TOPICS

RENAL DIALYSIS

The kidneys cleanse the blood and remove excess fluid, minerals, and waste products; they also produce hormones necessary for strong bones and blood cell production, all vital functions. There are several causes of kidney failure, but whatever the reason, the consequences are the same—harmful wastes build up in the body, blood pressure rises, excess fluid is retained, and red cell production decreases. Acute kidney failure can cause death in only a few days if left untreated. In some cases acute kidney failure responds to treatment, and kidney function is regained. Chronic kidney failure, also called *chronic renal insufficiency*, leads to kidney failure more slowly. When a patient reaches the point where 85% to 90% of kidney function has been lost, treatment is required.

The two major treatments for kidney failure (end-stage kidney disease) are dialysis and kidney transplant. Dialysis is used to treat acute kidney failure and to treat patients with chronic kidney failure while they wait for a suitable kidney donor organ. In many cases, patients never receive a transplant but remain on dialysis for years.

Dialysis attempts to replace the function of the failed kidneys by using artificial means to remove harmful wastes, salts, and fluids. Two types of dialysis are used, *hemodialysis* and *peritoneal* dialysis. Hemodialysis is used to treat acute kidney failure; chronic kidney failure can be treated with hemodialysis or peritoneal dialysis. With both types of dialysis, the patient's condition must be closely monitored by frequent physical examinations and laboratory tests. Dialysis patients must follow a careful, restricted diet low in sodium, phosphorus, potassium, and fluid intake. Vitamin and mineral supplements are required because of diet limitations and loss of vitamins and minerals during dialysis.

Hemodialysis

In hemodialysis, blood from a patient's vein is slowly passed through a *dialyzer* that removes wastes and extra fluid. The dialyzer, also called an artificial kidney, is a canister containing special membrane filters (Diagram 1). A permanent *fistula* or graft connecting a vein to an artery is surgically created beneath the patient's skin. A dialysis machine pumps blood from this fistula or graft to the dialyzer (Diagram 2). Blood remains on one side of the membrane filters, and a fluid called a **dialysate** is constantly pumped around the other side of the dialyzer membranes, drawing wastes and excess fluid from the blood across the membranes into the dialysate. The wastes and excess fluid are carried away as the dialysate leaves the dialyzer, and the cleansed blood is returned to the body. Hemodialysis is a slow process, taking 4 to 5 hours, and must be done three to four times a week. Most patients go to a dialysis center for treatment; some patients are trained to perform hemodialysis at home.

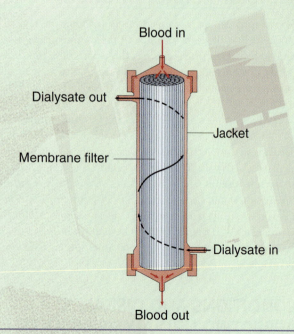

DIAGRAM 1 Dialyzer

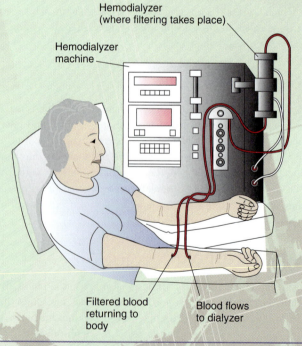

DIAGRAM 2 Patient undergoing hemodialysis

(continued)

CURRENT TOPICS

Peritoneal Dialysis

The **peritoneum** is the membrane that lines the walls of the abdominal cavity, creating a peritoneal space or cavity. In peritoneal dialysis, the peritoneal cavity is used as the exchange container and the peritoneal membrane acts as a filter. The patient's abdomen is filled with a dialysate (usually containing dextrose) using a soft tube called a catheter (Diagram 3). The dialysate pulls wastes and extra fluid from the blood into the peritoneal cavity by diffusion. After a few hours, the dialysate fluid containing this waste and excess fluid, is drained and discarded. More dialysate fluid is then pumped into the cavity to begin another exchange. A typical schedule calls for four exchanges a day, each with a dwell time (time the dialysate is in the peritoneal cavity) of 4 to 6 hours. Peritoneal dialysis can be the *ambulatory* type that does not require a machine and allows the patient to remain mobile. In other cases, a cycler machine fills and drains the abdomen while the patient sleeps. Both types require that a catheter be permanently placed in the abdomen to carry the dialysis solution into and out of the abdomen. Peritoneal dialysis gives the patient more freedom and independence.

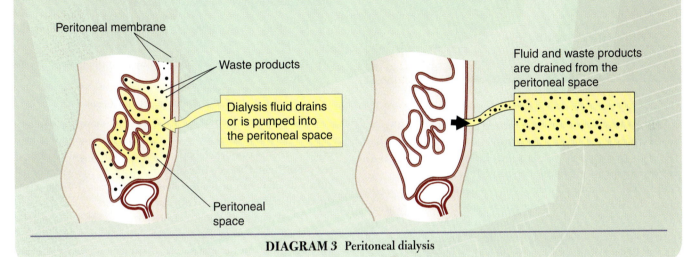

DIAGRAM 3 Peritoneal dialysis

parts of the body affects kidney function or urine composition. Disease can cause changes in the:

- Urine volume
- Urine color
- Urine transparency or clarity
- Urine odor
- Cells present in urine
- Chemical constituents of urine

Urinary Tract Infections

Urine stored in the urinary bladder is normally sterile. Urinary tract infections (**UTIs**) most commonly occur in the urethra and can be caused by bacteria, yeasts (fungi), or protozoan parasites. Untreated bacterial infections can spread to the urinary bladder, causing **cystitis**. In severe cases, the kidney can become involved, resulting in **pyelitis**, an inflammation or infection of the renal pelvis, or **pyelonephritis**, an inflammation or infection of the renal pelvis and the kidney.

Diseases of the Kidneys

Kidney disease can be mild or severe and acute or chronic. Chronic kidney disease is often far advanced by the time it is discovered because kidney failure does not occur until a large percentage of the nephrons are nonfunctional. When kidney function decreases, toxic products such as urea, uric acid, and creatinine accumulate in the blood. Kidney failure can be treated by dialysis (see Current Topics) or kidney transplant. Some examples of diseases of the kidneys include glomerulonephritis, polycystic kidney disease, and tubular necrosis (Table 5-3).

Glomerulonephritis

Glomerulonephritis (GN) is an inflammation of the glomeruli, usually due to deposition of antibodies or immune complexes in the glomeruli, causing glomerular damage. Glomerulonephritis can develop as a result of infection somewhere in the body, autoimmune diseases, or systemic diseases in which capillary damage occurs (since the glomeruli are made of capillaries). Damage to glomerular capillaries results in inefficient filtering; protein and

TABLE 5-3. Examples of conditions and diseases that can affect urinalysis results

KIDNEY DISEASES
Glomerulonephritis
Polycystic kidney disease
Tubular necrosis

SYSTEMIC DISEASES AFFECTING KIDNEY FUNCTION
Diabetes mellitus
Hypertension
Atherosclerosis
Autoimmune diseases
Nephrotic syndrome
Malignancies

OTHER CONDITIONS
Urinary tract infections

blood cells may be present in urine, and excess body fluid accumulates, causing edema and hypertension.

Post-streptococcal GN is a well-known but infrequently occurring type of glomerulonephritis. It is a complication of untreated or incompletely treated group A hemolytic *Streptococcus* throat or skin infection. The glomerular damage in post-streptococcal GN is caused when immune complexes, which form in response to the infection, become deposited in the glomeruli causing inflammation and interfering with glomerular function. All group A streptococcal infections should be treated promptly with antibiotics to avoid the possibility of complications. When symptoms associated with post-streptococcal GN are treated, the condition may subside after a few months. However, in some cases the condition can progress to chronic renal failure.

Polycystic Kidney Disease

Polycystic kidney disease is an inherited condition in which glomerular function is lost because of formation of multiple cysts in the kidneys.

Tubular Necrosis

Tubular necrosis can occur when the blood supply to the kidney is diminished, or upon exposure to, or ingestion of, substances that are **nephrotoxic** (toxic to kidney cells). The capacity of the tubules to concentrate urine is affected in this condition.

Systemic Diseases Affecting Urinalysis Results

Systemic diseases that can cause abnormal urinalysis results include diabetes mellitus, hypertension, atherosclerosis, autoimmune diseases, nephrotic syndrome, and malignancies (Table 5-3). Uncontrolled diabetes, prolonged hypertension, and autoim-

mune diseases such as lupus erythematosus can cause glomerular damage. Nephrotic syndrome is a complex condition associated with circulatory disorders and is characterized by tissue edema and protein in the urine. Malignancies developing in the urinary system can cause obstruction, abnormal urinalysis results, or the appearance of malignant cells in the urine.

SUMMARY

A normal functioning urinary system is necessary for good health. The kidneys are responsible for the formation and excretion of urine, the principal way the body gets rid of waste products and excess fluid. Urine excretion provides a means of regulating the body's state of hydration and the blood concentration of ions such as sodium, potassium, and other small molecules. Three processes are involved in urine formation:

- Filtration of waste products, salts, and excess fluid from the blood

- Reabsorption of water and solutes from the glomerular filtrate

- Secretion of ions and molecules into the urine

Although most think of urine production as the primary function of the kidneys, the kidneys also produce hormones necessary for strong bones, blood pressure control, and red blood cell production. Diseases or conditions that interfere with normal kidney function can be life-threatening if not treated. Kidney failure can be treated by dialysis or organ transplant.

Tests such as the ones performed in the routine urinalysis provide an indication of an individual's metabolism and general state of health. An understanding of kidney function and urine composition helps laboratory personnel understand and interpret routine urinalysis results.

REVIEW QUESTIONS

1. Name the organs of the urinary system.

2. Draw a kidney and label the parts.

3. What are the four major functions of the kidneys?

4. Draw a nephron and label the parts; state the function associated with each part.

5. Explain how urine is formed.

6. What components are in urine?

7. What are the three parts of a routine urinalysis?

8. List three hormones produced by the kidneys, and state the function of each.

9. List three hormones that influence kidney function, and explain their function.

10. Name three conditions or diseases of the urinary system that can affect urinalysis results.

11. Name three systemic diseases that can affect urinalysis results.

12. Explain why dialysis can be used as a treatment for kidney failure.

13. Define Bowman's capsule, cortex, cystitis, dialysate, distal convoluted tubule, glomerular filtrate, glomerulonephritis, glomerulus, kidney, loop of Henle, medulla, nephron, nephrotoxic, peritoneum, proximal convoluted tubule, pyelitis, pyelonephritis, renal hilus, renal pelvis, renal threshold, renal tubule, tubular necrosis, ureter, urethra, urinary bladder, urine, and UTI.

STUDENT ACTIVITIES

1. Complete the written examination for this lesson.

2. Select five urine solutes listed in Table 5-1. Consult an anatomy/physiology text and find out what determines the urine concentration of each solute. That is, is it secreted from a portion of a renal tubule, filtered by the glomerulus, or partially reabsorbed in a portion of the renal tubule?

WEB www ACTIVITIES

1. Use the Internet to search for information on kidney diseases, using reliable sources such as medical school Web sites, research institutes such as the National Institutes of Health, or nonprofit kidney disease associations.

2. Use the Internet to find information on one of the following diseases: polycystic kidney disease, post-glomerulonephritis, nephrotic syndrome, lupus erythrematosus, hypertension, or diabetes mellitus. Report on how the disease affects kidney function.

3. Use the Internet to search for information about kidney transplantation. Find out why it would be performed, how donor kidneys are obtained, and what criteria must be met for the patient and the donor.

Collection and Preservation of Urine

LESSON OBJECTIVES

After studying this lesson, the student will:

- Explain the importance of the proper collection of urine specimens.
- List four types of urine specimens and explain when each might be required.
- State the normal 24-hour urine volumes for adults, children, and newborns.
- Explain why a preservative is required for some urine specimens.
- Instruct patients on how to collect a midstream urine specimen.
- Instruct patients on how to collect a clean-catch urine specimen.
- Instruct a patient on how to collect a 24-hour urine specimen.
- Explain how collecting urine specimens for drug screening differs from collecting specimens for routine urinalysis.
- Discuss the importance of quality assessment in the collection and handling of urine specimens.
- Explain safety precautions that must be observed when handling urine specimens.
- Define the glossary terms.

GLOSSARY

anuria / absence of urine production; failure of kidney function and suppression of urine production

clean-catch urine / a midstream urine sample collected after the urethral opening and surrounding tissues have been cleansed

midstream urine / a urine sample collected from the mid-portion of a urine stream

nocturia / excessive urination at night

oliguria / decreased production of urine

polyuria / excessive production of urine

random urine specimen / a urine specimen collected at any time, without regard to diet or time of day

INTRODUCTION

The proper collection, labeling, and handling of urine specimens are the first steps leading to reliable urine test results. The type of specimen required for a urine test depends on the nature of the test that is ordered. A different type of specimen is required for quantitative chemical tests, such as a test for urine calcium, than is required for a routine urinalysis.

Since urine specimens are usually collected by the patient, it is important that the patient be given specific instructions on how to properly collect the urine specimen. Urine specimens must sometimes be transported to a laboratory for testing, so it is also important that collection site, transporting, and receiving laboratory personnel understand transport requirements and limitations. This lesson explains the various types of urine specimens that are used for urine tests and describes the proper urine collection and handling procedures for each.

TYPES OF URINE SPECIMENS

The type of urine specimen required varies according to the type of test to be performed. Common types of urine specimens submitted for laboratory analysis are:

- Random urine specimen
- Fasting or first morning urine specimen
- Clean-catch urine specimen
- Timed urine specimen
- Twenty-four-hour urine specimen

All urine specimens except 24-hour urine specimens, should be collected by the midstream procedure. A **midstream urine** specimen is one in which the patient collects only the middle portion of the urine flow.

Specimens for Routine Urinalysis

The preferred specimen for most routine urine testing is the *first morning specimen.* This specimen is normally more concentrated and usually has an acid pH that helps preserve any cells present. The first morning specimen can be used as a *fasting* specimen if it is collected before the patient has eaten. Most routine urinalysis specimens, however, are **random urine specimens**—specimens obtained at any time without regard to food intake.

Timed Specimens

For certain tests, timed specimens are required. For example, in one screening test for diabetes, urine collected 2 hours postprandial (after eating) is tested for glucose.

Clean-Catch Specimens

The **clean-catch urine** collection procedure is required when urine is to be cultured for microorganisms. The procedure for collecting a clean-catch urine is described in detail in this lesson. Occasionally, urine specimens for culture or routine analysis must be collected by catheterization, a procedure not normally performed by laboratory personnel. The urine culture procedure is explained in Lesson 7-8.

Twenty-Four-Hour Urine Specimens

Quantitative urine tests require a *24-hour urine specimen.* These tests are used primarily to assess kidney function and are usually performed in large hospital or reference laboratories. Protein, creatinine, urobilinogen, and calcium are just a few examples of analytes that can be measured in 24-hour urine specimens. Results are expressed as analyte units per 24 hours. Instructions for collecting 24-hour urine specimens are given in this lesson.

HANDLING AND PRESERVING URINE SPECIMENS

Urine Containers

Several types of containers are available for collecting urine specimens. Random and first morning specimens can be collected in clean, lidded, disposable containers large enough to hold at least 50 mL. For clean-catch specimens, urine containers must be sterile (Figure 5-5). Large, opaque containers capable of holding 4 L or more are provided to patients for collecting 24-hour urine specimens (Figure 5-6). These containers usually contain preservatives.

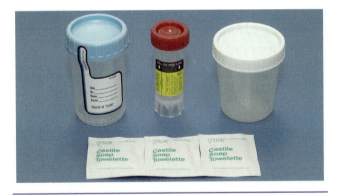

FIGURE 5-5 Clean-catch urine collection kits

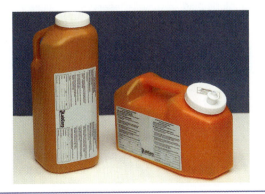

FIGURE 5-6 Two types of 24-hour urine specimen containers

Labeling Urine Specimens

Urine specimens must be labeled clearly with the patient's name, as well as the date and time of collection. Labels must be on the container, not just on the lid.

Storage of Urine Specimens

Urine specimens, for all tests except 24-hour tests, should be examined within 1 hour of collection. If this is not possible, deterioration of the specimen can be prevented by storing urine in the dark, in a lidded container, at 4°C to 6°C for up to 4 hours.

Test results can be affected by the way urine specimens are handled after collection. When urine remains at room temperature for an extended time, any bacteria present will multiply rapidly. This can increase the urine pH and cause the specimen to develop an unpleasant, ammonia-like odor. A delay in testing can also increase the decomposition of urine sediment components such as casts and cells.

Preservation of Urine Specimens

Urine specimens that cannot be refrigerated or that have to be mailed or transported over a long distance can have preservatives added to them. The addition of a preservative retards the growth of bacteria and slows the destruction or decomposition of other urine components.

The preservative used must be one that will not interfere with the tests that have been ordered. Some commonly used urine preservatives are hydrochloric acid (HCl), sulfuric acid, sodium hydroxide (NaOH), sodium carbonate, and boric acid (Table 5-4). Containers for 24-hour urine specimens often have preservatives added before the urine is collected. *No preservative of any kind should be added to urine for bacteriological culture.*

TABLE 5-4. Common urine preservatives and their uses

PRESERVATIVE	USE
Sulfuric acid	Preserves calcium
Hydrochloric acid	Preserves for calcium, magnesium, and phosphorus tests
Sodium carbonate	Preserves porphyrins, urobilinogen
Sodium hydroxide	Preserves myoglobin
Boric acid	Preserves creatinine, uric acid, protein, steroids, and glucose
Refrigeration	Use for tests for protein, barbiturates, and drug abuse screen

PROCEDURES FOR COLLECTING URINE SPECIMENS

Safety Precautions

 Standard Precautions must be observed by all personnel. All urine specimens must be submitted in clean, nonleaking containers; otherwise, they should not be accepted for testing by laboratory personnel. Personal protective equipment (PPE) such as gloves, face protection, and a buttoned, fluid-resistant laboratory coat should be worn when working with specimens. Splashes and the creation of aerosols must be avoided when pouring or discarding urine. Spills of urine must be wiped up with laboratory disinfectant. Sinks used for discarding urines should be flushed with water and appropriate laboratory disinfectant. Patients who must collect 24-hour urine specimens should be given the material safety data sheet (MSDS) information or written instructions for safe handling of any preservative in the collection container.

Quality Assessment

 Specimens must be collected, labeled, transported, and stored following the institution's standard operating procedures (SOPs). Careful, complete instructions must be given to patients so they understand how to correctly collect the specimen. Written instructions must be understandable to all patients and should be available in non-English versions. Specimen labeling must be accurate and complete. Containers (not lids) should be labeled with the patient's name, date, time, and method of collection. Specimens must be delivered to the testing site, and logged in with time received, as soon as possible after collection so that testing can be done within the accepted time limits. Specimens that cannot be tested within an hour of collection should be stored in the dark with lid on at 4°C to 6°C until tested.

Midstream Urine Samples

Specimens for routine urinalysis should be collected by the midstream method. The patient should be instructed to begin voiding into the toilet and then to interrupt the urine stream to collect only the middle portion of the urine stream in the specimen container. Using this method prevents contaminating the specimen with epithelial cells, microorganisms, or mucus from the urethra. This method is used for first morning, fasting, random, and timed specimens.

Clean-Catch Urine Samples

A clean-catch urine specimen is required if urine is to be cultured for bacteria. If the specimen is also to be used for routine urinalysis, the culture must be set up first to avoid any chance of compromising specimen sterility during the routine urinalysis procedure.

Hospitals and physician offices will provide the patient with a kit containing towelettes and a sterile urine container (Figure

5-5). Patients should be instructed to cleanse the urethral opening and carefully collect the urine specimen using the mid-stream collection method. Instructions, written or pictorial and understandable to all patients, must be available and should also be posted in the restroom near the toilet.

Instructions to the Male Patient

The male patient should retract the penis foreskin (if not circumcised), using a towelette. A second towelette should be used to cleanse the urethral opening with a single stroke directed from the tip of the penis toward the ring of the glans. The towelette should then be discarded and the cleansing procedure repeated using two more towelettes.

The patient should begin to void into the toilet. The urine stream should be interrupted to collect only the middle portion of the urine flow in the supplied container.

After the specimen has been collected, the lid should be placed securely on the container, avoiding touching the inside of the container or the lid. The information on the label should be completed and attached to the specimen container.

Instructions to the Female Patient

The female patient should position herself comfortably on the toilet seat and swing one knee to the side as far as possible. She should spread the outer vulval folds (labia majora) using a towelette and wipe the inner side of one inner fold (labium minora) with a towelette, using a single stroke from front to back. The towelette should then be discarded and a second towelette used to repeat the procedure on the opposite side. A third towelette should be used to cleanse the urethral opening with a single front-to-back stroke.

The patient should then begin to void into the toilet. The urine stream should be interrupted to collect only the middle portion of the urine flow in a container. Touching only the outside of the container and the lid, the patient should close the container securely, complete the label, and attach it to the container. If the patient has vaginal discharge, a clean tampon should be inserted before collection to decrease the possibility of specimen contamination.

Drug Screens

Urine drug screens can be required in a number of situations, such as participation in athletic events, job applications, or cases of suspected drug abuse. Although a random urine specimen is used for drug screens, much documentation is required to guarantee the reliability of the collection procedure and the identity of the person submitting the specimen. Each laboratory that handles specimens for drug abuse screening must follow a written protocol, which will be detailed in the laboratory's SOP manual. Chain-of-custody of the specimen must be documented; this is to safeguard against possible tampering and to guarantee the specimen's integrity. Some requirements likely to be included in a protocol for urine drug-screen collection are:

- Photo identification verified
- Signed consent of patient/donor obtained

- Use of special collection kits provided to the patient by the laboratory
- Inspection of bathroom before and after collection, with a monitor stationed outside during collection
- Urine temperature measured and recorded immediately after collection
- Specimen labeled in presence of donor, sealed in outer container, and secured under lock until transported to testing agency.

Twenty-Four-Hour Urine Specimens

The collection procedure for a 24-hour urine specimen must be followed carefully for test results on the specimen to be meaningful. The laboratory must provide to the patient a collection container and verbal and written instructions describing how to properly collect the specimen.

Specimen Containers

The laboratory must provide a 3 to 4 L capacity collection container with appropriate preservative for the test to be performed (Figure 5-6). Laboratory personnel should consult the SOP manual for a list of tests that can be performed on 24-hour urines, the preservative (if any) required for each, and the temperature at which the specimen should be stored during the 24-hour collection period. Most tests suggest storing the specimen at 4°C to 6°C (refrigerated). If preservative is used, the patient should be provided written safety information, such as the MSDS, explaining any hazards associated with exposure to the preservative.

Instructions to the Patient

Twenty-four-hour urine specimens must contain all the urine excreted by the patient in a 24-hour period. Collection usually begins at a designated morning hour, for example, 8 AM. The patient should be instructed to completely empty the bladder by voiding into the toilet at 8 AM on the day collection begins. *This urine is not included in the 24-hour collection.* The patient should then collect ALL urine produced until 8 AM the following morning. Urine can be collected in a small container and then carefully transferred to the large 24-hour urine container. At 8 AM on the day after collection began (24 hours later), the patient should empty the bladder and add this urine to the 24-hour container. The container should then be delivered to the laboratory. An example of a patient instruction card is shown in Figure 5-7.

Measuring Urine Volume

When a routine urinalysis is performed, the volume of the specimen is usually not recorded. However, the volume of a 24-hour urine specimen must be carefully measured and recorded because the volume measurement is used in calculating the test results.

The specimen volume is measured using a large graduated cylinder, and the urine is returned to its container. The total volume must be recorded on the specimen label and the accompanying requisition form.

Instructions for 24-Hour Urine Collection

Patient Name_____   Date_____

Your physician has ordered a 24-hour urine test. For this test, urine is usually collected from the morning of one day until the same time the next day (for example, from 8 AM one day to 8 AM the following day). It is important that you carefully follow these instructions:

1.   To begin the collection, *void into the toilet* as usual and note the time. DO NOT SAVE THIS URINE.

2.   Collect ALL urine the next time you void, and ALL urine after that for 24 hours. Each time you urinate, collect the urine into a specimen cup and transfer the entire amount to the 24-hour container given to you.

3.   At 24 hours from the beginning of the test (the morning of the second day), empty your bladder and add this urine to the 24-hour container.

4.   Bring all the urine in the collection container to the laboratory the morning of the second day.

Additional instructions:
- Time the test to end on a day when the laboratory is open to receive the specimen
- Keep the 24-hour urine container tightly capped during the collection period
- Once urine collection begins, store the 24-hour urine container:
  - ☐ At room temperature
  - ☐ In the refrigerator

If you have any questions about this procedure, please contact the laboratory at 555-1234.

FIGURE 5-7   Sample patient instruction card for collecting a 24-hour urine specimen

TABLE 5-5. Reference ranges for 24-hour urine volumes

AGE	VOLUME (mL/24 HOURS)
Newborn	20–350
One year	300–600
Ten years	750–1,500
Adult	750–2,000

Reference Ranges for 24-Hour Urine Volumes

Several factors influence urine volume. These include fluid intake, diet, fluid lost in exhalation and perspiration, hormone levels, and the status of renal and cardiac functions. Excessive production of urine is called **polyuria**. **Oliguria** is insufficient production of urine, and **anuria** is absence of urine production. The term **nocturia** refers to excessive production of urine at night.

The volume of urine normally excreted in 24 hours varies according to age. Newborns produce between 20 and 350 mL in 24 hours. By the age of one year, 300 to 600 mL/24 hours is normal. For 10-year-olds, the 24-hour urine volume can range from 750 to 1,500 mL. Adults produce from 750 to 2,000 mL in 24 hours, with 1,500 mL being average (Table 5-5).

SAFETY Reminders

- Use Standard Precautions when handling urine specimens.
- Use appropriate work practice controls when handling urine preservatives.
- Wear gloves, eye protection, and buttoned, fluid-resistant laboratory coat.
- Avoid creating splashes or aerosols when disposing of urine specimens.
- Clean all spills with surface disinfectant.

PROCEDURAL Reminders

- Be sure the patient understands the collection procedure for the test that has been ordered.
- Check to see that the specimen is correctly labeled with patient's name, time and date of collection, and any other information required by the laboratory.
- Keep the lid on urine specimens until testing is performed.
- Store urine specimens at 4°C to 6°C for up to 4 hours if testing cannot be performed within 1 hour of collection.
- Culture clean-catch specimens *before* performing routine urinalysis.

C R I T I C A L   T H I N K I N G

A hospital laboratory employee working in urinalysis received a specimen for routine urinalysis at 2 PM. The collection time on the specimen label was 9:30 AM the same day. What would be the appropriate action for the laboratory employee?

C A S E   S T U D Y

On Thursday morning, Mr. Strickland, a healthy-appearing 62-year-old patient, brought a 24-hour urine specimen to the laboratory. He related that he had begun the collection on Wednesday morning and had just completed collection that morning. Alice, the laboratory technician, measured the urine volume and found it to be 550 mL.

1. This 24-hour urine volume is:
   a. Within the reference range
   b. Greater than the reference range
   c. Less than the reference range
2. The correct procedure for Alice to follow is:
   a. The urine volume is acceptable; Alice should forward the required volume of urine to chemistry for the 24-hour test to be performed.
   b. The urine volume is suspect, and Alice should question Mr. Strickland about how he collected the specimen.
   c. The urine volume is suspect, and Alice should call Mr. Strickland's physician's office and inquire whether any known condition could affect his urine volume.
   d. Both b and c are correct.

SUMMARY

The examination of a patient's urine can yield many results helpful to the physician in diagnosis and treatment. However, reliable laboratory test results cannot be achieved without properly collected specimens, and urine specimens are no exception. Requirements for urine collection differ slightly, depending on the test that is to be performed. A midstream specimen is preferred for all tests except 24-hour tests because external skin contaminants are minimized. First morning, random, and clean-catch specimens should all be collected midstream. When bacterial culture is to be performed, the urine specimen must be a clean-catch specimen. Urine collected over a 24-hour period is required for some quantitative chemical tests.

Collection procedures for all urine tests are detailed in the laboratory's SOP manual and must be strictly followed. Adherence to quality assessment guidelines for specimen collection, labeling, handling, transport, and storage ensures that the laboratory receives an acceptable specimen. Standard Precautions must be followed when handling urine as with all other body fluids.

REVIEW QUESTIONS

1. Why is proper urine collection important?
2. How is a clean-catch urine collected?
3. When is a clean-catch urine required?
4. What is a midstream urine specimen?
5. Describe the procedure for collecting a 24-hour urine specimen.
6. When is a urine preservative necessary?
7. Name three commonly used urine preservatives.
8. What is the major disadvantage of using preservatives in urine?
9. What is the normal 24-hour urine volume for newborns? One-year-olds? Adults?
10. How can improper collection of urine affect urinalysis test results?
11. Why is the first morning specimen preferred for routine urinalysis?
12. How does urine collection for drug screening differ from urine collection for routine urinalysis?
13. Why might a 24-hour urine test be ordered?
14. Define anuria, clean-catch urine, midstream urine, nocturia, oliguria, polyuria, and random urine specimen.

STUDENT ACTIVITIES

1. Complete the written examination for this lesson.
2. Design cards instructing male and female patients in collecting clean-catch urine specimens.
3. Practice giving instructions to male and female patients for collecting clean-catch urine samples, using the patient instruction cards.
4. Practice instructing a patient in the collection of a 24-hour urine specimen.

WEB ACTIVITIES

1. Use the Internet to find information about 24-hour urine tests from Web sites of hospitals or reference laboratories. Find out which 24-hour urine tests require the following preservatives: sodium hydroxide, hydrochloric acid, sodium carbonate, and boric acid.
2. Find MSDS information for each of the preservatives listed in Web Activity 1. For each, list the precautions that should be given patients who have containers with these preservatives.

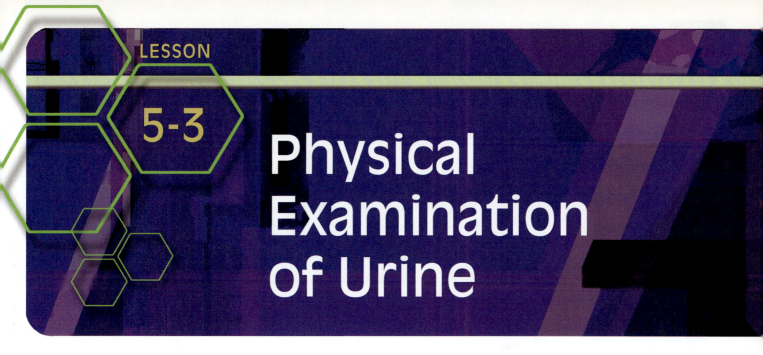

Physical Examination of Urine

LESSON OBJECTIVES

After studying this lesson, the student will:

- Name the physical characteristics of urine evaluated during a routine urinalysis.
- List three causes of abnormal urine odor.
- Explain why normal urine is yellow.
- List three abnormal urine colors and give a cause for each.
- List two conditions that can affect the appearance or transparency of urine.
- Explain what determines the specific gravity of urine.
- Demonstrate proper use of the urinometer and refractometer.
- Perform a physical examination of urine.
- Define the glossary terms.

GLOSSARY

hematuria / the presence of blood in the urine

ketones / a group of chemical substances produced during increased fat metabolism; ketone bodies

melanin / a dark pigment of skin, hair, and certain tumors

myoglobin / a pigmented, oxygen-carrying protein found in muscle tissue

opalescent / having a milky iridescence

porphyrins / a group of light-sensitive, pigmented, ringed chemical structures that are required for the synthesis of hemoglobin

refractometer / an instrument for measuring the refractive index of a substance

specific gravity / the ratio of the weight of a solution to the weight of an equal volume of distilled water; a measurement of density

turbid / having a cloudy appearance

urinometer / a float with a calibrated stem used for measuring specific gravity of urine; hydrometer

urochrome / the yellow pigment that gives urine its color

INTRODUCTION

A routine urinalysis consists of three parts—the physical, chemical, and microscopic examinations. This lesson covers the physical examination; the chemical and microscopic examinations are covered in Lessons 5-4 and 5-5.

The physical examination is the first part of the urinalysis performed and includes observing urine color and transparency and measuring the specific gravity. An example of a laboratory requisition form for a routine urinalysis is shown in Figure 5-8. The physical examination of urine is the easiest and quickest part of a routine urinalysis and can

---

Tri-Cities Family Health Clinic
Urinalysis Laboratory Request Form

Patient _____ Date_____

Ordering Physician_____

☐ Routine Urinalysis with Microscopic
☐ Dipstick Urinalysis
☐ Urine Culture and Sensitivity
☐ Other _____

Specimen Collection Time _____   ☐ a.m.   ☐ p.m.
Laboratory Log-in Time   _____   ☐ a.m.   ☐ p.m.

Results		**Reference**
Color	_____	yellow to amber
Transparency	_____	clear
Specific Gravity	_____	1.005-1.030

Dipstick:		
Glucose	_____	negative
Bilirubin	_____	negative
Ketone	_____	negative
Blood	_____	negative
pH	_____	4.5 – 8.0
Protein	_____	negative-trace
Urobilinogen	_____	0.2-1.0 mg/dL
Nitrite	_____	negative
Leukocyte	_____	negative

Microscopic:		
WBC/HPF	_____	0-4
RBC/HPF	_____	0-4
Epith. Cells	_____	occas, squamous
Casts	_____	occas, hyaline
Bacteria	_____	none
Mucus	_____	
Amorphous Sediment	_____	
Crystals	_____	
Type	_____	
Other	_____	

Tech: _____
Date: _____
Time: _____

FIGURE 5-8 Example of a urinalysis request form

be performed while the urine specimen is being prepared for other procedures.

PHYSICAL CHARACTERISTICS OF URINE

The physical characteristics of urine noted during urinalysis are color, transparency or clarity, specific gravity, and odor.

Color

The normal color of urine ranges from pale yellow to amber. Variations in color can be caused by diet, medications, physical activity, and disease (Table 5-6). Urine color can sometimes provide a clue to certain diseases or conditions.

Yellow Urine

The pigment that produces the normal yellow-to-amber color of urine is **urochrome**. As the urine concentration varies, so will the color intensity. Dilute urine samples are pale; more concentrated urine samples are darker yellow or amber.

Red Urine

The abnormal color seen most frequently in urine is red or red-brown. Cloudy red urine can be due to **hematuria**, the presence of blood. Clear red urine can be due to the presence of hemoglobin or **myoglobin**, a pigmented protein found in muscle tissue. Red blood cells, hemoglobin, and myoglobin form a red-brown color in acidic urine. **Porphyrins** can cause the urine to be red or wine-red.

Brown or Black Urine

Hemoglobin will become brown in acidic urine that has been standing. The presence of **melanin**, a dark pigment, will also cause urine to become dark or black on standing. This can occur in patients with advanced melanoma, a tumor of melanin-producing cells.

Yellow-Brown or Green-Brown Urine

Bilirubin or bile pigments cause urine to be dark yellow-brown or green-brown. Urine specimens containing these substances can form a yellow-green foam when shaken. Bilirubin can be present in the urine of patients with hepatitis.

Transparency (Clarity)

Fresh normal urine is usually clear immediately after voiding. As the urine reaches room temperature, or after refrigeration, it can become **turbid**, or cloudy. Depending on the pH of the urine, this cloudiness can be due to amorphous urates or phosphates (Table 5-7). The transparency of urine can give clues to possible problems. Clear urine usually has normal microscopic results; any abnormalities in a clear specimen are usually detected in the chemical examination. The cause of a cloudy or turbid urine specimen usually becomes evident during the microscopic examination.

Turbidity or cloudiness in a freshly voided urine sample can be an indication of disease. Four common causes of turbid urine are white and red blood cells, epithelial cells, and bacteria. Red blood cells in urine give it a cloudy, red appearance. Mucus in the urine also causes a cloudy appearance. Fats or lipids cause urine to appear **opalescent** (milky).

TABLE 5-6. Abnormal urine colors and their causes

COLORS CAUSED BY FOOD OR MEDICATIONS

Color	Cause
Red	Beets, rhubarb (in alkaline urine)
Yellow-orange	Carrots, vitamins, some antibiotics
Green, blue-green	Drugs such as amitryptiline
Brown-black	Methyldopa, metronidazole

COLORS CAUSED BY DISEASE STATES

Color	Cause
Red, red-brown	Red blood cells, hemoglobin, myoglobin
Wine-red	Porphyrins
Brown-black	Melanin, homogentisic acid, hemoglobin (in acid urine)
Dark yellow-brown or green-brown	Bilirubin, bile pigments

TABLE 5-7. Conditions affecting the transparency of urine

NORMAL URINES

Transparency	Causes
Hazy	Mucus (females), talcum powder, squamous epithelial cells
Cloudy	Calcium oxalate, uric acid crystals, amorphous phosphates, amorphous urates

ABNORMAL URINES

Transparency	Causes
Cloudy-red	Red blood cells
Turbid or cloudy	White blood cells, bacteria, yeasts, renal epithelial cells, lipids
Opalescent, milky	Fats, lipids

Odor

Normal, recently voided urine has a characteristic aromatic and not unpleasant odor. Changes in urine odor can be due to disease, diet, or the presence of microorganisms. Although urine odor is not usually reported on the urinalysis form, it is a noticeable property that can alert the technologist to possible abnormalities or improper handling of the urine specimen.

The odor of urine from a patient with uncontrolled diabetes is described as fruity. This is due to the presence of **ketones**, products of fat metabolism. Other metabolic diseases can also cause an unusual urine odor. *Phenylketonuria* (PKU), an inherited condition in which the amino acid phenylalanine is not metabolized, causes urine to have a mousy or musty odor. All newborns are tested for PKU because mental retardation will result if the condition is allowed to go untreated. *Maple syrup urine disease* is a rare metabolic condition in which the urine has the odor of maple syrup. This condition is evident in the first weeks of life of affected infants.

If urine is allowed to remain unrefrigerated for a few hours, any bacteria present can break down urea to form ammonia; the resulting urine odor is similar to ammonia. A recently voided sample of urine with a foul, pungent odor suggests urinary tract infection.

Foods such as garlic and asparagus can also produce an abnormal urine odor. Although urine odor may be striking in certain instances, odor alone is not a reliable enough characteristic to use in making a diagnosis.

Specific Gravity

The **specific gravity** (sp. gr.) of a solution is the ratio of the weight of the solution compared to the weight of an equal volume of distilled water at the same temperature. Stated another way, the specific gravity is the density of a solution compared to the density of distilled water, which is 1.000.

The range of specific gravity for normal urine is 1.005 to 1.030, with most samples falling between 1.010 and 1.025 (Table 5-8). Specific gravity is highest in the first morning specimen, which usually has a specific gravity greater than 1.020. The specific gravity of urine estimates the concentration of solutes such as urea, phosphates, chlorides, proteins, and sugars in the urine. The specific gravity is an indicator of renal tubular function; it is used to assess the ability of the kidneys to reabsorb essential chemicals and water from the glomerular filtrate.

TABLE 5-8. Physical characteristics of normal urine

CHARACTERISTIC	NORMAL URINE
Transparency	Clear
Color	Pale yellow to amber
Specific gravity	1.005 to 1.030

Darker urine samples are usually more concentrated than pale urine samples. Patients who are dehydrated may have highly concentrated urine with high specific gravity.

PERFORMING A PHYSICAL EXAMINATION OF URINE

Safety Precautions

 Standard Precautions must be observed when handling urine and all other body substances. Gloves, face protection, and other appropriate personal protective equipment (PPE) must be worn. Since some infectious agents, such as the hepatitis virus, can be present in urine, all urine specimens must be handled with caution to prevent possible exposure of laboratory personnel. Specimens can be discarded in a sink, followed by water and disinfectant, but the creation of aerosols or splashes must be avoided. Urinometers must be disinfected with surface disinfectant after use. Refractometers should be disinfected by placing a small amount of 10% chlorine bleach solution on the surface of the glass plate and cover and wiping dry.

Quality Assessment

 Only properly collected specimens should be accepted for testing by laboratory personnel. Specimens that cannot be tested immediately after collection can be refrigerated for up to 4 hours. Before testing, urines should be allowed to reach ambient temperature (21°C to 25°C) and should be mixed well by gentle swirling. Refractometers and urinometers must be checked at specified intervals with distilled water (specific gravity, 1.000) and control solutions, and the results should be documented.

Specimen Preparation

Physical characteristics are best observed by examining a urine sample immediately after voiding before the sample is refrigerated. If the urine cannot be examined within 1 hour after collection, it can be refrigerated at 4°C for up to 4 hours but should be allowed to reach room temperature before the urinalysis is performed.

Procedure

The urine specimen is mixed well by gentle swirling, a portion is poured into a clear tube, and the urine is observed for color and transparency. The specific gravity of the urine is measured, and the urine is then used for chemical and microscopic examination. The physical characteristics of normal urine are given in Table 5-8.

Color and Transparency

Urine color is observed and recorded as pale (or straw), yellow, amber, or other. The urine should be observed for transparency (clarity) using good light. Transparency is usually reported as clear, hazy (slightly cloudy), cloudy (turbid), or milky (opalescent).

Measurement of Specific Gravity

Specific gravity can be measured with a urinometer, refractometer, or reagent strip. The urinometer method requires 20 to 50 mL of urine, depending on the size of the urinometer. The refractometer method requires only a drop of urine. Measurement of specific gravity with a reagent strip is included in Lesson 5-4, Chemical Examination of Urine.

Urinometer Method. Well-mixed urine is poured into a special glass cylinder, and the **urinometer**, a weighted float with a calibrated stem, is placed in the urine with a slight spinning motion (Figure 5-9). The specific gravity is read at the urine's meniscus on the float's stem. The urinometer will float high in a concentrated sample (high sp. gr.) and will sink lower in a dilute sample (low sp. gr.). A disadvantage of this method is the large urine volume required and the need to disinfect cylinder and urinometer.

Refractometer Method. A **refractometer**, sometimes called a *total solids meter* (TS meter), measures specific gravity optically by measuring the refractive index of the urine. The refractive index is the ratio of the speed of light in air to the speed of light in a solution.

To use the refractometer, one drop of well-mixed urine is placed on the glass plate and the cover is gently closed (Figure 5-10). While one looks through the ocular, the specific gravity is read directly from a scale that converts refraction to specific gravity (Figure 5-11).

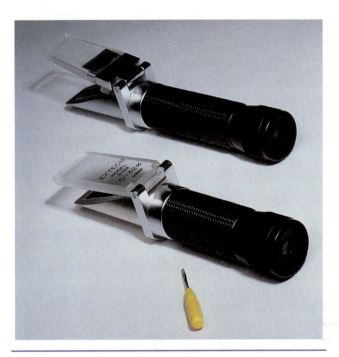

FIGURE 5-10 Refractometers

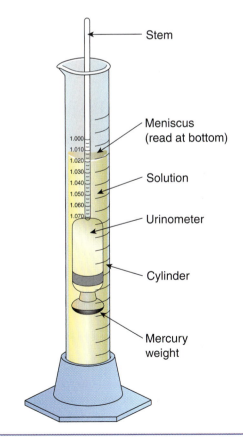

FIGURE 5-9 Urinometer used for specific gravity measurement

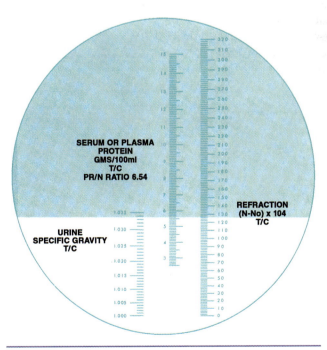

FIGURE 5-11 Refractometer scale showing a specific gravity reading of 1.034. The small scale (lower left) is used to read the urine specific gravity (*Courtesy of Leica, Inc., Buffalo, NY*)

SAFETY Reminders

- Review safety precautions before performing procedure
- Observe Standard Precautions when handling urine specimens and other body fluids.
- Wear gloves, face protection, and other appropriate PPE.
- Wipe up all urine spills with surface disinfectant.
- Use appropriate exposure control methods when handling and discarding urine specimens to avoid potential exposure to infectious agents.

PROCEDURAL Reminders

- Review quality assessment section before performing procedure.
- Test only properly collected specimens.
- Allow refrigerated specimens to reach room temperature before testing.
- Mix urine gently and thoroughly before making physical observations.
- Test refractometer or urinometer daily with distilled water and urine control

CASE STUDY 1

A urine specimen from a 48-year-old woman was received in the urinalysis laboratory at 9 AM. The specimen label indicated the urine was collected that morning at 8:30 AM, and the laboratory log-in time was 8:46 AM. While preparing the specimen for urinalysis, the technician noticed that the urine had a strong, unpleasant odor and was very cloudy.

What could be the cause of these findings?

CASE STUDY 2

A urine specimen submitted from a patient suffering from severe vomiting and diarrhea was a dark amber color.

1. This color is most likely due to:
   a. Myoglobin in the urine
   b. White blood cells in the urine
   c. High specific gravity of the urine
   d. Bilirubin in the urine
2. Explain your answer.

SUMMARY

The physical examination of urine includes observations of color, transparency, and odor, and measurement of specific gravity. The results of the physical examination of urine often confirm or explain chemical or microscopic results. Abnormalities in the physical characteristics of urine can also provide significant clues to renal or metabolic disease. However, variations in characteristics such as color or transparency do not always reflect pathologic changes. Sometimes these variations are caused by incorrect handling of the specimen, such as improper storage temperature or delay in examination. Standard Precautions must be observed when performing physical examination of urine.

REVIEW QUESTIONS

1. What observations are included in the physical examination of urine?

2. Name three metabolic conditions in which abnormal urine odor can occur.

3. If a urine smells like ammonia, what should be suspected?

4. What gives urine its normal color?

5. Name four abnormal urine colors and list a possible cause for each.

6. What is the normal transparency of urine?

7. What are three causes of cloudy urine?

8. What is the normal specific gravity of urine?

9. What kidney function is reflected by urine specific gravity?

10. Define hematuria, ketones, melanin, myoglobin, opalescent, porphyrins, refractometer, specific gravity, turbid, urinometer, and urochrome.

STUDENT ACTIVITIES

1. Complete the written examination for this lesson.

2. Practice performing physical examinations of several urine specimens as outlined in the Student Performance Guide, using the worksheet.

3. Obtain several urine samples. Compare the specific gravities of lighter-colored urines with those of darker-colored urines.

4. Divide a urine sample. Put one part in the refrigerator; place the other part on the counter at room temperature. Observe each for transparency changes and odor changes at the end of 1 hour, 2 hours, or more.

W E B 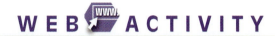 A C T I V I T Y

Report on one topic from this list: myoglobinuria, porphyria, pyuria, glomerulonephritis, or tubular necrosis. Use the Internet to search for information on your topic. Report on the condition, listing causes, symptoms, and expected findings in the physical portion of the urinalysis (urine color, transparency, and specific gravity).

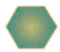

Student Performance Guide

LESSON 5-3 Physical Examination of Urine

Name _____ Date _____

INSTRUCTIONS

1. Practice the procedure for performing a physical examination of urine following the step-by-step procedure and using the worksheet.

2. Demonstrate the procedure for the physical examination of urine satisfactorily for the instructor, using the Student Performance Guide. Your instructor will determine the level of competency you must achieve to obtain a satisfactory (S) grade.

NOTE: Consult manufacturers' directions before using instruments or performing tests.

MATERIALS AND EQUIPMENT

- gloves
- face protection or acrylic safety shield
- antiseptic
- clear plastic conical centrifuge tubes
- test tube rack
- recently collected urine sample
- disposable transfer pipets
- refractometer and/or urinometer
- distilled water
- urinalysis worksheet or report form (p. 498)
- laboratory tissue or paper towels
- biohazard container
- surface disinfectant
- urine control solutions

PROCEDURE

Record in the comment section any problems encountered while practicing the procedure (or have a fellow student or the instructor evaluate your performance).

S = Satisfactory
U = Unsatisfactory

You must:	S	U	Comments
1. Assemble equipment and materials. Put on face shield or place acrylic safety shield in position			
2. Wash hands and put on gloves			
3. Obtain a recently collected urine specimen. If specimen has been refrigerated, allow it to reach room temperature before proceeding with tests. (Perform procedure behind shield if not wearing face protection)			
4. Record the specimen identification on the worksheet (or report form)			
5. Mix the urine gently by swirling and pour approximately 10 mL into a clear, conical centrifuge tube			

463

You must:	S	U	Comments
6. Observe the color of the urine and record on the worksheet			
7. Notice the odor of the urine. If unusual, record in comment section			
8. Observe and record the transparency of the urine			

9. Measure specific gravity using the refractometer:
  a. Place one drop of distilled water on the glass plate of the refractometer and close gently
  b. Look through ocular and read the specific gravity from the scale. For water, the specific gravity should read 1.000. (If it does not, calibrate with the screwdriver provided with the refractometer)
  c. Clean the glass plate, place one drop of urine control solution on the plate and close gently
  d. Look through the ocular, read the specific gravity from the scale, and record the control value
  e. Clean the glass plate with disinfectant and dry with a laboratory tissue
  f. Repeat steps 9c through 9e with a urine specimen, and record the result on the worksheet			

10. Measure specific gravity using the urinometer. (If urinometer is not available, go to step 11)
  a. Pour 40 to 50 mL of distilled water into the glass cylinder (approximately three-fourths full)
  b. Insert urinometer, with gentle spinning motion
  c. Read the specific gravity from the scale on the stem of the urinometer when it stops spinning and record (Specific gravity of water should be 1.000)
  d. Rinse equipment and dry with laboratory tissue and repeat 10a through 10c with a urine specimen and record the result
  e. Disinfect urinometer and cylinder			

11. Discard urine sample properly or save specimen for chemical examination, Lesson 5-4			
12. Disinfect and clean equipment and return to proper storage			
13. Clean work area with disinfectant			
14. Remove and discard gloves into biohazard container			
15. Wash hands with antiseptic			

Evaluator Comments:

Evaluator _____ Date _____

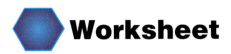 **Worksheet**

LESSON 5-3 Physical Examination of Urine

Name _____ Date _____

Specimen I.D. _____

OBSERVATION	RESULT	NORMAL CONTROL	ABNORMAL CONTROL	REFERENCE VALUES
1. Transparency (appearance)	_____ clear	_____	_____	clear
	_____ hazy (slightly cloudy)	_____	_____	
	_____ cloudy (turbid)	_____	_____	
	_____ milky (opalescent)	_____	_____	
	_____ other	_____	_____	
2. Color:	_____	_____	_____	pale yellow to amber
3. Specific gravity:	_____	_____	_____	1.005–1.030

Comment: _____

_____

_____

_____

_____

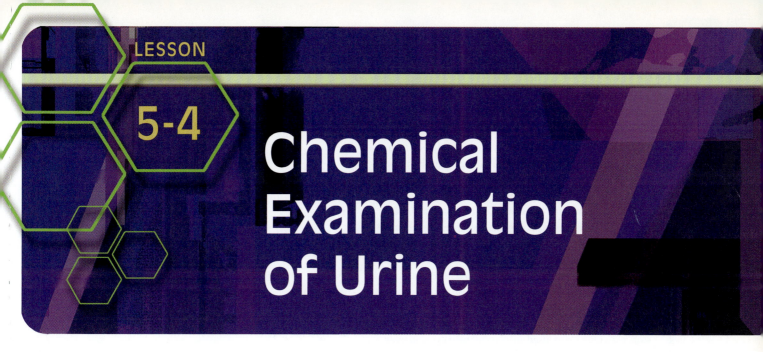

Chemical Examination of Urine

LESSON OBJECTIVES

After studying this lesson, the student will:

- Name 10 urine chemical tests routinely performed by reagent strip and explain the principle of each.
- Give the reference values for the 10 urine chemical tests.
- Explain the specimen requirement for the chemical examination of urine.
- Explain the importance of quality assessment procedures in the chemical examination of urine.
- Use a reagent strip for the chemical examination of urine and interpret the results.
- List a condition that can cause an abnormal result in each of the chemical tests routinely performed on urine.
- Perform the copper reduction test on urine.
- Discuss the safety precautions that must be observed in chemical testing of urine.
- Perform confirmatory tests for protein, ketones, and bilirubin in urine.
- Define the glossary terms.

GLOSSARY

albumin / the most abundant protein in normal plasma; a homogeneous group of plasma proteins that are made in the liver and help maintain osmotic balance

bilirubin / a product formed in the liver from the breakdown of hemoglobin

chromogen / a substance that becomes colored when it undergoes a chemical change

glycosuria / glucose in the urine; glucosuria

hematuria / presence of blood in the urine

ketonuria / ketones in the urine

microalbumin / small amount of albumin in urine, not detectable by routine reagent strip

microalbuminuria / condition in which small amounts of albumin are present in the urine

proteinuria / protein in the urine, usually albumin

urobilinogen / breakdown product of bilirubin formed by the action of intestinal bacteria

UTI / urinary tract infection

INTRODUCTION

Several biochemical tests can be performed quickly and easily on urine using reagent strip methods. Reagent strip analysis is called the chemical, biochemical, or analyte analysis of urine. Chemical testing by reagent strip is included in a routine urinalysis. It can also be ordered as a test to be performed alone, without the urine physical and microscopic examinations. Chemical analysis of urine by reagent strip method is a CLIA-waived procedure.

Reagent strips, thin plastic strips with reagent pads attached, are used by dipping the reagent strip in urine and observing chemical reactions on each reagent pad within a specified time. Reagent strips are available in a variety of types. Two common brands of urine reagent strips are the Multistix line (Siemens Medical, formerly Bayer Corp.) and Chemstrip (Roche Diagnostics Corp.).

One reagent strip can test for as many as 10 different substances while others are available that test for only one or two substances or analytes. Strips used in routine urinalysis usually include tests for acid-base balance (pH), protein, bilirubin, blood, nitrite, ketones, urobilinogen, glucose, leukocyte esterase, and sometimes specific gravity.

The results of chemical analysis of urine provide information on the patient's carbohydrate metabolism, kidney and liver function, and pH balance. In some situations, urine chemical test results are critical to diagnosis. This lesson presents the principles and methods of chemical analysis of urine using reagent strips. Procedures for performing the test for reducing sugars and confirmatory tests for protein, ketones, and bilirubin are also given.

PRINCIPLES OF URINE CHEMICAL TESTS BY REAGENT STRIP

Urine reagent strips, sometimes called dipsticks, are single-use plastic strips to which reagent pads have been attached. Each reagent pad contains chemicals required for a specific chemical reaction.

When the strips are dipped into a urine specimen, the chemicals within the reagent pads react rapidly with substances in the urine to form color changes in the pads (Figures 5-12 and 5-13).

In routine urinalysis, the reagent strips commonly used test up to 10 parameters:

- Glucose
- Bilirubin
- Ketones
- Blood
- pH
- Protein
- Urobilinogen
- Nitrite
- Leukocyte esterase
- Specific gravity

Basic principles of the biochemical reactions involved in each of the 10 tests above are discussed briefly in this section. However, since reagent strip manufacturers might use slightly different biochemical detection methods in their strips, the manufacturer's instructions must be consulted to determine the proper procedure for, and the specific chemical principles of, the test strip being used.

Glucose

The presence of detectable glucose in urine is called **glycosuria**, and indicates that the blood glucose level has exceeded the renal threshold for glucose. This condition can occur in diabetes mellitus and in gestational diabetes. The presence of glucose in urine can be an indication that diabetes is not under good control.

The reagent strip is specific for glucose and will not react with other sugars. The glucose reagent pad contains the enzymes glucose oxidase and peroxidase plus a **chromogen**, a substance that produces a color in the chemical reaction. These enzymes react with glucose in the urine to change the color of the reagent pad. The intensity of the color formed is proportional to the glucose concentration. Normal urine is negative for glucose by the reagent strip method.

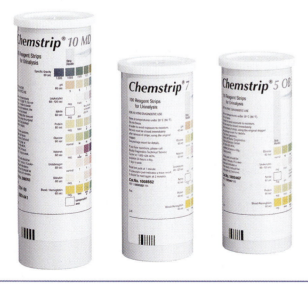

FIGURE 5-12 Chemstrip urine reagent strips
(*Courtesy Roche Diagnostics Corp., Indianapolis, IN*)

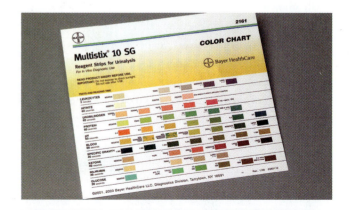

FIGURE 5-13 Bayer Multistix 10 SG color chart for urine reagent strips

Bilirubin

Bilirubin is the primary bile pigment. Bilirubin is a hemoglobin breakdown product formed in the liver from senescent (old) red blood cells. When bilirubin is present in urine, it can indicate liver disease, bile duct obstruction, or hepatitis. The test for bilirubin is based on coupling bilirubin with a diazonium salt in the reagent pad to form a purple-brown color. Direct light causes decomposition of bilirubin so specimens should be protected from light until testing is completed to prevent false-negative results. Normal urine contains no detectable bilirubin by the reagent strip method.

Ketones

When the body burns fat rather than sugar for energy, a group of molecules called ketones are produced. Ketones include acetone, acetoacetic acid, and beta-hydroxybutyric acid. In uncontrolled diabetes, starvation, or prolonged dieting or fasting, ketones are excreted into the urine, a condition called **ketonuria**. The reagent strip pads for ketones detect acetoacetic acid and/or acetone.

The ketone test is based on the reaction of ketones with sodium nitroferricyanide in the ketone reagent pad, causing the formation of a dark pink to maroon color. Since ketones evaporate at room temperature, urine should be kept tightly capped and refrigerated if it cannot be tested promptly. Normal urine is negative for ketones when tested by reagent strip.

Blood

The presence of blood in the urine is called **hematuria**. It can occur in conditions such as infection, trauma to the urinary tract, bleeding in the kidneys, glomerular damage, or tumor. Blood cells can also contaminate urine due to menstruation, or trauma from catheter insertion. The blood reagent pad detects both hemoglobin and intact red blood cells. In the presence of either, a color forms because of the peroxidase-like action of hemoglobin in the red blood cells reacting with chromogen and peroxide in the reagent pad. The resulting color ranges from orange through green to dark blue. Intact red blood cells can cause a spotty appearance on the reagent pad. Myoglobin will also cause a positive reaction on the reagent strip. Normal urine is negative for blood by reagent strip method.

pH

The pH is a measure of the degree of acidity or alkalinity of the urine. A pH below seven indicates an acid urine; a pH above seven indicates alkaline urine. The pH of urine changes with diet, medications, kidney disease, and metabolic diseases such as diabetes mellitus. Indicator dyes such as methyl red and bromthymol blue in the pH reagent pad form colors from yellow-orange for acid urine to green-blue for alkaline urine. Normal, freshly voided urine has a pH range of 4.5 to 8.0.

Protein

The condition in which an increased amount of protein is present in the urine is called **proteinuria**. Proteinuria is an important indicator of renal disease but can also be caused by vigorous exercise or conditions such as urinary tract infection, commonly called **UTI**. Positive tests for protein in urine are usually due to the presence of **albumin**, the most abundant plasma protein. Since the protein reagent pad is not a good detector of globulins, the protein sulfosalicylic acid turbidity test, discussed later in this lesson, should be used if proteins other than albumin are suspected.

The reagent strip test for protein is based on the principle that proteins can alter the color of some acid-base indicator dyes without changing the pH. The protein reagent pad is kept at pH 3 with a buffering dye such as tetrabromphenol blue. At the constant acid pH, the development of any green color on the reagent pad is due to the presence of protein (albumin) and is usually reported using a plus system (Neg, 1+, 2+, 3+, 4+). Colors range from yellow for negative to yellow-green or green for positive, depending on the amount of protein present. Normal urine is negative or contains just a trace of protein by the reagent strip method.

Urobilinogen

Urobilinogen is a bilirubin degradation product that is formed by the action of intestinal bacteria. Urobilinogen can be increased in hepatic disease or hemolytic disease. The urobilinogen reagent pad contains chemicals that react with urobilinogen to form a pink-red color, based on the Ehrlich aldehyde reaction. Since urobilinogen is unstable in light and in acidic urine, negative results on routine specimens are not considered significant. The reagent strip method can detect urobilinogen in concentrations as low as 0.1 mg/dL (0.1 EU, Ehrlich unit). The urobilinogen level is normally 0.1 to 1.0 mg/dL (or 0.1 to 1.0 EU/dL) of urine by the reagent strip method.

Nitrite

Gram-negative bacteria produce enzymes that convert urinary nitrate (a normal urine constituent) to nitrite. Nitrite reacts with chemicals in the nitrite reagent pad to form a pink color. A positive nitrite test is an indication of possible bacterial UTI. However, since not all bacteria can convert nitrates, a negative result is possible in the presence of infection. Examples of organisms that frequently cause UTI and cause a positive nitrite test are *Escherichia coli, Klebsiella, Proteus,* and *Pseudomonas.* Normal urine is negative for nitrite by the reagent strip method.

Leukocyte Esterase

Granular leukocytes, primarily neutrophils, contain an enzyme called leukocyte esterase. The presence of this enzyme in urine indicates the presence of leukocytes in urine, usually due to infection or inflammation in the urinary tract. The esterase enzyme reacts with esterase substrate in the leukocyte esterase reagent pad to form a purple color. The color intensity is proportional to the number of leukocytes present. Normal urine is negative for leukocyte esterase by the reagent strip method.

Specific Gravity

The specific gravity of urine reflects the kidneys' ability to concentrate urine. The specific gravity reagent pad contains an indicator that changes color from blue-green to green to yellow-green depending on the urine ion concentration. Specific gravities between 1.000 and 1.030 can be measured. Alkaline urines can give a false low value and should be checked by another method. The normal specific gravity of urine is 1.005 to 1.030 by reagent strip method.

REFERENCE VALUES BY REAGENT STRIP

Normal urine, when tested with a reagent strip, is negative for glucose, ketone, bilirubin, bacteria (nitrite), leukocyte esterase, and blood (see Table 5-9). Normal urine may be negative for protein or contain a trace of protein. Normal, recently voided urine usually has a pH of 4.5 to 8.0 and a specific gravity between 1.005 and 1.030.

Positive or abnormal results should be confirmed according to laboratory policy. Some test results are confirmed by retesting with a single analyte strip or a different brand of strip. Other results must be confirmed using nonreagent strip confirmatory tests. Positive leukocyte esterase or nitrite tests should be confirmed by microscopic examination of urine sediment.

SINGLE ANALYTE AND SPECIAL REAGENT STRIPS

Reagent strips that test only for one or two constituents of interest, such as glucose or ketones, are useful in certain cases. Examples of these are Diastix and Clinistix, which can be used at home to monitor urine glucose. The Ketostix strips only test for ketones, and the Keto-Diastix strips test for ketones and glucose on the same strip.

The Multistix PRO line of strips is particularly useful for detecting or monitoring kidney disease and complications from diabetes mellitus. The strips measure creatinine levels as well as protein, allowing calculation of the protein:creatinine ratio, a value that previously was only possible by testing a 24-hour urine. Clinitek Microalbumin strips detect **microalbumin**, protein in the urine in amounts too small to be detected with a routine urine reagent strip. **Microalbuminuria**, the condition in which very small amounts of albumin are present in the urine, is an indicator of early renal disease or damage and can occur as a complication of diabetes.

PERFORMING CHEMICAL TESTS BY REAGENT STRIP

Directions for the use of reagent strips and a color comparison chart are included with each vial. These instructions must be followed precisely for accurate results. The instructions also give information about potential causes of interference for each test on the strip. The technician should be familiar with these before performing the test and reporting results.

Safety Precautions

 Standard Precautions must be used when performing all urinalysis procedures. Since urine is a body fluid, all urine specimens must be considered potential biological hazards. Urine specimens often require more handling than other laboratory specimens, such as swirling to mix and pouring. An acrylic safety shield or face shield should be used to prevent splashes to the eyes or other mucus membranes. Gloves must be worn and hands must be washed with antiseptic after gloves are removed.

Care must be taken to avoid spills, splashes, and creation of aerosols. In addition, the test for reducing substances and some confirmatory tests present chemical hazards because they require the use of acids or caustic reagents. Chemical-resistant gloves should be worn when performing the Clinitest or protein confirmatory test. The rules of the institution must be followed for specimen disposal.

Quality Assessment

Adherence to a comprehensive quality assessment (QA) program ensures that the results from the chemical analysis of urine are reliable. The QA program must encompass all procedures, from specimen collection to reporting results.

Specimen Collection and Storage

It is essential that specimens be collected and labeled correctly, stored properly, and tested within the required time limits to prevent deterioration of urine components. A recently collected midstream specimen is preferred. Testing should be performed within 1 hour of collection. If the test cannot be performed within this time, the specimen can be refrigerated up to 4 hours.

TABLE 5-9. Reference values for urine chemical tests using reagent strips

SUBSTANCE TESTED	REFERENCE VALUE
Glucose	Negative
Bilirubin	Negative
Ketones	Negative
Blood	Negative
pH	4.5–8.0
Protein	Negative to trace
Urobilinogen	0.1 to 1.0 mg/dL
Bacteria (nitrite)	Negative
Leukocyte esterase	Negative
Specific gravity	1.005 to 1.030

Refrigerated specimens should be allowed to reach room temperature before testing. Because some urine components are volatile, labile, or light-sensitive, specimens should remain tightly covered and in the dark until tested.

Reagent Strips

Although reagent strip testing appears quick and easy, many factors must be kept in mind to ensure that reported results are valid. Individual manufacturer's directions for proper storage, use, timing of reactions, and interpretation of results must be followed since these can vary with the brand of strip used. Reagent strips must be stored at room temperature in their original air-tight container and protected from light, heat, and moisture. Strips must not be used after the expiration date and are used only once and then discarded. Specimens must be mixed well before using the reagent strip to be sure the reagent pads will be exposed to any solid components that may settle out, such as blood cells. Since manual tests are interpreted visually using a color comparison chart, technicians must pass a color blindness test before being allowed to perform and report manual urine reagent strip results.

Urine Controls

The reliability of urine test materials such as reagent strips and confirmatory test reagents is validated by using urine chemistry controls. Examples of urine control solutions are qUAntify by Hematronix, Inc. and KOVA-Trol from Hycor Biomedical, Inc. Urine controls should be run and results recorded at least once each shift (or day) that urine tests are performed. Commercial normal (negative), low abnormal, and high abnormal controls should be used. In addition, controls must be run when a new container of strips is opened and any other time the technician has reason to question the strip integrity. The results of these controls must be within the manufacturer's stated ranges before patient results can be reported. When the control results fall outside the specified ranges, the control should be retested using a new reagent strip. If that result is also out of range, a strip from a new vial and/or a new control should be tested. Patient results should not be reported until the discrepancy's cause is identified.

Manual Method

Testing is performed by quickly dipping a reagent strip into recently collected, well-mixed urine (Figure 5-14A). The excess urine is removed by touching the edge of the urine container with the strip as it is withdrawn from the urine. Timing of reactions should begin at this point. The edge of the strip should be quickly blotted on absorbent paper and the test areas observed at the manufacturer's specified time intervals. The color changes on the reagent pads must be visually compared to the color chart provided with the strips and the results recorded (Figures 5-13 and 5-14).

Reagent Strip Readers

Many laboratories use strip readers to interpret the results of urine reagent strip tests (Figures 5-15 and 5-16). These readers

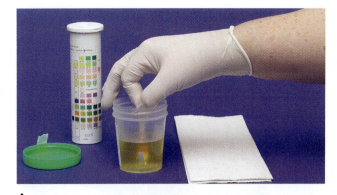

A

B

C

FIGURE 5-14 Chemical testing of urine by reagent strip: (A) hold the reagent strip by the top end and dip the strip into the urine specimen; (B) remove the strip from the urine, blot edge of strip to remove excess urine, and begin timer; (C) read reactions at appropriate time intervals by comparing reagent pad colors to color chart

contain reflectance photometers that detect the colors formed on the reagent pads when urine reacts with the various reagents. The technician can read the results from the instrument display screen or the results can be printed out. Reagent strip readers reduce errors caused by incorrect timing of reactions or incorrect interpretation of colors.

Some reagent strip readers are semi-automated or automated and can process several patient samples in a short time. These readers are ideal for higher volume POLs, hospital laboratories, and reference laboratories. One example

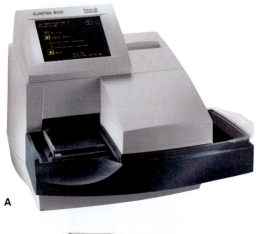

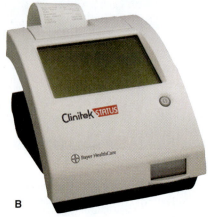

FIGURE 5-15 Clinitek urine strip readers for high and low volume laboratories: (A) Clinitek 500; (B) Clinitek Status (*Courtesy Bayer HealthCare Diagnostics Division, Norwood MA*)

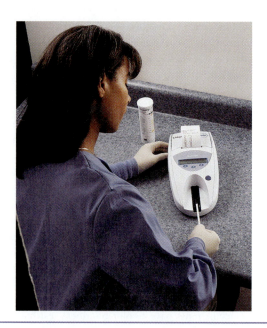

FIGURE 5-16 Urysis 1100 Analyzer (*Courtesy Roche Diagnostics Corp., Indianapolis, IN*)

is the Clinitek 500 (Figure 5-15A, from Bayer Healthcare Diagnostics Division, now Siemens Medical Solutions Diagnostics). The Clinitek 500 uses a handheld barcode reader to identify the specimen and to determine the urine color and clarity. Samples can be processed every 7 seconds and results can be uploaded to the central laboratory computer system. In semi-automated readers such as the Criterion II from Roche Diagnostics, the technician applies the urine to the reagent strip and places the strip in the tray. The technician enters the patient identification and the urine color and clarity into the database. The strip is then taken into the reader and the colors of the chemical reactions or endpoints are measured by reflectance photometry. The results are printed out when the analysis is complete. Another reagent strip reader, the Clinitek Status, can also read microalbumin reagent strips and hCG cassettes (Figure 5-15B).

To use the simplest reagent strip readers, the technician applies the urine to the reagent strip and inserts the strip into the reader. The test strip results are displayed on a screen or printed out. This type of reader is ideal for POCT and low-volume POLs. The Urisys 1100 Analyzer from Roche Diagnostics is an example of this type of reader (Figure 5-16).

PERFORMING THE COPPER REDUCTION TEST—CLINITEST

The copper reduction test is a chemical test that detects reducing sugars, including glucose, fructose, lactose, and galactose. Other substances, such as penicillin, salicylates, ascorbic acid, and cephalosporins, can give false-positive reactions with this test when present in large quantity. The Clinitest tablet contains the reagents required for the copper reduction test.

Historically, the Clinitest was used to estimate glucose in urine of individuals with diabetes. However, with the development of glucose-specific reagent strips, this method is no longer used for glucose. The copper reduction test is now used as a simple way to screen patient urine for reducing sugars other than glucose, as when screening newborns for *galactosuria*. Because the glucose pad on reagent strips is specific for glucose alone, other reducing sugars such as galactose are not detected.

To perform the Clinitest, 5 drops of urine and 10 drops of water are added to a large heat-resistant test tube (Figure 5-17). The Clinitest tablet is placed in the diluted urine, and the color is observed while the tablet effervesces or boils. If a reducing sugar is present in the urine, the color changes from blue to green and then to orange, depending on the amount of reducing substance present. When the reaction is complete, the color of the liquid is compared to the color chart included with the Clinitest tablet vial, and the results are recorded (Figure 5-17). The 2-drop Clinitest is performed in the same manner as the 5-drop method except that 2 drops of urine are used and the color reaction is compared to the 2-drop color chart.

Manufacturers' safety recommendations should always be followed when performing the Clinitest method. Care must be taken to avoid injury from heat or caustic products generated during the reaction. The test tube opening should be kept pointed away from the face, and face protection should be worn to prevent splashes on the face or into the eyes.

PERFORMING CONFIRMATORY TESTS

Sometimes it is necessary to measure chemicals in urine by methods other than reagent strips. These other methods are called confirmatory tests because their most common use is to confirm a positive (or negative) result obtained using the reagent strip.

Confirmatory tests are more time-consuming and require more reagents and equipment than the reagent strip method. Three commonly performed confirmatory tests are for protein, ketones, and bilirubin.

Protein

Most simple confirmatory tests for urine protein involve treating a portion of the urine with an acid to cause the protein to precipitate and therefore become visible. The amount of precipitate formed is roughly proportional to the concentration of protein present. Precipitate is graded as negative, trace (slightly cloudy), 1+ (turbid), 2+ (turbid with granulation), 3+ (granulation and flocculation), or 4+ (clumps). Dilute acetic or sulfosalicylic acids can be used to precipitate the protein.

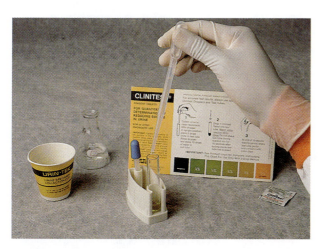

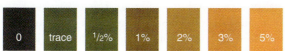

FIGURE 5-17 Clinitest for reducing sugars and example of color chart (Note: Do not use this chart to read results, use chart that comes with tablets.)

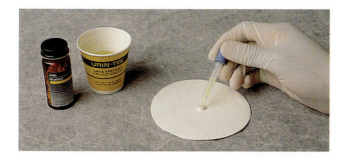

FIGURE 5-18 Acetest for urine ketones

Ketones

The Acetest is a test for ketones and is available in tablet form. The tablet test is based on the same principle as the reagent strip test. If ketones are present in urine, a drop of urine added to the tablet will produce a purple color (Figure 5-18). Serum or plasma can also be tested for the presence of ketones using Acetest tablets. Strips such as Ketostix or Ketodiastix are also used to confirm the presence of ketones in urine.

Bilirubin

The Ictotest is a specific test for bilirubin and is four times as sensitive as the reagent strip method. The test uses a tablet and absorbent mat. A few drops of urine are placed on the mat, the tablet is placed on the moist area, and water is dropped on the tablet. If bilirubin is present, a purple color will develop on the mat within 60 seconds (Figure 5-19).

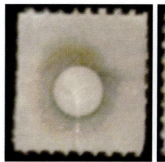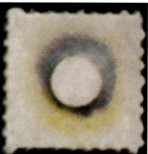

Weak positive   Strong positive

FIGURE 5-19 Ictotest for bilirubin; both tests shown are positive for bilirubin

SAFETY Reminders

- Review safety section before beginning procedure.
- Use Standard Precautions when handling all urine specimens.
- Use care in performing the Clinitest procedure because of the heat that is generated and the caustic nature of the reagent.
- Wipe up spills promptly and disinfect area.
- Avoid creating aerosols or splashes when transferring or discarding urine specimens.

CASE STUDY

Chemical analysis of a patient's urine using a reagent strip gave negative protein and negative glucose results. However, using a separate microalbumin reagent strip, the result was positive. Earlier in the day, the urine controls gave the expected results with both types of reagent strips.

1. Is there a discrepancy in the patient's test results obtained with the two strips?
2. Should the urine chemistry controls be rerun?
3. What is the most likely explanation for the results?

CRITICAL THINKING

Megan received two specimens for routine urinalysis. She poured a portion of each specimen into a conical centrifuge tube, recorded the transparency and color, and measured the specific gravity of each. She was then interrupted and had to leave the urinalysis bench. While Megan was away, one of her coworkers centrifuged the urine for her to prepare it for microscopic examination and left a note stating what had been done. Megan returned and performed chemical testing on the centrifuged specimens. Specimen A had pH 6, specimen B had pH 6.5, and both were negative for the remaining tests. Specimen B had a moderate amount of visible sediment at the bottom of the centrifuge tube. Which is the correct action for Megan? Explain your answer.

1. Which is the correct action for Megan?
   a. Repeat reagent strip test on both tubes of urine.
   b. Report the reagent strip results and proceed to the microscopic examination.
   c. Retest only specimen B using well-mixed, uncentrifuged urine.
   d. Retest both specimens using well-mixed, uncentrifuged urine.
2. Explain your answer.

PROCEDURAL Reminders

- Review quality assessment section before beginning procedure.
- Collect and store urine specimens properly to preserve components such as bilirubin and ketones.
- Store reagents and reagent strips according to manufacturer's directions.
- Do not allow reagent strip pads or the reagent tablets to touch anything other than the specimen tested.
- Test reagent strips with negative and positive controls on each day of use.
- Observe and record color changes at the appropriate time intervals.

SUMMARY

The chemical analysis of urine is one part of the routine urinalysis. Chemical tests of urine became greatly simplified with the development of urine reagent strips, single-use strips that contain multiple test areas. Reagent strip tests are performed manually or by reagent strip reader. Confirmatory tests for protein, ketones, or bilirubin are used to validate positive or questionable results for these components. Clinitest tablets are used to detect the presence of reducing sugars other than glucose in urine. For reliable results, urine control solutions must be run as directed by the policy of the institution, and manufacturers' instructions for using strips and reagents must be followed.

The chemical examination of urine is frequently performed and provides valuable information for the diagnosis and treatment of certain diseases and conditions. Abnormal chemical test results are sometimes the first indication of a problem in the kidneys or other body systems and can sometimes aid in confirming or ruling out a diagnosis.

REVIEW QUESTIONS

1. Name 10 chemical tests routinely performed on urine using the reagent strip method.

2. Explain how a reagent strip is used.

3. What type of urine specimen is preferred for chemical testing?

4. Name three confirmatory tests performed on urine.

5. For each of the following, name a condition that can cause the substance to be increased in the urine: protein, ketones, glucose, bilirubin, nitrite, and microalbumin.

6. Name a method of measuring urine protein other than the reagent strip method.

7. What is the purpose of the Clinitest? What does it detect?

8. Explain how controls are used in urine testing.

9. What are the advantages of using a urine strip reader?

10. How can handling and storage of specimens influence the results of chemical tests?

11. What safety precautions should be used when performing urine tests?

12. Define albumin, bilirubin, chromogen, glycosuria, hematuria, ketonuria, microalbumin, microalbuminuria, proteinuria, urobilinogen, and UTI.

STUDENT ACTIVITIES

1. Complete the written examination on this lesson.

2. Practice performing chemical examinations on several urine specimens as outlined in the Student Performance Guide, using the worksheet.

3. Compare the results of the physical examination of a urine sample with the chemical examination results. Are they as expected? If protein is present in a sample, is specific gravity also high? If blood is positive on a reagent strip, was it visible in the physical examination?

4. Compare the package inserts of two brands of urine reagent strips. Determine the principles of each reagent pad test and note which tests from the two manufacturers are based on the same chemical principles.

5. Administer a color blindness test to a fellow student.

WEB ACTIVITIES

1. Find information about two urine strip readers on the Internet. Compare their capabilities: sampling methods, strips used, calibration methods, process times, etc. Can the instruments read reagent strips for microalbumin?

2. Use the Internet to find information on myoglobin. Find out what conditions can cause myoglobinuria (myoglobin in the urine) and what reagent strip reactions indicate presence of myoglobin.

3. Use the Internet to find tests for color blindness. How many types of color blindness are there?

Student Performance Guide

LESSON 5-4 Chemical Examination of Urine

Name _____ Date _____

INSTRUCTIONS

1. Practice the procedure for performing a chemical examination of urine following the step-by-step procedure and using the worksheet.

2. Demonstrate the procedure for the chemical examination of urine satisfactorily for the instructor using the Student Performance Guide. Your instructor will determine the level of competency you must achieve to obtain a satisfactory (S) grade.

NOTE: Consult reagent package inserts for manufacturers' specific instructions before performing tests

MATERIALS AND EQUIPMENT

- acrylic safety shield
- gloves
- face shield or protective eyewear
- antiseptic
- recently collected urine specimens
- urine control solutions (normal and abnormal)
- various types of reagent strips with color charts
- paper towels or laboratory tissues
- timer
- reagent strip reader (optional)
- clear, conical disposable plastic centrifuge tubes
- forceps
- centrifuge
- disposable heat-resistant test tubes, 13 × 100 mm and 16 × 125 mm
- test tube racks
- test tube clamp
- disposable transfer pipets
- distilled water
- 20% (or 3%) sulfosalicylic acid
- Clinitest tablets
- Acetest tablets and filter paper
- Ictotest tablets and absorbent pads
- worksheet
- urinalysis report form
- surface disinfectant
- biohazard container
- sharps container

PROCEDURE

Record in the comment section any problems encountered while practicing the procedure (or have a fellow student or the instructor evaluate your performance).

S = Satisfactory
U = Unsatisfactory

You must:	S	U	Comments
1. Assemble equipment and materials. Put on face protection or position acrylic safety shield on work area			
2. Wash hands and put on gloves			
3. Obtain urine specimen and urine control solutions. If specimen has been refrigerated, allow it to reach room temperature before proceeding. Mix specimen by gentle swirling (working behind safety shield or wearing face protection)			
4. Perform reagent strip test: a. Dip reagent strip into well-mixed urine, moistening all pads b. Remove strip from urine immediately and tap on container edge to remove excess urine; quickly blot *edge* of strip on absorbent paper. Begin timing as strip is withdrawn from urine c. Observe reagent pads and compare colors to color chart at appropriate time intervals d. Record results on urinalysis worksheet e. Discard reagent strip into biohazard container f. Repeat 4a through 4e using urine to control solution(s)			
5. Retest the urine specimen using a reagent strip reader following the manufacturer's instructions for the instrument. Compare the manual test results with those from the strip reader. If no strip reader is available, go to step 6			
6. Perform sulfosalicylic acid test for protein: a. Centrifuge 5 mL of urine b. Place 4 mL of clear supernatant (from 6a) into a test tube c. Add 3 drops of 20% sulfosalicylic acid. (Alternatively, add 4 mL of 3% sulfosalicyclic acid to 4 mL of urine using a larger test tube) d. Mix thoroughly and estimate the amount of turbidity after 10 minutes e. Record results on worksheet as: negative (no turbidity or cloudiness), trace (slight cloudiness), 1+ (turbid), 2+ (turbid with granulation), 3+ (granulation and flocculation), or 4+ (clumps)			

You must:	S	U	Comments

7. Perform Clinitest for reducing substances:
   a. Place a 16 × 125 mm heat-resistant test tube into a test-tube rack
   b. Place 5 drops of urine into the test tube
   c. Place 10 drops of distilled water into the test tube and gently mix tube contents
   d. Drop a Clinitest reagent tablet into the urine-water mixture using forceps
   e. Observe color while allowing tablet to effervesce or boil until boiling stops, without touching the test tube
   f. Wait 15 seconds after boiling stops, hold tube with test tube clamp, and mix tube contents gently. Compare color of liquid to color chart (tube will be hot and opening should be kept pointed away from your face)
   g. Record results on worksheet as negative, $\frac{1}{4}$%, $\frac{1}{2}$%, $\frac{3}{4}$%, 1%, or 2% or more
   h. Repeat 7a through 7d using urine control solution(s)			

8. Perform Acetest for ketones:
   a. Place an Acetest tablet on a clean piece of white paper towel or filter paper
   b. Place 1 drop of urine on top of the tablet
   c. Compare color of tablet to color chart at 30 seconds
   d. Record results on worksheet as negative or positive
   e. Repeat 8a through 8d using urine control solution(s)			

9. Perform Ictotest for bilirubin:
   a. Place 10 drops of urine on an Ictotest mat
   b. Place an Ictotest reagent tablet on the moistened area of the mat
   c. Apply 2 drops of water to the tablet
   d. Observe test for 60 seconds and interpret results: When elevated amounts of bilirubin are present in urine, a blue to purple color forms on the mat within 60 seconds. The rapidity of the color formation and the color intensity are proportional to the amount of bilirubin in the urine. A pink or red color is a negative result
   e. Record results on worksheet as negative or positive
   f. Repeat 9a through 9e using urine control solutions			

10. Dispose of urine specimen properly, avoiding splashes or retain specimen for microscopic examination			

You must:	S	U	Comments
11. Dispose of test tube and contents properly, avoiding splashes			
12. Discard used materials into appropriate biohazard containers			
13. Clean work area with surface disinfectant			
14. Remove gloves and discard into biohazard container			
15. Wash hands with antiseptic			

Evaluator Comments:

Evaluator _____ Date _____

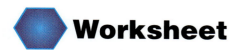 **Worksheet**

LESSON 5-4 Chemical Examination of Urine

Name _____ Date _____

Specimen I.D. _____

REAGENT STRIP	RESULT OBSERVED	REFERENCE VALUES
Glucose	_____	negative
Bilirubin	_____	negative
Ketones	_____	negative
Blood	_____	negative
pH	_____	4.5 to 8.0
Protein	_____	negative, trace
Urobilinogen	_____	0.1 to 1.0 mg/dL (or EU/dL)
Nitrite	_____	negative
Leukocyte esterase	_____	negative
Specific gravity	_____	1.005 to 1.030

Reducing Substances   (Circle Result)

Clinitest	negative	¼%	½%	¾%	1%	2% or more

Confirmatory Test Results   (Circle Result)

Protein (sulfosalicylic acid)	negative	trace	1+	2+	3+	4+
Ketones (Acetest)	negative	positive				
Bilirubin (Ictotest)	negative	positive				

Comment: _____

_____

_____

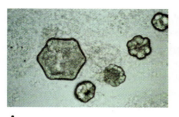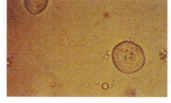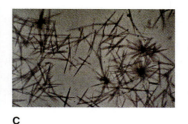

A   B   C

FIGURE 5-23 Abnormal crystals in urine: (A) cystine; (B) leucine; (C) tyrosine
(*Courtesy Hycor Biomedical Inc., Garden Grove CA, and Bayer Healthcare, Norwood MA*)

Abnormal Crystals in Urine

Abnormal crystals can occur in the urine of patients with certain metabolic diseases or after administration of low solubility drugs such as sulfa drugs. Some abnormal crystals are cystine, tyrosine, leucine, cholesterol, hippuric acid, and sulfa (Table 5-12 and Figure 5-23). Abnormal crystals are not frequently seen but, when present, are usually in acid urine.

- Cystine—Cystine forms colorless, refractile, flat, hexagonal crystals, often with unequal sides. Presence of these crystals in urine indicates disease such as *cystinuria*, a condition in which the amino acid cystine is not reabsorbed by the kidney (Figure 5-23A).

- Leucine—Leucine crystals are refractile, oily-appearing spheres. They can be yellow-brown in color and have concentric striations. Presence of these crystals in urine is an indication of liver disease or damage (Figure 5-23B).

- Tyrosine—Tyrosine forms fine needles arranged in sheaves. Presence of these crystals indicates liver disease or damage (Figure 5-23C).

- Cholesterol—Cholesterol crystals are colorless, flat plates with notched or broken corners.

- Sulfa—Sulfa crystals are now rarely seen because of the increased solubility of newer sulfa drugs. When seen, they appear as bundles of needles with striations.

- Hippuric acid—Hippuric acid is a byproduct of the breakdown of benzoic acid and is found in small amounts in normal urine. It is also formed when xylene and toluene are metabolized. Levels of hippuric acid can be used to monitor workplace exposure to these solvents or to monitor substance abuse, such as glue sniffing. When levels of hippuric acid rise, crystals can form in the urine. These appear as colorless, slender needles or prisms.

- Radiographic media—Occasionally crystals are present in urine for a brief period following intravenous radiographic studies or retrograde cystograms that use diatrizoate dyes. These crystals usually appear as flat, colorless plates or slender rectangles. When present, they can cause urine specific gravity to be abnormally high (greater than 1.040).

Other Substances in Urine Sediment

Mucus from the urinary tract lining and contaminants such as fibers, hair, starch or talc granules, and oil droplets sometimes are present in urine sediment (Figure 5-24). These substances must be recognized and should not be confused with clinically significant substances in the sediment. Mucus, when seen, is reported; contaminants or artifacts are not.

PERFORMING THE MICROSCOPIC EXAMINATION OF URINE SEDIMENT

The procedure for microscopic examination of urine and the policy for reporting results must be standardized for each laboratory according to equipment and supplies that are available in the particular laboratory.

TABLE 5-12. Abnormal crystals in urine sediment	
CRYSTAL	**MICROSCOPIC APPEARANCE**
Cholesterol	Colorless flat plates with notched or broken corners
Cystine	Colorless, hexagonal plates
Hippuric acid	Colorless to yellow needles or prism-like structures
Leucine	Yellow-brown spherical crystals showing concentric circles
Sulfa	Yellow to brown-green rosettes or bundles of needles
Tyrosine	Colorless to pale yellow sheaves of needles

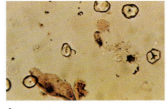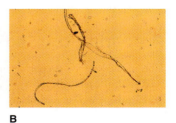

A   B

FIGURE 5-24 Other substances in urine:
(A) starch granules; (B) cotton fibers

Safety Precautions

Because urine is a biological fluid, Standard Precautions must be followed when preparing urine sediment for microscopic examination. Appropriate personal protective equipment (PPE), including gloves and face protection, must be worn during specimen handling, preparation, and evaluation. The creation of splashes or aerosols must be avoided. Safety guidelines for the use of the centrifuge must be followed (see Lessons 1-5 and 1-9). The use of microscope slides with beveled corners will decrease the likelihood of injury or glove tears when handling slides. Sediment slides must be discarded in a sharps container.

Quality Assessment

Each laboratory procedure manual will describe the procedure for microscopic examination of urine, including the volume of urine to be used for each microscopic exam, the length and force of centrifugation, the volume used to resuspend sediment, and the counting and reporting methods. These guidelines must be followed by all technicians performing the examinations in order to minimize individual differences in technique.

Because urine sediment components deteriorate rapidly, stable controls for urine microscopy are more difficult to produce than are controls for biochemical tests. However, controls such as KOVA-Trol from Hycor contain stabilized red and white blood cells. These controls can be used to check technicians' recognition of blood cells in urine specimens. Each level of control should be tested at least daily or once each shift in which the tests are performed. All control results must be recorded.

Specimen Collection and Handling

The preferred specimen is a midstream early morning specimen. The use of midstream specimens prevents contamination of the specimen with epithelial cells and microorganisms. Early morning specimens are usually more concentrated, which increases the chances of finding certain sediment components. In addition, concentrated urines protect some sediment components from deterioration. Red and white blood cells and epithelial cells can be damaged or destroyed in dilute urines, causing the numbers of these components to appear falsely decreased. All urine specimens should be examined as soon as possible after collection to prevent cellular deterioration and multiplication of any bacteria present.

Preparing the Sediment

The procedure for preparing urine sediment must be standardized within each laboratory. Typically, procedures use 10, 12, or 15 mL of well-mixed urine. The urine is poured into a conical centrifuge tube and centrifuged at $400g$ for 5 minutes. The supernatant is then carefully removed by pouring or pipeting. By gently tapping the tip of the tube, the sediment is resuspended in the urine remaining in the tube (0.5 to 1.0 mL). One drop of the suspension is pipetted onto a glass microscope slide and covered with a coverglass.

Several commercial systems are available that standardize the procedure for preparing and examining sediment and thus eliminate variation in technique among technicians. Urisystem by Fisher Scientific, KOVA System by Hycor Biomedical, and CenSlide 2000 by StatSpin, Inc., are examples of such systems (Figures 5-25, 5-26, and 5-27). These systems include centrifuge tubes, pipets, and plastic slides designed to ensure that a standard amount of urine is centrifuged and a standard amount of sediment is examined. Most systems also include an optional urine stain to make it easier to identify sediment components.

Counting Sediment Components

Counting and reporting methods can differ slightly among laboratories; therefore, the method used must always be that of the laboratory where the test is being performed. A microscope equipped with phase contrast optics is preferred for observing urine sediment. However, if a conventional light microscope is used, the light level can be decreased and the condenser lowered to provide more contrast and make it easier to see elements such as casts.

The sediment slide is examined using the low power objective (10×) to count elements that are few in number, such as casts. The high-power objective (40×) is used to identify and count red and white blood cells, epithelial cells, yeasts, bacteria, and crystals, and to identify casts. For each component, 10 to 15 consecutive microscopic fields are scanned and the numbers of each component present in each field are recorded.

Reporting Results

White blood cells, red blood cells, and epithelial cells are reported as the number of cells per high power field (HPF) and are usually reported as a range, such as 0–2, 2–4, 4–8, etc. (Tables 5-13 and 5-14). To determine the number to report, the total number of a component seen in all microscopic fields examined is divided by the total number of fields examined.

For example, 10 HPF fields were counted and the numbers of red blood cells seen in the 10 fields were 2, 4, 0, 1, 3, 2, 0, 1, 2,

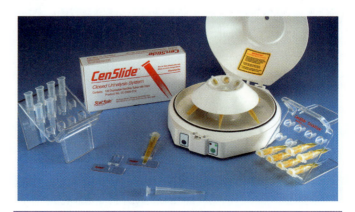

FIGURE 5-25 Stat-Spin CenSlide standardized urinalysis system (*Photo courtesy of StatSpin Inc., Norwood, MA*)

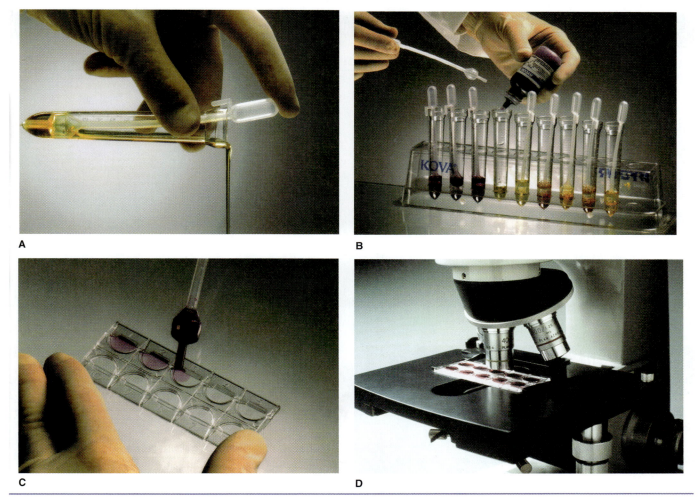

FIGURE 5-26 Using the KOVA system for standardized urinalysis: (A) pour off supernatant
from centrifuged urine; (B) stain the sediment (optional); (C) load the slide chamber using the KOVA pipet;
(D) observe microscopically (*Courtesy Hycor Biomedical Inc., Garden Grove, CA*)

and 4. The total number of red blood cells seen (19) should be
divided by the total number of fields counted (10) to give an average of 1.9 red blood cells per HPF. Using the ranges given earlier,
this would be reported as *0–2 RBCs/HPF*.

When a component is not seen in every field, it can be
reported as rare (only one seen per five fields) or occasional (only
one seen per one to three fields). Casts are reported as number of
casts per low power field (LPF). Casts should also be identified as
hyaline, granular, or cellular. Table 5-14 lists the reference values
for urine sediment.

Microorganisms such as yeasts and *Trichomonas* should be
reported, if seen. Bacteria are usually reported only if large numbers are seen in a recently collected urine sample that has been
properly collected. Bacteria are reported as neg, 1+, 2+, 3+, or 4+.

Mucus and crystals should be reported if seen, and crystals
should be identified. Mucus is usually reported as negative, 1+, 2+,
3+, and 4+. Spermatozoa are reported according to laboratory policy.

Once the microscopic examination is complete, the results
of the physical and chemical examination of the specimen should

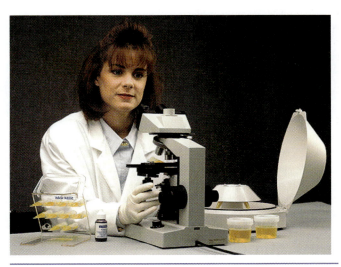

FIGURE 5-27 Using the CenSlide urinalysis system
(*Courtesy of StatSpin Inc., Norwood, MA*)

TABLE 5-13. Example of a typical method of counting and identifying components of urine sediment

SEDIMENT COMPONENT	IDENTIFY USING:	COUNT USING:	REPORT:
Red blood cells	HP	HP	Average # / HPF
White blood cells	HP	HP	Average # / HPF
Epithelial cells	HP	HP	Average # / HPF
Casts	HP	LP	Average # / LPF
Bacteria/yeasts	HP	HP	0–4+*
Mucus	HP	HP	0–4+
Crystals	HP	—	Type present

0 = none seen in 10 fields
Rare = only 1 seen per 5 fields
Occasional = only 1 seen per 1–3 fields
HP = high power objective; HPF = high power field
LP = low power objective; LPF = low power field
* Usually only reported when large numbers are present in fresh urine

TABLE 5-14. Reference values for components of urine sediment

COMPONENT	REFERENCE VALUE
Red blood cells/HPF	0–4
White blood cells/HPF	0–4
Epith/HPF	Occasional (may be higher in females)
Casts/LPF	Occasional, hyaline
Bacteria	Negative
Yeasts	Negative
Mucus	Negative to 2+
Crystals	Types present vary with pH (crystals such as cystine, leucine, tyrosine, and cholesterol are considered abnormal)

HPF = high power field
LPF = low power field

TABLE 5-15. Correlation of microscopic examination of urine sediment with physical and chemical urinalysis results

MICROSCOPIC FINDINGS	EXPECTED RESULTS	
	PHYSICAL	CHEMICAL
White blood cells*	Turbid	+ protein
		+ nitrite*
		+ leukocytes*
Red blood cells**	Turbid, red color	+ blood
Large numbers of epithelial cells	Turbid	—
Casts	Clear to turbid	+ protein
Normal crystals	Turbid	pH acid to alkaline
Bacteria	Turbid	+ nitrite

*In cases of bacterial infection, may also see bacteria
**Red blood cells may not be seen if hemolysis has occurred

be reviewed to confirm that the microscopic examination results agree or correlate with the physical and chemical tests (Table 5-15). For instance, if the chemical strip test was positive for leukocyte esterase, it would be expected that increased numbers of white blood cells would be seen in the microscopic examination.

Urine Analyzers

Several semi-automated analyzers are available for urinalysis. These instruments have the advantages of processing large num-

bers of samples rapidly, improving standardization, and decreasing clerical errors. One fully automated analyzer is the IRIS iQ200 Urinalysis System manufactured by International Remote Imaging Systems, Inc. The iQ200 performs the physical, chemical, and microscopic parts of routine urinalysis by linking together modules that perform each part of the examination.

The technologist loads a well-mixed, bar-coded aliquot of urine into a sample tray on the analyzer. Physical and chemical examinations are performed first. The instrument mixes the sample again and robotically dispenses urine onto pads of a reagent strip. The reactions are read colorimetrically at the appropriate times. Urine color is determined spectrophotometrically, transparency is determined using a turbidimeter, and specific gravity is read using an internal refractometer. The specimen is then moved to the microscopy analyzer. There the sample passes through a flow cell where 500 digital images are taken of each sample. Using particle recognition software, 12 urine sediment components can be identified and categorized into 14 categories based on characteristics such as size, shape, texture, and contrast. The categories are red blood cell, white blood cell, white blood cell clump, hyaline cast, unclassified cast, crystals, squamous epithelial cell, nonsquamous epithelial cell, yeast, bacteria, mucus, sperm, amorphous, and unclassified. Before results are reported, abnormal results are visually confirmed by a technologist using a video screen. Images are archived and can be viewed at any time; the images also can be used for teaching.

The UF-50 and UF-100i by Sysmex use laser flow cytometry to differentiate among, and determine numbers of, formed elements in urine sediment (Figure 5-28). This urine sediment analyzer operates similarly to hematology flow cytometry analyzers, which are discussed in Lesson 2-13. As stained sediment components flow through the analyzer, measurements are made of fluorescence, scatter, and impedance, providing identification and classification of 10 components. A specimen having unusual results is flagged, and the results are confirmed microscopically by the technician.

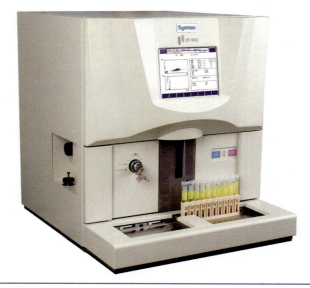

FIGURE 5-28 Sysmex UF 100i fully automated urine analyzer (*Courtesy Sysmex America, Inc., all rights reserved*)

TABLE 5-16. Correlation of urine sediment components with a physiologic condition such as strenuous exercise and some disease states

| | CONDITION/DISEASE | | | |
COMPONENT	STRENUOUS EXERCISE	ACUTE CYSTITIS	GLOMERULONEPHRITIS	CHRONIC END STAGE KIDNEY DISEASE
White blood cells	0–1×	4×	2×	1–2×
Red blood cells	0–1×	2×	4×	1–2×
Bacteria	0	+	0	±
Renal epithelial cells	0	0	1×	1–2×
Hyaline casts	3–4×	1×	1–2×	2×
Granular casts	1×	0	1–2×	1–2×
White blood cell casts	0	0	1–2×	1–2×
Red blood cell casts	0	0	4×	1–2×

X denotes a fold increase over reference range. For example, in glomerulonephritis, a two-fold increase (2×) over the normal amount of white blood cells may be seen.
0 = count of cells or casts does not exceed reference range
± = small amount present
+ = present
1× = one-fold increase over normal
2× = two-fold increase over normal
3× = three-fold increase over normal
4× = four-fold increase over normal

SAFETY Reminders

- Review safety section before beginning procedure.
- Use Standard Precautions when handling urine specimens.
- Wipe the work area promptly with surface disinfectant if spills occur and when work is finished.
- Use proper safety procedures when operating the centrifuge.
- Avoid creating splashes or aerosols when pouring urine from the centrifuge tube and discarding specimen.
- Discard slides in a biohazard sharps container.

PROCEDURAL Reminders

- Review quality assessment section before beginning procedure.
- Follow standard operating procedure in preparing urine sediment.
- Adjust the microscope light, iris diaphragm, and condenser of the microscope to give the best contrast of urine sediment.
- Use the fine adjustment to continually focus up and down to facilitate finding components, especially casts.
- Differentiate yeasts from red blood cells by performing the acetic acid test.

CASE STUDY

A complete urinalysis was performed on a fresh, random specimen. The results are given below.

Physical Test	Patient Results	Microscopic Exam	Patient Results
clarity	slightly turbid	WBC	6–8/HPF
color	yellow	RBC	10–15/HPF
SG	1.015	epith cells	0–2/HPF
		casts	rare/HPF
Chemical Test	**Patient Results**	bacteria	neg
pH	6.4	yeasts	neg
protein	1+	crystals	none seen
glucose	neg		
ketone	neg		
bilirubin	neg		
blood	neg		
urobilinogen	neg		
nitrite	neg		
leuk. esterase	1+		

1. Which chemical and microscopic results show a discrepancy?
   a. + leukocyte esterase and 6–8 white blood cells/HPF
   b. negative blood and 10–15 red blood cells/HPF
   c. 1+ protein and 6–8 white blood cells/HPF
   d. neg nitrite and 6–8 white blood cells/HPF
2. What follow-up test(s) would be appropriate to resolve the discrepancy?

SUMMARY

xamination of urine sediment is an important part of the routine rinalysis and is considered by many to be the single most impor- nt test in the diagnosis of renal disease (Table 5-16). Experience required to become proficient in the microscopic identification urine sediment components. Because there are few controls r urine sediment, it is very important that each laboratory andardize the technique of sediment preparation and count- g and reporting procedures. Standardizing these procedures is ade easier by the use of commercial urinalysis systems such as riSystem and KOVA System as well as semi-automated and fully tomated urine analyzers.

Reproducibility of results is important when tests are per- rmed by different technicians. For example, patients with acute chronic kidney disease may have urinalysis performed fre- ently to monitor the course of the disease and/or the effective- ss of treatment. When standardized procedures are followed h every patient sample, clinicians can be assured that changes urinalysis results are not due to technical variation but are reli- e indicators of the patient's condition.

REVIEW QUESTIONS

What is the preferred urine specimen for microscopic exami- nation of urine sediment?

How is urine sediment prepared for a microscopic examina- tion?

Why are microscopic urine tests important?

Why is it important to wear gloves and avoid splashes when handling urines?

What happens to cells in dilute urine samples?

6. What is the advantage of a standardized urine system such as the KOVA System or UriSystem?

7. Name four types of cells that can be seen in urine sediment.

8. Explain how casts are formed.

9. Name eight crystals that can be seen in normal urine sedi- ment.

10. List the normal values for red blood cells, white blood cells, casts, and bacteria in urine sediment.

11. The following numbers of white blood cells were observed in 15 consecutive HPFs when performing microscopic examination of urine sediment: 6, 5, 6, 2, 7, 1, 3, 4, 8, 6, 9, 7, 6, 5, and 8. How should the white blood cells be reported for this specimen?

12. Define amorphous, cast, flagellum, hyaline, protozoa, sedi- ment, supernatant, and yeast.

STUDENT ACTIVITIES

1. Complete the written examination for this lesson.

2. Practice identifying components of urine sediment using visuals provided by the instructor.

3. Practice performing a microscopic examination on one or more urine specimens as outlined in the Student Performance Guide, using the worksheet or report form.

4. Compare the results of the examinations with results obtained by fellow students or the instructor.

5. Compare the microscopic results with the chemical test results. Do they correlate?

6. Draw three components that were found in the urine sedi- ments. Are they normal components of urine?

WEB ACTIVITIES

1. Use the Internet to search for information on glomerulonephritis, nephritis, and cystitis. Discuss the urine sediment components you might expect to see in each condition.

2. Use the Internet to find images of urine sediment components. Make your own reference atlas of sediment components from online images. (Be sure that you do not violate any copyrights. Most Web sites allow personal use of images.)

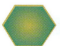

Student Performance Guide

Lesson 5-5 Microscopic Examination of Urine Sediment

Name _____   Date _____

INSTRUCTIONS

1. Practice preparing and examining urine sediment following the step-by-step procedure and using the worksheet.

2. Demonstrate the procedure for preparing and examining urine sediment satisfactorily for the instructor, using the Student Performance Guide. Your instructor will determine the level of competency you must demonstrate to obtain a satisfactory (S) grade.

NOTE: Follow instructions on the package insert for the system being used

MATERIALS AND EQUIPMENT

- gloves
- face shield or acrylic safety shield
- antiseptic
- recently collected urine samples
- urine sediment controls
- centrifuge
- microscope
- worksheet or urinalysis report form
- biohazard container
- sharps container
- timer (if centrifuge lacks timer)
- visuals depicting various components of urine sediment or prepared slides of urine sediment
- commercial standardized urinalysis system or the following materials:
  - microscope slides
  - cover glasses
  - disposable pipets
  - conical graduated centrifuge tubes
- surface disinfectant

PROCEDURE

Record in the comment section any problems encountered while practicing the procedure (or have a fellow student or the instructor evaluate your performance).

S = Satisfactory
U = Unsatisfactory

You must:	S	U	Comments
1. Assemble equipment and materials, wash hands and put on gloves. Practice microscopic identification of urine sediment using visuals or prepared slides			
2. Put on face shield or position acrylic safety shield on work area			
3. Obtain a urine sample or a urine sediment control			
4. Pour 10 to 15 mL of well-mixed urine into a clean conical centrifuge tube (or tube from standardized system)			

You must:	S	U	Comments
5. Place filled tube in centrifuge, insert balance tube, and close lid			
6. Centrifuge urine at 1500 to 2000 rpm (400 g) for 5 minutes			
7. Remove tube from centrifuge after rotor stops spinning			
8. Pipet or pour off supernatant urine, leaving approximately 0.5 mL of urine in tube (follow system instructions if applicable)			
9. Resuspend urine sediment by tapping the bottom of the tube			
10. Place 1 drop of resuspended urine onto a clean glass slide or into chamber provided with the system			
11. Place coverglass over drop of urine if using glass slide			
12. Place slide on microscope stage and focus using low-power (10×) objective, low light, and lowered condenser			
13. Scan 10 to 15 low-power fields, count the number of casts per field, and record the average (Divide the total number of casts seen by the # of fields counted)			
14. Rotate the high-power (40×) objective into position (raise condenser or increase light if necessary)			
15. Identify the type(s) of casts present and record			
16. Scan 10 to 15 fields on high power			
17. Count the number of red blood cells, white blood cells, and epithelial cells per high-power field and record the average for each cell type			
18. Observe the sample for the presence of microorganisms, crystals, or mucus, and record if present. If crystals are present, identify type			
19. Complete the urinalysis report form or worksheet			
20. Discard specimen tube and pipet appropriately, avoiding aerosol formation			
21. Discard slide in sharps container			
22. Clean and return equipment to proper storage			
23. Clean work area with surface disinfectant			
24. Remove and discard gloves appropriately			
25. Wash hands with antiseptic			
26. Use unlabeled illustrations or pre-prepared slides of urine sediment provided by the instructor to identify components of sediment not seen on slides			

Evaluator Comments:

Evaluator _____ Date _____

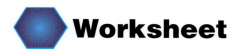 **Worksheet**

LESSON 5-5 Microscopic Examination of Urine

Specimen I.D. _____   **Date** _____

White blood cells: _____ / HPF

Red blood cells: _____ / HPF

Epithelial cells: _____ / HPF

Casts: _____ / LPF

  Type present _____

Yeasts: (circle result)   negative 1+ 2+ 3+ 4+

Bacteria: (circle result)   negative 1+ 2+ 3+ 4+

Mucus: (circle result)   negative 1+ 2+ 3+ 4+

Amorphous deposits: _____ none seen _____ present

Crystals: _____ none seen _____ present

  Type: _____

REFERENCE VALUES

0–4

0–4

occasional (higher in females)

occasional, hyaline

negative

negative

negative to 2+

Tech/Student _____   **Date** _____

Routine Urinalysis Report Form

LESSON 5-5 Microscopic Examination of Urine

Specimen I.D. _____ Date _____

Physical Examination

		REFERENCE VALUES
Transparency:	_____ clear	clear
	_____ hazy (slightly cloudy)	
	_____ cloudy (turbid)	
	_____ milky (opalescent)	
	_____ Other	
Color:	_____	pale yellow to amber
Specific gravity:	_____	1.005–1.030

Chemical Examination – Reagent Strip

		REFERENCE VALUES
Glucose	_____	negative
Bilirubin	_____	negative
Ketones	_____	negative
Blood	_____	negative
pH	_____	4.5–8.0
Protein	_____	negative, trace
Urobilinogen	_____	0.1–1.0 mg/dL urine
Nitrite	_____	negative
Leukocyte esterase	_____	negative
Specific gravity	_____	1.005–1.030

Reducing Substances (circle result)

Clinitest   negative $^1/_4$% $^1/_2$% $^3/_4$%   1%   2% or more

Confirmatory Test Results (circle results)

Protein (sulfosalicylic acid):   negative   trace   1+   2+   3+   4+

Ketones (Acetest):   negative   positive

Bilirubin (Ictotest):   negative   positive

Comment: _____

Microscopic Examination

		REFERENCE VALUES
White blood cells:	_____ / HPF	0–4
Red blood cells:	_____ / HPF	0–4
Epithelial cells:	_____ / HPF	occasional (higher in females)
Casts:	_____ / LPF	occasional, hyaline

Type present: _____

Yeasts: (circle result)	negative	1+	2+	3+	4+	negative
Bacteria: (circle result)	negative	1+	2+	3+	4+	negative
Mucus: (circle result)	negative	1+	2+	3+	4+	negative to 2+

Crystals: _____ none seen _____ present

Type: _____

Amorphous deposits: _____ none seen _____ present

Other observation   _____

Tech/Student _____   **Date** _____

5-6

Urine hCG Tests

LESSON OBJECTIVES

After studying this lesson, the student will:

- Explain why modern pregnancy tests are designed to detect human chorionic gonadotropin (hCG).
- Discuss how solid-phase immunochromatographic assays are used to detect hCG.
- Perform a test for urinary hCG and report the results.
- Discuss possible causes of false-positive and false-negative results in urine hCG tests.
- Discuss factors that must be considered when interpreting hCG test results.
- Explain the differences between internal and external controls in urine hCG tests.
- List safety precautions to observe when performing urine hCG tests.
- Explain the importance of quality assessment procedures in performing urine hCG tests.
- Define the glossary terms.

GLOSSARY

agglutination inhibition / interference with, or prevention of, agglutination

ectopic pregnancy / development of fetus outside the uterus; extrauterine pregnancy

EIA / enzyme immunoassay

human chorionic gonadotropin (hCG) / the hormone of pregnancy, produced by the placenta; also called uterine chorionic gonadotropin, uCG

implantation / attachment of the early embryo to the uterus

teratogenic / relating to a substance capable of causing birth defects or interfering with normal fetal development

trophoblastic / relating to embryonic nutritive tissue

INTRODUCTION

Urine pregnancy tests are based on the detection of the **human chorionic gonadotropin (hCG)** hormone in urine. HCG is also called uterine chorionic gonadotropin, or uCG. HCG is produced by the placenta shortly after fertilization and reaches detectable levels in urine and serum about 1 week after **implantation**, attachment of the early embryo to the uterine lining. Levels of hCG continue to rise during the first trimester of pregnancy, making it an excellent marker for pregnancy.

Tests for hCG are used when pregnancy is suspected and to rule out pregnancy before surgery or before prescribing birth control pills. Pregnancy should also be ruled out before prescribing therapies or procedures known to be **teratogenic**, that is, capable of damaging a fetus or interfering with fetal development. These include X-ray studies, chemotherapy drugs, and certain other medications and antibiotics.

Urine tests for hCG are designed to be sensitive, to be easy to perform and interpret, and to give rapid results. Many kits are CLIA-waived if performed using urine. Some are intended for home use and can be purchased in pharmacies or drug stores. Whether kits are designed for home or clinical use, the tests are based on immunochemical detection of hCG. Results of home tests should be confirmed by testing performed by a laboratory using appropriate controls. All positive hCG tests should be confirmed by a physical examination.

EVOLUTION OF PREGNANCY TESTS

Testing urine for pregnancy is one of the oldest documented tests and is mentioned in Egyptian papyri over 3,000 years old. A woman's urine was placed on plant seeds, and if the seeds germinated or grew, the woman was predicted to be pregnant; if the seeds did not grow, she was declared not pregnant. In the Middle Ages and through later centuries, urine characteristics such as color and clarity, or the reaction of urine with wine, were used to predict pregnancy. It was not until the 1890s, that scientists and physicians described the importance of certain internally secreted chemicals to the workings of the body, and named these chemicals *hormones*. However, even as the twentieth century began, physical symptoms such as morning sickness were still the most reliable predictors of pregnancy.

In the first half of the twentieth century, scientists began to unravel some of the mysteries of human reproduction. In the 1920s, a substance was described that promoted ovarian growth, and it was recognized that a specific hormone was present only in pregnant women—the hormone we now know as hCG. The 1930s brought development of bioassays (assays using live animals) that required injection of a woman's urine into rabbits, frogs, or rats. If the injected urine contained the pregnancy hormone, ovulation would be stimulated in the animal, a condition that could only be determined by sacrificing the animal and examining the tissue. In practice, these assays were not always reliable.

The isolation of sex hormones in the late 1950s provided the foundation for development of the first nonanimal assay for pregnancy—a hemagglutination inhibition tube assay that was an early type of immunoassay. Although the test was not very sensitive and many substances could cause false reactions, results were available within several hours rather than days. In the 1960s, research to understand antibodies, hormones, and other biochemicals continued, providing information used to improve test methods. A radioimmunoassay for hCG was developed during this decade, but cross-reactivity was still a problem because purified hormones and specific antibodies were not yet available.

Hemagglutination Inhibition and Radioimmunoassay

Beginning in the 1970s, increased attention was given to prenatal health care and to early testing for pregnancy. A 2-hour test was developed that could detect hCG just a few days after a missed menstrual period. This test was an improvement of the original hemagglutination inhibition tube test, but false-positive reactions still occurred. Meanwhile researchers, primarily at the National Institutes of Health (NIH), discovered molecular characteristics of hCG and were able to develop specific antibodies against the antigenic hCG beta subunit. A breakthrough came when a radioimmunoassay (RIA) using these antibodies was developed that was specific for hCG even in the presence of other hormones.

Home Pregnancy Tests

In 1976, the manufacturer of the e.p.t (early pregnancy test) requested Food and Drug Administration (FDA) approval to sell the kit for home use, and by the end of 1977, the test was available in pharmacies. Ads for e.p.t., as well as other home pregnancy tests also having FDA approval, began appearing in women's magazines. These home tests were still tube tests using the hemagglutination inhibition principle and required several steps to perform, but the tests had greater specificity than earlier tests.

Rapid Tests for hCG—Latex Agglutination Inhibition and EIA

Through the 1970s and 1980s, as women were encouraged to take an active role in their reproductive health, pregnancy tests continued to be improved. The first rapid slide tests for hCG were developed, based on the principle of **agglutination inhibition** (Figure 5-29). The tests were very sensitive (detected low levels of hCG) and specific (few false reactions), and results could be available in minutes rather than hours. In a two-step reaction, urine was reacted with anti-hCG antibodies. Then hCG-coated latex particles were added to the mixture. If hCG was in the urine, it would bind to the anti-hCG, thus preventing the anti-hCG from agglutinating the hCG-coated latex particles. Therefore, *absence of agglutination* was a positive reaction. If hCG was not present, agglutination occurred, and was reported as a negative result (Figure 5-29).

In the 1990s, pregnancy tests based on modified enzyme immunoassays **(EIAs)** were developed for both home and clinical use. These tests were called solid-phase EIAs, membrane EIAs, or solid-phase chromatographic immunoassays and are the test methods currently used. Principles of EIAs and chromatographic immunoassays are also described in Lessons 4-1 and 4-5.

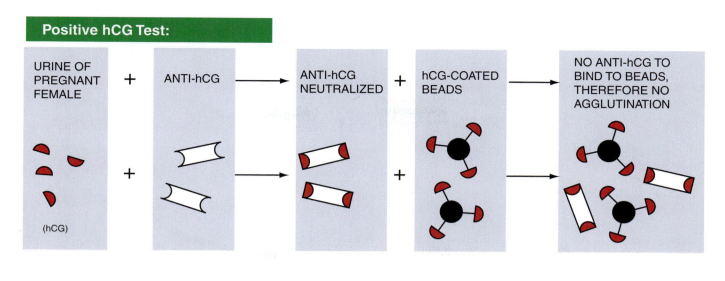

Positive hCG Test:

URINE OF PREGNANT FEMALE + ANTI-hCG → ANTI-hCG NEUTRALIZED + hCG-COATED BEADS → NO ANTI-hCG TO BIND TO BEADS, THEREFORE NO AGGLUTINATION

(hCG)

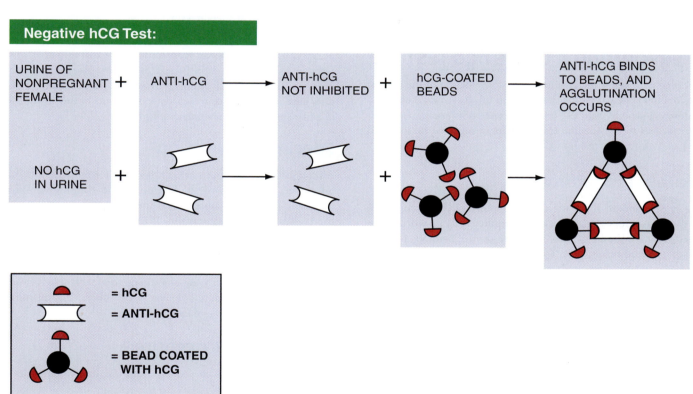

Negative hCG Test:

URINE OF NONPREGNANT FEMALE + ANTI-hCG → ANTI-hCG NOT INHIBITED + hCG-COATED BEADS → ANTI-hCG BINDS TO BEADS, AND AGGLUTINATION OCCURS

NO hCG IN URINE +

= hCG
= ANTI-hCG
= BEAD COATED WITH hCG

FIGURE 5-29 Principle of agglutination inhibition test for hCG

Many of the hCG tests currently used in clinical laboratories can be used with urine or serum, but the urine procedures are the only ones that are CLIA-waived. Most tests use a plastic cassette or cartridge containing reactants such as specific antibodies, chromogens, and other reagents such as internal controls immobilized in an absorbent membrane. The operator is only required to add urine to the cassette. When the urine containing hCG is applied, it migrates through the membrane contacting the various reagents and produces easy-to-read colored reactions in the *result* area of the test unit (Figure 5-30).

The results are available in minutes and appear as colored lines, bars, or symbols such as + or −.

To make results of home tests even more unequivocal, in 2003 the Clear-Blue Easy digital test was approved. In this test, rather than colored lines, the results are displayed in word form, *pregnant* or *not pregnant*.

Bayer Corporation (now Siemens Medical), a manufacturer of urine reagent strips, also makes an hCG test that can be read on the Clinitek Status reagent strip reader. This is a CLIA-waived test when performed using the strip reader.

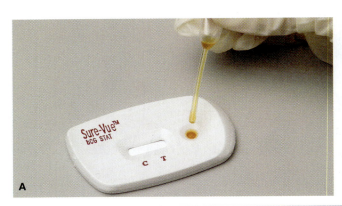
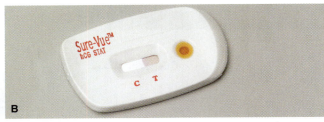
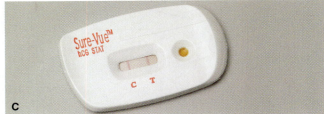

FIGURE 5-30 Examples of positive result in membrane EA pregnancy test: (A) urine is added to well; (B) sample is allowed to react; (C) reactions are observed at specified time

PERFORMING A URINE hCG TEST

Several companies manufacture hCG tests for use in the clinical laboratory. The procedure described in this lesson is intended to present a general principle of hCG detection in urine. The package inserts of the specific test kit being used must be followed when performing a test for hCG.

Safety Precautions

Standard Precautions must be observed and appropriate personal protective equipment (PPE) worn when performing urine hCG tests. Exposure control methods must be used to avoid urine spills, splashes, or aerosol formation. After testing, the used kit materials must be discarded into a biohazard container. Specimens should be discarded or stored temporarily according to laboratory procedure.

Quality Assessment

Specimen I.D. must be verified and the institution's privacy policy and guidelines for reporting hCG test results must be followed. The manufacturer's instructions must be rigorously followed for the kit in use, including:

- Specimens must be collected, stored, and used following manufacturer's directions
- Kits must be stored and used at manufacturer's recommended temperatures
- Urine must not be tested using a kit designed only for use with serum
- Kits must not be used after the expiration date
- Reagents must not be interchanged with other kits
- Reactions must be interpreted and recorded accurately

Most test kits contain an internal or procedural control that is positive when proper technique and sufficient sample volume are used. If the internal control is negative, the test is invalid. A positive hCG urine control (containing 25 to 250 mIU/mL) and negative hCG urine control (0 mIU/mL) must also be run daily or as specified in the laboratory's procedure manual. Since hCG tests have different sensitivities, detection limits of the test in use must be considered when interpreting results.

Specimen Collection

Although any urine specimen can be used for most hCG tests, the preferred specimen is the first urine voided in the morning because it is the most concentrated specimen and should contain the highest hCG concentration. If the urine cannot be tested immediately, it can be stored for 24 to 48 hours; for some kits the urine can be stored frozen. A clear aliquot must be used for testing. Visible precipitate should be removed by centrifugation or allowing it to settle. Many test kits can be used with either serum or urine; other kits require only one or the other. Most quantitative tests must be performed using serum.

ICON 25 hCG Procedure

The ICON 25 hCG is an example of a qualitative chromatographic immunoassay for hCG. In this test, anti-hCG antibodies are immobilized in a membrane that is enclosed in a test cartridge. The membrane contains a test region and an internal procedural control region. Three drops of urine are added to the sample well of the cartridge. The urine migrates into the membrane by capillary attraction, and the test is read at 3 minutes. Any hCG in the urine binds to anti-hCG that is conjugated to a dye and immobilized in the test region. A colored line in the test region indicates the specimen is positive for hCG and presumptive for pregnancy. Absence of a colored line in the test region is a negative test. A positive procedural control is built in. If the test has been performed properly, a colored line will always form in the control region (Figure 5-31). Absence of a control line invalidates the test. The procedural control serves primarily to check technique. Positive and negative hCG controls must still be used with kits to ensure kit reliability.

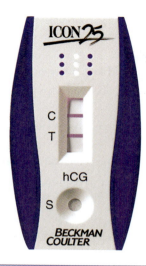

FIGURE 5-31 Illustration of positive result with ICON 25 hCG test (*Courtesy Beckman Coulter, Fullerton, CA*)

Reporting hCG Results

Results should be reported following the policy of the institution, and patient privacy rights must be protected. The usual reporting method is to report the test as positive or negative for hCG, not for pregnancy. Urine hCG tests are only presumptive for pregnancy, and positive hCG tests should be confirmed by physical examination and by ruling out other possible interfering conditions.

Significance of hCG Test Results

HCG appears in the urine and serum about 1 week after implantation, and the level rises during early pregnancy. By the first missed menstrual period, the hCG level can exceed 100 mIU/mL. By the 10th or 12th week of pregnancy, hCG levels are greater than 100,000 mIU/mL. The hCG level begins to decline about the third month of pregnancy and is not detectable within a few days after delivery.

Many tests are designed to detect hCG levels as low as 25 mIU/mL in urine and can often be positive before a menstrual period is missed. However, early in a pregnancy, urine hCG can be below test sensitivity levels, causing a (false) negative test result. Therefore, negative tests should be repeated on a first morning specimen after a few days to a week, if symptoms still warrant.

Conditions other than pregnancy can cause elevated hCG levels and (false) positive reactions in hCG tests. These include

trophoblastic disease, such as *choriocarcinoma*, and nontrophoblastic disease, such as breast, ovarian, and testicular tumors. Quantitative hCG tests performed on serum can be useful in diagnosing and following the course of these diseases as well as in diagnosing ectopic pregnancy (pregnancy outside the uterus) or suspected spontaneous abortion. Presence of hCG in urine should not be used to diagnose pregnancy unless other conditions have been ruled out and clinical findings support a pregnancy diagnosis.

SAFETY Reminders

- Review safety precautions section before beginning procedure.
- Use Standard Precautions when performing test.
- Wipe up spills with surface disinfectant.
- Discard specimens and used kits appropriately.

PROCEDURAL Reminders

- Review quality assessment section before beginning procedure.
- Follow manufacturer's directions for kit use.
- Keep urine specimens refrigerated and test within specified time limit.
- Store test kits at manufacturers' recommended temperatures.
- Use appropriate control solutions to verify that kits are working properly.
- Do not use kits or controls after expiration date.
- Interpret and report test results carefully, following institution's policy.

CASE STUDY

A patient brought a urine specimen to the clinic for hCG testing. She reported that she had performed a home pregnancy test earlier that day on this same specimen and the results were negative, even though she felt sure that she was pregnant. The technician tested the specific gravity of the urine and found it to be 1.007.

1. Is the patient pregnant?
2. What advice should be given the patient?

SUMMARY

Modern pregnancy tests are based on immunological detection of hCG in the urine or serum of pregnant females. The tests can detect hCG as early as a week or two after conception. Today's hCG tests give rapid results, and most require little expertise to perform. Many urine hCG test kits are CLIA-waived, and several are available over-the-counter for home use.

All manufacturers' directions for specimen requirements, kit storage and use, and interpretation of results must be followed. Positive and negative controls must be used to validate kit performance and technician competency. The patient's right to privacy must be protected, and technicians must follow their institution's policy regarding the reporting of test results. Laboratory personnel must interpret urine hCG test results carefully, as the results reported will have certain consequences. For example, it is important that results are interpreted correctly and reported accurately when a patient is to receive a treatment that has the potential to cause damage to a fetus, such as X-ray or drug therapy. Trophoblastic disease and certain types of cancers are sometimes associated with hCG production and can cause positive hCG tests.

REVIEW QUESTIONS

1. What hormone is detected in pregnancy tests? Where is the hormone produced?

2. What is the preferred specimen for urine hCG tests?

3. What specimen is used for quantitative tests?

4. When does hCG first appear in pregnancy? When does it disappear?

5. Explain the principle of agglutination inhibition, which was used in the first rapid slide pregnancy tests.

6. Describe the design of chromatographic immunoassays for hCG.

7. What safety precautions must be observed when performing hCG tests?

8. What is the purpose of an internal or procedural control?

9. Why are external controls required if internal controls are present?

10. What conditions can cause a positive hCG test?

11. What can cause a false-negative hCG test?

12. What action should be recommended to a woman who thinks she is pregnant but the urine hCG test is negative?

13. Define agglutination inhibition, ectopic pregnancy, EIA, human chorionic gonadotropin, implantation, teratogenic, and trophoblastic.

STUDENT ACTIVITIES

1. Complete the written examination for this lesson.

2. Practice performing a test for hCG as outlined in the Student Performance Guide.

3. Survey what over-the-counter pregnancy (hCG) test kits are available and compare the major features of each.

WEB ACTIVITIES

1. Use the Internet to find the names and manufacturers of five CLIA-waived urine hCG test kits. Locate the manufacturers' Web sites and look for package inserts or other descriptions of the principle and procedure for each kit. Make a table showing differences and similarities among the five kits, including principle of test design, endpoint reaction, types of internal controls, sensitivity level, specimen required, quantitative or qualitative, etc.

2. Download a package insert for an hCG test other than one discussed in this lesson. Write a procedure for performing the hCG test.

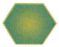 # Student Performance Guide

LESSON 5-6 Urine hCG Tests

Name _____   Date _____

INSTRUCTIONS

1. Practice performing a urine hCG test following the step-by-step procedure.

2. Demonstrate the urine hCG test procedure satisfactorily for the instructor, using the Student Performance Guide. Your instructor will determine the level of competency you must achieve to obtain a satisfactory (S) grade.

NOTE: Procedures given here for the ICON 25 hCG test and for other test kits are general. Always consult and follow the manufacturer's instructions that accompany the kit being used.

MATERIALS AND EQUIPMENT

- face shield and/or acrylic safety shield
- gloves
- antiseptic
- urine specimen
- timer
- surface disinfectant
- biohazard container
- ICON 25 hCG test kits or other rapid hCG test kits:
  - kits should include instructions, test units, and dispensers and may include hCG-positive and hCG-negative urine controls.
- hCG-negative urine control (if not in kit)
- hCG-positive urine control (if not in kit)

PROCEDURE

Record in the comment section any problems encountered while practicing the procedure (or have a fellow student or the instructor evaluate your performance).

S = Satisfactory
U = Unsatisfactory

You must:	S	U	Comments
1. Put on face protection or position acrylic safety shield on work surface. Wash hands and put on gloves			
2. Perform the ICON 25 hCG procedure following the steps below. (If a different hCG test kit is used go to step 3) a. Obtain test units, controls, timer, urine specimen, and test instructions b. Allow urine, test device, and controls to reach room temperature c. Open the pouch and place the test device on a level surface d. Use the disposable dropper to dispense 3 drops of urine into the sample well e. Start the timer			

You must:	S	U	Comments

f. Read the results in 3 minutes. The background must be colorless before results are read
   g. Interpret and record the test results:
      1) A red line should appear in the internal control (C) area indicating proper technique. Absence of the red *C* line invalidates the test
      2) A red line appearing in the test (T) area is a positive test for hCG
      3) Absence of a red line in the test (T) area is a negative test for hCG
   h. Repeat steps 2b through 2g using both hCG-positive and hCG-negative urine controls			

3. Perform a urine hCG test following the manufacturer's instructions
   a. Obtain test units, controls, timer, urine specimen, and package insert for the test kit used
   b. Open test unit and place on level surface
   c. Apply specified volume of urine to the test unit and start timer
   d. Observe color development after specified time interval. Verify that internal control(s) displays correct reaction
   e. Record results, consulting manufacturer's package insert to interpret test results
   f. Repeat steps 3b through 3e using both hCG-positive and hCG-negative urine controls			

4. Discard disposable supplies in biohazard container			
5. Dispose of specimen as instructed			
6. Clean work area with surface disinfectant			
7. Remove gloves and discard in biohazard container			
8. Wash hands with antiseptic			

Evaluator Comments:

Evaluator _____ Date _____

UNIT 6

Basic Clinical Chemistry

UNIT OBJECTIVES

After studying this unit, the student will:

- Discuss the importance of clinical chemistry.
- Identify 15 frequently performed clinical chemistry tests and explain the significance of each.
- Explain the importance of the proper collection and handling of specimens for clinical chemistry.
- Describe three technologies used in chemistry analyzers.
- Discuss the role of point-of-care testing in health care.
- Explain the principles of clinical chemistry tests for glucose and hemoglobin A1c.
- Explain the principles of clinical chemistry tests for cholesterol and triglycerides.
- Explain the principles of clinical chemistry tests for electrolytes.

UNIT OVERVIEW

Clinical chemistry is the branch of laboratory medicine that uses chemical analysis to study the level of various body constituents during health and disease. These chemical tests are usually performed on blood samples, but urine and other body fluids are also analyzed. The test results are used by the physician to diagnose disease, institute treatment, and follow the disease's progress. The physician also uses the results to counsel the patient in preventive medicine.

The study of body chemistry has a long history; as far back as Hippocrates, certain physicians emphasized chemical analysis in patient care. Early testing was performed on urine and feces because of the ease of collecting these specimens. These early tests were qualitative in nature in that they could only detect whether or not a constituent was present. As analytical methods improved, it became possible to quantitate, or measure, how much of a substance was present. The results of analyses of some constituents performed by crude methods over 100 years ago compare very well with results obtained today using sophisticated methods.

This unit is an introduction to some basic theories and principles of clinical chemistry. To understand the basis of the chemical tests discussed in this unit and the significance of test results, the student or health care worker must have a fundamental knowledge of human physiology. A review of organ systems and functions may be appropriate before studying this unit.

Lesson 6-1 introduces the topic of clinical chemistry and the relationships between the values of certain blood components and the state of health or disease of the individual. Lesson 6-2 presents general information about collecting and processing specimens for clinical chemistry tests.

The increase in testing in physician office laboratories (POLs) has resulted largely from the development of small, portable, affordable instruments that can perform a variety of tests. Lesson 6-3 presents the basic theory and operation of a few of these instruments. Lesson 6-4 discusses point-of-care testing (POCT), also called bedside or near-patient testing. Since blood glucose is one of the most frequently requested chemistry tests, Lesson 6-5 presents information about glucose metabolism, methods of glucose analysis, and hemoglobin A1c.

Lesson 6-6 explains the importance of cholesterol and triglycerides and gives a procedure for their measurements. Lesson 6-7 explains the functions of electrolytes and methods and instruments for measuring electrolytes. Since quality assessment procedures are used throughout clinical chemistry, it may be appropriate to review Lesson 1-7, Quality Assessment, before beginning this unit.

READINGS, REFERENCES, AND RESOURCES

Bishop, M. L., et al. (Eds.) (2004). *Clinical chemistry: principles, procedures, correlations* (5th ed.). Baltimore: Lippincott Williams & Wilkins.

Burtis, C. A., et al. (Eds.) (2005). *Tietz textbook of clinical chemistry and molecular diagnosis* (4th ed.). Philadelphia: W. B. Saunders Company.

Burtis, C. A., & Ashwood, E. R. (Eds.) (2001). *Tietz fundamentals of clinical chemistry* (5th ed.). Philadelphia: W. B. Saunders Company.

CHOLESTECH. Manufacturer's package insert. Hayward, CA: Cholestech LDX (2004).

Clinical Laboratory Improvement Act of 1988. (Feb. 28, 1992). *Federal Register*, vol. 7, no. 40.

Daniels, R. (2003). *Delmar's manual of laboratory and diagnostic tests*. Clifton Park, NY: Thomson Delmar Learning.

Henry, J. B. (Ed.) (2006). *Clinical diagnosis & management by laboratory methods* (21st ed.). Philadelphia: W. B. Saunders Company.

Hill, B. (2005). Accu-Chek advantage: Electrochemistry for diabetes management. In *currentseparations.com*, Vol. 21, No. 2.

Kaplan, L. E., et al. (Eds.) (2003). *Clinical chemistry: theory, analysis and correlation* (4th ed.). St. Louis: C. V. Mosby.

McClatchey, K. D. (Ed.) (2002). *Clinical laboratory medicine* (2nd ed.). Philadelphia: Lippincott Williams & Wilkins.

METRIKA. Professional package insert. (2003). Sunnyvale, CA: Metrika, Inc.

Nagy, H., et al. (2005). *Case-based pathology and laboratory medicine.* Ames, IA: Blackwell Publishers.

Sacher, R. A., et al. (2000). *Widmann's clinical interpretation of laboratory tests* (11th ed.). Philadelphia: F. A. Davis Company.

Venes, D., et al. (Eds.) (2005). *Taber's cyclopedic medical dictionary* (20th ed.). Philadelphia: F. A. Davis Company.

Wadsworth, H. M., et al. (2001). *Modern methods for quality control and improvement* (2nd ed.). New York: Wiley.

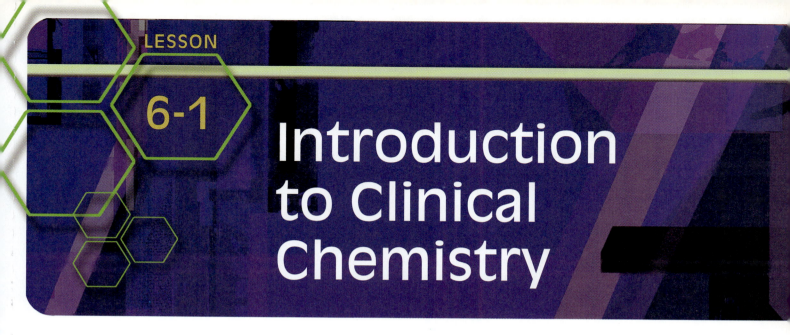

Introduction to Clinical Chemistry

LESSON OBJECTIVES

After studying this lesson, the student will:

- Discuss the history of clinical chemistry.
- List six body fluids tested in clinical chemistry.
- List 15 constituents commonly assayed in a chemistry profile.
- Explain the significance or function of each of the constituents commonly included in a chemistry profile.
- List the normal or reference values for 15 constituents measured in a chemistry profile.
- Explain how reference ranges are established and how they are used by the laboratory and physician.
- Define the glossary terms.

GLOSSARY

alanine aminotransferase (ALT) / an enzyme present in high concentration in the liver and that is measured to assess liver function; also called SGPT

albumins / the most abundant protein in normal plasma; a homogeneous group of plasma proteins that are made in the liver and help maintain osmotic balance

alkaline phosphatase (ALP or AP) / an enzyme widely distributed in the body, especially in the liver and bone

analyte / a chemical substance that is the subject of chemical analysis

anion / a negatively charged ion

aspartate aminotransferase (AST) / an enzyme present in many tissues, including cardiac, muscle, and liver, and that is measured to assess liver function; also called SGOT

bilirubin / a product formed in the liver from the breakdown of hemoglobin

BUN / blood urea nitrogen; a test measuring urea in blood

cation / a positively charged ion

creatine kinase (CK) / an enzyme present in large amounts in brain tissue and heart and skeletal muscle and that is measured to aid in diagnosing heart attack

creatinine / a breakdown product of creatine that is normally excreted in the urine

electrolytes / the cations and anions important in maintaining fluid and acid-base balance

gamma glutamyl transferase (GGT) / an enzyme present in liver, kidney, pancreas, and prostate, and that is measured to assess liver function

globulins / a heterogeneous group of serum proteins with varied functions

513

gout / a painful condition in which blood uric acid is elevated and urates precipitate in joints

HDL cholesterol / high-density lipoprotein fraction of blood cholesterol; *good* cholesterol

homeostasis / the tendency toward steady state or equilibrium of body processes

hypercalcemia / blood calcium levels above normal

hyperlipidemia / excessive amount of fat in the blood

hyperthyroidism / excessive functional activity of the thyroid gland; excessive secretion of thyroid hormones

hypoalbuminemia / marked decrease in serum albumin concentration

hypocalcemia / blood calcium levels below normal

hypothyroidism / thyroid function deficiency

lactate dehydrogenase (LD or LDH) / an enzyme widely distributed in the body and that is measured to assess liver function

LDL cholesterol / low-density lipoprotein fraction of blood cholesterol; *bad* cholesterol

lipids / any one of a group of fats or fat-like substances

thyroid stimulating hormone (TSH) / a hormone synthesized by the anterior pituitary gland and that regulates the activity of the thyroid gland; thyrotropin

thyroxine / a thyroid hormone, commonly called T_4

triglycerides / the major storage form of lipids; lipid molecules formed from glycerol and fatty acids

triiodothyronine / one of the thyroid hormones, commonly called T_3

uric acid / a breakdown product of nucleic acids

VLDL cholesterol / very low density lipoprotein fraction of blood cholesterol

INTRODUCTION

Chemical constituents in a healthy body are in a delicate balance or equilibrium, that is influenced by both internal and external factors. This equilibrium or steady state is referred to as **homeostasis**.

A change in concentration of a chemical constituent will usually trigger a reaction to bring the concentration back to the equilibrium state. For example, when the blood glucose level rises after a meal, the pancreas releases insulin to bring the blood glucose concentration down to a normal level.

In the clinical chemistry laboratory, tests are performed on blood and other body fluids. These fluids are analyzed for the presence or absence of certain substances or for the level or amount of the substances. The tests can be for **analytes**, or substances, that have a biological function, nonfunctional metabolites or waste products, substances that indicate cell damage or disease, or drugs or toxic substances. The test results are compared with normal, or reference, values, those found in a healthy body.

Physicians use the results of clinical chemistry tests to aid in the diagnosis, treatment, and prevention of disease. Interpretation of test results is based on understanding the physiological and biochemical processes occurring in health and in disease.

Test results must be reliable so the physician can have confidence in basing diagnosis and treatment on test findings.

Reliability is ensured when specimens are collected, handled, and stored properly until tests can be performed; when specimens are analyzed using correct procedures and appropriate quality assessment measures; and when results are calculated and reported accurately.

This lesson contains information about routine clinical chemistry tests often included in chemistry profiles. Included are the expected (reference) ranges for each component and a brief rationale for performing the tests.

CHEMISTRY PROFILES

Blood chemistry tests can be organized into the categories of routine and special. The routine tests are those that are frequently ordered, such as a single test for glucose or a chemistry profile. A chemistry profile, also called a complete metabolic profile, is a group of tests performed simultaneously on a patient specimen to provide an assessment of the patient's general condition. The physician can use the results of the chemistry profile, in conjunction with the physical examination, to assess the overall health of the patient.

Tests included in a routine chemistry profile reflect the state of carbohydrate and lipid metabolism, as well as kidney, thyroid, liver, and cardiac function (Figure 6-1). Profiles or panels that assess one particular biological system, such as renal or liver

CURRENT TOPICS

HISTORY OF CLINICAL CHEMISTRY

The development of analyzers for use in clinical chemistry has been fairly recent, but physicians have been using chemistry for centuries. Recorded accounts say that urine specimens were tested as early as 400 BC. Before that time, physicians in Egypt and Mesopotamia diagnosed patients by listening to internal body sounds and palpating areas of the body. However, methods for the poor and middle classes often included ritual sacrifice of animals and examination of their organs for diagnosis and treatment of the humans.

In ancient Greece around 300 BC, Hippocrates, a physician often called the *Father of Medicine*, began attributing all disease to abnormalities in the body fluids. His methods included tasting the patient's urine, listening to the lungs, and observing the patient's appearance. He also made the connection between the appearance of blood and pus in the urine to the presence of disease. In AD 50 a physician in Ephesus described hematuria (blood in the urine). Urine analysis continued to be at the forefront of medicine through the middle ages.

In the 1600s the microscope was invented, allowing scientists to study structures such as plant cells. During this century the circulation of blood throughout the body by the heart was described. Also during this time a method of precipitating urine protein by heat and acid was discovered.

In the late 1700s, advances were made in the study of diabetes when it was proved that sugar was responsible for the sweetness of urine of diabetic patients. The first tests for sugar in the urine, using yeasts, were also developed. It was not until about 1850 that laboratory medicine became more accepted, and even up to the 1890s, most laboratory tests were performed by physicians using a microscope in their homes or offices.

By 1918 the inspection criteria of the American College of Surgeons required hospitals to have an adequately equipped and staffed laboratory. In the 1920s almost half of U.S. hospitals had laboratories. By this time, several methods for determining urine analytes had been developed, many by Otto Folin. In addition, he did important work on epinephrine, uric acid, ammonia, nonprotein nitrogen (NPN) and protein in blood and established the relationship of uric acid, NPN, and blood urea nitrogen (BUN) to renal function. One reagent he developed, Folin Ciocalteau, is still used today for protein determination. During this same period, clinical methods for measuring phosphorus and magnesium in serum were introduced.

In the 1930s, methods were developed for the clinical determination of alkaline phosphatase, acid phosphatase, serum lipase, serum and urine amylase, and blood ammonia. Also a refractometer was first used for measuring protein in urine. Beckman Instruments, a company that was to play a large part in laboratory science, was founded, and introduced the first pH meter to measure the acidity or alkalinity of fluids.

The 1940s brought more developments such as photoelectric colorimeters to read color reactions of chemistry analyses and vacuum collection tubes for blood. In addition, the College of American Pathologists and the American Association of Clinical Chemistry, two organizations important to clinical chemistry, were formed.

In 1950, in a move that made tracking quality control easier, Levey and Jennings adapted the Shewhart QC chart for use in the clinical laboratory. Methods to measure several enzymes were developed. These were useful to indicate the site of organ or tissue damage. In the late 1950s, a method was developed to directly measure blood triglycerides. A landmark invention, the *Auto-Analyzer,* was introduced by Technicon Corporation, and flame photometry was applied to automated methods of clinical analysis.

The 1960s were years of rapid development in technology. In one year alone, Perkin-Elmer introduced the atomic absorption spectrophotometer for determination of calcium and magnesium, the laser was developed, and the first mechanical pipetter, the Auto Dilutor, was put into use. Also in this decade, Becton Dickinson introduced the disposable needle and syringe, disk storage for computers was developed by IBM, and the first random-access analyzer for clinical chemistry was introduced by DuPont.

The inventions of the 1960s set the stage for the rapid progression of clinical chemistry instrumentation that continues today. New technologies and methods are constantly being introduced. Analyzers have evolved from being large and difficult to operate to counter-top analyzers or handheld analyzers that are simple enough to be used at home by the patient.

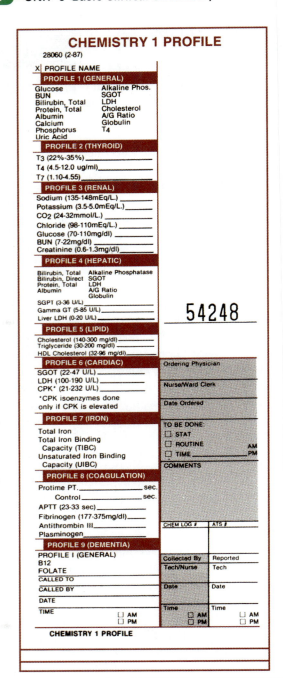

FIGURE 6-1 An example of a laboratory requisition form for clinical chemistry

TABLE 6-1. Examples of chemistry panels

PANEL/PROFILE	ANALYTES ASSAYED
Kidney (renal)	Glucose, BUN, creatinine, electrolytes
Lipid	Triglycerides, total cholesterol, LDL and HDL cholesterol fractions
Thyroid	T_3, T_4, thyroid stimulating hormone (TSH)
Cardiac	Creatine kinase, AST
Liver (hepatic)	Total protein, albumin, bilirubin, enzymes (alkaline phosphatase, gamma glutamyl transferase, alanine aminotransferase, aspartate aminotransferase, lactate dehydrogenase)

Types of Specimens for Chemical Analysis

Specimens that can be submitted for chemical testing include blood and urine, and, less commonly, cerebrospinal fluid (CSF) and synovial, pleural, or pericardial fluids. Lesson 6-2 explains the proper methods of collecting and handling blood for routine chemical analysis. Fluids such as synovial, pericardial, or CSF are collected by the physician.

Specimens for most chemistry tests require only routine handling, but some require special attention. Before specimen collection, it is important to know which tests will be performed so the specimen will be collected and processed appropriately.

Units of Measure

Clinical chemistry test results are usually reported in metric units or SI units (International System of Nomenclature). Commonly used units are milligrams (mg) or micrograms (μg) per deciliter (dL), millimoles per liter (mmol/L), or, in the case of enzymes, enzyme activity units per liter (U/L).

Reference (Normal) Ranges

The reference (or normal) range of a substance is determined by measuring the level of the substance in a portion of the general population and applying statistical methods to the data. For instance, when establishing the reference range for total protein, a hospital might test 100 random samples from the patient population and calculate the mean value and the standard deviation (s.d.) of the set of values. The reference range is then determined by adding (and subtracting) two standard deviations ($\pm$ 2 s.d.) to the mean. So a total protein reference range of 6 to 8 g/dL is established when the mean value is 7 g/dL and the s.d. is 0.5 mg/dL. Patient results are then compared to

function, are also performed. Examples of chemistry panels are listed in Table 6-1. Tests such as routine profiles are performed in batches at least once daily in the laboratory. Many chemistry analyzers are capable of performing chemistry profiles on hundreds of patient samples per hour.

Tests that are ordered less frequently, such as hormone or certain drug levels, may be performed only two or three times each week and are sometimes referred to as special tests. These tests are usually requested when a particular diagnosis is suspected or treatment must be monitored.

this reference range when the results are reported to the physician. Laboratory reports indicate which results fall outside the reference range, but leave it to the physician to determine the significance of these results. (See Lesson 1-7 for a more complete explanation of quality assessment, quality control, and reference ranges.)

Based on the laws of probability, it is expected that, in the general population, one value of every 20 sampled (5%) will fall outside the reference range, but usually only slightly higher or lower. So, a single test slightly outside the reference range might not be significant. However, if this happens, the physician will usually want to retest at a later time.

The reference ranges of many substances differ according to patient age or gender, time of day, time elapsed after a meal, or drugs or medications a person may be taking. Reference ranges can also differ slightly according to the population sample's geographical area and the methods of analysis. Types of analyzers in use and testing methods are not standardized among different laboratories. This means each laboratory must establish its own reference ranges and will supply its reference range when a test result is reported. Reference values for common chemical tests, given in Table 6-2, are those for an adult male using commonly accepted testing methodologies. However, it is important that both physician and patient evaluate test results using reference ranges supplied by the laboratory that performed the test, rather than a general or theoretical reference range from a book.

There are times when the reference range is not the most important consideration, for instance, when cholesterol is tested. Although the high end of the cholesterol reference range is 250 mg/dL, the *recommended* level for good heart health is below 200 mg/dL. There are also some tests for which a reference range is not relevant, such as measuring blood levels of a drug in an unconscious patient. The result will be interpreted in terms of the effect the drug would be expected to have at that level, given the patient's age, size, and physical condition, as well as other factors.

TABLE 6-2. Table of clinical chemistry reference values*

SUBSTANCE MEASURED	CONVENTIONAL UNITS	SI UNITS
Alanine aminotransferase (ALT)	3–30 U/L	3–30 U/L
Albumin	3.8–5.0 g/dL	38–50 g/L
Alkaline phosphatase (AP)	20–130 U/L	20–130 U/L
Aspartate aminotransferase (AST)	10–37 U/L	10–37 U/L
Bicarbonate (HCO_3^-)	22–28 mEq/L	22–28 mmol/L
Bilirubin (Total)	0.1–1.2 mg/dL	2–21 μmol/L
Bilirubin, direct	0–0.3 mg/dL	0–6 μmol/L
BUN	8–18 mg/dL	2.9–6.4 mmol/L
Calcium	8.7–10.5 mg/dL	2.18–2.63 mmol/L
Chloride	98–108 mEq/L	98–108 mmol/L
Cholesterol (Total)	140–250 mg/dL	3.6–6.5 mmol/L
	(desirable level <200 mg/dL)	
Creatine kinase (CK)	30–170 U/L	30–170 U/L
Creatinine	0.7–1.4 mg/dL	62–125 μmol/L
Gamma glutamyl transferase (GGT)	3–40 U/L	3–40 U/L
Glucose	70–110 mg/dL	3.9–6.2 mmol/L
Iron	65–165 μg/dL	11.6–29.5 μmol/L
Lactate dehydrogenase (LD)	110–230 U/L	110–230 U/L
Phosphorus	3.0–4.5 mg/dL	0.96–1.44 mmol/L
Potassium	3.5–5.4 mEq/L	3.5–5.4 mmol/L
Sodium	135–148 mEq/L	135–148 mmol/L
Thyroid stimulating hormone (TSH)	0.35–5.0 μIU/mL	0.35–5.0 mIU/L
Total protein	6.0–8.0 g/dL	60–80 g/L
Triglycerides	10–190 mg/dL	0.11–2.15 mmol/L
Uric acid	3.5–7.5 mg/dL	0.21–0.44 mmol/L

* All reference ranges listed are for serum.

ANALYTES COMMONLY TESTED IN A CHEMISTRY PROFILE

Protein

Proteins are essential components of cells and body fluids. They are formed from chains of amino acids. Some amino acids are made by the body, while others must be provided by dietary protein.

Two major groups of serum proteins are the **albumins** and the **globulins**. Albumins comprise approximately 60% of total serum proteins; globulins, about 40%.

The albumins are made in the liver and are homogeneous in structure. They serve as transport proteins and help maintain fluid balance in the body.

The globulins are a heterogeneous group of molecules. Antibodies, blood coagulation proteins, enzymes, and proteins that transport iron are all serum globulins.

Total Serum Protein

The total serum protein concentration is normally 6.0 to 8.0 g/dL (60-80 g/L) and represents the sum of many different proteins. Total protein values can provide information about the state of hydration, nutrition, and liver function, as most serum proteins are made in the liver. Protein is most commonly measured in serum, but it can also be measured in both urine and CSF, where the concentration is normally low. Total serum protein can be measured chemically or using a refractometer.

Albumin

The reference range for serum albumin is 3.8 to 5.0 g/dL (38-50 g/L). Decreased levels of albumin, or **hypoalbuminemia**, can occur in liver disease, starvation, impaired amino acid absorption, increased protein catabolism, and protein loss through the skin, kidneys, or gastrointestinal tract.

Albumin-to-Globulin Ratio

Total serum protein and albumin are usually measured in a sample simultaneously and globulin is computed from the difference (total protein – albumin = globulin). A ratio of albumin to globulin (A/G ratio) can be computed and reported.

Electrolytes

In clinical chemistry, the term **electrolytes** refers to the major **cations**, *sodium* (Na^+) and *potassium* (K^+), and the major **anions**, *chloride* (Cl^-) and *bicarbonate* (HCO_3^-). These four ions have a great effect on hydration and acid–base (pH) balance, as well as heart and muscle function. Electrolyte measurement is included in most routine chemistry profiles and renal profiles.

Sodium is the cation with the highest serum concentration, having a reference range of 135 to 148 mmol/L (mEq/L). The reference range for serum potassium is 3.5 to 5.4 mmol/L (mEq/L). Chloride is the anion with the highest serum concentration; the reference range for serum chloride is 98 to 108 mmol/L (mEq/L). The serum bicarbonate reference range is 22 to 28 mmol/L (mEq/L).

Mineral Metabolism

Minerals are necessary for good health. Calcium, phosphorus (phosphate), and iron are examples of minerals often measured in chemistry profiles. Calcium and phosphorus are necessary for proper bone and tooth formation. Calcium is also required for blood coagulation. Iron is essential for hemoglobin production and is an integral component of some enzymes.

Calcium

The reference range for serum calcium is 8.7 to 10.5 mg/dL (2.18 to 2.63 mmol/L). Of all the minerals in the body, calcium is present in the highest concentration. Approximately 99% of the body's calcium is bound in calcium complexes in the skeleton and is not metabolically active. Only unbound calcium ions are metabolically active and are measured in the calcium assay.

Calcium is required for proper blood coagulation and for normal neuromuscular excitability. The calcium balance is influenced by vitamin D_3, parathyroid hormone, estrogen, and calcitonin. These control dietary absorption of calcium, calcium excretion by the kidneys, and calcium movement in and out of bone.

Hypercalcemia, an increased level of blood calcium, occurs in parathyroidism, bone malignancies, hormone disorders, excessive vitamin D_3, and acidosis. It can cause calcium to be deposited in soft organs, leading to complications such as kidney stones.

Decreased levels of blood calcium, or **hypocalcemia**, can be life-threatening and should be reported to the physician immediately. Low calcium levels can be due to hypoparathyroidism, vitamin D_3 deficiency, poor calcium absorption due to intestinal disease, and kidney disease.

Phosphorus

The reference range for serum phosphorus is 3.0 to 4.5 mg/dL (0.96 to 1.44 mmol/L). Most phosphorus in the body is in the form of inorganic phosphate. Approximately 80% is in bone and the rest is mostly in high-energy compounds such as adenosine triphosphate (ATP). Phosphorus levels are influenced by calcium and certain hormones. Children have higher phosphorus levels than adults because they have higher levels of growth hormone.

Iron

Serum iron is normally 65 to 165 µg/dL (11.6 to 29.5 µmol/L). Iron is essential for hemoglobin synthesis. Iron is absorbed from dietary sources and is highly conserved by the body. In blood, iron is transported by *transferrin*, a serum protein. Iron levels differ with age, gender, and time of day, being higher in the AM than in the PM.

Iron deficiency can lead to anemia. The deficiency can be due to insufficient iron in the diet, poor iron absorption, impaired release of stored iron, or increased iron loss due to bleeding. Serum iron levels can be elevated with hemolytic anemias, increased iron intake, or blocked synthesis of iron-containing compounds, such as occurs in lead poisoning.

Kidney Function

Proper kidney function is necessary for water and electrolyte balance. The kidneys eliminate waste products, help maintain water and pH balance, and produce certain hormones. Substances are excreted into and reabsorbed from urine to help maintain homeostasis. The serum and plasma concentrations of certain substances such as creatinine, BUN, and uric acid are altered in certain kidney diseases.

Creatinine

The reference range for serum creatinine is 0.7 to 1.4 mg/dL (62 to 125 µmol/L). **Creatinine** is a waste product of creatine phosphate, a substance stored in muscle and used for energy. Creatinine is excreted by the kidney. When renal function is impaired, blood creatinine levels rise, but more than 50% of kidney function must be lost before this happens.

Creatinine levels are not affected by diet or hormone levels. Increases occur when there is impairment of urine formation or excretion, which occurs in renal disease, shock, water imbalance, or ureter blockage.

BUN

The reference range for serum BUN is 8 to 18 mg/dL (2.9 to 6.4 mmol/L). In mammals, surplus amino acids are converted to urea and excreted by the kidneys. This surplus is measured as **BUN**, or blood urea nitrogen.

The BUN concentration is influenced by diet, hormones, and kidney function. Therefore, BUN level is not as good an indicator of kidney disease as is the creatinine level.

BUN levels can be low during starvation, pregnancy, and a low-protein diet. Increased BUN concentration can occur during a high-protein diet, after administration of steroids, and in kidney disease.

Uric Acid

The reference range for serum uric acid is 3.5 to 7.5 mg/dL (0.21 to 0.44 mmol/L). **Uric acid** is formed from the breakdown of nucleic acids and is excreted by the kidneys. It has low solubility and tends to precipitate as uric acid crystals, or urates.

Uric acid measurement is principally used to diagnose and treat **gout**, a disease in which uric acid precipitates in tissues and joints, causing pain. Uric acid levels can also increase after massive radiation or chemotherapy because of increased cell destruction.

Liver Function

The liver is both a secretory and excretory organ and has numerous metabolic functions. The liver functions in carbohydrate metabolism, synthesizing glycogen from glucose. Most plasma proteins are made in the liver, including albumin, lipoproteins, transport proteins, and blood coagulation proteins such as fibrinogen. The liver is also important in lipid metabolism and is one source of cholesterol.

The liver is a storage site for iron, glycogen, vitamins, and other substances. Other functions include destruction of old cells by phagocytosis and the detoxification of many substances.

Significant liver function must be lost or impaired before some laboratory tests show abnormality. Numerous tests are used to estimate liver function. Most are not specific for a particular disease but only reflect liver tissue damage or liver dysfunction.

Bilirubin

The reference ranges for bilirubin are total serum bilirubin, 0.1 to 1.2 mg/dL (2.0 to 21.0 µmol/L), and direct bilirubin, 0 to 0.3 mg/dL (0 to 6 µmol/L). **Bilirubin**, a waste product from the breakdown of hemoglobin, is formed in the liver and excreted in the bile. In the liver, most bilirubin becomes bound to a glucuronide and is then excreted into the bile—this is called *conjugated* or *direct bilirubin*. Bilirubin that is not conjugated is called *indirect bilirubin*. Total serum bilirubin equals direct bilirubin plus indirect bilirubin. Bilirubin assays usually measure both total and direct bilirubin. Indirect bilirubin is then calculated from those two numbers.

Bilirubin is measured to screen for or to monitor liver or gall bladder dysfunction. Since bilirubin levels are normally low, only increases in serum bilirubin are significant. Bilirubin can be increased when there is excessive destruction of hemoglobin such as in the hemolytic anemias, impaired excretion by the liver such as in biliary obstruction or gall bladder disease, or impaired bilirubin processing as in hepatitis.

Liver Enzymes

A rise in serum enzymes generally reflects injury to tissue, since most enzymes are intracellular. Some enzymes are widely distributed in many body tissues, whereas others are found in only a few tissues. The measurement of enzyme levels is not always specific for damage to a particular organ but is most helpful when used with other tests, clinical symptoms, and patient history.

Enzymes used to assess liver function include **alkaline phosphatase (ALP), lactate dehydrogenase (LD), gamma glutamyl transferase (GGT)**, and the aminotransferases **alanine aminotransferase (ALT)** and **aspartate aminotransferase (AST)**.

Alkaline Phosphatase. ALP, also called AP, is widely distributed in the body, especially in bone and the liver ducts. Serum AP levels can greatly increase with liver tumors and lesions and can show a moderate increase with diseases such as hepatitis. The reference range of serum AP is 20 to 130 U/L.

Aminotransferases. Liver tissue is rich in the aminotransferase enzymes. When liver cells are injured, these enzymes are released. Serum concentrations of these enzymes change with time, rising during acute liver disease and falling as recovery occurs. Generally, only one enzyme need be measured, as levels tend to mirror each other.

AST was formerly called serum glutamic oxaloacetic transaminase (GOT or SGOT). It is present in many tissues, particularly cardiac, muscle, and liver. It is elevated after myocardial infarction, as well as in liver disease. The reference range of serum AST is 10 to 37 U/L.

ALT was formerly called serum glutamic-pyruvic transaminase (GPT or SGPT). Levels are low in cardiac tissue and high in liver tissue. This enzyme usually rises higher than AST in liver disease, with moderate increases (up to 10 times normal) in cirrhosis, infections, or tumors, and increases up to 100 times normal in viral or toxic hepatitis. The reference range of serum ALT is 3 to 30 U/L.

Gamma Glutamyl Transferase.

GGT is found in kidney, pancreas, liver, and prostate tissue. GGT can be more helpful than AP in determining liver damage because GGT remains normal in bone disease. It is more useful than AST because it remains normal in muscle disorders. GGT measurement is often used to monitor recovery from hepatitis. The reference range of serum GGT is 3 to 40 U/L.

Lactate Dehydrogenase.

LD, also called LDH, is widely distributed in tissue. The LD level increases in blood during liver disease and following myocardial infarction. Hemolysis of a blood sample will cause increased LD levels in the serum because of LD release from red blood cells. The reference range of serum LD is 110 to 230 U/L.

Cardiac Function

Creatine kinase (CK) is an enzyme measured to help diagnose myocardial infarction. CK is present in large amounts in muscle and the brain, but in small amounts in organs such as the liver and kidneys. Following heart attack, CK is released from the damaged heart muscle. The serum CK level peaks in about 24 hours, reaching five to eight times the upper limit of normal. It falls rapidly back to normal levels within 3 to 4 days. Serum CK levels also increase following skeletal muscle damage and brain injury. The reference range for serum creatine kinase is 30 to 170 U/L.

Lipid Metabolism

Lipids are synthesized in the body from dietary fats. The most commonly measured lipids are cholesterol and triglycerides. These are of interest primarily because of their association with cardiovascular disease (CVD).

Cholesterol and Cholesterol Fractions

Cholesterol is present in all tissues, and serum concentrations tend to increase with age. Elevated cholesterol levels can increase the risk of coronary artery disease. It is recommended that total serum cholesterol levels be maintained below 200 mg/dL (reference range is 140 to 250 mg/dL). Cholesterol fractions such as **LDL** (low-density lipoprotein) **cholesterol, HDL** (high-density lipoprotein) **cholesterol**, and **VLDL** (very low density lipoprotein) **cholesterol**, are also measured.

Triglycerides

Serum triglyceride reference levels range from 10 to 190 mg/dL (0.11 to 2.15 mmol/L). **Triglycerides** are the main form of lipid storage in humans, comprising approximately 95% of fat (adipose) tissue. Triglycerides are transported in the plasma bound to lipoproteins, molecules composed of lipid and protein. The group of lipoproteins called *chylomicrons* carry most of the plasma triglycerides. Increased blood levels of triglycerides cause the plasma to have a milky appearance. Blood to be tested for triglycerides should be collected when the patient has been fasting for 12 to 14 hours, such as in the morning before breakfast. **Hyperlipidemia** is the condition of having high blood levels of triglycerides.

Carbohydrate Metabolism

The reference range for serum glucose is 70 to 110 mg/dL (3.9 to 6.2 mmol/L). Glucose metabolism is largely regulated by insulin, which is produced by the pancreas. It is also influenced by other hormones such as growth hormone, glucagon, and cortisol. Glucose is a commonly tested blood constituent.

Thyroid Function

The thyroid gland synthesizes hormones that stimulate metabolism by increasing protein synthesis and oxygen consumption by the tissues. Thyroid hormones are synthesized from iodide and the amino acid tyrosine. In the blood, more than 99% of thyroid hormones are bound to serum proteins and are metabolically inactive. Graves' disease is an example of a disease caused by **hyperthyroidism**, excessive secretion of thyroid hormones. **Hypothyroidism**, decreased thyroid function, causes a condition called myxedema.

The two major thyroid hormones are **thyroxine**, also called T_4, and **triiodothyronine**, also called T_3. Measurement of thyroid hormones is usually not included as part of a routine chemistry profile. Thyroid profiles or endocrine panels will include measurement of free or total T_4, free or total T_3, and **thyroid stimulating hormone (TSH)** levels. TSH is an anterior pituitary hormone that regulates thyroid gland activity. The reference range for TSH is 0.35 to 5.0 µIU/mL (mIU/L). Levels of thyroid hormones vary according to age and the reference ranges can be different depending on the particular assay method. Thyroid hormones are usually measured using immunological techniques.

LESS COMMONLY ORDERED CLINICAL CHEMISTRY TESTS

Dozens of available tests have not been mentioned here. Many are special tests that measure hormones such as insulin, growth hormone, adrenocorticotropic hormone (ACTH), or follicle-stimulating hormone (FSH). Others measure vitamins, trace minerals, isoenzymes, and metabolic products. Such tests often require special specimen collection as well as special instruments and expertise. A clinical chemistry text should be consulted for more information.

SUMMARY

Assays performed in the clinical chemistry department provide a wealth of information about the status of a patient's health. Numerous tests are available that give information about cardiac, renal, and liver function as well as the state of lipid and carbo-

CASE STUDY 1

A clinic patient had total protein and albumin assays performed on his blood. When the physician was given the test results, total protein 6.5 g/dL and albumin 3.0 g/dL, she asked the technician to calculate the A/G ratio.

1. What results are used to calculate the A/G ratio?
2. What is this patient's globulin value?
3. Calculate the patient's A/G ratio.
4. The patient's results are:
   a. Both within the reference ranges
   b. Both below the reference ranges
   c. Both above the reference ranges
   d. Normal for total protein and low for albumin

CASE STUDY 2

Dr. Talbot ordered the following chemistry tests for a patient: Creatine kinase, AST, and cholesterol fractions.

Which of the following do you think Dr. Talbot suspects?
a. Heart disease
b. Renal disease
c. Liver disease
d. Thyroid disease

hydrate metabolism. In addition, many specialized tests such as hormone assays and drug assays are performed in the clinical chemistry department. The majority of clinical chemistry assays are performed using instrumentation. Quality assessment programs, that include everything from specimen collection and handling to assay procedure and results reporting, must be followed to ensure reliable, high-quality test results.

REVIEW QUESTIONS

1. What are the two most commonly tested body fluids in clinical chemistry?

2. What three enzymes are useful in diagnosing liver disease?

3. Give the reference ranges for 15 constituents included in a chemistry profile. Explain the significance of variations from reference range for each constituent.

4. What three tests can be useful in diagnosing kidney disease?

5. What enzyme is most useful in diagnosing myocardial infarction?

6. Name the four electrolytes commonly measured in serum.

7. What are the two major types of serum proteins and what are their functions?

8. How are reference ranges established? How are they used by the physician?

9. Define alanine aminotransferase, albumins, alkaline phosphatase, analyte, anion, aspartate aminotransferase, bilirubin, BUN, cation, creatine kinase, creatinine, electrolytes, gamma glutamyl transferase, globulins, gout, HDL cholesterol, homeostasis, hypercalcemia, hyperlipidemia, hyperthyroidism, hypoalbuminemia, hypocalcemia, hypothyroidism, lactate dehydrogenase, LDL cholesterol, lipids, thyroid stimulating hormone, thyroxine, triglycerides, triiodothyronine, uric acid, and VLDL cholesterol.

STUDENT ACTIVITIES

1. Complete the written examination for this lesson.

2. Ask what tests are included in chemistry panels in a nearby hospital or laboratory. Find out the laboratory's reference ranges and compare them to those in this lesson.

3. Tour a clinical chemistry laboratory in your area.

WEB ACTIVITIES

1. Use the Internet to find the Web site of a university medical center or commercial reference laboratory. Find three types of chemistry panels available and list the analytes included in each panel.

2. Use the Internet to find an example of a high-volume chemistry analyzer for processing chemistry profiles. Write a short report on the analyzer; include the technology used, test menu, and number of samples processed per hour.

Specimen Collection and Processing for Clinical Chemistry

LESSON OBJECTIVES

After studying this lesson, the student will:

- List six body fluids tested in clinical chemistry.
- Explain the importance of obtaining a quality specimen for clinical chemistry testing.
- Name five problems associated with blood collection and processing that could cause erroneous test results.
- Explain safety precautions that must be followed during specimen collection, handling, and processing.
- Discuss quality assessment procedures involved in specimen collection, processing, and handling.
- Define the glossary terms.

GLOSSARY

anticoagulant / a chemical that prevents blood coagulation

cerebrospinal fluid (CSF) / the fluid surrounding the spinal cord and bathing the ventricles of the brain

diurnal / having a daily cycle

lipemic / having a cloudy appearance due to excess lipid content

pericardial fluid / the fluid within the pericardial cavity

plasma / the liquid portion of blood in which blood cells are suspended; the straw-colored liquid remaining after blood cells are removed from anticoagulated blood

pleural fluid / the fluid in the space between the pleural membrance of the lung and the inner chest wall

serum / the liquid obtained from blood that has been allowed to clot

synovial fluid / a viscous fluid secreted by membranes lining the joints

INTRODUCTION

The clinical chemistry department performs tests on blood and other body fluids, such as urine; **cerebrospinal fluid (CSF)**; and **pleural**, **synovial**, and **pericardial fluids**. Collecting blood specimens for testing in the central laboratory is usually the responsibility of the laboratory. Blood collection can be performed by laboratory technicians or phlebotomists.

Special attention must be paid to the type of specimen required for each test and to the handling and processing of the specimen. Laboratory analyses can only produce useful results if they are performed on a specimen that has been properly collected and maintained in an appropriate environment until the test is performed. This lesson describes procedures for collecting and processing blood specimens for clinical chemistry. Lesson 5-2 describes collection procedures for urine specimens. Other body fluids are usually collected by the physician. A review of blood-collection procedures (Lesson 1-12 and 1-13) may be helpful before studying this lesson.

TYPES OF BLOOD SPECIMENS FOR CHEMICAL ANALYSIS

Blood for chemical analysis can be capillary, venous, or sometimes arterial (for blood gas measurements). Some analyzers and methods can use whole blood, serum, or plasma for testing; other analyzers or methods may require one particular type of specimen, such as heparinized plasma.

Serum

Serum is the specimen used for most clinical chemistry tests. **Serum** is the fluid portion that remains after blood has been allowed to clot. It is obtained by collecting blood in a tube without anticoagulant, allowing the blood to clot, centrifuging the clotted sample, and removing the liquid (serum). Blood can also be collected in serum separator tubes that contain a substance that forms a barrier between the serum and cells during centrifugation (Figure 6-2).

Plasma

Plasma is obtained by removing the liquid portion of anticoagulated blood following centrifugation. When either plasma or serum are to be used for testing, the liquid must be removed from the blood's cellular portion as soon as possible after collection. This prevents the exchange of substances between the cellular and liquid portions, which could alter test results.

Whole Blood

Whole blood can be obtained by capillary puncture or venipuncture. Whole blood obtained by capillary puncture must be used immediately after collection. Blood from venipuncture must be

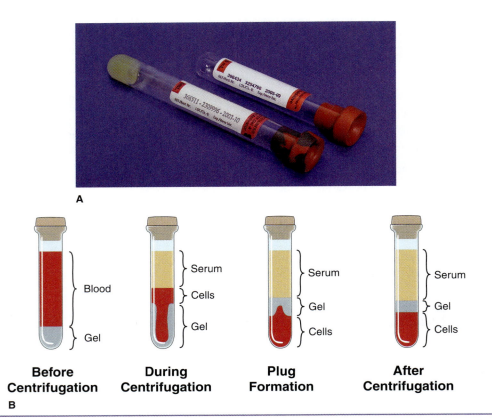

FIGURE 6-2 Serum collection tubes: (A) left, serum separator tube with red and gray stopper, and right, red top clot tube; (B) illustration of separation of serum from cells during centrifugation of serum separator tube

collected in an **anticoagulant**, such as heparin or EDTA, to prevent clotting. The tube of whole blood must be mixed well immediately before testing. Detailed procedures for collecting blood by venipuncture and information on anticoagulants are given in Lesson 1-13.

COLLECTING AND PROCESSING BLOOD SPECIMENS FOR CHEMICAL ANALYSIS

Collection procedures for capillary or venous blood should be followed as outlined in the laboratory's procedure manual. Strict attention must be paid to the specimen requirements for the test(s) ordered.

Safety Precautions

Accidental exposure to blood and body fluids is more likely to occur during collection and processing of specimens than during specimen analysis. Standard Precautions must be observed at all times. Appropriate personal protective equipment (PPE), including gloves, face protection, and a buttoned fluid-resistant laboratory coat, should be worn. Frequent handwashing and changing of gloves are required.

Several safety collection devices that eliminate the need for recapping used needles are available, such as quick-release needles, needles with safety shield, and needles that blunt on exit from the vein. Patient rooms, blood-collection stations, and phlebotomy trays should be equipped with disposal containers so that used sharps can be immediately discarded.

Sometimes specimens must be collected from a patient who is suspected of having a contagious disease. The phlebotomist or technician must remain up-to-date on specific procedures that must be used with each transmission-based precaution category. Lesson 7-2 discusses these in detail.

Uncapping of vacuum tubes containing specimens presents the potential hazards of aerosol creation, splatters, and tube breakage. Several safety devices have been developed to eliminate these problems. Plastic vacuum tubes should be used whenever possible. Through-the-stopper samplers available on many analyzers and some sample-processing instruments prevent the aerosol potential created by uncapping tubes. Whenever possible, available safety devices must be incorporated into laboratory procedures.

Quality Assessment

The quality of the specimen is of utmost importance. Specific instructions for type and volume of specimen required, the collection procedure, and the processing method is included in every laboratory's procedure manual for each test performed in that laboratory (or for which they collect a specimen). Table 6-3 gives examples of suggested specimen collection tubes; some are shown in Figure 6-3.

Before a specimen is collected, the patient must be identified. Specimens must be labeled immediately after collection, while the phlebotomist is still in the patient's presence. The

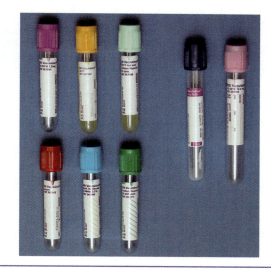

FIGURE 6-3 Assortment of vacuum collection tubes

TABLE 6-3. Uses of vacuum collection tubes according to additive and stopper color

STOPPER COLOR	ADDITIVE OR ANTICOAGULANT	USED FOR
Red	None	Serum, blood chemistries, blood banking
Red/gray	Polymer gel/silica activator	Serum separation, blood chemistries
Green	Lithium heparin	Whole blood, plasma, blood chemistries
Gray	Glycolytic inhibitor + anticoagulant	Glucose determination
Royal blue	None or sodium heparin	Trace metals
Lavender, pink	EDTA	Whole blood, hematology, blood banking
Blue	3.2% or 3.8% sodium citrate	Coagulation tests
Yellow	ACD solution	Blood banking studies
Black	Buffered sodium citrate	Westergren ESR

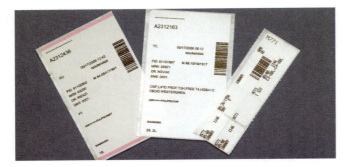

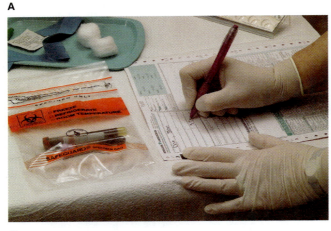

FIGURE 6-4 Specimen labeling and transport: (A) illustration of bar-coded specimen labels; (B) specimen transport bag

TABLE 6-4. Examples of some criteria that must be met for a specimen to be acceptable for testing
■ Label must be complete (name, date, time of collection, person collecting) and attached in the proper place
■ Blood specimens must be free of hemolysis
■ Anticoagulated blood specimens must be free of clots
■ Specimens must be delivered to the laboratory within the specified amount of time after collection
■ Outer surfaces of specimen containers must have no visible contamination
■ Specimens must be stored properly until the time of testing
■ Blood specimens cannot be drawn from a site above an intravenous line
■ Specimens collected in anticoagulant must have the proper blood:anticoagulant ratio

label should include patient name and identification number, the date and time of collection, and the phlebotomist's initials. Many laboratories use bar-coded labels generated at the same time the test is requisitioned (Figure 6-4A). Analyzers read the bar-code when the tube is inserted into the instrument and code the patient's identification to the test result, reducing transcribing errors.

The laboratory procedure manual includes a list of specific criteria that must be met in order for a specimen to be accepted for testing. Table 6-4 lists some of these criteria. Tests requiring special collection procedures will have additional criteria for acceptability. Failure to meet these criteria will cause the specimen to be rejected, necessitating another one being collected, which can be traumatic for the patient and is time-consuming for the laboratory. Therefore every effort must be made to ensure that all requirements are met before collecting the specimen.

Collection of Difficult Specimens

Special care must be used when collecting specimens from patients where venipuncture can be difficult, such as children and the elderly. In these cases the specimen must be collected in a manner to ensure that specimen quality is not compromised. When patients have an intravenous (IV) line, the specimen must be collected from a different arm or from a vein below the i.v. insertion. The laboratory's procedure manual will contain specific instructions for specimen collection in these cases.

Timing of Specimen Collection

Some body fluid constituents are affected by meals, medications, or the time of day. Each test procedure contains specimen-collection and handling instructions that must be strictly followed.

Most blood constituents do not change significantly after eating, so blood used to test for these can be collected at any time. However, concentrations of constituents such as glucose, triglycerides, and cholesterol will change after eating, and specimens for these tests are usually collected when the patient is fasting, generally in the morning before breakfast.

Specimens collected from patients with lipid metabolism disorders or shortly after a patient has eaten may appear lipemic. Since **lipemic** serum or plasma is milky or cloudy, it can interfere with certain tests, particularly those that use photometry.

In some diseases, certain blood constituents follow patterns of increase or decrease that make the collection time very important. For example, creatine kinase, an enzyme measured to detect heart attacks (myocardial infarctions), rises rapidly after a heart attack and falls back to normal levels in the 3 to 4 days following the attack. If this enzyme is not measured during this critical period, a heart attack can go undiagnosed.

Diurnal variation, changes with the time of day, can occur with certain blood constituents such as iron and corticosteroids. It is important, therefore, to note the collection time of specimens for these tests and to consider this when interpreting test results.

Some drug or medication blood levels will fluctuate depending on the dosage time. Some tests for therapeutic drug monitoring must be done at set intervals before or after administering medication.

Specimen Transport

The specimen transport method is determined by the distance the specimen must travel and the type of transport systems available. Specimens for point-of-care testing (POCT) require no transport, one of the benefits of POCT.

The phlebotomist or nursing staff can transport specimens to a nearby room or another floor or hospital wing for testing. Many hospitals have pneumatic tube systems for rapid delivery of specimens to the central laboratory in special leak-proof, impact-resistant containers.

Sometimes couriers transport specimens to another laboratory, perhaps in a different city. Specimens can also be shipped to a reference laboratory for testing. Regardless of the transport methods used, specimens must be packaged in secure containers to protect carriers from contamination (Figure 6-4B). They must also be transported in an environment that meets biosafety regulations and protects the quality of the specimen.

Specimen Storage and Preservation

For most routine tests to be performed within 1 hour, the specimen can remain at room temperature until testing. However, if testing is to be delayed for a few hours, samples should be refrigerated at 4°C. Some enzyme tests require specimens to be frozen immediately after collection to prevent the loss of enzyme activity.

Most specimens can be stored in capped test or collection tubes until testing. However, certain specimens require special handling. For example, bilirubin is degraded by light, so specimens should be stored in the dark.

Problems Associated with Specimen Collection and Processing

Reliable test results can only be obtained if the technologist has a proper specimen to work with (Table 6-4). Improperly collected or handled specimens can cause erroneous test results. It has been estimated that 50% to 70% of laboratory time is spent on specimen sample preparation. Therefore, it becomes extremely important that it is done correctly the first time. Some problems to be avoided are:

Hemolysis

Blood that is hemolyzed during collection or processing cannot be used for most analyses. The destroyed red blood cells will release substances such as hemoglobin, enzymes (LD and AST), potassium (K^+), and other intracellular components into the serum, resulting in a sample that does not represent the patient's true status. Hemolysis can be caused by overcentrifugation, excessive turbulence of the sample (shaking, etc.), freezing of cells, or poor venipuncture technique.

Hemoconcentration

Hemoconcentration can occur if the tourniquet is left on too long (more than 1 to 2 minutes) during venipuncture. This causes blood stasis within the vein, resulting in some blood constituents becoming concentrated (Lesson 1-13).

Overcentrifugation

Blood collected to obtain serum should remain undisturbed for 20 to 30 minutes, to allow clotting to occur. It is then centrifuged according to the laboratory procedure manual, to separate serum from blood cells. Serum should be removed from the tube as soon as possible after centrifugation (unless blood was collected in a serum separator tube). To obtain plasma, the anticoagulated specimen can be centrifuged immediately after collection. Serum and plasma must be removed from cells before freezing, since freezing will cause cell lysis.

Evaporation

Specimens should remain capped until they are tested. Evaporation will occur in uncapped specimens, resulting in concentration of some constituents. Gas escape or exchange can also occur, and can alter values such as acid–base (pH) balance or bicarbonate (HCO_3^-) concentration.

Microbial Contamination

Clean pipets or pipet tips should be used to transfer each sample. Sample cups must be clean and dry to avoid contaminating or diluting the samples. Bacterial contamination of specimens must be avoided.

Anticoagulant Contamination

When multiple blood samples are obtained using a vacuum-collection system, the order of draw is important. Serum collection tubes must be filled before tubes that contain anticoagulant.

CASE STUDY

Ms. Tan came to the laboratory for blood tests because her physician suspected renal disease. The tests ordered were serum BUN, creatinine, and electrolytes. The blood specimen was obtained and processed. When the laboratory technician received the serum to perform the tests, he noticed that the serum had a reddish tinge.

1. Was there a problem with this serum sample? If so, what?
2. What conditions could cause this to happen to a serum specimen?
3. Is the sample acceptable for use in performing the BUN, creatinine, and electrolyte tests?

SUMMARY

The tests performed in the chemistry laboratory reveal much about the patient's health status. The physician or other health care provider uses the results to make decisions about diagnosis, treatment, or prevention of disease. The quality of the specimen can be compromised at any point from collection through analysis. Therefore, the facility must have quality assessment procedures in place for collection, processing, and analysis of specimens. These must include positive identification of the patient, correct specimen collection, proper handling after collection, and utmost attention to the analytical process. Specimens must be collected in the appropriate tube or container. Separation of serum or plasma from cells should be done within the time limit specified by the test procedure. Standard Precautions must be observed in all steps of collection and processing for the protection of the patient and workers.

REVIEW QUESTIONS

1. What are the most commonly tested body fluids?
2. Explain how to collect blood for procedures requiring serum.
3. Explain how to collect blood for procedures requiring plasma.
4. Explain the differences between serum and plasma.
5. What safety measures must be observed to avoid accidental needlesticks?
6. What PPE must be worn when collecting and processing specimens?
7. Name two types of tubes (stopper color) that can be used to collect serum.
8. How can the timing of specimen collection affect test results?
9. What can cause hemolysis of a specimen? How will test results be affected if hemolysis occurs?
10. Discuss why quality assessment procedures are important in collecting and processing specimens for clinical chemistry.
11. Define anticoagulant, cerebrospinal fluid, diurnal, lipemic, pericardial fluid, plasma, pleural fluid, serum, and synovial fluid.

STUDENT ACTIVITIES

1. Complete the written examination for this lesson.
2. Visit a clinical laboratory and obtain information about the specimen-collection and processing section. Find out who is responsible for collecting, transporting, and processing specimens. Request permission to see the specimen collection section of the procedure manual.

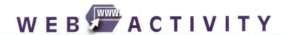

WEB ACTIVITY

Select 10 clinical chemistry tests from Table 6-2 (Lesson 6-1). Use the Internet to find specimen collection and handling requirements for each test. Make a table showing the collection requirements for the tests.

6-3

Chemistry Instrumentation in the Physician Office Laboratory

LESSON OBJECTIVES

After studying this lesson, the student will:

- Explain the major differences between instruments used in small and large laboratories.
- Discuss the reasons for the increase in testing in small laboratories.
- List factors that should be considered when purchasing an instrument.
- Explain Beer's law and the principles of photometry.
- Discuss the basic differences among photometers, reflectance photometers, and ion-selective analyzers.
- Explain what is meant by solid-phase technology.
- Explain the importance of observing all safety precautions when using instrumentation.
- List components that must be included in instrumentation quality assessment programs.
- Discuss the importance of regular instrument maintenance and using controls.
- Define the glossary terms.

GLOSSARY

absorbance (A) / a logarithmic expression of the amount of light absorbed by a substance containing colored molecules; optical density (O.D.)

amperometry / the technology that uses electrodes and electrode potential to measure electron generation

Beer's law / a mathematical relationship that demonstrates the linear relationship of concentration to absorbance and that forms the basis for spectrophotometric analysis

ion-selective electrode / an electrode manufactured to respond to the concentration of a specific ion

monochromator / a device that isolates a narrow portion of the light spectrum

percent transmittance (%T) / the percentage of light that passes through a solution

reflectance photometer / an instrument that measures the light reflected from a colored reaction product

solid-phase chemistry / an analytical method in which the sample is added to a strip or slide containing, in dried form, all the reagents for the procedure

spectrophotometer / an instrument that measures intensities of light in different parts of the light spectrum

INTRODUCTION

Automation makes it possible for clinical laboratory analyses to be performed much more rapidly and more precisely than when done manually. When analysis time is reduced, the *turn-around time* (TAT)—time elapsed between ordering a laboratory test and the physician receiving the results—is also usually reduced. Shortened TAT allows for more rapid diagnosis and treatment.

Analysis speed and the ability to analyze several patient samples at one time are especially important in larger laboratories, such as those in hospitals. These laboratories process hundreds of samples daily. The use of automation increases the productivity of these larger laboratories. However, automation also has a place in the smaller clinical laboratory and in physician office laboratories (POLs).

This lesson presents a few examples of instruments available for the smaller laboratory with a brief discussion of the principles of operation and examples of the tests each can perform. The instruments mentioned were chosen because they are in use in many laboratories and they present different principles of operation.

CURRENT TRENDS IN INSTRUMENTATION

Instrumentation technology is in a continuous state of change. Updated and improved instruments are constantly being brought to market. In the past, as the volume of testing increased, the major instrument manufacturers concentrated on developing larger and more diversified instruments designed to meet the needs of larger laboratories.

In recent years, however, a revolution has taken place in the technology of clinical laboratory instrumentation. Improved electronic, computer, and chemical technology have made it possible for manufacturers to drastically reduce the size of many instruments. This has happened at the same time that we have experienced a major change in health care delivery, where more diagnostic procedures are provided at point of care and home testing by the patient is on the increase. These smaller instruments are well suited for the limited space in most POLs. Several instruments are available for patient home use, such as blood glucose meters.

Physician Office Laboratories

The number of tests performed in POLs has increased in recent years. The availability of testing in the physician's office can be a benefit, especially to the very ill or elderly patient. Tests most often performed include complete blood counts, prothrombin time, urine dipstick, blood glucose, and blood cholesterol.

The tests performed are regulated by the Centers for Medicare and Medicaid Services (CMS), formerly the Health Care Financing Administration (HCFA), and come under the Clinical Laboratory Improvement Amendments (CLIA) regulations. POLs are subject to inspection. The laboratory owner or director must obtain a copy of the CLIA regulations and imple-

ment them or hire a clinical consultant to ensure compliance with the laws.

To be in compliance, laboratories are required to run controls and keep records of the results. Since January 1994, laboratories have been required to enroll in proficiency testing programs, depending on the test complexity performed. If acceptable results are not obtained on proficiency samples, the CMS can prohibit the laboratory from performing certain tests until the deficiencies are corrected.

Point-of-Care Testing

One goal in critical care areas of the hospital is to cut down on the TAT for laboratory results. Point-of-care testing (POCT) enables the instrument to be near the patient, perhaps at the bedside. Tests usually performed are those for which the results may affect the patient's immediate well-being and treatment. These include blood glucose, blood urea nitrogen, blood gases, electrolytes, and coagulation tests.

Trained laboratory personnel or nursing staff may perform the tests, and testing is regulated by the CMS. Controls must be run and records kept of the results. Proficiency testing by an approved agency must also be performed.

CHOOSING AN INSTRUMENT FOR THE LABORATORY

Many factors must be considered before purchasing an instrument for the laboratory. First, the decision must be made concerning which and how many tests need to be performed. This decision can be based on the patient population being served, which tests would be most helpful to the physician, and availability of personnel to perform the testing.

Other considerations are cost per test, ease of operation, and maintenance costs. The cost may be more than expected if an inexpensive instrument requires expensive reagents and supplies. The purchase price should be compared to the lease price. Although lease prices sometimes seem more expensive, they often include maintenance and automatic instrument replacement when newer models are available.

The most important factor in choosing an instrument is the quality of results. An instrument that produces unreliable results is detrimental to patient care.

SAFETY AND INSTRUMENTATION

 The operation, maintenance, and repair of laboratory instruments expose workers to biological, physical, and chemical hazards. Standard Precautions must be observed at all times. Care must be taken when handling controls that are made from biological materials. Parts of the instrument that come in contact with specimens and controls must be disinfected regularly. Instruments that incorporate safe technologies, such as through-the-cap sampling, can decrease exposure hazards to workers.

Instruments must be properly installed and grounded as recommended by the manufacturer to avoid electrical shocks. The outside case should never be removed except by a person trained in maintenance and repair. Removal of the case can expose wiring and other parts that could cause injury or death if touched. Dangling metal jewelry is especially dangerous, since it could inadvertently contact an electrical part.

Technicians must observe all MSDS and chemical label warnings to prevent injury from hazardous chemicals. Some chemical hazards can be reduced by using self-contained reagent packs or cassettes and commercially prepared reagents.

Technicians should carefully follow instructions for operating and maintaining battery-powered instruments, such as those used in POCT. The battery type must be the one recommended by the manufacturer. Used batteries must be disposed of properly.

QUALITY ASSESSMENT PROGRAMS AND INSTRUMENTATION

 Most clinical laboratory analyses are performed using instruments. The instrument aspirates the sample, performs the analysis programmed for the sample, and prints the results with little input from humans during the analysis. Because of this, automated methods are generally more precise and accurate than are manual methods, since variation in operator technique is reduced.

Each laboratory or testing site must have in place a quality assessment program that encompasses everything from specimen collection and patient identification to testing, reporting, and charting results. Documentation of employee training is also included. Although many of today's instruments appear simple to use, personnel must complete training for each instrument before they are allowed to report patient results. As new modules or accessories become available, personnel must be trained in their operation, care, and maintenance.

Quality checks must be in place to ensure appropriate specimen collection and processing. These quality checks continue as the instrument is turned on and readied for use. It must be verified that the correct reagents or reagent test units are being used and that the expiration dates are valid. All patient identification information must be entered properly. Regulatory organizations and manufacturers have requirements for temperature and barometric pressure readings for certain instruments.

When required maintenance and upkeep procedures are performed on a regular basis, analyzers provide reliable results. The manufacturer's operating manual for the instrument in use must be consulted for maintenance procedures. Some instruments are almost maintenance free; others require more frequent maintenance. A notebook or log containing a record of all instrument maintenance and repair must be kept.

Most manufacturers have quality control products, such as calibrators and normal and abnormal controls, for use with their instruments. In most cases these standard and control solutions should only be used with the indicated instrument and the appropriate analysis. The institution's policies must be strictly followed regarding acceptable standard deviation and the actions required when trends or shifts in control values are identified. If careful attention is given to these details, the results from an instrument will be valid and give an accurate view of patients' conditions.

Although many instruments operate on similar principles, the manufacturer's protocol for each particular instrument must be followed. Reagents, test strips, cartridges, and other supplies must be used only with analyzers for which they are approved.

BASIC PRINCIPLES OF INSTRUMENTATION

Most clinical laboratory instruments used in small laboratories are discrete analyzers, meaning that tests are performed by applying each patient sample to its own test cartridge, cassette, or reagent strip. After the patient sample is applied to the test unit, the instrument must detect and quantitate the endpoint of the reaction. This is accomplished in different ways, depending on instrument design. Four principles of instrumentation used in benchtop or portable analyzers and discussed in this lesson include:

- Photometry
- Reflectance photometry
- Ion-selective electrodes
- Electrochemical technology

Photometry

Photometers are instruments that measure light intensity and are used to determine the concentration of colored solutions. This determination is made by passing a beam of light of a specific wavelength through the solution contained in a glass or plastic cell called a cuvette. The portion of light that passes through the colored solution is detected by a photoelectric cell. This light is the **percent transmittance (%T)**. The light that does not pass through is absorbed by the colored solution and is measured as **absorbance (A)** units. The more concentrated the solution, the greater its absorbance and the less its transmittance. For most colored solutions, the absorbance increases proportionally with the concentration (Figure 6-5). These solutions are said to follow **Beer's law**. Several clinical analyzers contain simple or modified photometers. These usually operate at only one or a few preset wavelengths.

Spectrophotometers

Spectrophotometers are sophisticated photometers. They vary in external design, but the principles are the same, whether they are stand-alone instruments or are included as a part of an analyzer (Figure 6-6). A light source in the spectrophotometer provides a beam of light that passes to a **monochromator** with a diffraction grating that disperses the light into a spectrum. A narrow slit isolates a beam of monochromatic (one wavelength) light selected by the operator according to the analysis being performed. The monochromatic light is directed through the cuvette containing a colored solution. The light that passes through is detected by a photoelectric cell, which converts it to an electrical current that is measured and converted to a digital readout. This information can be presented as either absorbance (A) or percent transmittance (%T).

Photometers

Clinical analyzers which use principles of photometry include the HemoCue analyzers (Figure 6-7A) and the Cholestech GDX (Table 6-5). HemoCue makes handheld glucose and hemoglobin analyzers. Special clear disposable cuvettes contain the reagents required for a specific analysis. Blood samples are collected directly into the cuvette and reagents within the cuvette lyse the blood cells creating a clear, colored solution. The cuvette is inserted into a chamber in the analyzer. After the sample interacts with the reagent in the cuvette, the photometer measures the light passing through the solution and converts this to conventional or SI units. Calibration of the analyzer can be electronic or by use of a control cuvette that is an optical interference filter. Cholestech GDX uses a single wavelength spectrophotometer to measure hemoglobin A1c (see Lesson 6-6).

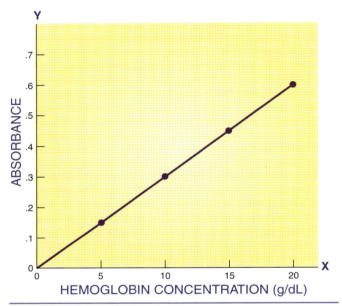

FIGURE 6-5 Illustration of a standard curve showing relationship of absorbance to concentration

Reflectance Photometry

Reflectance photometers measure light of a specific wavelength that is *reflected* by a colored product. This reflected light is detected by a photocell, and the information is converted into the appropriate units. Reflectance photometry is incorporated into several small clinical analyzers that use *solid-phase technology,* such as the Cholestech LDX (Figure 6-7B and Table 6-5).

Solid-Phase Technology

In **solid-phase chemistry** analyzers, the reagents are in dried form in the test unit. Solid-phase chemistry analyzers can often use whole blood as the sample. The blood sample is applied directly to the reagent strip, slide, or cartridge that contains all of the reagents needed for the analysis (Figure 6-8). The reagents are in multiple layers, with each layer having a specific function. The area where the reagents are located is called the *test area* or *reagent pad.* The test cartridges or strips have features that filter out the red blood cells, leaving only plasma to mix with the test reagents. The resulting color of the final product is detected by reflectance photometry. The color intensity is measured and converted to the correct units for the test being performed.

Chemistry analyzers that combine solid-phase technology with reflectance photometry include the Ortho Vitros DT 60 II and the urine strip analyzers such as the Criterion II (Figure 6-9).

In the Ortho VITROS DT 60 II system, each test procedure is contained on a dry reagent slide. The slide is placed into the sample drawer where the instrument reads the magnetic code on the slide to determine which test is to be performed. The patient sample is dispensed onto the test slide. The colored product produced by the reaction is automatically measured by a reflectance photometer inside the instrument. The Ortho Vitros DT 60 II can perform more than 30 different test procedures, including blood glucose, total cholesterol and cholesterol fractions, creatinine, bilirubin, amylase, and hemoglobin.

Urine strip analyzers also operate by reflectance photometry. The reagent strip pads change colors depending on the composi-

TABLE 6-5. Examples of chemistry analyzers suitable for the small laboratory and point-of-care testing, the technologies used, and their test capabilities

TECHNOLOGY	EXAMPLE	TEST CAPABILITIES
Electrochemical/amperometry	ACCU-CHEK (Roche Diagnostics)	blood glucose
	FreeStyle (Abbott Laboratories)	
Photometry	HemoCue Analyzers (HemoCue, Inc.)	Hb, blood glucose
	COBAS Integra 400 Plus (Roche Diagnostics)	blood chemistries
	Cholestech GDX	HbA1c
Reflectance photometry with solid-phase technology	Urine reagent strip readers	urine chemistries
	Ortho Vitros DT 60	blood chemistries
	Cholestech LDX	lipids, ALT, AST
Ion-selective electrodes	COBAS Integra 400 Plus, i-STAT, NOVA 14+, NOVA CCX	electrolytes

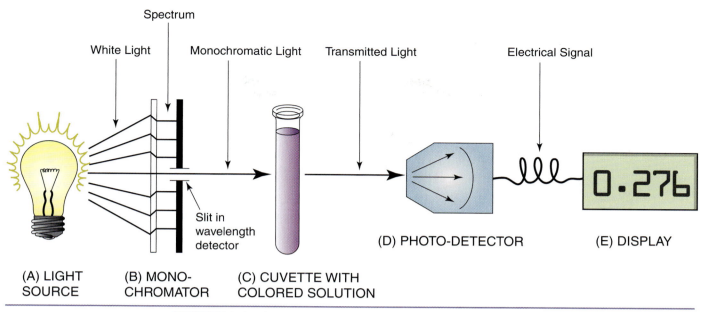

FIGURE 6-6 Diagram of the internal parts of a spectrophotometer

tion of the urine. These color changes are detected by the analyzer and the results are displayed or printed.

Ion-Selective Electrodes

Electrodes are probes that measure ions in solution. A common use of electrodes in clinical chemistry is to measure hydrogen ion concentration using a pH meter. **Ion-selective electrodes** selectively measure a particular ion in the presence of other ions. So a pH electrode is an ion-selective electrode for hydrogen (H^+).

Two electrodes are required for an analysis. One electrode contains a known concentration of the ion to be measured and is called the *reference electrode*. The other electrode, which is responsive only to the ion being measured, is exposed to the unknown solution. The difference between the concentration of ions in the reference electrode and the ions in the unknown solution causes an electrical potential to develop. This potential across a membrane in the electrode is proportional to the difference between the two concentrations. A microprocessor converts this voltage into a number representing the concentration of the ion in the unknown solution. Because each ion-selective electrode is responsive to a specific ion, the sodium (Na^+) electrode, for example, will measure only Na^+ ions present in a sample. The technology of ion-selective electrodes is used in many clinical instruments and is particularly useful for

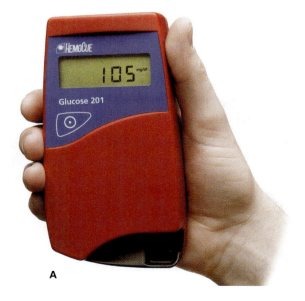

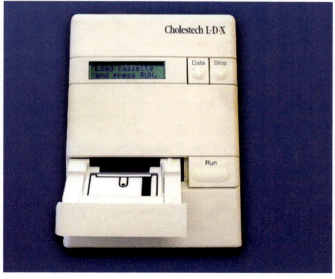

FIGURE 6-7 (A) HemoCue Glucose 201 Analyzer (*Courtesy of HemoCue, Inc., Lake Forest, CA*); (B) Cholestech LDX

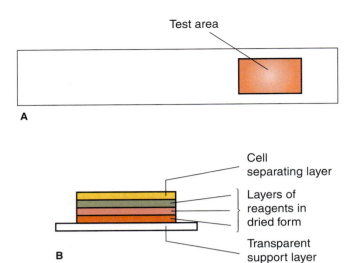

Test area

A

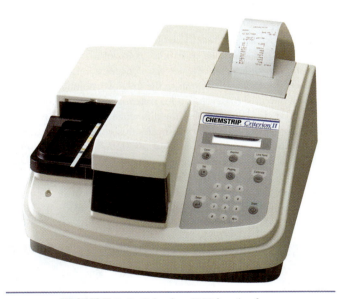

Cell separating layer

Layers of reagents in dried form

Transparent support layer

B

FIGURE 6-8 Illustration of the composition of a solid-phase reagent strip: (A) top view of a strip, showing reagent test area; (B) expanded side view of a test area, showing the layers

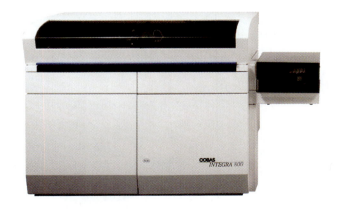

FIGURE 6-9 Criterion II Urine Analyzer
(*Courtesy Roche Diagnostics Corp., Indianapolis, IN*)

measuring electrolytes. Analyzers using ion-selective technology include Nova's Critical Care Xpress and 12⁺ analyzers and the COBAS INTEGRA 400 Plus (Figure 6-10).

Nova Analyzers

Nova Biomedical manufactures several analyzers that use ion-selective electrode technology and are suitable for use in smaller laboratories and critical care areas. The Nova 12⁺ has a test menu that includes Na^+, potassium (K^+), chloride (Cl^-), glucose, BUN (blood urea nitrogen), and hematocrit. It can analyze more than 50 samples per hour and, depending on the test, requires up to 200 μL of whole blood, serum, plasma, or urine. The small size of the instruments is made possible because of the compact size of the electrodes. Nova Biomedical also markets a line of analyzers called

Critical Care Xpress for use in POCT areas such as emergency departments. The instruments in the series can perform different combinations of blood gas, electrolyte, and hematocrit analyses.

Control solutions are run in the same manner as patient samples on most of the Nova chemistry analyzers. However, their Stat Profile Critical Care Xpress analyzer has an automated onboard quality control system. Special QC packs containing tri-level controls are loaded into the instrument. The instrument analyzes these packs at preset intervals, and the data are automatically stored. If the controls are not within limits, an audible alarm can alert the technician or an optional feature can put a lockout on the instrument until the problem is corrected. An additional feature is the SmartCheck automated maintenance program that ensures the instrument is operating correctly.

COBAS INTEGRA Analyzers

The COBAS INTEGRA analyzers (Figure 6-10) combine a *mix tower* with an ion-selective electrode analyzer. The mix tower is used to assure that sample and reagents are thoroughly mixed together. With the optional ion-selective electrode module, Na^+, K^+, and Cl^- ions can be measured directly. In addition, the instruments have menus of up to 72 tests including routine chemistries, HbA1c, and assays of drugs of abuse (Table 6-5). The COBAS 400 can process up to 400 samples per hour, depending on the combination of tests chosen.

Electrochemical Technology

Several handheld analyzers such as glucose meters are based on electrochemical technology. Other terms used for this technology include *amperometry* and *coulometry*. Analyzers using this technology include Roche Diagnostics' ACCU-CHEK meters, the FreeStyle glucose meters by Abbott Laboratories, and Medtronic Minimed's Paradigm Link glucose monitor. Analyzers using electrochemical technology incorporate electrodes that measure electrons generated when the sample and reagents react.

Some models of ACCU-CHEK glucose meters (Figure 6-11) use the principle of **amperometry**. Patient samples are applied to disposable biosensors, strips that look similar to other

FIGURE 6-10 The COBAS INTEGRA 800 chemistry analyzer (*Courtesy Roche Diagnostics Corp., Indianapolis, IN*)

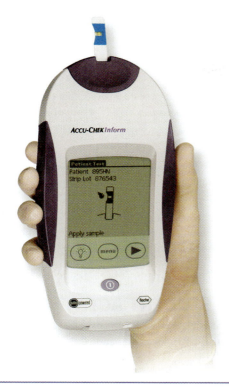

FIGURE 6-11 ACCU-CHEK Inform glucose meter (Courtesy *Roche Diagnostics Corp., Indianapolis, IN*)

reagent strips. These biosensors, in addition to containing reagents for the chemical reactions, also contain electrodes called electrochemical sensors. When the sample interacts with the reagents in the biosensor strip, the current (electrons) generated is detected by the meter and converted into glucose units.

SAFETY Reminders

- Follow Standard Precautions when using, maintaining, and repairing instruments.
- Always read the manufacturer's operating manual when operating or repairing an instrument.

PROCEDURAL Reminders

- Always follow the operating manual when using an instrument.
- Follow all quality assessment procedures.
- Understand the quality control and maintenance requirements of the instrument.
- Never use reagents or supplies for one instrument in another.
- Call the manufacturer's technical service department if a problem cannot be resolved.
- Attend training sessions offered by the instrument manufacturer.

CRITICAL THINKING

Dr. Sharma, a physician in a small group clinic, ordered a triglyceride test on a patient, and wanted the results before the patient left the clinic. Latitia, who worked in the clinic laboratory, prepared to perform the test. She calibrated the chemistry analyzer used for triglycerides and found it to be working correctly. However, Latitia found that, although the triglyceride controls had not expired, the reagent packs for the analyzer had expired the previous week.

1. Latitia should:
   a. go ahead and run the patient sample since the reagent packs had expired so recently
   b. use a triglyceride reagent pack from another analyzer to perform the test
   c. inform Dr. Sharma that the test cannot be run until in-date reagent packs are obtained for the analyzer
   d. run the controls and, if they are acceptable, perform the patient test
   e. perform the patient test, but only report the results if they are in the reference range
2. Discuss the choices above and justify your answer.
3. What laboratory policies should have been in place that would have prevented Latitia's dilemma?

SUMMARY

Using chemistry analyzers in smaller laboratories or POLs can be a real convenience for the patient and physician. Many types of chemistry analyzers are available. Factors to consider in choosing an analyzer include reliability of results, the number and kinds of tests to be performed, and the patient population. Purchase price, reagent costs, ease of operation, and maintenance requirements also should be considered. In addition, current users of instruments being considered should be contacted to discuss reliability, accuracy and precision, and quality of technical support. Training sessions offered by the manufacturer or distributor should be attended if possible or, preferably, a representative can come to the laboratory to train everyone who will be using the instrument. Quality assessment and quality control programs must be maintained for each instrument.

REVIEW QUESTIONS

1. Explain why instruments used in small laboratories might be different from those used in larger laboratories.

2. What has brought about increased testing in POLs?

3. What are the basic differences between photometers and reflectance photometers?

4. Explain solid-phase technology.

5. What is the principle of the ion-selective methods?

6. Discuss the principles of photometry.

7. Why is a regular instrument maintenance program important?

8. Discuss the importance of a quality assessment program for chemistry analyzers.

9. What safety hazards are associated with using instrumentation?

10. What is the advantage of an analyzer that can use whole blood specimens instead of only serum or plasma?

11. Explain how instrumentation affects TAT and why this is important.

12. Explain why the information in a maintenance logbook would be important when a problem arises with an instrument.

13. Define absorbance, amperometry, Beer's law, ion-selective electrode, monochromator, percent transmittance, reflectance photometer, solid-phase chemistry, and spectrophotometer.

STUDENT ACTIVITIES

1. Complete the written examination for this lesson.

2. Tour a small laboratory to observe the operation of some chemistry analyzers.

3. Ask at a local POL what analyzers are used there and what quality assessment procedures are performed.

4. Visit a health fair or a cholesterol screening event to observe the analyzers used.

5. Using the information from this lesson and an analyzer available in the laboratory, complete the worksheet accompanying this lesson.

WEB 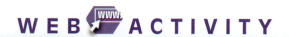 ACTIVITY

Using the Internet, find the Web site of a manufacturer mentioned in this lesson. Select a chemistry analyzer not mentioned in this lesson, and report on its principle of operation and test capabilities.

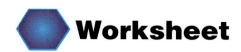 **Worksheet**

LESSON 6-3 Chemistry Instrumentation in the Physician Office Laboratory

Read the manufacturer's operating manual (or laboratory procedure manual) for an analyzer available in the laboratory and answer the following questions:

1. What is the name of the instrument? _____

2. What technology is used? _____

3. What kinds of test units are used with the instrument? _____

4. List two test procedures that can be performed using this instrument.

   _____

5. How is the instrument prompted or programmed for the test to be performed?

6. How are control solutions used with this instrument?

7. Has a Levey-Jennings chart been constructed for the procedures run on this instrument? _____

   Are values plotted daily? _____

8. What specimen(s) can be used for the analyses performed on this instrument?

   _____

9. Are maintenance and repair records kept in a logbook? _____

10. List in order the steps for performing a specific analysis using this instrument.

Student/Tech Name _____ **Date** _____

6-4

Point-of-Care Testing

LESSON OBJECTIVES

After studying this lesson, the student will:

- Explain what is meant by point-of-care testing (POCT).
- Discuss the benefits of POCT.
- Discuss safety procedures that must be followed in POCT.
- Explain why compliance with a quality assessment program is important in POCT.
- Name the health care professionals who are part of the POCT team.
- List five test procedures commonly performed as POC tests.
- Name three common POCT sites.

INTRODUCTION

Testing at point of care (POC) is a way of bringing laboratory testing to the patient, rather than sending patients or patient specimens to the laboratory. POCT has been made possible in part by the development of small, portable analyzers that give rapid test results. These analyzers are easy to use, give reproducible results, and require little maintenance.

POCT began when blood glucose monitors were developed for home use by diabetics. No special expertise was required to operate these first monitors, and the glucose test could be performed using a drop of capillary blood. Patients could have daily access to rapid test results and could use these results for adjusting their insulin dosage, diet, or activity levels.

In the 1990s, technological advances in instrument design mushroomed. Today, numerous small, sophisticated, but easy-to-use analyzers are available that can perform hematology, urinalysis, coagulation, chemistry, microbiology, and immunological tests. These analyzers are being used in a variety of settings to provide rapid laboratory testing. In addition, rapid immunological tests that require no instrument have been developed and are used at the point of care. Some of these, such as pregnancy test kits, are also available over the counter.

BENEFITS OF POCT

Rapid Results

The immediate benefit of near-patient testing, or POCT, is that laboratory test results can be obtained quickly, decreasing turnaround time (TAT). This benefits patients, health care workers, and the health care system (Table 6-6). Patients can receive required therapy more quickly, which can be especially important for critically ill patients. POCT programs in hospitals can lead to shorter hospital stays, owing to the rapid availability of test results.

Less Trauma–More Patient Participation

Another benefit is that these testing methods are less traumatic, requiring only a drop or two of capillary blood. Patients also feel

TABLE 6-6. Benefits of point-of-care testing (POCT) programs
Improved turnaround time (TAT) of test results
Increased patient participation in health care
Less traumatic testing method
Smaller specimen required
Shorter hospital stays
More rapid therapy intervention
Improved cooperation and communication among all members of health care team
Reduced errors in specimen handling and processing
Reduced need for specimen transport

TABLE 6-7. Departments and agencies involved in decision making in point-of-care testing (POCT) programs	
Clinical laboratory	Infection control
Nursing staff	Safety officer
Medical staff	Administration

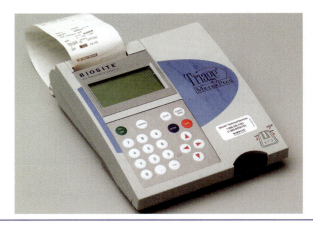

FIGURE 6-12 Triage MeterPlus
(*Courtesy Biosite, Inc., San Diego, CA*)

a greater sense of participation in their own care, usually learning of the test results immediately, since the test is performed in their presence.

Multiskilled Personnel

An additional benefit of POCT is that diverse groups of health care workers can be easily trained to perform the tests. This is because of simple-to-use rapid test kits and the ease of operation and low maintenance requirements of POC analyzers. For instance, in the physician office laboratory (POL), the medical assistant is often trained to take a patient's physical measurements such as blood pressure and pulse, as well as to perform laboratory tests such as measurements of glucose and cholesterol and urine chemical analysis.

Reduced Errors

The potential for errors is also decreased in POCT because the specimen need not be labeled, transported to the laboratory, or processed before testing—all opportunities for mishandling, mislabeling, or degrading a specimen.

POCT also provides increased communication and cooperation among the laboratory staff, nursing staff, and patients, enhancing the quality of care.

WHO IS INVOLVED IN POCT?

Good POCT programs require a multidisciplinary team effort among physicians and laboratory, nursing, and other hospital medical staff (Table 6-7). Nurses, medical assistants, emergency medical technicians, licensed practical nurses, or physicians can perform testing that has traditionally been done by laboratory personnel. The laboratory's usual role in POCT is to provide technical assistance, data management, quality assessment, compliance monitoring, and personnel training.

POINT-OF-CARE TESTING SITES

POCT programs are quite varied. They can be classified as hospital-based or nonhospital-based.

Hospital Point-of-Care Testing

Hospital POCT programs are usually geared toward providing service to critically ill patients in critical care units, emergency departments, surgical suites, and cardiac units. These patients benefit from quick action by the medical team, which is facilitated by having rapid test results. One example of a hospital POCT program is the use of bedside analyzers that measure glucose, clotting time, and electrolytes in the emergency department, critical care units, and surgery (Figure 6-12). These analyzers are calibrated and maintained by laboratory personnel, who provide procedure manuals, technical assistance, training of nursing staff, and assessment of the training. A POCT coordinator is responsible for reviewing and analyzing QC data, ensuring compliance with accreditation agencies, coordinating staff training, and serving as a liaison between nursing service and the laboratory.

Nonhospital Point-of-Care Testing Programs

POCT is also used in POLs, nursing homes, screening centers such as blood donation centers and health fairs, physical examinations for insurance or employment, and homes (Figure 6-13).

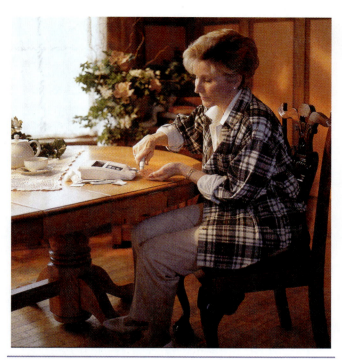

FIGURE 6-13 Patient performing at-home coagulation testing (*Courtesy Roche Diagnostics Corp., Indianapolis, IN*)

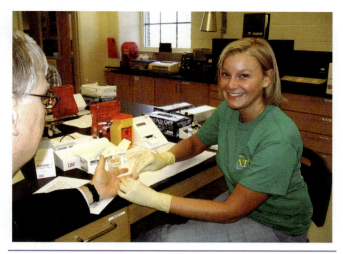

FIGURE 6-14 Cholesterol testing at a health fair

POCT programs outside the hospital have a different purpose from hospital programs. In nonhospital settings, rapid results are usually not critical to patient immediate care, but the on-site testing saves time and costs for the patient as well as the health care provider.

Nonhospital POCT programs are designed to provide a small menu of laboratory tests in a convenient, cost-effective, and efficient way. These tests are important in preventive medicine and can be used to screen for anemia, cardiovascular disease risk, and kidney disease, as well as to monitor and provide information for managing oral anticoagulant therapy or conditions such as diabetes.

Screening Programs

An example of a nonhospital POCT program is a 1-day cholesterol screening program that offers cholesterol tests and heart attack risk assessment. Volunteer health care personnel perform rapid cholesterol tests on capillary blood using portable cholesterol analyzers (Figure 6-14). Maintenance, calibration, and quality control of these analyzers are performed at the central laboratory facility before and after the screening event so that minimal control procedures are required during the screening event. Cholesterol results are available so those tested can decide whether or not to consult their physician.

Physician Office Laboratories

Another example of a nonhospital POCT program is a POL that offers tests such as hemoglobin, blood glucose, urine dipstick, and prothrombin time. These rapid tests can be performed by medical assistants or nursing staff before the patient sees the phy-

sician. The results are available for the physician to use in making decisions concerning further patient treatment or follow-up. This is much more efficient than sending patients to a laboratory for tests, waiting for the results, and calling or having the patients come back later to learn their test results.

Most POLs use CLIA-waived analyzers or test kits that require few routine maintenance and quality control procedures. However, procedure manuals and documentation of maintenance and quality control procedures are required, even though they may be minimal compared to those required for more complex analyzers. A laboratory professional may be employed as a consultant to provide periodic review of procedures and technical assistance.

COMPONENTS INCLUDED IN A POINT-OF-CARE TESTING PROGRAM

Whether a POCT program is large-scale or small, there are several components that must be incorporated into the program. These include:

- Compliance with regulatory agencies
- Safety program
- QA program
- Personnel training and assessment
- Technical support
- Data management

Compliance with Regulatory Guidelines

The primary law that regulates POCT is CLIA '88. This law describes the standards that must be met for all testing procedures used in diagnosing and treating human disease. To receive federal Medicare and Medicaid funds, laboratories must obtain a CLIA certificate granting permission to perform certain tests.

CURRENT TOPICS

ESTABLISHING A POINT-OF-CARE TESTING PROGRAM

Enhancement of the quality of patient health care should be the primary consideration behind establishment of a POCT program. The Joint Commission (JC), has created National Patient Safety Goals (NPSG) to ensure POCT patient safety. POCT programs are not beneficial if test results are not reliable or are not evaluated and acted upon quickly. The health care facility must maintain a high-quality program, meet all regulatory requirements, and train and assess testing personnel.

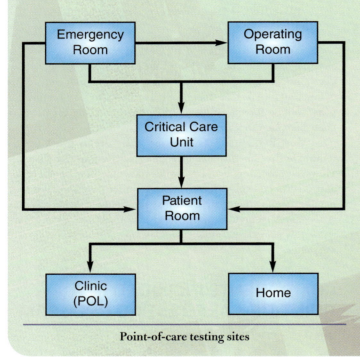

Point-of-care testing sites

POCT can be performed in the emergency department, operating room, critical care unit, patient hospital room, a clinic or POL, or the patient's home (see diagram). Several factors must be incorporated into any successful testing program:

- Testing protocols should be *standardized* across all sites.
- Excellent *communication* is required among testing sites and with the central laboratory.
- All personnel involved should consider themselves to be on a *goal-oriented team*.
- There should be constant program *improvement*, including problem solving and incorporation of new methodologies.
- *Networking* with others in the field and with manufacturers' technical representatives is important.
- Keeping up with *current research* into trends, such as new QA methods, is vital.
- *Connectivity* is essential; this could include automatic documentation of data, electronic posting of POCT data into medical records, and integration of POCT results into the overall patient care pathway (such as with results from the main laboratory).
- *Data management* is facilitated using computers incorporated into many analyzers.
- Most of all, a *positive attitude* is required. POCT personnel must be willing to be cross-trained to perform laboratory work in addition to their other duties.

Each POCT site must be self-managed and responsible for its operation. A self-inspection worksheet is helpful for that. Even though the central laboratory may train those performing the tests, the overall responsibility for compliance lies with the individual site and its CLIA director.

Safety Precautions

   Occupational Safety and Health Administration (OSHA) and Centers for Disease Control and Prevention (CDC) guidelines must be followed to prevent exposure of health care personnel and patients to chemical, physical, and biological hazards. Written safety rules that encompass Standard Precautions must be included in all procedure manuals and must be followed rigorously.

Quality Assessment

A POCT program must be able to provide accurate, reliable test results. This is assured by having a comprehensive QA program in place. QA includes procedures that ensure the quality of the test procedure from beginning (test requisition) to end (interpretation and reporting of results). Instrument calibration, up-to-date procedure manuals, testing of control sera or reagents, participation in a proficiency testing program, comprehensive documentation, and employee training and assessment are all part of a QA program. For many instruments and kits used for POCT, the burden of performing frequent controls is lessened because internal controls are included in many instruments and kits. Central laboratories that operate POCT sites must also assure that the values obtained at the POCT sites are equivalent to the values obtained in the central laboratory.

Training and Assessment

Depending on the type of POCT program, personnel can be trained by the laboratory or by a technical representative of the instrument manufacturer. Testing personnel must be trained and their competence verified before they can be permitted to test patient specimens. Periodic review and documentation of personnel performance is required. Participation in a proficiency testing program is one method of assessing performance.

Technical Support

Laboratories running POCT programs must either have a director on site or employ a qualified laboratory consultant who is available to provide technical assistance. Technical support is also available through instrument manufacturers, usually through a hotline or local service representative.

Data Management

Data management at POCT sites can be simple or complex. In a POL, test results are usually written directly on the patient's chart or an instrument printout is inserted into the chart. In a hospital POCT program, the data management system can be sophisticated. Testing personnel may have bar-coded identification badges that must be used to have access to an analyzer. In this way, only personnel who have proven competency in performing the procedure are permitted to operate the instrument. The analyzers can also be linked directly to the laboratory information system (LIS), with results transferred electronically to the laboratory as soon as they are generated.

SUMMARY

Although POCT is not the answer for all situations, it can be an important component of health care. Careful studies must be done to determine if a POCT program should be implemented and what the scope of the program should be. Improved patient care should be the most important goal. POCT programs must be constantly monitored to ensure they are achieving their goal and that test results are of the highest quality.

Many test procedures have been adapted to POCT use (Table 6-8). Some provide important data useful in acute care

---

TABLE 6-8. Tests commonly performed at point-of-care testing (POCT) sites

Hematology tests
- Hemoglobin
- Hematocrit

Coagulation tests
- Activated clotting time
- Prothrombin time
- Activated partial thromboplastin time
- D-dimer

Chemistry tests
- Cholesterol
- Electrolytes
- Blood glucose
- Cardiac panel
- Fecal occult blood
- BUN (Blood urea nitrogen)
- Creatinine
- Hemoglobin A1c

Urine tests
- Urine dipstick
- Pregnancy (hCG)
- Microalbumin

Microbiology/immunology tests
- Rapid strep
- Infectious mononucleosis
- HIV
- Influenza
- *Helicobacter pylori*

CRITICAL THINKING

Community Hospital has decided to develop several POCT sites both inside and outside the hospital. The plan calls for establishing active POCT programs in the hospital emergency department and intensive care unit, and in one site in a free clinic. All sites would be supplied with the same instruments to perform the same menu of tests. The laboratory manager has agreed for an educator in the laboratory to train all employees for the three sites in the operation and maintenance of the instruments. However, the physician/director of the free clinic also wants to be trained so that he can train personnel who perform the testing at his site. In addition, he wants to perform quality assessment and keep QA records at his site.

1. Explain why it is preferable for the same person to train all the employees.
2. If the physician performs the QA and keeps all the records, is the laboratory responsible for his results?

facilities, such as electrolyte analysis, activated clotting time assay, and assays for heart attack assessment. Others are more useful in health-screening situations or physician offices. These include hemoglobin, hematocrit, cholesterol, urine dipstick, rapid strep tests, pregnancy tests, prothrombin time, and fecal occult blood tests.

REVIEW QUESTIONS

1. What are four benefits of a POCT program?

2. Name five departments that participate in POCT programs.

3. What technological developments have made POCT possible?

4. How do hospital POCT programs differ from nonhospital programs?

5. Name two hematological tests often performed at point of care.

6. Name four chemistry tests often performed at point of care.

7. Discuss the importance of quality assessment in POCT programs.

8. Why is it important for one department to be responsible for training all POCT technicians?

9. What is the primary law that regulates POCT?

10. What safety precautions must be observed when performing POCT?

STUDENT ACTIVITIES

1. Complete the written examination for this lesson.

2. Inquire about a POCT program in a hospital near you. Find out what tests are performed, who performs them, and how QA is accomplished.

3. Find POCT programs that are in place in your community and comment on the benefits they provide.

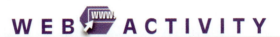

WEB ACTIVITY

Select two tests from Table 6-8. Use the Internet to find information about a test kit or small analyzer that would be appropriate for POCT for each test. Report on the test method, training required, specimen required, TAT, and reliability of results.

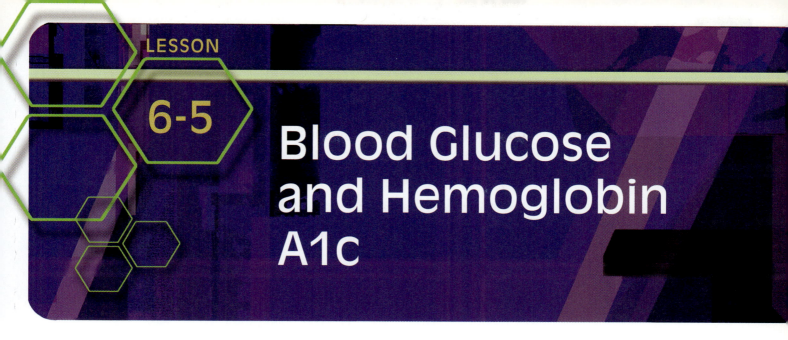

LESSON 6-5

Blood Glucose and Hemoglobin A1c

LESSON OBJECTIVES

After studying this lesson, the student will:

- Explain the function of glucose in the body.
- Describe factors that affect blood glucose levels.
- Name two disorders of glucose metabolism.
- Explain the collection requirements for blood glucose specimens.
- Explain the principles of glucose test methods.
- Explain the purpose of a postprandial glucose test.
- Explain how a glucose tolerance test is performed.
- State the reference values for fasting blood glucose, 2-hour postprandial glucose, and glucose tolerance tests.
- Perform a blood glucose measurement using a glucose analyzer.
- Explain the relationship of hemoglobin A1c (HbA1c) to blood glucose.
- Discuss the importance of measuring HbA1c.
- Perform a test for HbA1c.
- Discuss the importance of quality assessment programs for glucose and HbA1c testing.
- Discuss safety precautions that must be observed when performing tests for glucose and HbA1c.
- Define the glossary terms.

GLOSSARY

chromogen / a substance that becomes colored when it undergoes a chemical change

diabetes mellitus / a disorder of carbohydrate metabolism characterized by a state of hyperglycemia due to insulin deficiency

glucagon / the pancreatic hormone that increases blood glucose concentration by promoting the conversion of glycogen to glucose

glucose dehydrogenase / an enzyme that converts glucose to gluconolactone and that is used in glucose analytical methods

glucose oxidase / an enzyme that converts glucose to gluconic acid and that is used in glucose analytical methods

glycated hemoglobin (GHb) / see hemoglobin A1c

glycogen / the storage form of glucose found in high concentration in the liver

glycolysis / energy production as a result of the metabolic breakdown of glucose

545

hemoglobin A1c (HbA1c) / hemoglobin modified by the binding of glucose to the beta globin chains of hemoglobin; also called glycated or glycosylated hemoglobin

hexokinase / an enzyme that converts glucose to glucose-6-phosphate and that is used in glucose analytical methods

hyperglycemia / blood glucose concentration above normal

hypoglycemia / blood glucose concentration below normal

insulin / the pancreatic hormone essential for proper metabolism of blood glucose and maintenance of blood glucose levels

oral glucose tolerance test (OGTT) / analysis of blood glucose at timed intervals following ingestion of a standard glucose dose

peroxidase / an enzyme that converts hydrogen peroxide to water and oxygen

postprandial / after eating

INTRODUCTION

Glucose, the major carbohydrate in blood, is used for energy by the body's cells. Blood glucose is one of the most frequently performed clinical chemistry tests.

Two disorders of glucose metabolism are (1) **diabetes mellitus**, in which there is increased blood glucose, called **hyperglycemia**, and (2) **hypoglycemia**, (decreased blood glucose), as can be seen in deficiencies of adrenocorticotropic hormone (ACTH) or growth hormone.

The glucose test is most often used to aid in diagnosing and managing diabetes, or in managing hypoglycemia. This lesson presents information about glucose metabolism, diagnosis and management of diabetes, and methods of glucose analysis.

MECHANISMS REGULATING BLOOD GLUCOSE LEVELS

Although the body has many metabolic pathways that involve glucose, certain hormones keep blood glucose within a fairly narrow range.

Insulin

Insulin, a hormone produced by the pancreas, *lowers* blood glucose by increasing cellular uptake of glucose and increasing the rate of **glycolysis**. Glycolysis is a cellular process that produces energy by the metabolic breakdown of glucose. Insulin also increases the rate of conversion of glucose to **glycogen**, the short-term storage form of glucose.

Other Hormones

Hormones such as growth hormone, epinephrine, cortisol, and **glucagon** act in a variety of ways to *increase* blood glucose concentration. These hormones are sometimes called insulin antagonists, because their action is opposite to the action of insulin.

DIAGNOSTIC TESTS FOR DIABETES AND HYPOGLYCEMIA

Most health care providers now use the fasting glucose value to diagnose diabetes. However, some health organizations recommend performing an **oral glucose tolerance test (OGTT)** for diagnosis. The OGTT is more expensive and time-consuming, and some patients do not tolerate the glucose beverage that must be consumed. The fasting glucose can be performed on a very small sample of blood with the results obtained while the patient is still in the physician's office. The speed of analysis and the relative low cost of the fasting glucose make it the test of choice for screening patients for diabetes.

Fasting Blood Glucose

A fasting blood glucose is performed on a blood sample taken when the patient has not eaten for a specified period of time. A fasting specimen is usually obtained before breakfast after the patient has gone without food for at least 8 hours.

Oral Glucose Tolerance Test

The OGTT has been used to diagnose diabetes mellitus as well as hypoglycemia. However, the traditional OGTT is performed infrequently because the test can range from 3 to 5 hours, requiring the patient to remain in the laboratory waiting area and be carefully supervised. For the test, a fasting blood glucose sample is drawn and a urine sample is obtained from the patient. Next the patient consumes a beverage containing a standard glucose dose (usually 50, 75, or 100 mg). Blood and urine samples are subsequently collected at set intervals (typically 30 minutes and 1, 2, and 3 hours) after the beverage has been consumed. Glucose is measured in the blood samples, and urine glucose is estimated using a urine dipstick. The OGTT can be used to confirm the diagnosis of diabetes in a patient with an elevated fasting glucose.

CURRENT TOPICS

DIABETES

Diabetes mellitus, commonly called diabetes, is a chronic disease in which the body either produces insufficient insulin or is unable to use insulin properly. It is a very serious disease because insulin is the hormone that enables the body to convert food into energy. Insulin *unlocks* the cells of the body to allow glucose to enter and become fuel for the cells. When glucose is not used by the cells, it accumulates in the blood, causing a condition called hyperglycemia. When allowed to continue over the long-term, hyperglycemia causes damage to blood vessels, tissues, and organs.

Type 1 diabetes results from insufficient insulin or lack of insulin and usually appears in children and young adults. Type 2 diabetes results when the body fails to properly use insulin and usually appears later in life, although an increased incidence in adolescents is now being seen. The latter condition is known as *insulin resistance.* Two additional conditions are *gestational diabetes* and *prediabetes.*

Gestational diabetes occurs in about 4% of pregnant women. Prediabetes is the condition in which the blood glucose is above normal but still below the level of being considered diabetic.

The American Diabetes Association (ADA) recently estimated that while approximately 15 million people in the United States have been diagnosed with diabetes, there are probably at least 6 million who have the disease but are unaware of it. It is estimated that clinicians are diagnosing about 800,000 new cases of type 2 diabetes each year. People in the undiagnosed group can have diabetes for up to 10 years without being aware of it until they suffer its complications. Diabetes causes damage to small blood vessels resulting in problems in the kidneys, the eyes, and extremities such as feet and toes, and is a major cause of cardiovascular disease. Early diagnosis is very important because proper management of diabetes can lessen, postpone, or even prevent many of these complications.

TABLE 6-9. Glucose reference values*

TEST	GLUCOSE CONCENTRATION	
	mg/dL	mmol/L (SI)
Fasting		
Serum	70–110	3.9–6.1
Whole blood	60–100	3.3–5.6
Plasma	66–105	3.7–5.9
Two-hour postprandial (serum)	≤110	≤6.1
Oral glucose tolerance (serum)		
Fasting	70–110	3.9–6.1
1 hour	20–50 above fasting	1.1–2.8 above fasting
2 hour	5–25 above fasting	0.3–1.4 above fasting
3 hour	fasting level or below	fasting level or below

* Values vary slightly among laboratories, depending on test method used

---

It is often used to obtain a true picture of glucose metabolism in pregnant women who have higher than normal fasting glucose levels.

Diabetes can often be diagnosed by modifying the glucose tolerance test and using just two glucose measurements—the fasting blood glucose and a glucose measurement 2 hours after the glucose dose. However, patients suspected of having hypoglycemia are usually required to undergo the entire test and often have blood glucose tested for 5 to 6 hours following the glucose dose.

Patients undergoing OGTT should be monitored carefully for adverse reactions.

Two-Hour Postprandial Glucose

A 2-hour **postprandial** test is a measurement of glucose 2 hours after the patient has eaten. Postprandial tests are most reliable if the patient is tested following a standard glucose dose (50 to 100 g) such as in the 2-hour OGTT rather than a random meal.

GLUCOSE REFERENCE VALUES

Fasting Glucose

The reference (normal) fasting blood glucose value for serum is 70 to 110 mg/dL (Table 6-9). Plasma values are about 5% lower than serum and about 10% to 15% higher than whole blood values. The ADA has recently recommended that fasting plasma glucose values ≥126 mg/dL be interpreted as indicating hyperglycemia.

Oral Glucose Tolerance Test

A patient with normal metabolism of glucose should have a normal fasting serum glucose level (70 to 110 mg/dL); a 1-hour level of 90 to 160 mg/dL; a 2-hour level less than 140 mg/dL, and a 3-hour level at or below the fasting level (Table 6-9).

Two-Hour Postprandial

The 2-hour postprandial serum glucose value is normally less than 140 mg/dL.

Critical Glucose Values

In the clinical laboratory, test results that are extremely high or low are called *critical values, alert values,* or *action values,* meaning immediate action is required by laboratory staff to alert physicians and/or nursing staff of the results. Every laboratory has a list of critical values for various tests and a written procedure to follow when a test result falls into this category.

In the case of glucose, a patient is considered to be hypoglycemic if the glucose falls below 50 mg/dL. Glucose <40 mg/dL is considered a critical value. Hypoglycemic patients can experience fainting, weakness, confusion, or lack of coordination and may lapse into unconsciousness if left untreated (Table 6-10).

An extremely high glucose level can lead to diabetic coma and requires immediate treatment to reduce the glucose level. Blood glucose exceeding 400 mg/dL is considered dangerously high. Symptoms of hyperglycemia include confusion, lethargy, extreme thirst, weak pulse, dry skin, and nausea (Table 6-10). Each laboratory must establish the critical glucose values that require immediate action.

DIABETES MANAGEMENT

Home Glucose Meters

Good diabetes management is important for preventing or delaying microvascular complications. Meters for patient use in monitoring blood glucose levels were first introduced in the 1970s.

TABLE 6-10. Critical glucose values and symptoms that can accompany them

HYPOGLYCEMIA <40 mg/dL	HYPERGLYCEMIA >400 mg/dL
Faintness	Confusion
Weakness	Coma
Hunger	Nausea
Diaphoresis	Intense thirst
Visual disturbances	Ketoacidosis
Palsy	Dry flushed skin
Confusion	Weak pulse
Personality changes	

Note: Patient may not experience all symptoms

CURRENT TOPICS

BLOOD GLUCOSE REFERENCE RANGES VERSUS RECOMMENDED BLOOD GLUCOSE LEVELS

The blood glucose reference range is the laboratory's acceptable range of glucose values obtained from statistical analysis of glucose values in the general population. This reference range is shown on a facility's laboratory report form (Table 6-9). Reference ranges can differ slightly from laboratory to laboratory, depending on the type of specimen analyzed. Serum glucose can be as much as 5% higher than plasma glucose, while whole blood glucose is slightly lower than plasma glucose.

Recommended blood glucose values differ from blood glucose reference ranges. Recommended values are the *ideal* glucose levels recommended by organizations such as the ADA and are used in the differential diagnosis of diabetes. The recommended glucose value has changed significantly in recent years. The ADA recommendations (as of 2005) for diagnosing diabetes/hyperglycemia are that:

■ Patients with a fasting plasma glucose (FPG) < 100 mg/dL be considered *nondiabetic*

■ Patients with FPG from 100 through 125 mg/dL be considered *prediabetic* due to *impaired fasting glucose* (IFG) and

■ Patients with an FPG ≥ 126 mg/dL be considered *hyperglycemic* and should have follow-up testing.

Since then, meter accuracy, precision, and ease of use have improved. It is recommended that all diabetic patients use a home glucose monitoring system regularly.

Hemoglobin A1c

The patient's ability to keep blood glucose levels within acceptable ranges can be assessed by periodic measurement of **hemoglobin A1c**, also called **glycated hemoglobin**.

What is HbA1c?

Hemoglobin (Hb) is present in all red blood cells and is the molecule that transports oxygen from the lungs to the tissues. The major hemoglobin is Hb A. After glucose is absorbed from the gastrointestinal tract and enters the circulation, it is taken up by cells for energy. During periods of high blood glucose levels, glucose molecules enter red blood cells and bind to hemoglobin, forming HbA1c, also called glycated hemoglobin. The amount of HbA1c is proportional to the amount of glucose in the blood. Since the half life of red blood cells is approximately 60 days, the level of HbA1c is related to the average amount of glucose in the blood for that period of time. In reality the HbA1c more closely represents levels over the previous 2 to 4 weeks.

Why is HbA1c measured?

The fasting glucose level indicates how well the patient has glucose under control at the time the specimen is taken. The HbA1c value tells the physician how tightly the patient has controlled the blood glucose level over a period of time. Recent studies have shown that HbA1c is the single best test for evaluating the risk of damage to nerves and to the small blood vessels of the eyes and kidneys. This damage leads to the complications of diabetes, such as blindness and kidney failure. Clinical trials have shown that reducing the HbA1c level in diabetics and maintaining it below 7% will prevent the development of, or further progression of, complications from diabetes (Table 6-11). This is true for both type 1 and type 2 diabetes. Several instruments can quickly measure HbA1c (Figure 6-15); some

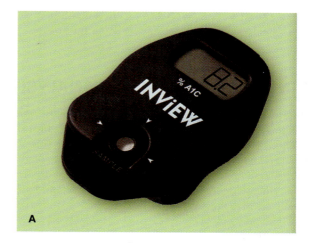

A

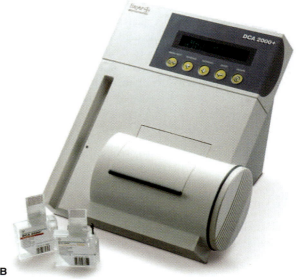

B

FIGURE 6-15 Hemoglobin A1c analyzers: (A) Metrika A1c Now Inview system (*Courtesy Metrika, Inc., Sunnyvale, CA*); (B) DCA 2000+ analyzer (*Courtesy Bayer Healthcare Diagnostics Division, Norwood, MA*)

TABLE 6-11. Relationship between hemoglobin A1c percentages and average blood glucose values

HEMOGLOBIN A1c (%)	AVERAGE WHOLE BLOOD GLUCOSE (mg/dL)	AVERAGE PLASMA GLUCOSE (mg/dL)	INTERPRETATION
4	61	65	Normal (nondiabetic) range (4%-5%)
5	92	100	
6	124	135	
7	156	170	Target for good diabetes control (6%–7%)
8	188	205	Action required (8%–12%)
9	219	240	
10	251	275	
11	283	310	
12	314	345	

of these are CLIA-waived. Additionally, some home glucose meters calculate HbA1c from the average of the glucose values in memory.

PRINCIPLES OF GLUCOSE ANALYSIS

Most glucose testing methods use the enzymes **glucose oxidase**, **hexokinase**, or **glucose dehydrogenase** to measure glucose concentration. These enzyme tests are simple, quick, and specific for glucose and have been adapted for use in many types of glucose analyzers both large and small. In general, tests that use hexokinase or glucose dehydrogenase are more specific and have less interferences than those using glucose oxidase.

Glucose Oxidase Method

The glucose oxidase method of analysis is a two-step reaction. Glucose is converted to gluconic acid and hydrogen peroxide (H_2O_2) in the presence of glucose oxidase and oxygen. The resulting concentrations of gluconic acid and H_2O_2 are proportional to the amount of glucose originally present. In the second part of the reaction, in the presence of the **peroxidase** enzyme and a **chromogen**, the H_2O_2 is converted to water (H_2O) and the chromogen produces a color:

$$(1)\ \text{Glucose} + H_2O + O_2 \xrightarrow{\text{Glucose Oxidase}} \text{Gluconic acid} + H_2O_2$$

$$(2)\ H_2O_2 + \text{Chromogen} \xrightarrow{\text{Peroxidase}} 2\,H_2O + \text{Color formation}$$

The color intensity is proportional to the amount of H_2O_2 (and thus the amount of glucose) and can be measured using photometry.

Hexokinase Method

The hexokinase method is also a two-step reaction. This method has advantages over the glucose oxidase method, primarily because fewer substances interfere and safer reagents are used. In the first step, hexokinase forms glucose-6-phosphate (G6P) from glucose. In the second step, G6P is converted to 6-phosphogluconate (6PG) by the enzyme glucose-6-phosphate dehydrogenase (G6PD) with the production of NADPH:

$$(1)\ \text{Glucose} + \text{ATP} \xrightarrow{\text{Hexokinase}} \text{G6P} + \text{ADP}$$

$$(2)\ \text{G6P} + \text{NADP} \xrightarrow{\text{G6PD}} \text{6PG} + \text{NADPH}$$

NADPH absorbs ultraviolet light at 340 nm. This absorbance can be measured using a spectrophotometer. The increase in absorbance due to NADPH in the solution is proportional to the glucose concentration in the original reaction.

Glucose Dehydrogenase Method

Both the HemoCue and ACCU-CHEK meters use the enzyme glucose dehydrogenase (GDH) to convert glucose to gluconolactone. This method has few interferences. However, the meters use different detection methods.

PERFORMING BLOOD GLUCOSE AND HbA1c MEASUREMENTS

Safety Precautions

 Standard Precautions must be followed when performing blood glucose measurements. Appropriate personal protective equipment (PPE) must be worn when obtaining the blood specimen and performing the test. All test materials must be discarded in appropriate biohazard containers.

Quality Assessment

The manufacturer's instructions must be followed for the particular analyzer used. With all instruments, it is important to use consistent, correct technique to avoid variations in results. Test materials, such as reagent strips or cuvettes, that are made for a particular instrument must be used only with that instrument.

Glucose controls purchased from instrument manufacturers should be used to check instrument performance. Control tests and calibration checks must be performed daily before patient samples are run and anytime results are questionable. Control tests let the technician know that the test strips, cuvettes, or cartridges and the analyzer are working properly and that technique is adequate.

Control tests use solutions of known concentrations of glucose that react similarly to blood when used with the test cuvette or strip. The controls are available in normal, low, and high concentrations and are used in the same manner as a blood sample.

When control tests are performed, the control results on the display screen should be recorded and compared to the values printed on the control bottle or package insert. If the results are within the acceptable range, the patient specimen can be analyzed. If not, the control tests must be repeated using new test strips and being certain that correct technique is used. If the controls are still out of the acceptable range, the strips or controls could be defective and a new lot or control should be tested. If an out-of-range result is obtained with the new lot of strips or new control, there may be an instrument problem and the operating manual should be consulted. Patient specimens must not be analyzed until the instrument and strips are working properly as indicated by the control tests. A log of control test results must be kept. In this way, any deterioration of the test system can be noted early and corrective action taken.

Specimen Collection

Glucose measurement can be performed on whole blood, plasma, serum, urine, or cerebrospinal fluid. The laboratory requisition will specify whether the specimen can be random or must be a fasting specimen.

Blood cells metabolize glucose and, if left in contact with serum or plasma, rapidly lower the specimen's glucose concentration, causing a false low glucose value. If serum or plasma is used, it must be separated from the blood cells as soon as possible after collection. If separation will be delayed, blood can be collected in tubes (gray top) containing a glycolytic inhibitor.

If whole blood glucose is to be measured, the test should be performed immediately following capillary puncture, or on blood collected in a suitable anticoagulant, such as EDTA or heparin. The anticoagulant must be one that will not interfere with the glucose analysis method being used.

Glucose Analyzers

Glucose analyzers use enzymatic methods to measure glucose. Some analyzers measure only glucose, are simple to use, give rapid results, and are appropriate for point-of-care testing (POCT), physician office laboratory (POL), and even home use. Analyzers used in larger laboratories measure glucose as part of a profile. Most glucose analyzers use either photometry or electrochemical principles (Lesson 6-3).

Photometry

The HemoCue Blood Glucose System is an example of an analyzer that uses photometry to measure blood glucose (Figure 6-16). The system includes a small handheld analyzer and disposable clear microcuvettes that contain the glucose enzyme reagent. The self-filling microcuvette automatically draws up 5 μL of blood from a capillary puncture into the reaction chamber; it is then inserted into the analyzer. The glucose concentration in mg/dL or mmol/L is displayed in 45 to 240 seconds. This system is ideal for POLs and POCT because of its calibration stability and the minimal operator training required. Data management programs are available with the HemoCue.

Electrochemical Technology/ Amperometry

Electrochemical technology, or amperometry, is a technology that uses electrodes to detect current (electrons) generated during a chemical reaction. Several glucose meters, including ACCU-CHEK Advantage (Roche Diagnostics), FreeStyle (Abbott Laboratories), and Medtronic Paradigm Link glucose meter (Figure 6-17) use

this technology. In these meters, electrodes measure the reaction of glucose with glucose dehydrogenase (GDH). A biosensor strip is inserted into the meter and the blood sample is applied to the strip. The GDH enzyme within the strip reacts with glucose in the blood specimen to form gluconolactone, causing a release of electrons. The sensor in the meter detects voltage changes resulting from the electron release, and converts this electrical signal into glucose concentration, which is displayed on the meter screen.

Some glucose meters are designed for home use. Others, such as the ACCU-CHEK Inform, are designed for POCT and can interface with hospital or laboratory computer systems, allowing storage and retrieval of patient and QC data.

Determining HbA1c

Glycated hemoglobin (GHb), more commonly called HbA1c or just A1c, can be measured using one of several analyzers such as the Cholestech GDX, Bayer DCA 2000+ or Metrika A1cNow Inview System (Figure 6-15). The CLIA-waived Cholestech GDX uses affinity chromatography to measure both glycated and nonglycated hemoglobin in a 10 μL blood sample. The results are converted to the percentage of A1c in the sample and are available in less than 5 minutes. The A1cNow Inview measures the A1c in less than 5 minutes using just 5 μL of fingerstick or venous blood. The method is CLIA-waived and can be performed at home or in point-of-care situations.

The DCA 2000+ uses monoclonal antibody to analyze whole blood samples for HbA1c. Blood is collected from a finger puncture into a capillary holder supplied with the analyzer. The sample-filled holder is inserted into the reagent cartridge. The analyzer's calibration is verified by sliding the reagent cartridge through the slot and past the integral bar-code reader. The reagent cartridge containing the specimen is then inserted into the DCA 2000+ through the door. A pull-tab on the cartridge is removed to release buffer into the patient sample and the analysis is initiated when the instrument door is closed. Results are available within 5 minutes and are displayed on the analyzer. The DCA 2000+ can also analyze urine specimens for microalbumin, creatinine, and albumin/creatinine ratio using the appropriate cartridge (Figure 6-15B).

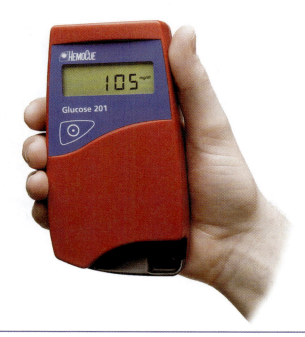

FIGURE 6-16 HemoCue Glucose 201 Analyzer
(*Courtesy of HemoCue Inc., Lake Forest, CA*)

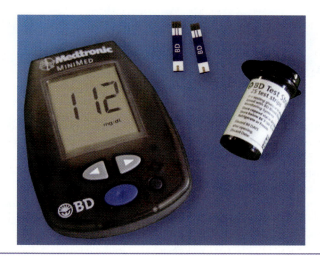

FIGURE 6-17 Medtronic Paradigm Link glucose meter
(*Courtesy A. Estridge, Los Angeles, CA*)

CASE STUDY 1

Jose has had insulin-dependent diabetes for 12 years. His physician measures his HbA1c every 3 months. Jose's latest HbA1c was 6.7.

His physician:
a. will be concerned because the HbA1c is so high
b. will compliment Jose on good management of his glucose
c. will advise Jose to decrease his insulin dosage
d. will order the test repeated because the results do not make sense

CASE STUDY 2

Mrs. Simpson had the first morning appointment with Dr. Mitchell for her yearly physical. Before seeing the doctor, the nursing assistant drew blood for some routine chemistry tests. The laboratory called Dr. Mitchell's office, and reported that Mrs. Simpson's glucose test result was 140 mg/dL.

Dr. Mitchell's nursing assistant should:
a. call Mrs. Simpson and tell her she has diabetes
b. interrupt the doctor because the glucose is above the panic value
c. look on Mrs. Simpson's chart to see if she was fasting when the blood specimen was collected
d. not worry about it and just chart the glucose results

SAFETY Reminders

- Review safety precautions before beginning procedure.
- Follow Standard Precautions when performing glucose measurements.
- Clean and disinfect the instrument before returning it to storage.

PROCEDURAL Reminders

- Review QA section before beginning procedure.
- Follow manufacturers' directions for the instrument and reagents used.
- Use appropriate controls and calibrators and record the results on the quality control log sheets.
- Use a specimen appropriate for the test method.
- Be sure reagents and test packs or strips are not used past their expiration dates.

SUMMARY

The measurement of the amount of glucose in the blood is an important analysis for the diagnosis and treatment of diabetes. A fasting glucose level can help to either rule out or diagnose diabetes and to indicate how well the patient is controlling the blood glucose level. Other glucose tests such as the 2-hour postprandial or OGTT also can add much information about the state of glucose metabolism in the patient.

The HbA1c test is of great value in the control of diabetes and its complications. The HbA1c result gives an estimate of the average blood glucose level over a period of several weeks. This information indicates how well the patient has been controlling the glucose level and guides the patient and physician in adjusting the diet, amount of exercise, or insulin dosage to achieve better blood glucose control.

Both the glucose level and the HbA1c can be analyzed in a few minutes using a small blood sample. Small handheld meters measure glucose using a variety of technologies. A number of analyzers can measure the HbA1c. Some glucose meters can calculate HbA1c from the glucose results stored in memory.

All Standard Precautions must be observed while performing these tests. The technician should wear appropriate personal protective equipment (PPE) and follow all safety recommendations of the meter manufacturers and of the facility where the test is performed. All QA procedures must be strictly followed to ensure the accuracy of the results obtained.

REVIEW QUESTIONS

1. What hormones influence glucose levels?

2. What is a storage form of glucose?

3. What are two major disorders of glucose metabolism?

4. Why must serum or plasma be separated from cells immediately following collection if the specimen is to be tested for glucose?

5. What is a 2-hour postprandial glucose test?

6. What is the reference value for fasting serum glucose?

7. Explain how the OGTT is performed.

8. Explain the glucose oxidase and hexokinase methods of analyzing glucose. What end product is measured in the glucose oxidase method? In the hexokinase method?

9. What is the purpose of using controls with glucose analyzers?

10. What is the final product measured in the GDH method?

11. What safety precautions must be observed when using glucose or HbA1c analyzers?

12. Discuss the importance of quality assessment procedures when performing glucose or HbA1c analysis.

13. What are two methodologies used in blood glucose analyzers? Explain how the end product is detected in each methodology.

14. Why is it important for diabetics to maintain blood glucose at or near reference levels?

15. What information is gained from the HbA1c test?

16. What is the difference between reference glucose values and recommended glucose values?

17. Give the ADA FPG recommendations for classifying nondiabetic, prediabetic, and hyperglycemic patients.

18. Define chromogen, diabetes mellitus, glucagon, glucose dehydrogenase, glucose oxidase, glycated hemoglobin, glycogen, glycolysis, hemoglobin A1c, hexokinase, hyperglycemia, hypoglycemia, insulin, oral glucose tolerance test, peroxidase, and postprandial.

STUDENT ACTIVITIES

1. Complete the written examination for this lesson.

2. Practice performing a glucose measurement as outlined in the Student Performance Guide, using the worksheet.

3. Practice performing the test for HbA1c as outlined in the Student Performance Guide and using the worksheet.

WEB ACTIVITIES

1. Use the Internet to explore the ADA Web site. Find brochures or resources available to diabetics. Request free information about diabetes management.

2. Use the Internet to find three drugs that are used to treat Type 2 diabetes. Explain how they work to control blood glucose.

3. Use the Internet to find information on inhaled insulin. Report on how it is used and who can benefit from it.

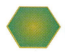

Student Performance Guide

LESSON 6-5 Blood Glucose and Hemoglobin A1c: Blood Glucose

Name _____ Date _____

INSTRUCTIONS

1. Practice the procedure for measuring glucose following the step-by-step procedure.

2. Demonstrate the procedure for measuring glucose satisfactorily for the instructor, using the Student Performance Guide. Your instructor will determine the level of competency you must achieve to obtain a satisfactory (S) grade.

MATERIALS AND EQUIPMENT

- gloves
- face shield and/or acrylic safety shield
- glucose meter such as HemoCue, ACCU-CHEK, FreeStyle, or other glucose analyzer
- test strips, cuvettes, or cartridges for glucose meter
- control solutions for glucose meter
- laboratory tissue
- capillary puncture materials
- antiseptic
- surface disinfectant
- biohazard container
- worksheet
- 70% alcohol and cotton balls, or alcohol swabs
- optional: micropipetter (0 to 100 μL) and tips
- sharps container

NOTE: The following is a general procedure for using a glucose analyzer. Consult the procedure manual for the instrument used and package inserts for specific instructions.

PROCEDURE

Record in the comment section any problems encountered while practicing the procedure (or have a fellow student or the instructor evaluate your performance).

S = Satisfactory
U = Unsatisfactory

You must:	S	U	Comments
1. Review operating instructions for the glucose analyzer			
2. Assemble materials and supplies			
3. Wash hands, put on face protection or position acrylic safety shield on work surface, and put on gloves			
4. Record instrument name, control ranges, control lot #, and test strip lot # on the worksheet			
5. Measure blood glucose using a glucose meter following steps 5a through 5h (to use HemoCue glucose analyzer go to step 6) a. Turn the meter on. Be sure the code on the display matches the code on the test strip vial			

You must:	S	U	Comments

b. Run the control tests following the manufacturer's instructions
   (1) Insert a test strip into the meter. Be sure the code matches the code on the test strip vial
   (2) Select control level (if applicable)
   (3) Mix contents of the control bottle; dispense 1 drop onto a paper towel and wipe the tip clean
   (4) Apply control to the test strip sample area
   (5) Read the result from the display when the test is complete, record result on worksheet, and discard the test strip into biohazard container. Check to see that the result is within the acceptable range
   (6) Insert a new strip and test the second control in the same manner (steps b1 through b5)
c. Insert a new test strip into the meter
d. Perform a capillary puncture on the patient and obtain a drop of blood
e. Touch the test strip to the drop of blood
f. When the test is complete, read and record the patient's glucose value
g. Discard the test strip into biohazard container
h. Turn off the meter and return it to storage			

6. Perform a blood glucose measurement using the HemoCue following steps 6a through 6k and manufacturer's instructions a. Turn on the analyzer b. Calibrate analyzer according to manufacturer's instructions c. Fill a cuvette with a glucose control solution following the manufacturer's directions d. Place the cuvette in the carrier and gently push it into the HemoCue. Read the value displayed and record. Verify that control is within acceptable range e. Discard cuvette f. Obtain a new cuvette g. Perform capillary puncture on patient h. Fill the cuvette from the capillary puncture. Do not allow air bubbles into the cuvette i. Place the cuvette in the carrier and gently push it into the HemoCue j. Read the patient's glucose value from the display and record k. Discard the cuvette into biohazard container l. Turn off the analyzer, wipe it with disinfectant, if necessary, and return it to storage			
7. Discard used capillary puncture materials into appropriate biohazard and sharps containers			
8. Disinfect work area with surface disinfectant			

You must:	S	U	Comments
9. Remove and discard gloves in biohazard container and wash hands with antiseptic			

Evaluator Comments:

Evaluator _____ Date _____

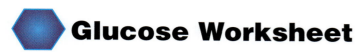

Glucose Worksheet

LESSON 6-5 Blood Glucose and Hemoglobin A1c

1. Instrument name: _____

2. Control test: Record lot numbers and acceptable ranges of glucose controls and reagent test unit. Record results of control test(s). If test(s) is within range, mark acceptable (A); if not, mark unacceptable (U).

Test Unit Lot # _____

Glucose Controls

	Lot No.	Acceptable Range	Control Results	A	U
Normal	_____	_____	_____	_____	_____
Abnormal	_____	_____	_____	_____	_____

Action taken if control test is unacceptable: _____

_____

_____

3. Patient test: Record the results below and compare with the appropriate reference range.

Patient I.D.	Test Result	Reference Ranges
_____	_____	Serum 70–110 mg/dL
_____	_____	Plasma 66–105 mg/dL
_____	_____	Whole blood 60–100 mg/dL

Student/Tech Name _____   Date _____

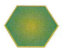

Student Performance Guide

LESSON 6-5 Blood Glucose and Hemoglobin A1c: HbA1c

Name _____ Date _____

INSTRUCTIONS

1. Practice the procedure for measuring HbA1c following the step-by-step procedure.

2. Demonstrate the procedure for measuring HbA1c satisfactorily for the instructor, using the Student Performance Guide. Your instructor will determine the level of competency you must achieve to obtain a satisfactory (S) grade.

MATERIALS AND EQUIPMENT

- gloves
- face shield and/or acrylic safety shield
- capillary puncture materials
- 70% alcohol and gauze or cotton balls
- antiseptic
- surface disinfectant
- biohazard container
- sharps container
- worksheet
- controls for HbA1c test (normal, low, high)
- DCA 2000+ with necessary supplies, including reagent cartridges and blood sampling devices, or other HbA1c analyzer with appropriate test packs and supplies

NOTE: The following is the general procedure for using the DCA 2000+. Consult the package enclosure for exact instructions or changes to the procedure. If a DCA 2000+ is not available, follow the instructions for the analyzer in use.

PROCEDURE

Record in the comment section any problems encountered while practicing the procedure (or have a fellow student or the instructor evaluate your performance).

S = Satisfactory
U = Unsatisfactory

You must:	S	U	Comments
1. Review the operating instructions for the DCA 2000+ analyzer (the screen will display all instructions)			
2. Assemble materials and supplies			
3. Wash hands and put on gloves and face protection			
4. Record the reagent cartridge Lot # and patient name on worksheet			
5. Obtain an HbA1c reagent cartridge and capillary holder for the DCA			
6. Assemble supplies for performing a capillary puncture			
7. Perform the capillary puncture			

You must:	S	U	Comments
8. Collect the 1 μL sample by touching the tip of the capillary holder to the drop of fingerstick blood			
9. Insert the sample into the cartridge by placing the sample-filled capillary holder into the reagent cartridge			
10. Verify the calibration by sliding the loaded reagent cartridge through the slot and past the analyzer's integral bar-code reader to automatically calibrate the instrument			
11. Open the door and insert the reagent cartridge into the DCA 2000+ analyzer			
12. Remove the pull tab on the cartridge to release the buffer			
13. Close the door on the analyzer to begin the analysis			
14. Read the result on the display when analysis is complete and record the results on the worksheet			
15. Analyze HbA1c controls, following steps 8 through 14 and using a new HbA1c cartridge and capillary holder for each control. Record control results on worksheet and complete remainder of worksheet			
16. Confirm that the controls are within the acceptable ranges before reporting the patient result. If an acceptable result is not obtained, consult the trouble-shooting guides in the operating manual			
17. Discard all contaminated materials and sharps into the appropriate containers			
18. Wipe the work surfaces with surface disinfectant			
19. Return all unused supplies to the storage area			
20. Clean any spills on the analyzer according to the manufacturer's instructions			
21. Remove gloves and wash hands with antiseptic			

Evaluator Comments:

Evaluator _____ Date _____

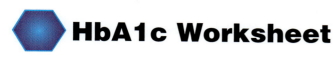 HbA1c Worksheet

LESSON 6-5 Blood Glucose and Hemoglobin A1c

1. Analyzer used _____

2. Reagent pack Lot # and expiration date _____

3. Controls (if applicable):

   Acceptable range for Normal control _____

   Acceptable range for High (HI) control _____

   Acceptable range for Low (LO) control _____

   Control values obtained:

   Normal _____   High _____   Low _____

4. Patient Test:

   Patient name/ID _____   Result _____

5. Compare the patient results with the reference ranges for HbA1c. Use Table 6-11 to interpret the results.

   _____

   _____

Student/Tech Name _____   Date _____

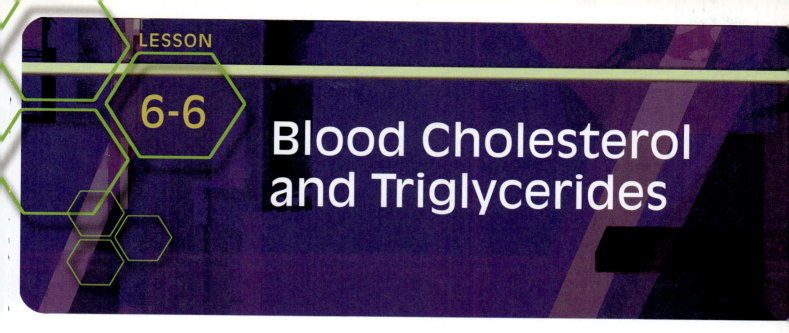

LESSON 6-6

Blood Cholesterol and Triglycerides

LESSON OBJECTIVES

After studying this lesson, the student will:

- Explain the functions of cholesterol in the body.
- Give the reference values for total cholesterol for males and females in each age group.
- Discuss the risks of elevated cholesterol levels.
- Explain the importance of HDL (high-density lipoprotein) and LDL (low-density lipoprotein) cholesterol.
- Give the mean reference values for HDL cholesterol for males and females in each age group.
- Explain how the risk factor for heart disease can be calculated from the HDL and LDL cholesterol values.
- Describe the function and structure of triglycerides.
- State the reference range for triglycerides.
- List the safety precautions that must be followed when performing blood lipid measurements.
- Discuss quality assessment and improvement policies that must be observed when measuring blood lipids.
- Perform a triglyceride determination.
- Perform a cholesterol determination.
- Define the glossary terms.

GLOSSARY

atherosclerosis / a form of arteriosclerosis in which lipids, calcium, cholesterol, and other substances deposit on the inner walls of the arteries

endogenous / produced within; growing from within

exogenous / originating from the outside

HDL cholesterol / high-density lipoprotein fraction of blood cholesterol; *good* cholesterol

LDL cholesterol / low-density lipoprotein fraction of blood cholesterol; *bad* cholesterol

myocardial infarction (MI) / heart attack caused by obstruction of the blood supply to or within the heart

triglycerides / the major storage form of lipids; lipid molecules formed from glycerol and fatty acids

INTRODUCTION

Measuring the total blood cholesterol level, along with the levels of cholesterol fractions, has become commonplace as the important role of cholesterol in coronary artery disease and other atherosclerotic conditions has become apparent. This lesson presents basic information about the biological sources and functions of cholesterol and triglycerides, as well as their relationship to good health. Total cholesterol, cholesterol fractions, and triglycerides are often included in a routine chemistry profile or are ordered as a lipid profile.

Many people know their cholesterol number and are aware of food especially high or low in cholesterol. Although most people have the test performed in a physician office laboratory (POL) or reference laboratory, cholesterol, and sometimes triglyceride, screening is increasingly being offered through health fairs and by employers, pharmacies, and others. Blood donation centers often measure donor cholesterol levels and report it to them. In addition, companies market over-the-counter (OTC) test kits that can estimate the blood cholesterol level and indicate if further testing is needed. This current availability of free or inexpensive blood lipid testing is a responsible reaction to the increased awareness of the importance of controlling blood cholesterol and triglyceride levels.

CHOLESTEROL

Structure and Biological Role

Cholesterol, a lipid sterol, is an important component of all body tissues. The chemical structure of cholesterol is shown in Figure 6-18. Cholesterol is a major constituent of all mammalian cell membranes, except those in red blood cells.

Since lipids have limited solubility in water, they help the cell membrane control the flow of water-soluble substances in and out of the cell. A relatively large amount of cholesterol is located in the skin, where it protects against the absorption of water-soluble substances. It also aids in protecting against damaging chemical agents, such as acids, and excessive water evaporation from the skin.

Another major function of cholesterol is to serve as a precursor to bile salts and steroid hormones. The sex hormones, adrenal

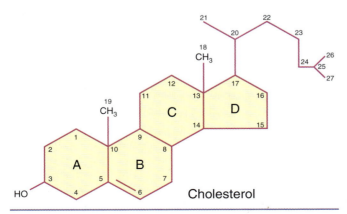

FIGURE 6-18 Structure of the cholesterol molecule

steroids, and bile salts are synthesized from cholesterol in specific cells of the ovaries, testes, adrenal gland, and liver.

Sources of Cholesterol

Cholesterol has two main sources. Certain body tissues, especially the liver, synthesize cholesterol. This is called **endogenous** cholesterol and is under genetic control. Everyone consumes at least some cholesterol. This dietary cholesterol is called **exogenous** cholesterol and is found in animal fats and egg yolks. People who eat a rich, fatty diet may develop dangerously increased blood cholesterol levels.

Pathology Associated with Increased Blood Cholesterol

When blood cholesterol levels remain elevated, a condition known as **atherosclerosis** can occur in which fat accumulates on the inner walls of blood vessels, narrowing the vessel opening. These deposits are especially likely to form on any damaged surface of a vessel wall. Although other fats (lipids) are found in these deposits, the major portion is cholesterol.

Once these deposits form, their rough edges can cause blood clots to develop. These clots can either damage the area in which they originate or travel to small vessels in vital organs such as the brain, heart, kidneys, or liver and cut off the blood supply to these organs. The result can be stroke, **myocardial infarction (MI)**, damage to other organs, or disease of the blood vessels.

Total Blood Cholesterol and Cholesterol Fractions

In the past, blood cholesterol was reported only as total cholesterol. Now it is more meaningful to measure total cholesterol and the fractions of cholesterol. The two fractions commonly measured are **HDL** (high-density lipoprotein) **cholesterol** and **LDL** (low-density lipoprotein) **cholesterol**. HDL and LDL cholesterol levels are genetically determined to some extent.

HDL transports cholesterol from the tissues to the liver to be broken down, mostly into bile acids. Because of this, HDL cholesterol is called *good* cholesterol. LDL transports cholesterol to the tissues to be deposited as fat. LDL cholesterol is sometimes referred to as *bad* cholesterol.

If the total cholesterol concentration is elevated in a patient, the physician uses the HDL and LDL values to determine the heart attack risk factor associated with the elevated cholesterol. Other factors, such as smoking and level of exercise, also influence the risk. When HDL is above the average value, it reduces the risk of MI, a type of heart attack, by as much as one-third.

Reference Values for Cholesterol

At birth, serum cholesterol ranges from about 50 mg/dL to 100 mg/dL. At one month, the levels approach 100 to 230 mg/dL and remain at those levels until the age of 20 to 21 years.

TABLE 6-12. Reference values for total blood cholesterol

AGE (YEARS)	RANGE* (mg/dL)	MALES (mg/dL) (MEAN)	FEMALES (mg/dL) (MEAN)
0–19	120–230	—	—
20–29	120–240	235	220
30–39	140–270	265	240
40–49	150–310	280	265
50–59	160–330	300	320

* The upper limits of ranges are not necessarily the desired levels, but represent levels found in the U.S. population.

TABLE 6-13. National Cholesterol Education Program (NCEP) recommended cholesterol levels

TEST	RANGE (mg/dL)	CLASSIFICATION
Total Cholesterol	<200	Desirable
	200–239	Borderline
	≥240	High
LDL cholesterol	<100	Optimal
	100–129	Near/above optimal
	130–159	Borderline high
	160–189	High
	≥190	Very high
HDL cholesterol	<40	Low
	>60	High

Cholesterol levels for adults are affected by age, diet, and gender. Even the patient's posture at collection can affect results; studies have shown that cholesterol values increase 10% to 20% in the nonresting patient compared to the resting patient. Estrogen seems to influence cholesterol levels, since in postmenopausal women the cholesterol level tends to increase.

Cholesterol reference values by age group are shown in Table 6-12. *These are not the recommended levels.* Organizations such as the American Heart Association and the National Cholesterol Education Program (NCEP) recommend that total cholesterol be kept below 200 mg/dL (Table 6-13). Cholesterol of 240 mg/dL or above is considered to present a high risk of heart disease. Cholesterol levels between 200 and 239 mg/dL are considered borderline. Reference ranges for HDL and LDL cholesterols are shown in Table 6-14.

Using Cholesterol Levels to Determine the Heart Attack Risk Factor

To determine the heart attack risk factor, the LDL/HDL ratio is calculated. The smaller the number, the less the risk.

As an example, a 45-year-old male (patient one) with an LDL cholesterol level of 140 mg/dL and an HDL cholesterol level of 70 mg/dL would have a lower risk of heart attack than a second male (patient two) of the same age and identical LDL level, but with an HDL of 30 mg/dL. The risk factor is calculated by dividing the LDL by the HDL (risk factor = LDL/HDL).

Patient one: $\dfrac{\text{LDL}}{\text{HDL}}$ = risk factor

$$\frac{140 \text{ mg/dL}}{70 \text{ mg/dL}} = 2$$

Patient two: $\dfrac{\text{LDL}}{\text{HDL}}$ = risk factor

$$\frac{140 \text{ mg/dL}}{30 \text{ mg/dL}} = 4.7$$

TABLE 6-14. Reference ranges for HDL and LDL cholesterol

AGE (YEARS)	HDL MALE RANGE (mg/dL)	HDL FEMALE RANGE (mg/dL)	LDL MALE AND FEMALE (mg/dL)
0–19	30–65	30–70	50–170
20–29	30–65	36–78	60–170
30–39	30–59	33–77	70–190
40–49	25–61	40–81	80–190
50–75	29–72	38–91	80–210

Therefore, in this comparison, patient one has a lower risk factor for heart attack than patient two, even though patient two has a lower total cholesterol level.

TRIGLYCERIDES

Structure and Function

Triglycerides, the most common form of fat in the body, also comprise the largest portion of fats in the diet. Any extra calories the body consumes are turned into triglycerides. The triglyceride molecule is composed of three chains of fatty acids combined with one molecule of glycerol. Triglycerides are a storage form of energy found in adipose tissue and muscle. Between meals they are gradually released and metabolized in response to the energy needs of the body.

CURRENT TOPICS

MANAGING BLOOD CHOLESTEROL

According to the American Heart Association, more than 107 million Americans (over one-third of the U.S. population) have cholesterol levels of 200 mg/dL or higher. Although cholesterol is required for normal cell function, it also contributes to the development of atherosclerosis, a condition in which cholesterol-containing deposits or plaques form within the arteries, reducing blood flow and potentially blocking arteries. This means that a significant portion of the population is potentially at risk for heart disease or stroke.

As part of a good preventive medicine program, individuals should have their cholesterol and triglycerides measured at an early age to establish baseline levels and then checked annually beginning in young adulthood. The goal should be to maintain blood lipid levels at or below the recommended levels (Tables 6-13 and 6-15). If one or more lipids are in the undesirable range, the physician can work with the patient to make changes to diet, medications, and/or lifestyle based on lipid levels and risk factors such as smoking, family history of heart disease, and high blood pressure.

Lifestyle Changes

The first steps to lowering total cholesterol levels are to begin an exercise program, lose weight, and modify the diet. Weight loss is usually accompanied by decreased cholesterol levels. When significantly overweight individuals lose several pounds, the decrease in cholesterol can be dramatic. Participation in a regular exercise program can help raise HDL cholesterol.

Changing to a diet low in cholesterol-rich foods can also result in lower cholesterol levels. However, since the body also produces endogenous cholesterol and that is under genetic control, low-cholesterol diets do not always lead to significantly lower blood cholesterol.

Statin Drugs

Several drugs are available that can lower cholesterol levels. The most widely used drugs belong to the class called statins. Statins interrupt production of cholesterol in the liver by blocking the enzyme needed for cholesterol production, as well as increasing the elimination of cholesterol from the body. Statins lower primarily LDL cholesterol and triglycerides, but statins also cause small increases in HDL cholesterol levels. Statins have been shown to reduce the incidence of MIs, strokes, and death and are known to provide several benefits in addition to lowering cholesterol. These include (1) reduced formation of new plaques; (2) reduction in the size of plaques that already exist; (3) stabilization of plaques, making them less prone to rupturing and forming clots; and (4) reduced inflammation, as early as 2 weeks after starting statin therapy.

In the past, most individuals were placed on statins because of high levels of cholesterol. Recent research shows, however, that although cholesterol reduction is important, heart disease is complex and other factors such as inflammation can play a role. Over one-third of individuals who have MIs do not have high blood cholesterol levels, yet most of them have atherosclerosis, indicating that high cholesterol levels are not always necessary for plaques to form. The goal of statin therapy is not only to reduce cholesterol but also to prevent MIs and stroke caused by atherosclerosis.

Other Drugs

Other classes of drugs are also used for lowering cholesterol, but with less frequency than the statins. These include resins and nicotinic acid. Resins act in the intestine to bind and dispose of cholesterol. Nicotinic acid (niacin) is effective in lowering LDL levels and raising HDL levels, but should not be combined with statin therapy. Other new drugs aimed at raising HDL levels and/or lowering triglyceride levels, such as clofibrate and gemfibrozil, have also recently been approved for use in treating hypercholesterolemia.

Side Effects of Cholesterol-Lowering Drugs

Cholesterol-lowering drugs can have side effects, so patients taking these drugs should see their physician on a regular basis. Although side effects in most individuals are mild, severe side effects can occur. Liver enzymes can rise to abnormal levels, so they must be monitored at regular intervals in individuals taking cholesterol-lowering drugs. Another rare but very serious side effect is damage to muscle, causing breakdown of muscle fibers, a condition called *rhabdomyolysis*. Undesirable interactions can also occur between cholesterol-lowering drugs and other prescription drugs, OTC products, and even certain foods, such as grapefruit. Therefore, it is important that patients inform their physicians of all medications, OTC products, and ingredients in their diet.

Triglyceride Reference Values

The reference (normal) value for triglycerides is less than 150 mg/dL (Table 6-15). Values from 150 to 199 mg/dL are considered borderline high. Values between 200 and 499 mg/dL are high. Triglyceride values of 500 mg/dL and greater are called very high.

Clinical Considerations

Triglyceride levels have long been thought to be a good predictor for the presence of or development of coronary heart disease (CHD). Levels greater than 200 mg/dL correlate with increased risk of CHD. However, an increased value can also indicate cirrhosis, familial hyperlipoproteinemia, hypothyroidism, or poorly controlled diabetes, especially in type 2 patients.

Some researchers now believe that an increased triglyceride value is not so much an indicator for CHD but is often part of a condition called *metabolic syndrome* that is closely related to insulin resistance. Associated with this syndrome are abdominal obesity, increased blood triglycerides, elevated blood pressure, elevated fasting glucose, and a low HDL value. The presence of metabolic syndrome increases the risk for coronary artery disease.

PERFORMING TESTS FOR CHOLESTEROL AND TRIGLYCERIDES

Techniques for measuring total serum cholesterol have been used for decades, but efficient, easy methods for measuring HDL and LDL cholesterols have been available only since about 1980. In the past, cholesterol was measured using chemical methods, which were time-consuming and used hazardous chemicals. Today's analyzers incorporate enzymatic methods for testing cholesterol, cholesterol fractions, and triglycerides. These methods are simpler, safer, and faster than chemical methods.

Measurement of triglycerides is a part of a lipid profile but is also offered separately in some screening situations. The analysis can be performed on either venous or capillary blood. Many point-of-care (POC) analyzers include triglyceride measurement in their menu of tests. Examples of analyzers that perform cholesterol and triglyceride measurements include the ACCU-CHEK Instant Plus (Roche Diagnostics) and the Cholestech LDX (Cholestech Corp.), shown in Figure 6-19.

TABLE 6-15. Reference (normal) value for triglycerides and interpretation of triglyceride levels

TRIGLYCERIDES (mg/dL)	INTERPRETATION
<150	Normal
150–199	Borderline high
200–499	High
≥500	Very high

Safety Precautions

 Standard Precautions must be observed while performing cholesterol and triglyceride tests. Control solutions are usually manufactured from human blood products and should be handled as if infectious. The technician must wear appropriate personal protective equipment (PPE). All contaminated materials must be discarded into appropriate biohazard containers. Manufacturer's instructions must be carefully followed to prevent personal injury or damage to the instruments. When tests are performed in screening situations such as in a mall, the same safety precautions must be observed that are required in medical facilities.

Quality Assessment

The type of specimen required for lipid tests depends on the test to be performed. The laboratory's procedure manual should be followed to determine the appropriate specimen (serum, plasma, whole blood). Tests for cholesterol and its fractions and for triglycerides are best measured on a fasting specimen.

Manufacturers of chemistry analyzers that perform lipid measurements provide calibrators and/or controls for use with their instruments. The controls are analyzed along with the patient samples. For analyzers that use reagent strips, the liquid control is applied to a separate strip in the same manner as a patient sample and is then analyzed in the instrument. This checks the reliability of the reagent strips, the function of the instrument, and the worker's technique. If control results are not within acceptable limits, the patient results cannot be reported until the problem is found and corrected. Only personnel who have been properly trained on the instrument in use should be allowed to perform lipid testing and report results.

Cholestech LDX

A compact instrument that can perform a lipid profile, plus glucose determination, is marketed by Cholestech Corporation (Figure 6-19). The Cholestech LDX System can be used to

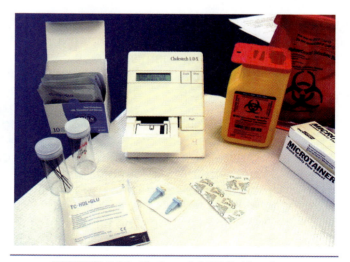

FIGURE 6-19 Cholestech LDX lipid analyzer

screen for risk of coronary disease in corporate wellness programs or community health fairs.

A capillary blood sample is collected and added to the sample well of the test cassette. Each cassette contains the reagents for a specific test or group of tests, such as total cholesterol; total cholesterol and HDL; or total cholesterol, HDL, and triglycerides. When a cassette performs more than one test, the portions of the sample are diverted into different test regions. The test cassette is inserted into the analyzer and the result is ready in less than 5 minutes.

PROCEDURAL Reminders

- Review QA section before beginning procedure.
- Use test kits or reagent strips only with the instruments for which they are intended.
- Follow manufacturer's instructions exactly.
- Pipet accurately to ensure good results.

SAFETY Reminders

- Review safety precautions before beginning procedure.
- Observe Standard Precautions when working with blood samples and standard and control solutions.
- Discard used sharps into a sharps container.
- Dispose of all biohazard waste in a biohazard container.
- Wipe work area with surface disinfectant when work is finished.
- Wash hands with antiseptic.

SUMMARY

In recent years, the role that lipids play in health has become recognized as increasingly important. Health care advocates are recommending that individuals know their blood lipid numbers so they can be active participants in maintaining a healthy lifestyle. With the development of rapid, easy-to-perform, and inexpensive test methods, cholesterol and triglyceride blood tests are now available to the general public through venues such as health fairs or pharmacies, precluding the need to go to a laboratory or doctor's office for screening tests.

Cholesterol and triglyceride levels are used for assessing risks for cardiovascular disease and for recommending treatment regimens. When blood lipids are elevated, the physician can prescribe medication, exercise, change in diet, or some combination of these. Studies indicate that keeping lipid levels at or below recommended levels will provide the possibility of living longer and healthier lives and decrease the incidence of heart disease and stroke.

CASE STUDY

Mr. Chen, 38 years old, attended a health fair at a local mall and had several tests performed. His lipid chemistry results were:

Total cholesterol	220 mg/dL
Total triglycerides	145 mg/dL
HDL cholesterol	50 mg/dL
LDL cholesterol	170 mg/dL

1. Compare Mr. Chen's results to the reference ranges and to desired levels. Are all of his values within the desirable ranges?
2. How can these values be used to calculate the risk factor for heart attack?
3. What is Mr. Chen's risk factor ratio?
4. Which lipid(s) should be targeted for reduction?

REVIEW QUESTIONS

1. What are the functions of cholesterol in the body?

2. What are the dangers of an elevated serum cholesterol?

3. Why are HDL and LDL cholesterol levels important?

4. What are the desirable levels of total cholesterol and LDL cholesterol as recommended by the NCEP? Are recommended values the same as reference values?

5. Increased levels of triglycerides are thought to be an indicator of what condition? Name one other condition that can be indicated by increased triglyceride levels.

6. How is the risk factor for heart disease calculated using HDL and LDL cholesterol values?

7. Discuss the function and importance of triglycerides.

8. Explain the value of using an OTC cholesterol test.

9. What drugs can be used to lower LDL cholesterol? What are some side effects?

10. Define atherosclerosis, endogenous, exogenous, HDL cholesterol, LDL cholesterol, myocardial infarction, and triglycerides.

STUDENT ACTIVITIES

1. Complete the written examination for this lesson.

2. If lipid screening is offered in your community, ask which method of analysis is being used.

3. If possible, determine which instruments are used in local POLs.

4. Have your blood lipids tested at a local health fair.

5. Practice performing cholesterol and triglyceride determinations as outlined in the Student Performance Guide, using whichever method is available.

WEB ACTIVITIES

1. Use the Internet to find online tools for assessing risk of heart disease or coronary artery disease. Use the calculators with these tools to assess your risk or that of a fellow student or family member for whom you have the needed information.

2. Use the Internet to find the NCEP Web site. Use their Risk Assessment Tool to estimate the 10-year risk of having a heart attack for you or a family member.

3. Use the Internet to access the National Heart, Lung, and Blood Institute section of the nih. gov Web site. Use the risk calculator to determine the risk factor for a non-smoking 62-year-old woman with total cholesterol of 200 mg/dL, HDL of 80 mg/dL, and systolic blood pressure of 115.

Student Performance Guide

LESSON 6-6 Blood Cholesterol and Triglycerides

Name _____   Date _____

INSTRUCTIONS

1. Practice the procedure for measuring blood cholesterol and triglycerides following the step-by-step procedure.
2. Demonstrate the procedure for measuring blood cholesterol and triglycerides satisfactorily for the instructor, using the Student Performance Guide. Your instructor will determine the level of competency you must achieve to obtain a satisfactory (S) grade.

NOTE: The following procedure is a general procedure for measuring blood lipids using an analyzer. Consult the manufacturer's instructions for the specific analyzer being used.

MATERIALS AND EQUIPMENT

- gloves
- face shield and/or acrylic safety shield
- blood-collecting supplies
- antiseptic
- marking pencil
- laboratory tissue
- calculator (optional)
- pipetter with disposable tips
- surface disinfectant
- biohazard container
- analyzer for performing cholesterol and triglyceride determinations, including test materials, controls, and standards
- Levey-Jennings charts
- sharps container

PROCEDURE

Record in the comment section any problems encountered while practicing the procedure (or have a fellow student or the instructor evaluate your performance).

S = Satisfactory
U = Unsatisfactory

You must:	S	U	Comments
1. Assemble equipment and materials			
2. Wash hands, put on face shield, and put on gloves			

3. Perform cholesterol/triglyceride measurement using an analyzer following steps 3a through 3j:
  a. Follow manufacturer's instructions for instrument start up
  b. Prepare controls or calibrator reagents
  c. Run appropriate controls or calibrator samples and record results
  d. Obtain correct patient specimen
  e. Choose appropriate test strip or pack for cholesterol or triglyceride determination			

You must:	S	U	Comments
f. Add patient sample to test unit g. Insert test strip or pack into instrument h. Ensure that correct test is displayed on instrument i. Wait for results to be displayed or printed out j. Record results			
4. For each test performed, plot the control values on a Levey-Jennings chart			
5. If the method is in control, report patient values			
6. Dispose of contaminated materials in appropriate biohazard container or sharps container			
7. Wipe work area with surface disinfectant			
8. Turn instrument OFF (or leave as manual instructs) and disinfect if required			
9. Remove gloves and discard in biohazard container			
10. Wash hands with antiseptic			

Evaluator Comments:

Evaluator _____ Date _____

6-7

Electrolytes

LESSON OBJECTIVES

After studying this lesson, the student will:
- Name the major cations and anions in body fluids.
- Name the four electrolytes routinely measured.
- Name the major intracellular electrolyte.
- List the major extracellular electrolytes.
- State the electrolyte reference ranges.
- Perform an electrolyte analysis and interpret the results.
- Describe safety precautions that must be observed when measuring electrolyte levels.
- Discuss how quality assessment policies affect electrolyte analysis.
- Define the glossary terms.

GLOSSARY

acidosis / an abnormal condition in which blood pH falls below 7.35

alkalosis / an abnormal condition in which blood pH rises above 7.45

hyperkalemia / blood potassium levels above normal

hypernatremia / blood sodium levels above normal

hypokalemia / blood potassium levels below normal

hyponatremia / blood sodium levels below normal

INTRODUCTION

Ions in body fluids are called electrolytes. Major ions include the positively charged cations, sodium, potassium, calcium, and magnesium, and the negatively charged anions, chloride, bicarbonate, and phosphate. However, a request for laboratory electrolyte measurement usually means the physician wants serum levels of four electrolytes—sodium (Na^+), potassium (K^+), chloride (Cl^-), and bicarbonate (HCO_3^-).

Proper electrolyte balance within the body's fluid compartments is essential to normal cellular functions. Electrolyte concentrations in body fluids are maintained within narrow ranges. The factors contributing to balanced electrolyte concentrations are complex. Homeostatic mechanisms regulate the distribution of fluid and ions within various body compartments, as well as their excretion.

Electrolyte imbalances occur when the blood concentration of an electrolyte is either too high or too low, affecting all organs and body systems. These imbalances can be life-threatening if not brought under control. Therefore, electrolyte measurement is often included in hospital point-of-care testing (POCT) programs and ordered as a STAT test, meaning it must be performed immediately.

This lesson provides a brief introduction to the functions of the four major electrolytes and to methods of measurement. Other ions such as calcium and phosphorus are discussed in Lesson 6-1.

FUNCTION AND CLINICAL SIGNIFICANCE OF ELECTROLYTES

Changes in electrolyte balance affect the function of all organ systems. In general, sodium influences body water distribution, blood volume, blood pressure, and fluid retention or loss. Potassium is important in maintaining normal muscular activity in the heart and skeletal muscle through transmission of electrical impulses. Bicarbonate, produced from carbon dioxide (CO_2) formation during cellular metabolism, is important in maintaining blood pH. In some illnesses, electrolyte balance is altered because of sudden fluid loss due to vomiting, diarrhea, or excessive urination. Such sudden imbalances can be harmful.

ELECTROLYTE REFERENCE RANGES

Electrolyte concentrations are expressed either in millimoles per liter (mmol/L), which are SI units, or as milliequivalents per liter (mEq/L). Since one mEq equals one mmol for monovalent ions such as electrolytes, the numerical value of an electrolyte is the same regardless which of the two units is used. Reference ranges for serum electrolytes are given in Table 6-16.

The electrolytes are distributed unequally between the intracellular (inside the cell) and extracellular (outside the cell) spaces. As shown in Figure 6-20 and Table 6-16, potassium is higher (↑) inside cells than outside cells. Sodium, chloride, and bicarbonate are in low concentrations (↓) inside cells and in higher concentrations (↑) outside cells.

Sodium

The reference range for serum sodium is 135 to 148 mmol/L (mEq/L). Sodium has an important influence on osmotic con-

centration and determines the extracellular fluid volume. Water moves back and forth across cell membranes to maintain proper sodium balance; rapid shifts in the water volume in cells can damage or destroy cells. Sodium concentration is influenced by aldosterone levels and kidney function.

Hypernatremia, increased concentration of sodium, occurs in dehydration, hyperadrenalism (Cushing's disease), and diabetes insipidus (a deficiency of antidiuretic hormone). **Hyponatremia**, decreased concentration of sodium, occurs in severe diarrhea, acidosis of diabetes mellitus, decreased aldosterone secretion (Addison's disease), and renal disease in which there is poor ion exchange in the tubules.

Potassium

The reference range for serum potassium is 3.5 to 5.4 mmol/L (mEq/L). Potassium is excreted by the kidney. Abnormally high or low levels of potassium should be reported immediately to the physician because levels outside normal limits can affect muscle function, particularly in the heart.

Hyperkalemia, increased serum potassium, can occur when potassium leaves cells rapidly and can occur in anoxia and acidosis. Increased potassium levels cause a decrease in muscle function and occur in decreased aldosterone secretion, circulatory failure (shock), and renal failure. **Hypokalemia**, decreased serum potassium, can be due to decreased intake of potassium, increased levels of aldosterone, or increased loss of potassium due to vomiting, diarrhea, or use of diuretics.

Chloride

Chloride is the anion with the highest extracellular concentration; the reference range for serum is 98 to 108 mmol/L (mEq/L). Chloride concentration varies inversely with bicarbonate (HCO_3^-). The concentration of chloride will increase in dehydration or in loss of CO_2 by hyperventilation (respiratory alkalosis). Decreased chloride concentration can occur in acidosis caused by uncontrolled diabetes, renal disease, and excessive vomiting.

Bicarbonate (CO_2 Content)

The bicarbonate anion is part of the blood buffer system that helps maintain a normal blood pH of 7.4; it is usually measured as total CO_2. The reference range for serum bicarbonate is 22 to

TABLE 6-16. Reference ranges for serum electrolytes	
ELECTROLYTE	**REFERENCE RANGE mmol/L (mEq/L)**
sodium (Na^+)	135–148
potassium (K^+)	3.8–5.5
chloride (Cl^-)	98–108
bicarbonate (total CO_2)	22–28

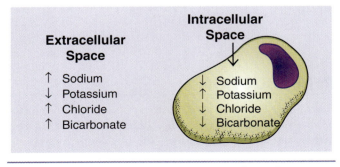

FIGURE 6-20 Relative intracellular and extracellular electrolyte concentrations

28 mmol/L (mEq/L). Carbon dioxide (CO_2) is constantly generated by metabolic processes. Combining CO_2 and water (H_2O) creates carbonic acid ($H_2CO_3^-$), which is converted to hydrogen ion (H^+) and bicarbonate:

$$H_2O + CO_2 \longrightarrow H_2CO_3 \longrightarrow H^+ + HCO_3^-$$

When the ratio of bicarbonate anion to carbonic acid changes, the pH changes. **Acidosis** occurs when the pH falls below 7.35 and can be caused by decreased HCO_3^- concentrations. **Alkalosis**, caused by increased HCO_3^- concentrations, occurs when the pH is greater than 7.45.

The bicarbonate concentration is rapidly affected by changes in respiration, the body's way of eliminating CO_2. Changes in lung function, such as pneumonia, or central nervous system (CNS) depression or stimulation due to drugs will affect HCO_3^- concentrations. Concentration changes can also occur in diabetic ketosis and renal failure.

Anion Gap

The anion gap (AG) is a mathematical calculation of the difference between the cation concentrations (sodium and potassium) and anion concentrations (chloride and bicarbonate) routinely measured in the electrolyte test. The cations not measured in the electrolyte test are calcium and magnesium; these average 7 mmol/L. The anions not measured in the electrolyte test are phosphate, sulfate, and anions of organic acids; these average 24 mmol/L.

The anion gap is calculated by the following formula:

$$([NA^+] + [K^+]) - ([Cl^-] + [HCO_3^-]) = AG \text{ (mmol/L)}$$

The normal anion gap is 10 to 17 mmol/L. If the sum of measured anions subtracted from the sum of measured cations is greater than 17 (mmol/L), this indicates an increase in unmeasured anions. Conditions that could cause this are acidosis, diabetic ketosis, starvation, or uremia.

METHODS OF MEASURING ELECTROLYTES

In the past, sodium and potassium were measured by atomic absorption spectrophotometry or flame photometry. Chloride was measured by titration or colorimetry, and CO_2 by manometry or colorimetry. Most analyzers today use ion-selective electrodes and PCO_2 electrodes that can be incorporated in compact instruments suitable for use in small laboratories (Figure 6-21). These analyzers can test serum, plasma, or whole blood, depending on their design. Principles of ion-selective electrodes are discussed in Lesson 6-3, Chemistry Instrumentation in the Physician Office Laboratory.

Safety Precautions

   Standard Precautions must be observed when performing any laboratory test using blood or other body substances. Gloves and other appro-

priate personal protective equipment (PPE) must be worn when obtaining the blood specimen and performing the test. Used test cartridges must be discarded in appropriate biohazard containers.

Quality Assessment

Manufacturer's instructions must be followed for the instrument used. All performance checks must be performed and documented as outlined in the procedure manual. Test cartridges or cassettes must be tested with abnormal and normal control sera or calibrators at required intervals. Patient specimens should be analyzed only after all quality control procedures have been successfully performed. Training of personnel must be documented, and competency must be verified.

Electrolyte Analyzers

Several small, portable electrolyte analyzers are available for use in POCT and POLs.

i-STAT Analyzer

The i-STAT analyzer, distributed by Abbott Laboratories, is an example of an instrument used in point-of-care testing (POCT) at critical care sites. It is a handheld analyzer with a test menu that includes sodium, potassium, chloride, and bicarbonate, as well as glucose, BUN, calcium, pH, hemoglobin, and hematocrit. Several parameters can be measured at one time using a sample size of only 2 or 3 drops of blood easily obtained from a capillary puncture and directly applied to a test cartridge. Test results are available within 2 to 3 minutes.

Electrolyte levels are measured by applying the patient's specimen to a single-use cartridge that also contains a calibration solution. The calibrator and the patient specimen are passed over miniaturized ion-specific electrodes within the cartridge that detect and measure the various electrolytes and correlate the results to values obtained with serum or plasma. Procedural checks within the instrument monitor the cartridge performance and user technique. Quality control cartridges inserted in the instrument monitor the electrical sensors. The i-STAT also contains data management capabilities that simplify reporting patient results and maintaining quality control records.

GEM Premier Plus

Instrumentation Laboratory's GEM Premier Plus is a blood gas and electrolyte analyzer that is useful in POCT sites such as intensive care units, emergency departments, and surgery suites. The analyzer can also measure the hematocrit and perform coagulation tests on whole blood. A computerized data management system allows central management of information generated by all units.

IRMA System

The IRMA TRUPOINT Blood Analysis System from International Technidyne Corp. (ITC) can be used at the bedside to measure electrolytes, blood gases, glucose, BUN, and hematocrit. The instrument measures Na^+, K^+, and Cl^-, but calculates the

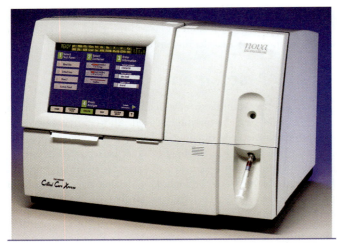

FIGURE 6-21 Nova CCX analyzer uses ion-selective electrode technology (*Courtesy NOVA Biomedical, Waltham, MA*)

and biosensors within the instruments. These electrodes are self-cleaning and essentially maintenance-free. The instruments aspirate the patient samples with an automatic sampling probe and complete a profile within minutes.

HCO_3^- value. The system has single-use cartridges, each with a self-contained calibrator for the specific analyte being tested.

Osmetech Optilion

The Optilion by Osmetech (formerly the AVL OPTI) has single-use cassettes, each with the ability to test up to eight different components in whole blood, plasma, or serum. The instrument uses optical sensor technology to read the results. Tests available include electrolytes, blood gases, and hemoglobin.

Nova Analyzers

The Nova 12$^+$, 16, and CCX analyzers provide chemistry profiles containing frequently ordered STAT chemistry tests. The analyzers are small enough to be portable on a cart and are useful both in intensive care units in large hospitals and in POLs (Figure 6-21). Most tests are performed using ion-selective electrodes

SAFETY Reminders

- Review safety precautions before beginning procedure.
- Follow Standard Precautions when handling specimens for chemical analysis.
- Discard all contaminated materials in appropriate biohazard containers.
- Treat all controls as if potentially infectious.

PROCEDURAL Reminders

- Review QA section before beginning procedure.
- Follow manufacturer's guidelines for proper specimen collection.
- Run appropriate normal and abnormal control sera or calibrators as required.
- Follow manufacturer's operating instructions.

CASE STUDY

Mr. Stein went to an urgent care clinic complaining of lingering "stomach flu," accompanied by severe bouts of diarrhea and vomiting. He also said he had almost fainted on the way to the clinic. When Dr. McCloud completed his physical examination, he ordered a laboratory test for serum electrolyte levels.

1. Mr. Stein's sodium levels would be expected to be:
   a. normal (within reference range)
   b. below normal (below reference range)
   c. above normal (above reference range)
2. Mr. Stein's potassium levels would be expected to be:
   a. normal (within reference range)
   b. below normal (below reference range)
   c. above normal (above reference range)
3. Explain why electrolytes are sometimes ordered as a STAT test.

SUMMARY

The measurement of electrolytes is an important analysis. The results can indicate or confirm problems in the ability of the body to maintain ion concentrations within the narrow ranges required for health. Changes in electrolyte balances can affect all organ systems. Electrolyte measurement is often ordered as a STAT test because electrolyte imbalances can be life-threatening. For test results to be of value, all quality assessment procedures must be strictly followed. Standard Precautions must be observed when collecting the sample, performing the analysis, and disposing of biohazardous materials.

REVIEW QUESTIONS

1. Name the four electrolytes commonly measured and state the reference range for each. Which are anions and which are cations?

2. Which electrolyte is most important in pH balance?

3. Which electrolyte is most important in maintaining fluid balance?

4. Which electrolyte has lower concentration in extracellular fluids than in the intracellular space?

5. What is the importance of potassium in the body?

6. What kind of blood specimens can be used to measure electrolytes?

7. Name four conditions that could cause electrolyte imbalance.

8. By what method are electrolytes measured in most analyzers?

9. What is the anion gap and what is the reference range? What ions other than the four major electrolytes influence the anion gap?

10. Discuss the safety precautions that must be observed when performing a test for electrolytes.

11. Why is it important to follow all the quality assessment policies of the institution when performing electrolyte analysis?

12. Define acidosis, alkalosis, hyperkalemia, hypernatremia, hypokalemia, and hyponatremia.

STUDENT ACTIVITIES

1. Complete the written examination for this lesson.

2. Perform measurement of electrolytes as outlined in the Student Performance Guide.

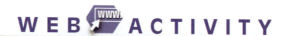

WEB ACTIVITY

Use the Internet to find a Web site where electrolyte results are matched to clinical symptoms. Report on the electrolyte results that might be seen in dehydration, dizziness, and confusion.

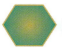 # Student Performance Guide

LESSON 6-7 Electrolytes

Name _____ Date _____

INSTRUCTIONS

1. Practice measuring electrolytes using an analyzer and following the step-by-step procedure.
2. Demonstrate the procedure for measuring electrolytes satisfactorily for the instructor, using the Student Performance Guide. Your instructor will determine the level of competency you must achieve to obtain a satisfactory (S) grade.

NOTE: The following is a general procedure for measuring electrolytes. The manufacturers' instructions for the specific method or analyzer being used must be consulted and carefully followed.

MATERIALS AND EQUIPMENT

- gloves
- face shield and/or acrylic safety shield
- serum or plasma specimens
- capillary blood-collection equipment
- previously collected whole blood, plasma, or serum
- i-STAT analyzer or other small analyzer capable of measuring electrolytes, including test cartridges and necessary controls
- quality control charts
- surface disinfectant
- biohazard container
- sharps container
- antiseptic

PROCEDURE

Record in the comment section any problems encountered while practicing the procedure (or have a fellow student or the instructor evaluate your performance).

S = Satisfactory
U = Unsatisfactory

You must:	S	U	Comments
1. Assemble equipment and materials. Put on face shield or position acrylic safety shield on work surface			
2. Wash hands and put on gloves			
3. Turn on instrument			
4. Perform quality control checks as directed by manufacturer and record results on quality control chart			
5. Obtain test cartridge or cassette			
6. Perform capillary puncture (or use previously obtained blood specimen)			
7. Apply specimen to test cartridge			

You must:	S	U	Comments
8. Insert cartridge into instrument			
9. Read and record test results			
10. Discard test cartridge in biohazard container			
11. Turn off instrument and store according to manufacturer's directions			
12. Discard all capillary puncture materials appropriately			
13. Clean work surface with surface disinfectant			
14. Remove and discard gloves and wash hands with antiseptic			

Evaluator Comments:

Evaluator _____ Date _____

UNIT 7

Basic Clinical Microbiology

UNIT OBJECTIVES

After studying this unit, the student will:

- Discuss the fields of study included in microbiology.
- Discuss the types of diseases caused by different groups of microorganisms.
- Explain why organisms are classified as normal flora, pathogens, or opportunistic pathogens.
- List some diseases that are considered emerging infectious diseases and explain why they are a threat to public health.
- List potential agents of bioterrorism, the diseases they cause, and the role of the clinical laboratory in dealing with them.
- Explain Standard Precautions and transmission-based precautions.
- Discuss basic culture techniques and culture media used in bacteriology.
- Prepare, stain, and microscopically observe bacterial smears.
- Describe the three basic types of bacterial morphology.
- Discuss growth requirements of some common bacteria.
- Perform a throat culture and a rapid test for group A *Streptococcus*.
- Perform a urine culture and colony count.
- Explain methods of bacterial identification and antibiotic susceptibility testing.
- Explain the importance of laboratory testing for sexually transmitted diseases.
- Discuss laboratory test methods for the detection of sexually transmitted diseases.
- Explain the importance and use of the fecal occult blood test.

UNIT OVERVIEW

Unit 7 is an introduction to clinical microbiology, including the microorganisms that cause disease and some of the laboratory tests to detect these organisms. The clinical laboratory's microbiology department isolates and identifies medically important bacteria, viruses, fungi, and parasites. The test methods presented in this unit emphasize bacteriological tests suitable for the smaller laboratory or physician's office. Advances in technology are providing an increased number of rapid, easy-to-use tests for bacteriology, virology, and parasitology.

Lesson 7-1 concentrates on history, background information, terminology, and knowledge about the different groups of organisms in microbiology and the diseases they cause. Infection control and the Centers for Disease Control and Prevention (CDC) categories of transmission-based precautions are discussed in Lesson 7-2.

Lessons 7-3 and 7-4 address two microbiology topics important to public health. Lesson 7-3 reviews emerging infectious diseases and discusses why these diseases are on the increase and how they pose a threat to public health. Lesson 7-4 addresses the topics of bioterrorism and biological weapons and the role of clinical laboratories in preparing for and investigating possible threat incidents.

In Lesson 7-5, growth requirements of various bacteria are presented, along with general culture techniques. The differences in primary, selective, and indicator media are described, as well as their uses. Safety in the microbiology laboratory and use of aseptic technique are emphasized.

The stained bacterial smear is important in identifying an organism. Lesson 7-6 details how to prepare a smear, perform a Gram stain, and examine the smear microscopically for Gram stain reaction and morphology.

Rapid tests for group A *Streptococcus*, which causes strep throat, are performed many times a day in most laboratories. The procedures for rapid strep tests as well as throat culture for group A strep are given in Lesson 7-7.

Lessons 7-8 and 7-9 describe how to perform a urine culture, colony count, bacterial identification, and antibiotic susceptibility test. Urine culture is one of the most frequently performed laboratory tests. Urine culture can be performed in the small laboratory as long as quality assessment measures are followed and qualified personnel are available.

Lesson 7-10 discusses sexually transmitted diseases (STDs) and the types of STD diagnostic tests available, including those suitable for the small laboratory.

The fecal occult blood test, discussed in Lesson 7-11, is used to screen for gastrointestinal disease and colorectal cancer. This test is often performed in the microbiology department.

READINGS, REFERENCES, AND RESOURCES

Ayliffe, G. A. J. & English, M. P. (2003). *Hospital infections*. London: Cambridge University Press.

Black, J. G. (2004). *Microbiology principles and explorations* (6th ed.). New York: John Wiley & Sons.

Burton, G. R. W. & Engelkirk, P. G. (2000). *Microbiology for the health sciences* (6th ed.). Philadelphia: Lippincott Williams & Wilkins.

Centers for Disease Control and Prevention (CDC) and National Institutes of Health (NIH) (1999). *Biosafety in microbiology and biomedical laboratories* (4th ed.). Washington, DC: U. S. Government Printing Office.

ColoScreen package insert. Beaumont, TX: Helena Laboratories.

Forbes, B. A., et al. (2002). *Bailey & Scott's diagnostic microbiology* (11th ed.). St. Louis: C. V. Mosby.

Gillespie, S. H. & Pearson, R. D. (Eds.) (2001). *Principles and practice of clinical parasitology*. New York: John Wiley & Sons.

Hemoccult and Hemoccult SENSA package insert. Fullerton, CA: Beckman Coulter, Inc.

Henry, J. B. (Ed.) (2006). *Clinical diagnosis and management by laboratory methods* (21st ed.). Philadelphia: W.B. Saunders Company.

ICON SC Strep package insert. Fullerton, CA: Beckman-Coulter, Inc.

Koneman, E. W. (2005). *Koneman's color atlas and textbook of diagnostic microbiology* (6th ed.). Philadelphia: Lippincott Williams & Wilkins.

Murray, P. R., et al. (Eds.) (2003). *Manual of clinical microbiology* (8th ed.). Washington, DC: American Society for Microbiology.

Shimeld, L. A. & Rodgers, A. T. (1999). *Essentials of diagnostic microbiology*. Clifton Park, NY: Thomson Delmar Learning.

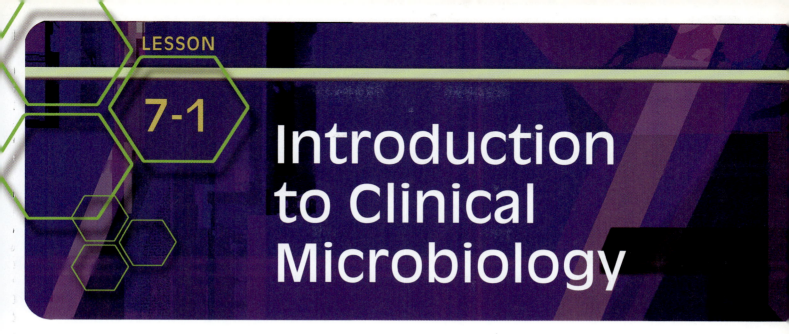

LESSON 7-1

Introduction to Clinical Microbiology

LESSON OBJECTIVES

After studying this lesson, the student will:

- List the fields of study included in microbiology.
- Discuss the microbiology department's organization and function in small and large laboratories.
- Discuss the differences among normal flora, pathogens, and opportunistic pathogens.
- Explain how infection occurs.
- Describe the three basic shapes of bacteria.
- Explain the importance of correct specimen collection.
- Discuss methods used to identify bacteria.
- Explain the functions of the parasitology laboratory.
- Explain how virology diagnostic procedures differ from bacteriology procedures.
- Discuss diagnostic methods used in mycology.
- Define the glossary terms.

GLOSSARY

aerobic / requiring oxygen

anaerobic / growing in the absence of oxygen

antibiotic susceptibility testing / determining the susceptibility of bacteria to specific antibiotics

bacillus / a rod-shaped bacterium

coccus / a spherical bacterium

colony / a defined mass of bacteria assumed to have grown from a single organism

communicable / able to be transmitted directly or indirectly from one individual to another

culture / growth of microorganisms in a special medium; the process of growing microorganisms in the laboratory

DNA / the nucleic acid that carries genetic information and that is found primarily in the nucleus of all living cells; deoxyribonucleic acid

fastidious bacteria / bacteria that require special nutritional factors to survive

fission / reproductive process in which the parent cell divides into two identical independent cells

Gram negative / designation for bacteria that lose the crystal violet (purple stain) and retain the safranin (red stain) in the Gram stain procedure

Gram positive / designation for bacteria that retain the crystal violet (purple stain) in the Gram stain procedure

Gram stain / a differential stain used to classify bacteria

host / the organism from which a parasite obtains nutrients and in which some or part of the parasite's life cycle is completed

hyphae / filaments of a mold that make up the mycelium

immunoassay / a diagnostic method using antigen-antibody reactions

infection / a pathological condition caused by growth of microorganisms in the host

medium / a substance used to provide nutrients for growing microorganisms

minimum inhibitory concentration (MIC) / minimum concentration of an antibiotic required to inhibit the growth of a microorganism

mycelium / mass of hyphae that makes up the vegetative body of molds

mycosis / infection caused by fungi

normal flora / microorganisms that are normally present at a specific site

opportunistic pathogen / a microorganism that causes disease in the host only when normal defense mechanisms are impaired or absent

pathogen / an organism or agent capable of causing disease in a host

progeny / offspring or descendants

RNA / the nucleic acid that is important in protein synthesis and is found in all living cells; ribonucleic acid

spiral bacteria / motile bacteria having a helical or spiral shape

zone of inhibition / in the antibiotic susceptibility test, the area around an antibiotic disk that contains no bacterial growth

INTRODUCTION

Microbiology is the study of organisms of microscopic size. Louis Pasteur first used the term in the 1860s. However, microorganisms were first observed in 1675 by Antony van Leeuwenhoek, a Dutchman. The term *microbe* was introduced in 1878 to refer to these organisms. Although the term *microorganism*, as commonly used, includes the bacteria, viruses, fungi, and parasites, viruses are not living organisms.

Clinical microbiology encompasses the study of viruses, fungi, bacteria, and parasites that cause disease in humans and other animals. Included are tests to isolate and identify these microorganisms. Table 7-1 lists the groups of organisms and terms used to describe their study.

In a large hospital laboratory or reference laboratory, each of these specialties might be in a separate department. However, a small laboratory may have a single microbiology department responsible for bacteriology, virology, parasitology, and mycology testing. In the physician office laboratory (POL), only the less complicated procedures are performed. Most parasitology, virology, and mycology specimens are sent to a reference laboratory for testing.

RULES OF NOMENCLATURE

All living things are classified according to international rules of nomenclature. Species of organisms are given two-part names, according to the rules of the binomial system of nomenclature. The first part is the name of the *genus* to which the organism belongs and is written with the first letter capitalized. The second, uncapitalized name is the *specific epithet*. It is never used without the genus name (or genus abbreviation) preceding it. The scientific names of organisms are underlined when hand-written and in italics in print, for example, *Staphylococcus aureus* (abbrev. *S. aureus*).

CLINICAL BACTERIOLOGY

General Characteristics of Bacteria

Bacteria are a large, diverse group of single-celled microorganisms. They usually multiply by **fission**, a process in which the parent body divides into two identical independent cells. A bacterium is a single organism. When many bacteria grow from a single organism they form a **colony**.

TABLE 7-1. Groups of microorganisms and the terms used for their study

MICROORGANISM	TERM
Bacteria	Bacteriology
Viruses	Virology
Fungi and yeast	Mycology
Parasites	Parasitology

Bacterial Morphology

Bacteria can be divided into three general groups by their morphology, or shape. The three types are **coccus** (round), **bacillus** (rod), and **spiral bacteria** (Figure 7-1). Certain kinds of cocci occur in pairs and are called diplococci. Some bacilli are filamentous, meaning they form multicelled, branching patterns.

Gram Stain Reactions

The **Gram stain** is a procedure that stains bacteria differentially according to the composition of their cell walls. A Gram stain is performed by applying crystal violet, Gram's iodine, a decolorizer, and a counterstain, safranin, to a bacterial smear. The complete procedure is described in Lesson 7-6. Bacteria that retain the crystal violet and appear blue-purple are called **Gram positive**. The bacteria that do not retain the crystal violet and stain pink-red with the safranin and are called **Gram negative**.

Growth Requirements

A **medium** is a substance used to provide nutrients for growing microorganisms. Many bacteria can grow on a common medium such as blood agar. However, other bacteria can grow only on a specialized medium and are called **fastidious bacteria**. **Aerobic** bacteria grow in the presence of oxygen while **anaerobic** bacteria live and multiply in the absence of oxygen. The growth of some types of bacteria is enhanced by growing them in an atmosphere of 5% to 10% carbon dioxide (CO_2). Examples of some common bacteria and their growth requirements are shown in Table 7-2.

Pathogenic Bacteria

Clinical bacteriology laboratories deal with the isolation and identification of bacterial **pathogens**, those bacteria capable of causing disease. Bacterial pathogens cause disease by overcoming the body's normal defenses and invading the tissues. The damage is caused by their growth in tissues or by the toxins they produce. This invasion is called **infection**. Diseases that can spread from person to person are called infectious or **communicable** diseases.

Pathogens make up only a small portion of the total population of bacteria. Most microorganisms are free-living, in soil or water. Some are natural inhabitants of the human body and are thus part of **normal flora**. Microorganisms that invade the body and cause illness only when the body's immune defenses are impaired or absent are called **opportunistic pathogens**.

The work of the bacteriology laboratory is to isolate the organism that has infected the patient. Once it has been isolated,

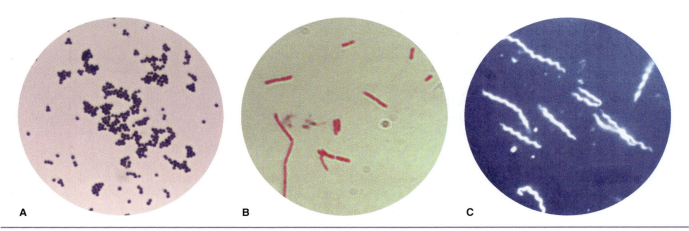

A   **B**   **C**

FIGURE 7-1 Three morphological types of bacteria: (A) cocci; (B) bacilli; and (C) spiral bacteria. Bacteria in A and B are Gram-stained; C is fluorescently stained

TABLE 7-2. Examples of some common bacteria and their growth requirements

ORGANISM	DISEASE	CULTURE MEDIUM	GROWTH CONDITIONS
Streptococcus	Strep throat	Blood agar	↓ O_2, 5–10% CO_2
Neisseria gonorrhoeae	Gonorrhea	Chocolate agar, modified Thayer-Martin (MTM)	↓ O_2, 5–10% CO_2
Staphylococcus	Infections, boils	Blood agar	O_2
Escherichia coli	Urinary tract infections	Blood agar, eosin methylene blue (EMB), MacConkey's (MAC)	O_2
Campylobacter sp.	Gastroenteritis	Campylobacter BAP medium	Anaerobic

the organism is subjected to various tests to help identify it. The next step is **antibiotic susceptibility testing** to determine which antibiotic will be most effective in treating the patient.

Bacteriological Procedures in the Small Laboratory

Bacteriology is an important part of the clinical laboratory. Isolating and identifying the organism causing a patient's illness is the first step in determining proper treatment.

Procedures performed in a small laboratory or POL usually include throat cultures or rapid strep tests, urine cultures, and, occasionally, *Neisseria gonorrhoeae* testing. The organism(s) in the specimen is grown, isolated, and either identified on site, or sent to a reference laboratory for identification.

Specimen Collection

Before bacteria suspected of causing an infection can be identified, a specimen must be collected and a culture set up. A **culture** is growth of the bacteria on a medium that provides nutrients to the microorganisms.

The results of a culture of bacteria from a patient specimen are only as reliable as the method used to collect and transport the specimen. Because cotton swabs are toxic to some bacteria, specimens must be collected on rayon or Dacron swabs. Organisms sensitive to drying must be immediately placed in special medium after collection or viability will be lost.

The health care provider who collects the specimen must be aware of the oxygen (O_2) requirements for various bacteria. If an anaerobic organism is kept in an aerobic atmosphere during transport to the laboratory, the organism can be killed; special anaerobic transport systems should be used. Likewise, if an aerobic organism is subjected to anaerobic conditions, the culture can fail to grow, causing a false negative culture result. For example, *Neisseria gonorrhoeae*, the cause of the sexually transmitted disease gonorrhea, has special growth requirements (Table 7-2). Therefore, immediately after collection, specimens suspected of containing *N. gonorrhoeae* must be inoculated to a special medium which is then placed in an atmosphere of reduced O_2 and increased CO_2.

Each facility's procedure manual will list media that should be used for culturing various types of specimens. The list will categorize media either by the type of bacteria suspected or by the specimen collection site, such as a wound. In addition, the reference laboratory should provide guidelines for the collection and transport of specimens to its laboratory.

Identifying Bacteria

Test methods to aid in bacterial identification include microscopic morphology, colony appearance, Gram and other stain reactions, growth on special media, biochemical reactions, gene probes, and antibody reactions (Table 7-3). Four common types of media used to isolate and identify bacteria are shown in Table 7-4.

Antibiotic Susceptibility Testing

Once the bacterium causing the patient's infection has been identified, the bacterial antibiotic susceptibility must be determined.

TABLE 7-3. Test methods used to identify bacteria

- Microscopic appearance
- Colonial morphology
- Selective or indicating media
- Gram and other stains
- Biochemical reactions
- Gene probes
- Antibody reactions

TABLE 7-4. Four common types of media used to isolate and identify bacteria

MEDIUM	USE
5% Sheep's blood agar (BA)	Supports growth of most Gram-positive and Gram-negative organisms, demonstrates hemolysis
Eosin methylene blue (EMB)	Supports growth of Gram-negative organisms, inhibits Gram-positive organisms, inhibits *Proteus* motility, demonstrates lactose and sucrose use
MacConkey's (MAC)	Supports growth of Gram-negative organisms, inhibits Gram-positive organisms, demonstrates lactose use
Chocolate agar	Provides heme to fastidious organisms *(Neisseria)*
Thayer-Martin (TM) and modified Thayer-Martin (MTM)	Chocolate agar with antibiotics added to suppress normal flora and contaminants

This can be accomplished by measuring the **zone of inhibition** around each antibiotic disk, which is the Bauer-Kirby method, or by finding the **minimum inhibitory concentration (MIC)** of various antibiotics.

The Bauer-Kirby method is performed on the solid surface of a special medium called Mueller-Hinton. This nonautomated procedure is interpreted visually. The MIC is determined by growing the organism in a special welled plate. Dilutions of various antibiotics are added to the growth wells. The minimum amount of antibiotic that inhibits the organism's growth is determined and is used by the physician as a guide to antibiotic choice.

PARASITOLOGY

Clinical parasitology involves studying and identifying parasites and parasitic diseases. Parasites are organisms that live in, on, and at the expense of, another organism called the **host** organism. Parasites can be unicellular (microscopic) or multicellular. They can be present in blood, bone marrow, intestinal tract, liver, spleen, skin, hair, or any organ system. To diagnose parasitic infections, the physician must recognize the symptoms and request the appropriate tests. Most smaller laboratories do not perform tests for parasites; instead they process specimens for transport to hospital, state, or reference laboratories for examination and parasite detection and identification. Table 7-5 lists specimens required for detection of some common parasites.

Intestinal Parasites

Roundworms, flukes, and hookworms, all of which are *helminths*, are common intestinal parasites. In addition, single-celled protozoa with amoeba or cyst forms can be found (Figure 7-2).

TABLE 7-5. Types of specimens required for parasite detection

ORGANISM	SPECIMEN
Trichomonas vaginalis	Urine, vaginal secretions, urethral discharge, prostatic secretions
Entamoeba histolytica	Feces
Giardia intestinalis	Feces
Cryptosporidium parvum	Feces
Enterobius vermicularis (pinworm)	Perianal swab
Necator americanus (hookworm)	Feces
Plasmodium (malarial parasite)	Blood
Toxoplasma	Tissue, blood

Intestinal parasites are discovered by examining stool specimens for ova and parasites (O & P). Intestinal worms release ova (eggs) that can be detected in stool specimens. Larvae (immature forms) or adults of some helminths can also be found. When protozoan parasites are suspected, the stool specimen is examined for cysts (nonmotile forms) and trophozoites (motile forms). To increase the likelihood of finding parasites, three stool specimens collected on separate days should be examined for O & P (Table 7-5). One test that is often performed in small laboratories is the the perianal swab or cellophane tape test for pinworm, a common parasite in the United States (see Lesson 8-2).

Stool Examination for Parasites

The O & P test includes microscopic examination of fecal wet mounts and a fixed, stained smear. The wet mount is useful for detecting protozoan motility and requires a fresh stool specimen (Table 7-5). A wet mount of the specimen is also examined after a concentration technique; this increases the likelihood of finding protozoan cysts and helminth eggs and larvae. The fixed, stained smear is for identifying and confirming intestinal protozoa. **Immunoassays** are also available to detect certain parasite antigens in stool specimens.

Preserving and Transporting Specimens

Specimens to be transported to a reference laboratory must be placed in special preservative solutions. The reference laboratory should provide collection vials containing a preservative such as a modified polyvinylalcohol (PVA).

Blood and Tissue Parasites

Examinations of blood and tissue for parasites are usually performed in large hospital laboratories or in a reference or state laboratory. In the United States, blood and tissue parasites are seen infrequently. However, worldwide the most common blood parasite is the malarial parasite, *Plasmodium* (Lesson 8-4). Blood parasites are discovered and identified by microscopic examination of specially stained blood smears. Although a small laboratory might

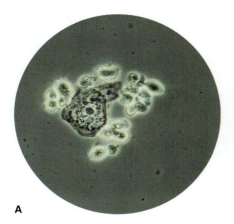
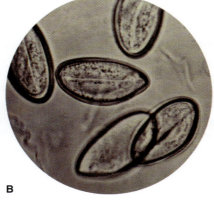
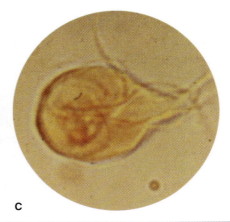

FIGURE 7-2 Examples of three common human parasites (not shown to scale): (A) unstained smear containing the flagellate *Trichomonas vaginalis* and squamous epithelial cells; (B) pinworm ova; and (C) unstained *Giardia* trophozoite (*From CDC, Atlanta, GA*)

not perform the actual malaria examinations, personnel must know how to prepare and stain thick and thin blood smears to send to the reference laboratory for examination. Tissue parasites are detected by examination of biopsy material. These specimens are usually prepared in the histology/cytology department.

Trichomonas vaginalis

A frequently-seen protozoan parasite is *Trichomonas vaginalis* (Figure 7-2A). It can be detected in vaginal or urethral discharge, prostatic secretions, or urine (Table 7-5). *Trichomonas* is recognized by its characteristic twitching motility when observed microscopically in a coverslip or well-slide preparation.

VIROLOGY

Virology is the study of viruses and the diseases they cause. Common viruses that cause disease are influenza viruses, rubella virus, mumps virus, measles virus, Epstein-Barr virus, and herpes viruses (Table 7-6). As a group, viruses are the most common cause of human infectious diseases. Some viruses are known to cause cancer.

TABLE 7-6. Common viruses, their abbreviations or acronyms, and the diseases they cause

VIRUS	ABBREVIATION OR ACRONYM	DISEASE
Herpes simplex virus, type 1	HSV-1	Cold sores, fever blisters
Herpes simplex virus, type 2	HSV-2	Genital herpes
Epstein-Barr virus	EBV	Infectious mononucleosis
Human papilloma virus	HPV	Warts, tumors, and cancer of genital tract
Hepatitis B virus	HBV	Hepatitis B
Hepatitis C virus	HCV	Hepatitis C
Rhinoviruses	–	Common cold
Influenza A,B,C		Influenza (flu)
Rubella virus	–	Rubella (German measles, 3-day measles)
Human immuno-deficiency virus	HIV	Acquired immuno-deficiency syndrome (AIDS)
Measles virus	–	Rubeola (red measles)

Characteristics of Viruses

Viruses are not considered living cells and can only replicate by invading a cell. Once inside the cell, they use the cell's replication processes to make more virus **progeny**, or offspring.

Each virus consists of a nucleic acid *core* and a protein coat called a *capsid*. Some have an additional component called an *envelope*. Living organisms contain both DNA and RNA, but a virus has only one or the other. **DNA** is the nucleic acid found primarily in chromosomes that carries genetic information. **RNA** is a nucleic acid responsible for protein synthesis. Because viruses are much smaller than bacteria and cannot be seen with a light microscope, electron microscopes are used to study them (Figure 7-3).

Diagnostic Testing in Virology

Interest in diagnostic clinical virology has increased dramatically because of the demand for more rapid diagnosis of viral diseases caused by influenza viruses, human immunodeficiency virus

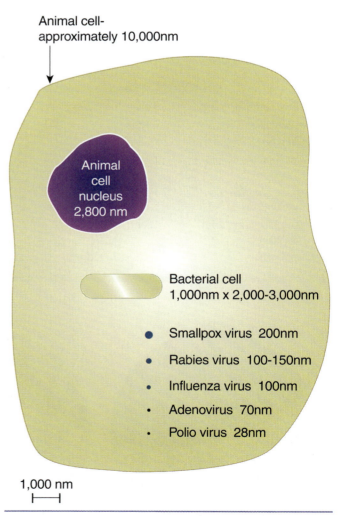

Animal cell- approximately 10,000nm

Animal cell nucleus 2,800 nm

Bacterial cell 1,000nm x 2,000-3,000nm

• Smallpox virus 200nm
• Rabies virus 100-150nm
• Influenza virus 100nm
• Adenovirus 70nm
• Polio virus 28nm

1,000 nm

FIGURE 7-3 Relative sizes of viruses compared to the size of a bacterial cell and an animal cell (Adapted from Brock, T.D. & Brock, K.M. (1973) *Basic microbiology and applications.* Englewood Cliffs, NJ: Prentice-Hall, Inc.)

(HIV), and human papilloma virus (HPV). In addition, increases in cases of hepatitis B and C, which can be chronic or fatal, have helped motivate development of improved laboratory tests for viral infection.

The standard method for isolating and identifying viruses has been cell culture, which is performed in large microbiology departments and in reference laboratories. Patient serum can also be tested for viral antibodies using enzyme immunoassays (EIAs). Table 7-7 lists the basic approaches to clinical virology testing. Rapid diagnostic kits are now available for several viral diseases. Many are CLIA-waived and are suitable for use in the smaller laboratory.

Small laboratories do not have the personnel and resources to perform most viral testing. However, they often collect and send specimens to the reference laboratory. A procedure manual listing available tests, collection methods, and transport media should be provided by the reference laboratory.

MYCOLOGY

Mycology is the study of fungi, a diverse group of microorganisms that exist in *mold* or *yeast* form. Most fungi are found in soil and on decaying plant matter. Of 250,000 known fungal species, only about 180 are considered capable of causing disease.

Characteristics of Molds

Molds have branching filaments called **hyphae** that make up the vegetative structure, the **mycelium**. They reproduce by forming spores (Figure 7-4A). Most molds are aerobic and grow in the range of 22°C to 30°C. They will grow on the usual bacteriological media, but their growth is so slow that bacteria usually overgrow them. One of the best media to select for growth of pathogenic fungi is Sabouraud's dextrose agar, which contains dextrose, maltose, and peptones. In addition, antibiotics can be incorporated to inhibit growth of bacteria and nonpathogenic fungi.

Characteristics of Yeast

Yeast cells are eukaryotic cells that are larger than bacteria. They are easily seen with the light microscope. The most common yeast shape is unicellular (one-celled) and oval. Yeasts usually reproduce by budding instead of forming spores (Figure 7-4B). There are about 350 known species of yeasts. Yeasts are used in fermentation processes such as beer and wine production and leavening of bread. Yeasts grow best with an abundant supply of oxygen and grow satisfactorily on common bacteriological media, as well as Saboraud's dextrose agar. Although yeasts are useful for food and other commercial purposes, there are some pathogenic yeasts and some that are opportunistic pathogens.

Fungal Diseases—Mycoses

Infection caused by a fungus is called a **mycosis** (pl., mycoses). The mycosis incidence is related to the degree of exposure to fungi in living conditions, occupation, and leisure activities, as well as to immune status. Table 7-8 lists some fungi and the diseases they cause.

Pathogenic fungi, which can infect any exposed individual, usually fall in the group called *dimorphic* fungi. This means that these fungi can grow in both yeast and mold forms, depending on culture conditions. In the environment, they are found as a mold form; when grown at body temperature, such as when infecting an animal or human, they are found in the yeast form. Three important pathogenic dimorphic fungi are *Blastomyces dermatitidis, Histoplasma capsulatum*, and *Coccidioides immitis*, the agent that causes San Joaquin Valley fever. Other fungi such as *Candida* and *Aspergillus* are opportunistic pathogens; they usually only cause serious disease in immunosuppressed (compromised) patients, such as HIV-infected patients. *Candida* can infect the mucous membranes of the mouth and vagina. The *dermatophytes*, the group of fungi that require keratin to grow, can infect hair, nails, and superficial skin. The fungi that cause ringworm and athlete's foot are dermatophytes.

Identifying Molds and Yeasts

Identification techniques for fungi depend on whether the organism is a mold or yeast. Molds are largely identified by macroscopic and microscopic study of their morphology and the spores they produce (Figure 7-4). Superficial yeast or dermatophyte infections can be detected by microscopic examination or culturing of skin scrapings or nail clippings. Yeast identification is based on culture and colonial morphology and on the results of biochemical reactions and the organism's ability to ferment certain sugars. *Candida albicans* can be identified by the development of pseudohyphae in a test called the *germ tube test*. Table 7-9 gives a simplified scheme for identifying molds and yeasts.

TABLE 7-7. Basic approaches to detecting viruses
1. **Cell culture:** Isolating and identifying the viruses in cell culture
2. **Direct detection:** Detecting the viral antigen in a clinical specimen
3. **Serodiagnosis:** Detecting antibodies to the virus

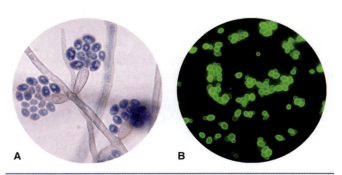

FIGURE 7-4 Reproductive forms of molds and yeasts: (A) spore-producing mold; (B) budding yeast cells stained with fluorescent stain *(Photos from CDC, Atlanta, GA)*

TABLE 7-8. Some common fungi and the diseases they cause

ORGANISM	DISEASE
Tinea species	Ringworm (dermatomycosis)
Candida	Thrush, vaginal infections (candidiasis)
Malassezia furfur	Pityriasis versicolor
Coccidioides immitis	Coccidioidomycosis (Valley fever)
Histoplasma capsulatum	Histoplasmosis
Aspergillus, Candida, Cryptococcus, and *Pneumocystis*	Involved in systemic infections (especially in immunocompromised patients)

TABLE 7-9. A simplified scheme for culturing and identifying molds and yeasts

ORGANISM	CULTURE CONDITIONS	METHOD OF IDENTIFICATION
Molds	Sabouraud's agar (22°C-27°C)	Macroscopic and microscopic appearance
Yeasts	Blood agar (37°C)	Fermentation of sugars, use of carbon or nitrogen compounds
		Germ tube test

SUMMARY

Microbiology is the study of a wide variety of agents, some helpful to man and some harmful. The bacteria, fungi, and parasites are named using international rules, so that scientists all over the world use the same nomenclature.

Humans have conquered many infectious diseases, mainly because of the discovery and use of antibiotics. However, we frequently hear of a new disease or discovery of a new microbe. Microorganisms and viruses can undergo rapid genetic change. An animal pathogen can become pathogenic to humans. A bacterium can become resistant to antibiotics. These discoveries lead to more microbiology research in academic institutions and pharmaceutical and research laboratories.

Each discovery causes a trickle-down effect in clinical laboratories. Eventually, if the organism is a pathogen, test methods are developed to detect it or antibodies to it. At the same time, methods to detect more commonplace causes of disease are always being improved and more automated methods are being introduced into the microbiology laboratory.

REVIEW QUESTIONS

1. When was the term microbiology first used?
2. What four areas of study are encompassed by clinical microbiology?
3. What are the functional differences between a small and large microbiology laboratory?
4. What is meant by the term normal flora?
5. What is a pathogen? An opportunistic pathogen?
6. How does infection occur?
7. Describe the three morphological types of bacteria.
8. What is a Gram stain?
9. What are the two morphological forms of fungi?
10. What is the difference between aerobic and anaerobic bacteria?
11. List the microbiological tests usually performed in a small laboratory.
12. How are viruses different from microorganisms? Name three viral diseases.
13. What type of specimen is required to detect malaria? To detect *Giardia*?
14. List seven test methods used to help identify bacteria.
15. Define aerobic, anaerobic, antibiotic susceptibility testing, bacillus, coccus, colony, communicable, culture, DNA, fastidious bacteria, fission, Gram negative, Gram positive, Gram stain, host, hyphae, immunoassay, infection, medium, minimum inhibitory concentration, mycelium, mycosis, normal flora, opportunistic pathogen, pathogen, progeny, RNA, spiral bacteria, and zone of inhibition.

STUDENT ACTIVITIES

1. Complete the written examination for this lesson.
2. Visit a microbiology laboratory in the community. Find out what types of tests are performed in the laboratory and which tests are sent to reference laboratories.
3. Interview an employee of a hospital microbiology laboratory.

WEB ACTIVITY

Use the Internet to find information on a disease caused by an agent from each microbiology category (bacteria, virus, fungus, and parasite). For each disease, report on the causative agent, disease symptoms, method of diagnosis, and treatment.

7-2

Infection Control and Transmission-Based Precautions

LESSON OBJECTIVES

After studying this lesson, the student will:

- Discuss the role of the hospital's infection control department.
- Explain why isolation techniques are used.
- List five exposure control methods that are included in Standard Precautions.
- List the three types of transmission-based precautions and explain the basis for each classification.
- Demonstrate proper handwashing technique.
- Demonstrate proper gowning technique.
- Demonstrate the proper method of putting on a mask.
- Demonstrate proper gloving technique.
- Demonstrate proper removal and disposal of mask, gown, and gloves.
- Define the glossary terms.

GLOSSARY

Airborne Precautions / a Centers for Disease Control and Prevention (CDC) isolation category designed to prevent transmission of infectious diseases, such as measles, that are spread by the airborne route

carrier / a person who harbors an organism, has no symptoms or signs of disease, but is capable of spreading the organism to others

Contact Precautions / a CDC isolation category designed to prevent transmission of diseases spread by close or direct contact

Droplet Precautions / a CDC isolation category designed to prevent transmission of diseases spread through the air over short distances

fomites / inanimate objects, such as bed rails, linens, or eating utensils, that may be contaminated with infectious organisms and serve as a means of their transmission

infection / a pathological condition caused by growth of microorganisms in the host

isolation / the practice of limiting the movement and social contact of a patient who is potentially infectious or who must be protected from exposure to infectious agents; quarantine

nonpathogenic / not normally causing disease in a healthy individual

nosocomial infection / an infection acquired in a hospital or health care facility

protective isolation / an isolation category designed to protect highly susceptible patients from exposure to infectious agents; reverse isolation

Standard Precautions / a set of comprehensive safety guidelines designed to protect patients and health care workers by requiring that all patients and all body fluids, body substances, organs, and unfixed tissues be regarded as potentially infectious

INTRODUCTION

The hospital's infection control department monitors contagious diseases within the hospital. This is accomplished by setting guidelines for managing contagious patients or patients who are highly susceptible to infection (have little resistance or immunity). This department also sets standards to ensure that patients do not acquire infections while in the hospital.

Every health care institution has an infection control program based on regulations and recommendations of agencies such as the Centers for Disease Control and Prevention (CDC); the Joint Commission (JC); the Association for Practitioners in Infection Control (APIC); and state regulatory agencies. One control method is **isolation**, which includes separating the infectious patient from other patients and limiting visitor and staff contact with that patient.

This lesson provides general guidelines for transmission-based precautions for laboratory personnel such as phlebotomists or others who must obtain blood from the patient in isolation, and who normally have only limited patient exposure. The student or technician must be sure to follow the particular institution's rules concerning these guidelines. Other texts should be consulted for guidelines for nursing personnel, who have more extensive patient contact.

CAUSES OF INFECTION

Microorganisms present in the environment and in and on the human body include bacteria, viruses, protozoa, and fungi. Most microorganisms are **nonpathogenic**, meaning they do not normally cause disease in a healthy individual. Microbes capable of causing disease are called pathogens.

Infection occurs when the body is invaded by a pathogenic agent that can, under favorable conditions, multiply and cause disease. Infections usually cause symptoms such as fever, redness, fluid accumulation, or pain. Three components must be present for infection to occur: (1) a source of microorganisms, (2) a susceptible person or host, and (3) a method of transmission from the source to the susceptible host (Table 7-10). The source can be an infected person or animal, the environment, or **fomites** (contaminated objects). The transmission method can be by:

- Direct contact
- Inhalation of dust or droplets containing microorganisms
- Inhalation of air droplets produced by coughing or sneezing

- Exposure to infectious body fluids
- Ingestion of contaminated water or food
- Vectors such as insects

TRANSMISSION-BASED PRECAUTIONS

In the past, each institution developed isolation procedures appropriate for its patient population, taking into consideration newly emerging diseases. In 1992, the CDC issued a set of guidelines called Universal Precautions to assist health care providers in reducing the risk of contracting or transmitting infectious diseases, particularly AIDS and hepatitis B.

In 1996, improvements were made in these guidelines. **Standard Precautions** were issued to augment and synthesize Universal Precautions with the techniques known as body substance isolation (BSI). Standard Precautions represent a comprehensive approach to protecting all health care providers, patients, and visitors from acquiring infectious diseases. Standard Precautions must always be observed along with the facility's exposure control plan and CDC safety regulations. The use of Standard Precautions prevents exposure to all blood and body fluids, whether known to be infectious or not. These precautions include:

- Using proper hand hygiene techniques
- Wearing gloves and buttoned fluid-resistant laboratory coat when handling all biological specimens, containers, and any potentially infectious materials
- Wearing eye and/or face protection if aerosols or splashes are likely or reasonably anticipated

TABLE 7-10. Methods of transmitting infection

Direct contact
Inhaling droplets produced by coughing or sneezing
Inhaling dust particles containing microorganisms
Exposure to infectious body fluids
Ingesting contaminated food or water
Exposure to disease vectors such as insects or rodents

TABLE 7-11. Current CDC transmission-based precautions and former isolation categories

CURRENT TRANSMISSION-BASED PRECAUTIONS	FORMER ISOLATION CATEGORIES
Droplet Precautions*	Contact isolation
Airborne Precautions*	Respiratory isolation
Contact Precautions*	Acid-fast bacillus (AFB) isolation
	Complete or strict isolation
	Reverse or protective isolation

* Used in addition to Standard Precautions

CONTACT PRECAUTIONS
In Addition to Standard Precautions

Visitors - Report to Nurses' Station Before Entering Room

BEFORE CARE	DURING CARE	AFTER CARE
1. Private room.	1. Limit transport of patient/resident to essential purposes only. Patient/resident must wear mask appropriate for disease. 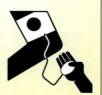	1. Bag linen to prevent contamination of self, environment, or outside of bag.
2. Wash hands.	2. Limit use of noncritical care equipment to a single patient/resident.	2. Discard infectious trash to prevent contamination of self, environment, or outside of bag.
3. Wear gown if soiling is likely.		3. Wash hands.
4. Wear gloves when entering room. Change after contact with infective material.		

FIGURE 7-5 Contact precautions, one category of transmission-based precautions (*Courtesy Brevis Corp.*)

■ Handling all sharps carefully and disposing of contaminated sharps in sharps containers

■ Cleaning up spills immediately with an appropriate disinfectant

In addition to issuing Standard Precautions, the CDC also simplified isolation guidelines. The former isolation classification scheme contained five categories: (1) contact isolation, (2) respiratory isolation, (3) acid-fast bacillus (AFB) isolation, (4) strict or complete isolation, and (5) reverse isolation, plus enteric precautions and drainage secretion precautions. These five categories were reduced to three *transmission-based precautions*, also called *expanded precautions*, classified according to the route of disease transmission. The transmission-based precautions are: (1) **Droplet Precautions**, (2) **Contact Precautions**,

and (3) **Airborne Precautions** (Table 7-11). These are used in addition to Standard Precautions when infectious disease is present or suspected. Transmission-based precautions and the former isolation categories are listed in Table 7-11.

Contact Precautions

Contact Precautions are used in addition to Standard Precautions when patients have diseases spread primarily by close or direct contact (Figure 7-5 and Table 7-12). The patient should be placed in a private room, if possible. Precautions used for this category are intended to protect health care workers against infection from contact with infectious material, such as wound or fecal material. Exposure could occur if the patient is incontinent or has diarrhea, an ileostomy, a colostomy,

TABLE 7-12. Transmission-based precautions and examples of illnesses and disease agents that require the precautions (adapted from the CDC)

Standard Precautions

Use for all patients

Airborne Precautions

Use in addition to Standard Precautions for illnesses transmitted by airborne droplet nuclei. Examples:

> Measles (rubeola)
>
> Tuberculosis
>
> Varicella

Droplet Precautions

Use in addition to Standard Precautions for illnesses transmitted by large-particle droplets. Examples:

Diphtheria	*Mycoplasma* pneumonia
Pertussis	Pneumonic plague
Invasive *Hemophilus influenzae*	Adenovirus
	Influenza
Invasive *Neisseria meningitidis*	Parvovirus B19
	Rubella
Mumps	
Streptococcal pharyngitis	

Contact Precautions

Use in addition to Standard Precautions for illnesses transmitted by direct contact. Examples:

Wound infections	Enteric infections
Respiratory syncytial virus	Skin infections
Colonization with multidrug-resistant bacteria	
Viral hemorrhagic infections	

or wound drainage not contained by a dressing. Since surfaces and items in the room can also be contaminated, the health care worker must wear gloves and gown and remove both before leaving the room to avoid transferring organisms outside the room. After glove removal, hands must be washed with an antimicrobial agent. Contaminated materials must be discarded in biohazard containers for disposal or disinfection.

Droplet Precautions

Droplet Precautions are used in addition to Standard Precautions when patients are infected with organisms easily transmitted through the air over short distances (Figure 7-6). Examples include mumps, pertussis (whooping cough), meningococcal pneumonia, and meningitis (Table 7-12). These patients should be in private rooms, if possible. Masks are required for those who come within 3 feet of the patient or upon entering the room, since the infectious agents are readily spread

by the patient's coughing or sneezing, a major mode of transmission for respiratory infections. Gloves and gown are also required.

Airborne Precautions

Airborne Precautions are used in addition to Standard Precautions when a patient is known to be, or suspected of being, infected with microorganisms transmitted by the airborne route (Figure 7-7 and Table 7-12). Persons entering the room of a patient with known or suspected infectious pulmonary tuberculosis must wear an N95 respirator (Figure 7-8). In addition, susceptible personnel should not enter rooms of patients known to have, or suspected of having, measles (rubeola) or chickenpox (varicella) unless an immune caregiver is not available. The patient must be in a private room with negative air pressure. The room must have six to 12 air changes per hour and room air must be discharged outside or recirculated through a HEPA filter.

Reverse or Protective Isolation

Earlier isolation classifications contained a category called reverse or **protective isolation** intended to protect immunosuppressed or otherwise susceptible patients. Current standards do not address protective isolation in a direct way. Individual hospitals continue to make it an unofficial category; signs are placed on the room doors of immunosuppressed patients. The signs direct health care workers and visitors to wear masks when entering the room if they have a cold or other contagious condition. Laboratory personnel should always clarify any questions about protective isolation by consulting with the floor nurse or the infection control officer.

COMPLYING WITH THE INSTITUTION'S EXPOSURE CONTROL PLAN

Laboratory personnel must observe their institution's exposure control plan and CDC's safety regulations, not only in the laboratory but also in patient rooms and all other health care situations. These procedures are discussed in depth in Lesson 1-6, Laboratory Safety: Biological Hazards. Personnel must observe Standard Precautions along with transmission-based (expanded) precautions. The types of transmission-based precautions can be combined for diseases that have multiple modes of transmission.

EXPOSURE CONTROL PRACTICES

Health care facilities provide specific instructions and necessary supplies outside the room of each patient requiring transmission-based precautions. Exposure control practices that must be used include hand hygiene and using protective barriers such as gloves, masks, and gowns.

Hand Hygiene

Hand hygiene is the single most important procedure in preventing the spread of infection. Studies show that the use of proper hand hygiene techniques reduces health-care–associated infec-

DROPLET PRECAUTIONS
In Addition to Standard Precautions

Visitors - Report to Nurses' Station Before Entering Room

BEFORE CARE	DURING CARE	AFTER CARE

BEFORE CARE

1. Private room. Maintain 3 feet of spacing between patient/resident and visitors.

2. Mask/face shield for staff and visitors within 3 feet of patient/resident.

DURING CARE

1. Limit transport of patient/resident to essential purposes only. Patient/resident must wear mask appropriate for disease.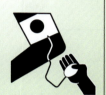

2. Limit use of noncritical care equipment to a single patient/resident.

AFTER CARE

1. Bag linen to prevent contamination of self, environment, or outside of bag.

2. Discard infectious trash to prevent contamination of self, environment, or outside of bag.

3. Wash hands.

FIGURE 7-6 Droplet Precautions, one category of transmission-based precautions (*Courtesy Brevis Corp.*)

AIRBORNE PRECAUTIONS
In Addition to Standard Precautions

Visitors - Report to Nurses' Station Before Entering Room

BEFORE CARE	DURING CARE	AFTER CARE

BEFORE CARE

1. Private room and closed door with monitored negative air pressure, frequent air exchanges, and high-efficiency filtration.

2. Wash hands.

3. Wear respiratory protection appropriate for disease.

DURING CARE

1. Limit transport of patient/resident to essential purposes only. Patient/resident must wear mask appropriate for disease.

2. Limit use of noncritical care equipment to a single patient/resident.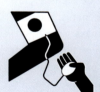

AFTER CARE

1. Bag linen to prevent contamination of self, environment, or outside of bag.

2. Discard infectious trash to prevent contamination of self, environment, or outside of bag.

3. Wash hands.

FIGURE 7-7 Airborne Precautions, one category of transmission-based precautions (*Courtesy Brevis Corp.*)

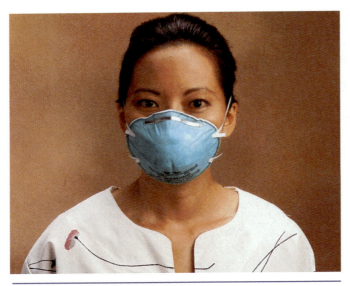

FIGURE 7-8 N95 respirator
(*Courtesy of 3M Company, St. Paul, MN*)

tions. Failure to use appropriate hand hygiene is considered the leading cause of health-care–associated infections and also contributes to the spread of drug-resistant organisms.

Several types and brands of antiseptic agents are available to use for handwashing or hand antisepsis. These agents include plain soaps, antimicrobial soaps, alcohol-based hand rubs, and chemical antiseptics. The alcohol-based hand rubs are available in several forms including rinses, gels, and foams. Several factors are considered by institutions when selecting hand hygiene products,

including the efficacy against a wide range of microorganisms, the willingness of workers to use the product, and the accessibility of the product.

Each hand hygiene product has its place in maintaining good hand hygiene. The effectiveness of hand hygiene techniques depends on the amount of antiseptic agent used, the duration of the hand cleaning procedure, and the type of product used. General recommendations for routine hand hygiene are:

- Hands should be decontaminated before and after all procedures

- Alcohol-based hand rubs or antimicrobial soap and water should be used for routine decontamination of hands in most clinical situations

- Visibly soiled hands should be washed with soap and water, followed by use of an antiseptic agent such as an alcohol-based rub

- Hands should be washed with soap and water before and after eating and after using a restroom

- Hands should be washed with water and antiseptic or antimicrobial soap after each 5 to 10 hand disinfections with an alcohol-based rub

- The institution's hand hygiene policy must be followed

Alcohol-Based Rub Technique

The alcohol-based product is applied to the palm of one hand and the hands are vigorously rubbed together, covering all surfaces of hands and fingers. This procedure is continued until all alcohol has evaporated and the hands are completely dry. Generally, an amount should be applied that would require at least 15 seconds to evapo-

CURRENT TOPICS

HEALTH CARE–ASSOCIATED AND NOSOCOMIAL INFECTIONS

Health care-associated infections are those that are acquired in health care settings by health care workers, patients, or others who enter health care settings. It is estimated that over 2 million health care–associated infections occur annually with 90,000 deaths.

Infections acquired by hospitalized patients or patients in hospital-like settings, such as long-term care facilities, are called nosocomial infections. In the United States, the incidence of nosocomial infections normally ranges from 5% to 10%. These infections can be acquired through contact with infected personnel, visitors, other patients, or contaminated equipment. One source of infection is contact with a carrier, a person who harbors an organism but feels well and displays no symptoms of infection. In addition, some patients who are admitted to health care facilities have an unrecognized infectious disease. Nosocomial infections usually present more problems than randomly acquired infections because:

- Hospitalized patients may already be more susceptible to infection.

- Invasive procedures such as surgery or indwelling catheters provide a portal to infection.

- Bacteria associated with nosocomial infections, such as *Staphylococcus aureus* and *Clostridium difficile*, are often drug-resistant, requiring treatment with less effective or more toxic drugs.

- Nosocomial infections generally require longer hospital stays, resulting in greater expense.

Through the use of good infection control practices, the incidence of health care–associated infections can be kept to a minimum. These practices include:

- Strict adherence to Standard Precautions

- Proper use of transmission-based precautions

- Immunization of health care workers against vaccine-preventable diseases

rate but the manufacturer's recommendations for the volume to use should be followed. One advantage of the alcohol-based rubs is that a sink is not required for hand decontamination.

Handwashing Technique

To wash hands with soap and water, hands should first be wet with warm or room temperature water, and an amount of product recommended by the manufacturer applied to the hands. The hands and wrists should be lathered and hands should be rubbed together vigorously for 15 to 30 seconds, covering all surfaces of the hands and fingers (Figure 7-9). Special attention should be given to cleaning fingernails and under rings. Hands should be held in a downward position and rinsed from the arm or wrist toward the tips of the fingers. The hands should be dried thoroughly with a disposable towel. Hand-operated faucets should be turned on and off using a clean disposable towel to avoid contaminating hands with organisms or substances that can be present on faucet handles. The use of hot water during handwashing should be avoided because repeated exposure to hot water can increase the risk of dermatitis.

Using Personal Protective Equipment

Standard Precautions require that personnel wear personal protective equipment (PPE) to protect against exposure to poten-tially infectious material. This PPE includes, but is not limited to, mask, gown, and gloves.

Masks

Masks should be put on after hands are washed, avoiding touching the skin with the hands. Masks can have ties for the upper neck and head or elastic bands to loop over the ears. Masks should be changed after being worn for 15 to 20 minutes.

Gowns

Laboratory coats should be removed before donning gowns. The gown should be touched only on the inside surface and should cover all clothing when tied (Figure 7-10). Gowns are removed by turning the inside of the gown to the outside and folding the contaminated outer side inward.

Gloves

A clean pair of gloves must be used for each patient. The gloves are put on by pulling the cuff or wrist area over sleeve ends of the gown so all skin or clothing is covered. It is best to avoid wearing sharp rings or jewelry that can puncture gloves.

Some special instances, such as reverse isolation, require sterile gloves. Sterile gloves are always used to handle sterile equipment or instruments.

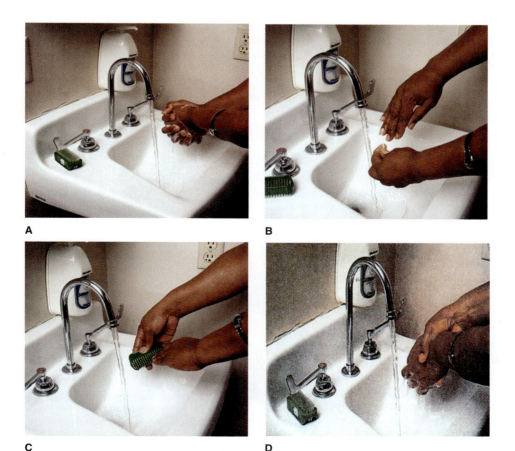

A **B** **C** **D**

FIGURE 7-9 Handwashing technique: (A) interlace the fingers to clean between them; (B-C) clean under the fingernails; and (D) rinse hands thoroughly, with the fingertips down

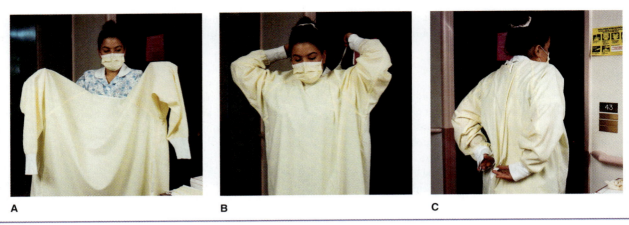

FIGURE 7-10 Putting on cover gown: (A) put on the gown outside the patient's room/unit by placing hands inside the shoulders; (B) slip fingers inside the neck-band and tie gown; (C) overlap the back edges of the gown so clothing is covered, and secure the waist ties

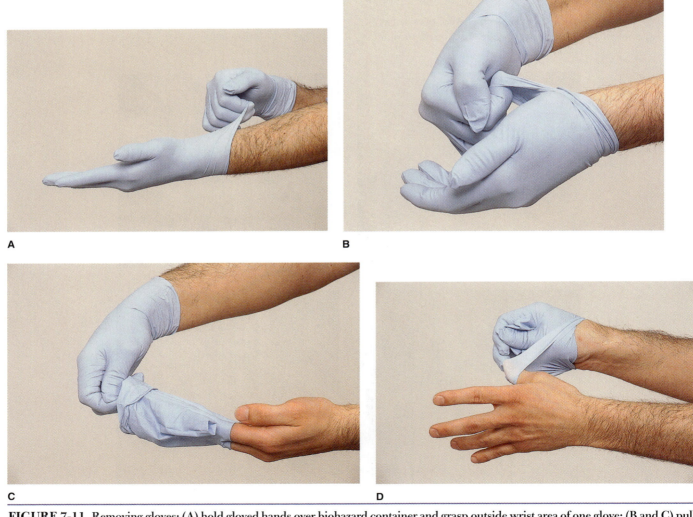

FIGURE 7-11 Removing gloves: (A) hold gloved hands over biohazard container and grasp outside wrist area of one glove; (B and C) pull the glove down over the hand, inside out, and discard into biohazard container; (D) insert bare fingers inside remaining glove cuff, pulling the glove inside out down over the hand, and taking care not to touch the outside of the glove. Discard glove into biohazard container

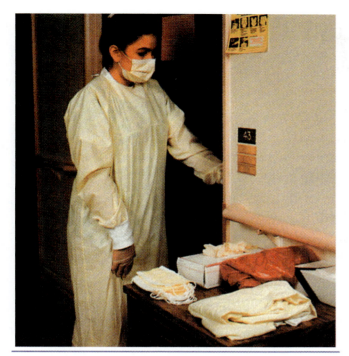

FIGURE 7-12 Laboratory professional wearing gown, gloves, and mask, entering the room of a patient requiring transmission-based precautions

Contaminated gloves are removed by grasping the cuff of one glove with the other gloved hand and pulling the glove off over itself. The removed glove is dropped into a biohazard container, and the second glove is removed and discarded in the same way, without touching the outer glove surface (Figure 7-11). Hands should always be decontaminated with antiseptic after glove removal.

The order in which PPE is put on and removed is important. A sequence of donning and removing PPE should be used that protects the wearer from becoming contaminated. Generally hands are cleaned with antiseptic and then gown, mask, eyewear or face protection, and gloves are donned in that order. The general order of removal is that gloves are removed first, and then the gown. Hands should then be cleaned with antiseptic before eyewear and mask are removed.

Entering and Exiting a Precaution Room

The procedure used for entering and exiting isolation rooms differs according to the type of precaution. In general, most personal protective equipment (PPE) is located on a cart outside the patient's room and is put on before entering (Figure 7-12).

Only items that will be used for the patient should be taken into the precaution room. Phlebotomists should leave trays and requisition slips outside the room to avoid having them become contaminated. Tourniquets and pens should be left in the room for future use.

When personnel exit the room, the used supplies should be left in a special disposal container usually located inside the room.

Exceptions to this procedure include protective isolation, where disposables are usually left in a container outside the room for disposal.

SUMMARY

Laboratory personnel must observe their institution's exposure control plan, not only in the laboratory but also in patients' rooms and all other health care situations. Standard Precautions must always be used to prevent exposure to all blood and body fluids, whether known to be infectious or not.

Transmission-based precautions must be used when a patient is suspected of having, or is known to have, a contagious disease or a condition that could expose caregivers or others to infectious agents. Transmission-based precautions protect health care workers, visitors, and patients. The disease or type of organism suspected and its mode of transmission determine which exposure control methods must be used, such as gowns, masks, or respirators. The institution's infection control department will have a written policy manual to follow when implementing transmission-based precautions.

REVIEW QUESTIONS

1. What is the function of the hospital's infection control department?
2. Why are transmission-based precautions used?
3. What are the three categories of transmission-based precautions? Give an example of a condition or disease requiring each type of precaution.
4. Explain the proper handwashing method. When is handwashing performed?
5. Explain the proper technique for putting on and removing a gown.
6. Explain how to put on and remove gloves.
7. What are five exposure-control methods used to prevent exposure to blood and body fluids?
8. How do Standard Precautions and transmission-based precautions differ? When are Standard Precautions used?
9. What exposure-control methods are used in each of the three categories of transmission-based precautions?
10. Define Airborne Precautions, carrier, Contact Precautions, Droplet Precautions, fomites, infection, isolation, nonpathogenic, nosocomial infection, protective isolation, and Standard Precautions.

STUDENT ACTIVITIES

1. Complete the written examination for this lesson.
2. Practice the procedures for proper handwashing and donning and removal of mask, gown, and gloves, as outlined in the Student Performance Guide.

WEB ACTIVITIES

1. Explore the Web sites of infection control organizations to see what publications, alerts, or regulatory information is available. One such site is *www.apic.org*.

2. Select a disease or condition from the list at the end of this section (or the instructor can assign a condition). Use the Internet to determine which (if any) of the transmission-based precautions should be used for the condition selected. If a disease was selected, use the Internet to research how the disease is transmitted. Outline a scheme, listing the proper precautions to use for a hospitalized patient with that condition. Include what PPE must be used, where the PPE should be located, and where and how used materials should be discarded.

Select a topic: Colostomy, chickenpox, tetanus, SARS, whooping cough, rubeola, HIV infection, West Nile virus, filovirus

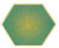

Student Performance Guide

LESSON 7-2 Infection Control and Transmission-Based Precautions

Name _____ Date _____

INSTRUCTIONS

1. Practice the procedures for hand hygiene and donning gown, mask, and gloves following the step-by-step procedure.
2. Demonstrate the procedures for hand hygiene and donning gown, mask, and gloves satisfactorily for the instructor using the Student Performance Guide. Your instructor will determine the level of competency you must achieve to obtain a satisfactory (S) grade.

NOTE: The following procedures are intended as general guidelines for laboratory workers who must have contact with patients in isolation. The appropriate institutional policy manual must be consulted for specific instructions.

MATERIALS AND EQUIPMENT

- sink for handwashing
- antiseptic soap
- alcohol-based antiseptic
- clean paper towels
- disposable masks and/or face shields
- disposable gowns
- disposable gloves (sterile gloves optional)
- disposal receptacle for used items
- biohazard bags or other plastic bags with materials for labeling

PROCEDURE

Record in the comment section any problems encountered while practicing the procedure (or have a fellow student or the instructor evaluate your performance).

S = Satisfactory
U = Unsatisfactory

You must:	S	U	Comments
1. Assemble equipment and materials			
2. Practice hand hygiene: a. Using antiseptic soap, perform steps a1 through a4: (1) Turn on warm water using a paper towel to turn the faucet handle, and discard the towel (2) Dispense antiseptic soap onto hands and rub fronts and backs of hands and between fingers vigorously for 1 to 2 minutes. (3) Rinse hands, holding them fingertips downward under warm running water (4) Use clean towel to dry hands and to turn off faucet. Dispose of towel, touching only the clean side			

You must:	S	U	Comments
b. Using alcohol-based antiseptic, perform steps b1 and b2: (1) Apply antiseptic to palm of hand and rub hands together vigorously for at least 15 seconds, covering all surfaces of hands and fingers (2) Continue procedure until all alcohol has evaporated and hands are completely dry			
3. Don gown: a. Slip arms into the sleeves of a gown, being careful to touch only the inside of gown b. Secure gown at neck and back of waist, being careful to cover your clothing completely			
4. Don mask: a. Pick up a mask and place it over your mouth and nose, being careful not to touch your face with your fingers b. Tie the ends of the mask around your head and neck			
5. Don gloves: a. Put on gloves, avoiding touching the outside of the gloves with your hands b. Pull the glove cuffs over the sleeves of your gown **NOTE:** If using sterile gloves, open the package, being careful not to touch the outside of the gloves. Pick up the right glove by the cuff and insert your right hand. Pick up and hold the left glove by inserting the fingertips of your gloved right hand into the cuff of the left glove. Insert your left hand into glove. Position glove cuffs over your wrists by using gloved fingertips to push cuff toward your elbow			
6. Remove the gloves by folding them down and turning them inside out. Discard gloves in receptacle for contaminated materials			
7. Remove gown by slipping hands back into gown sleeves, touching only the inside of the gown			
8. Fold the gown down over your arms inside-out and discard in appropriate receptacle			
9. Remove mask, touching only the ties			
10. Hold the mask by the ties and discard in proper receptacle			
11. Clean hands with antiseptic			
12. Leave the room using a clean paper towel to turn the door knob			

Evaluator Comments:

Evaluator _____ Date _____

7-3

Public Health Threats: I. Emerging Infectious Diseases

LESSON OBJECTIVES:

After studying this lesson, the student will:

- Explain what is meant by emerging infectious disease.
- List five factors that influence the emergence or re-emergence of disease.
- Discuss how emerging infectious diseases present a threat to public health.
- Name five emerging diseases and explain transmission, symptoms, precautions for caregivers, and treatment for each.
- Explain the role of the Laboratory Response Network in responding to emerging diseases.
- Explain how natural disasters can create a public health emergency.
- Define the glossary terms.

GLOSSARY

avian influenza / an infection of birds with one of the influenza A viruses; bird flu

biosafety level 4 (BSL-4) / a designation requiring the use of a combination of work practices, equipment, and facilities to prevent exposure of individuals or the environment to pathogens that can be transmitted by aerosol and that pose a high risk of life-threatening disease for which treatment or vaccine is not generally available

bovine spongiform encephalopathy (BSE) / a fatal, neurological disease of cattle caused by an unconventional transmissable agent called a prion; commonly called mad cow disease

Ebola virus / a highly infectious filovirus that causes a hemorrhagic fever

epidemic / disease affecting many persons at the same time, spread from person to person, and occurring in an area where the disease is not prevalent

epizootic / an outbreak of disease in an animal population

Laboratory Response Network (LRN) / a national network of laboratories coordinated by the CDC with the ability for rapid response to threats to public health

Marburg virus / a filovirus that causes a hemorrhagic fever

Mycobacterium tuberculosis / an acid-fast bacillus that causes tuberculosis

pandemic / widespread disease transmitted person to person and occurring over an entire country, continent, or even worldwide

SARS / the acronym for severe acute respiratory syndrome, a condition caused by a coronavirus

zoonotic / infection or disease that can be transmitted from vertebrate animals to humans

INTRODUCTION

Global pandemic, emerging infectious diseases, SARS, Ebola, bioterrorism, weapons of mass destruction, agroterrorism, small-pox, anthrax—these are terms that most of us either never worried about or, in some cases, never heard of until recent years. Photographs of citizens wearing surgical masks as they go about their daily life cause apprehension even to those thousands of miles away.

It is estimated that one-third of the 60 million deaths world-wide each year can be attributed to infectious diseases. Because of events happening around the world, the public health systems of every country must have plans for addressing potential threats caused by global disease, natural disasters, or terrorist events. These plans must include outfitting laboratories so that they have the ability to respond rapidly to a potential crisis and training first responders and primary health care providers, since these are the people who most often would have the first contact with affected individuals.

Recognizing the existence of several types of global threats, agencies such as the World Health Organization (WHO) are partnering with government health agencies around the world to plan, train, coordinate responses, and share information about disease outbreaks. It is imperative that governments provide the leadership, expertise, and funding to address these threats that could have significant clinical and public health consequences.

The agents recognized in recent years as presenting a danger to public health can be divided into two broad groups: *emerging infectious disease agents* and *bioterrorism agents*. In many cases the groups overlap. Emerging infectious diseases are diseases that have increased in humans or threaten to increase in the near future. Re-emerging diseases are those that were on the decrease for a time but have again become major health threats. This lesson introduces the topic of emerging infectious diseases, giving a brief summary of several agents of concern and outlining public health preparedness. Lesson 7-4 discusses potential agents of bioterrorism, as well as preparedness.

EMERGING INFECTIOUS DISEASES

In recent years the number of diseases classified as an emerging infectious disease has been on the increase. These diseases have gained our attention because they are usually associated with high morbidity and mortality, and no reliable preventive measure such as a vaccine exists. A variety of factors contribute to the emergence of these diseases. For most, it is not just one factor but a combination of factors such as environmental changes, global climate changes, natural disasters, movement of populations to more crowded living conditions, increase in international travel and trade, failures of public health policies or surveillance, and mutations or adaptations of pathogens (Table 7-13).

In some cases, the focus on a disease, such as SARS (severe acute respiratory syndrome), has occurred because it was newly recognized. In other cases, an animal disease has gained attention because of its potential to spread to humans, such as avian influenza and **bovine spongiform encephalopathy (BSE)**, commonly called mad cow disease. In still other cases, re-emergence of a pre-

TABLE 7-13. Factors that contribute to emergence or re-emergence of infectious disease

CAUSATIVE FACTOR	DISEASE EXAMPLE
Environmental change	Lyme disease, cholera
Population concentrations	dengue fever, polio
International travel/ commerce	cholera, hepatitis A, cyclosporiasis, antibiotic-resistant gonorrhea
Public health/policy failures	bovine spongiform encephalopathy (BSE), hepatitis B and C
Pathogen adaptation/ mutation	SARS, avian influenza, tuberculosis, infections with strains of antibiotic-resistant staph and strep
Natural disaster/flooding	cholera, hepatitis A

viously known pathogen gained attention because of mutations or changes in virulence or drug resistance, as has been the case with the tuberculosis bacterium.

Whatever the reason, we are seeing an emergence of infectious diseases that pose a threat to public health and, in some cases, have the potential to develop into a **pandemic**. Pandemics occur when a disease spreads to a wide area, sometimes even worldwide. Natural disasters such as the 2004 south Asia tsunami or the 2005 hurricanes in the United States also can create public health crises, causing increases in foodborne illnesses such as cholera due to contamination of water and food supplies or failure of wastewater treatment plants. Natural disasters such as floods also create environments favoring the growth and spread of insects and pathogens.

Because we are a global society, measures to control or prevent epidemics require new techniques and more attention. Several pathogens cause diseases that can be categorized as emerging infectious diseases. A sampling of these discussed in this lesson include SARS-associated corona virus, avian influenza virus, *Mycobacterium tuberculosis,* West Nile virus (WNV) and the hemorrhagic fever viruses (Ebola, Marburg, and Rift Valley viruses). In some cases, such as the Ebola, Marburg, and RVF viruses, these disease agents are also considered potential bioterrorism agents.

West Nile Virus

WNV, a member of the flavivirus family, was first isolated in 1937 in the West Nile district of Uganda (Figure 7-13). Until it surfaced in New York City in 1999, causing mortality in several types of birds, it had only been found in Asia, Africa, the Middle East, and Europe. WNV quickly became a cause of illness and mortality in humans, causing subclinical infection in the majority (80%) of

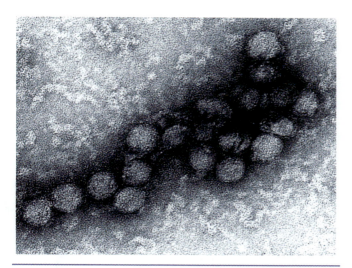

FIGURE 7-13 Electron micrograph of West Nile virus particles (*From CDC, Atlanta GA*)

TABLE 7-14. Viral hemorrhagic fevers (VHFs) grouped by virus family

ARENA VIRUSES

Lassa fever (Lassa virus)

Bolivian hemorrhagic fever (Machupo virus)

Argentine hemorrhagic fever (Junin virus)

Venezuelan hemorrhagic fever (Guanarito virus)

Brazilian hemorrhagic fever (Sabia virus)

FLAVIVIRUSES

Dengue

Yellow fever

Omsk hemorrhagic fever

FILOVIRUSES

Ebola hemorrhagic fever

Marburg hemorrhagic fever

BUNYAVIRUSES

Crimean-Congo hemorrhagic fever

Rift Valley fever

Hantavirus pulmonary syndrome

infected individuals, mild febrile illness or flu-like symptoms in about 20%, and severe encephalitis or meningitis in less than 1%. Elderly patients are at greatest risk for severe illness, which can cause permanent neurological damage or death.

West Nile infection is spread geographically by virus-infected migratory birds. Since 1999, the virus has spread over most of the United States and has also been documented in Canada, the Caribbean, and Mexico. In 2002 it caused the largest WNV **epidemic** and animal **epizootic** ever reported prior to that time, resulting in over 4,000 human cases with 284 deaths (all in the United States). In 2003, U.S. cases increased by greater than 100% over 2002, with almost 10,000 human cases reported.

The virus is normally transmitted by mosquitoes, but blood transfusion, transplacental transmission, organ transplantation, and breastfeeding-associated cases have all been documented. There is currently no specific treatment for WNV infection, and prevention is based on limiting mosquito exposure in enzootic and epidemic areas. Although an equine vaccine is available, as of early 2007 research was still ongoing to develop a human vaccine.

Viral Hemorrhagic Fevers

The viral hemorrhagic fevers (VHFs) are a group of febrile illnesses which have similar symptoms, ranging from mild to severe. Onset is often abrupt. Symptoms include fever, fatigue, and bleeding under the skin, internally, or from body orifices. These symptoms are caused by multiple organ damage, and especially vascular system damage. Some of the hemorrhages are life-threatening. Fatality rates vary according to which virus is involved, but range from less than 5% for some VHFs, to a 70% to 90% death rate from Ebola (Zaire) virus.

The VHFs are caused by RNA viruses in four families—arenaviruses, filoviruses, bunyaviruses, and flaviviruses (Table 7-14). These viruses are **zoonotic**, meaning they are found in vertebrate animals or arthropods. Of the known hosts/vectors, most

are rodents or arthropods. The reservoirs for some, such as Ebola virus and Marburg virus, remain unproven (Figure 7-14), but animals native to the African continent are believed to be a possible source. Although hemorrhagic fever viruses are found all over the globe, most are associated with a particular geographic area and host/reservoir. Therefore, only visitors or residents of a particular area would normally be susceptible to infection. However infection can also occur when exotic animals harboring the viruses are transported into a new area.

Once human disease occurs, some VHFs can be transmitted person to person. It is important to control disease spread by avoiding close physical contact with infected individuals and their body fluids. Infection control precautions for health care personnel include using personal protective equipment (PPE), disinfecting or disposing of all materials and equipment that contact the patient, and instituting airborne precautions when possible (Figure 7-14).

For the most part, there is no vaccine, cure, or treatment for VHFs, with the exception of yellow fever and Argentine fever. Prevention efforts focus on rodent and arthropod control measures, as well as discouraging cultural practices that bring populations in close contact with potential reservoirs. The viruses that cause the most severe hemorrhagic fevers are classified as **biosafety level 4 (BSL-4)** pathogens. Only a few laboratories worldwide have the BSL-4 facilities required to work with these pathogens (Figure 7-15). (Some hemorrhagic fever viruses, such as the dengue and yellow fever viruses are not considered BSL-4 pathogens.)

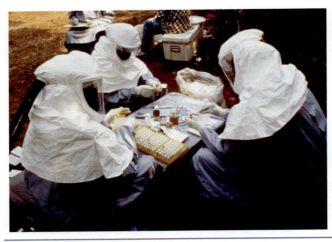

FIGURE 7-14 Centers for Disease Control and Prevention (CDC) and Zairian scientists collect animal samples during a 1995 Ebola outbreak near Kitwit, Zaire (*From CDC, Atlanta, GA*)

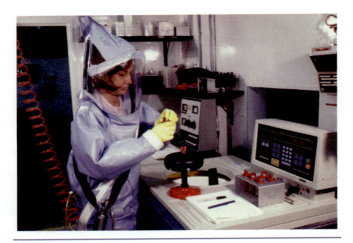

FIGURE 7-15 A Centers for Disease Control and Prevention (CDC) scientist wears a protective suit with helmet and face mask as she studies pathogens in the CDC BSL-4 laboratory (*From CDC, Atlanta, GA/Jim Gathany*)

Sporadic outbreaks of VHFs are expected to continue. To decrease morbidity and mortality from these diseases, improvements are needed in:

- Containment methods and facilities, especially in developing countries
- Antiviral drugs and supportive therapies
- Vaccine development
- Tools for rapid diagnosis
- Understanding the pathology of disease
- Understanding the ecology of the viruses and the natural reservoirs

Rift Valley Fever

RVF occurs in livestock and humans in Africa and Arabia. It is caused by a virus of the Bunyaviridae family and is normally trans-

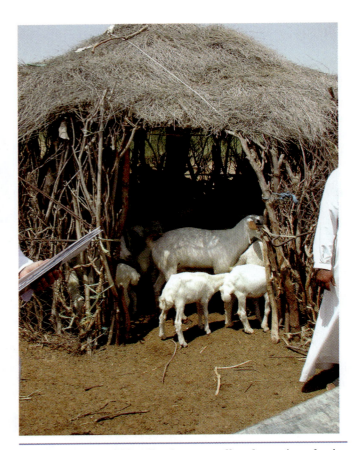

FIGURE 7-16 Rift Valley fever can affect domesticated animals such as these goats in Saudi Arabia. The disease can then be spread to humans after exposure to blood or body fluids of infected animals (*From CDC, Atlanta, GA*)

mitted by mosquitoes. Human outbreaks are usually associated with animal disease outbreaks and can occur in rural and urban areas (Figure 7-16). Infected individuals, who develop an acute, febrile form of the disease, can transmit the virus to other humans through aerosols. The virus has also been shown to be transmitted to humans by aerosols created in animal husbandry practices, or through livestock slaughtering. Infection rates can reach as high as one-third of a population. Most deaths are due to the development of a hemorrhagic fever. RVF is a much more severe disease than West Nile disease. Unlike West Nile disease, 90% of RVF patients are very ill, and the fatality rate is 10 times that of West Nile disease. The RVF outbreak in Kenya in the winter of 2006–2007 affected animals and humans, with a 25% to 30% human fatality rate.

RVF is considered a threat both as a natural emerging disease and as a potential biological weapon because it can be spread by aerosols as well as by the mosquito vector. RFV vaccines for livestock are available; however, military-developed human RFV vaccines are only at the research stage and quantities are limited. Antiviral drugs have not been effective and some have caused severe side-effects.

Ebola and Marburg Viruses

Two deadly viruses that have been in the news in recent years are the **Ebola** and **Marburg viruses** (Figures 7-17 and 7-18).

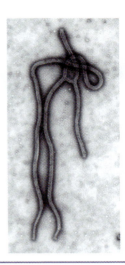

FIGURE 7-17 Electron micrograph of Ebola virus, a filovirus (*From CDC, Atlanta, GA/Cynthia Goldsmith*)

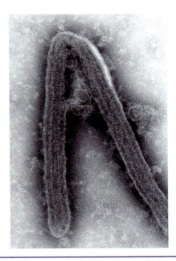

FIGURE 7-18 Electron micrograph of Marburg virus (*From CDC, Atlanta, GA/F.A. Murphy*)

Marburg and Ebola viruses are the only known filoviruses. These have caused several deadly outbreaks and also are considered to have potential as biological weapons. These viruses cause high mortality and morbidity, can be spread person to person, and are highly infectious in aerosol form. Four subtypes of Ebola have been identified, and three of the four have caused disease in humans. Through 2004, the WHO had documented 17 Ebola outbreaks in humans, totaling 1848 cases and 1287 fatalities, a fatality rate averaging 70%. A 2006 Ebola outbreak is believed to have killed more than 5000 gorillas in West Africa.

Ebola was first recognized in 1976 in the Democratic Republic of the Congo (formerly Zaire) (Figure 7-19). The initial route of infection remains unproven, but association with nonhuman primates has been suggested as a possibility. Once an individual becomes infected, secondary transmission of the virus can occur through direct exposure to blood or body secretions from that infected individual. Airborne transmission between humans has not been documented, although it has been docu-

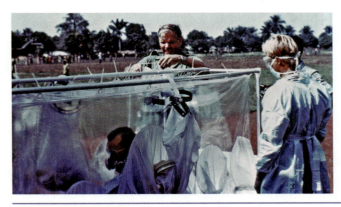

FIGURE 7-19 Evacuating a patient from a "hot zone." This 1976 photograph shows a scientist who became ill while surveying for Ebola virus. He is wearing a respirator inside an isolator and is being prepared for medical evacuation (*From CDC, Atlanta, GA/Lyle Conrad*)

mented between research animals in a primate quarantine facility in Reston, Virginia. Infection control measures, such as using Standard Precautions; wearing personal protective equipment (PPE) including gloves, gown, mask, eye protection; and decontamination of all materials and equipment that comes in contact with the patient is vitally important.

Although most outbreaks of Ebola and Marburg have been limited to their geographic region in Africa, the viruses have unintentionally been transported to other countries. In 1996, a health care professional who had been treating Ebola patients in Gabon traveled to South Africa and became ill. In the hospital the virus was transmitted to a nurse, who subsequently died. This secondary transmission can occur through close contact, exposure to infected body fluids or contaminated instruments, or inhalation of aerosolized virus particles.

Marburg virus has also been transported from its natural habitat. In fact, the virus was unknown until it was discovered in 1967 during simultaneous outbreaks among laboratory personnel in Marburg and Frankfurt, Germany, and Belgrade, Yugoslavia. These workers became infected by handling infected research monkeys that had been imported from Uganda. Since then small outbreaks have occurred periodically in Africa. Because the reservoir host is unknown, it is also not known exactly how the disease is contracted. However, once infected, secondary transmission to others can occur. The fatality rate is approximately 25%.

SARS

In 2002, news of fatalities associated with acute respiratory diseases surfaced in Asia. This disease came to be known as **SARS** (**s**evere **a**cute **r**espiratory **s**yndrome) and was found to be caused by a hitherto unknown variant of the coronavirus family (Figure 7-20). Members of the coronavirus family are responsible for the common cold. The SARS-associated coronavirus (SARS-CoV) is thought to have originated in the Guangdong Province of China. It was spread regionally and then to Hong Kong by a physician who treated patients for flu and then subsequently traveled to

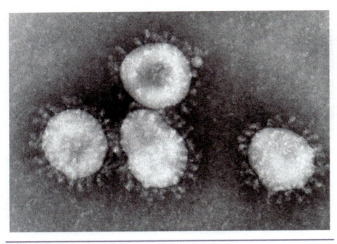

FIGURE 7-20 Electron micrograph of coronavirus, showing its characteristic crownlike (corona) appearance. The 2003 SARS outbreak was caused by a coronavirus (*From CDC, Atlanta, GA*)

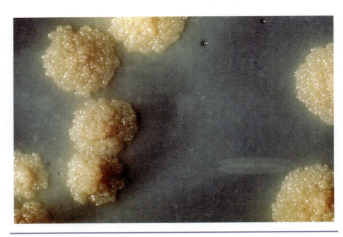

FIGURE 7-21 Colonies of *Mycobacterium tuberculosis* growing on special medium. Examination of colonial morphology is one component of identification (*From CDC, Atlanta, GA*)

Hong Kong. International travelers staying at the same hotel as this physician also became ill with SARS.

In the following weeks, SARS spread to parts of Asia, the Americas, and Europe, presumably through close contacts with air travelers, hospital workers, and relatives of infected individuals. In the first 9 months of the outbreak, over 8,000 cases of SARS were reported, with 774 deaths. Most cases occurred in China and southeast Asia; only eight confirmed cases were identified in the United States. In early 2004, several new cases of SARS were confirmed in China, causing public health officials to launch intense surveillance measures to detect spread of this virus. Symptoms of SARS include fever, headache and other body aches; respiratory symptoms such as cough; and pneumonia.

SARS was quickly recognized to be a highly contagious disease that spreads rapidly by person-to-person contact unless it is recognized early and strict infection control precautions are put in place. These include Standard Precautions, especially hand hygiene, droplet precautions, contact precautions, airborne precautions in a room with negative pressure, and use of an N-95 filtering respirator for all persons who enter the room.

Mycobacterium tuberculosis

Estimates are that, worldwide, 3 billion people are infected with *Mycobacterium tuberculosis*, the bacterium that causes tuberculosis, a disease of the lungs (Figure 7-21). In the last half of the twentieth century, cases of tuberculosis were cured by the use of new drugs developed against the organism. However, to obtain a cure, patients were required to take the drugs over a period of several months. It is believed that this prolonged exposure to antibiotics contributed to the emergence of multidrug resistant *M. tuberculosis* strains in the 1980s. As the incidence of immunosuppressive diseases such as AIDS has increased worldwide, the incidence of tubercu-

losis has also increased and has reached crisis levels in some parts of the world. Currently, in some places, 20% of the strains tested are antibiotic resistant. In sub-Saharan Africa, where infection with HIV is very high, 60% of the children and 70% of the adults who have tuberculosis also are infected with HIV. In 2006, an extensively drug-resistant form of tuberculosis (XDR-TB) emerged that has a very high mortality. The outlook for controlling this disease is sobering. Although *M. tuberculosis* was identified over 100 years ago, it is still a major cause of death, causing 1.75 million deaths in 2003.

Avian Influenza—H5N1

Influenza A viruses of several different types, strains, genetic differences, and pathogenicity levels can infect humans, swine, birds, horses, and other animals. The natural reservoir for these viruses is wild birds, and so it is called **avian influenza** or *bird flu*. Although wild birds do not necessarily become ill when infected, domestic poultry can become sick and die, especially when infected with a highly pathogenic form. Avian influenza viruses have been identified in human influenza cases that have high morbidity and mortality rates. The concern in medical and public health communities worldwide is that one of these avian influenza strains could cause a new global pandemic of influenza against which humans have little or no immunity.

Bird Flu Outbreaks

In early 2004, a widespread outbreak of H5N1 (highly pathogenic strain) avian influenza occurred in poultry across many Asian countries; 35 human cases were reported (Thailand and Vietnam) with 24 deaths. These cases occurred in persons with close association with poultry, and transmission was felt to be bird-to-human. New bird outbreaks of H5N1 influenza began again in late June 2004 across China and other parts of Asia, with sporadic human cases and more human deaths. Human mortality rates for H5N1 avian influenza infections are higher than in typical influenza cases caused by the usual human influenza strains. By February 2007 outbreaks of H5N1 avian influenza in wild birds and domestic poultry had been reported in most southeast Asian countries, several middle eastern countries, as well as Russia, Ukraine, Turkey, Romania, and England. Human cases with fatalities have been reported in several countries. In May 2006, the WHO confirmed that a cluster of cases of human H5N1 infections in Indonesia was caused by human-to-human transmission.

Prevention

Prevention has focused on eliminating infected poultry flocks and limiting human contact with infected birds. Importation of potentially infectious birds has been banned by most countries. Infection control precautions recommended by the CDC include Standard Precautions, contact precautions, eye protection, and airborne precautions. By early 2007, no vaccine against the H5N1 strain had been approved for human use, although trials began in mid 2005. The drug Tamiflu (oseltamivir) has been shown to be effective in some H5N1 infections. However, some H5N1 viral isolates have shown genetic changes and oseltamivir-resistant strains have emerged. H5N1 strains have been shown to be resistant to other antivirals (rimantidine, zanamivir, and amantadine) that are active against influenza A viruses.

IS PANDEMIC INFLUENZA A POSSIBILITY?

Pandemic influenza refers to a global influenza outbreak due to emergence of an influenza virus that can be transmitted from person to person and can rapidly spread worldwide. Pandemic flu may be a greater possibility today than ever before because of global travel. Whether or not H5N1 or another avian virus can cause a pandemic is uncertain. For this to happen, the virus would have to change abruptly, developing the ability to pass easily from person to person, before the general public could develop immunity. Public health agencies worldwide have the responsibility to be vigilant as influenza viruses undergo genetic changes and as infections in animal reservoirs spread. Since immunity to influenza is short-lived, influenza vaccinations must be given annually, and the vaccine mixture must be changed based on predictions of which virus outbreak might occur in the near future.

Although a viral pandemic might have a mortality of only 1% to 20%, that would produce a huge number of fatalities worldwide. During the 20th century, three pandemics occurred:

- 1918–1919—Spanish flu. This was caused by H1N1 influenza A virus and was the worst recorded in modern history, with more than 500,000 deaths in the United States and an estimated 50 million deaths worldwide.
- 1957–1958—Asian flu. This outbreak originating in China was caused by H2N2 influenza A virus. In the United States, 70,000 deaths were recorded.

- 1968–1969—Hong Kong flu. Caused by H3N2 influenza A virus, this outbreak resulted in 34,000 deaths in the United States.

Because human influenza viruses spread very efficiently from person to person, it may be almost impossible to prevent all influenza pandemics. Measures the general public and public health agencies can take to prevent disease spread include frequent handwashing; staying home when ill; closing schools and businesses when necessary; instituting travel restrictions; promoting vaccinations; increasing vaccine production; inclusion of new strains in vaccines; and stockpiling vaccines and antiviral drugs.

ROLE OF THE CLINICAL LABORATORY IN EMERGING DISEASES

Clinical laboratories must have a comprehensive plan in place for dealing with the appearance of a possible emerging infectious disease. In the United States, the CDC and state public health departments are the leaders in organizing and training personnel in how to deal with this possibility. The **Laboratory Response Network (LRN)** is a national network of laboratories organized by the CDC, Federal Bureau of Investigation (FBI), and Association of Public Health Laboratories. The LRN has the ability to respond rapidly to public health threats such as emerging diseases and acts of bioterrorism. Included in this network are federal laboratories such as the CDC, U.S. Department of Agriculture (USDA), and FDA laboratories; state and local public health laboratories; and veterinary, military, and environmental/water/food testing laboratories. The LRN also partners with international laboratories.

Three levels of laboratories have been designated as part of the LRN:

- National laboratories
- Reference laboratories
- Sentinel laboratories

The national laboratories include federal laboratories such as the CDC and USDA laboratories. These agencies are responsible for bioforensics and handling and characterizing highly infectious biological agents. The more than 140 reference laboratories have installed BSL-3 facilities and have the capability to perform confirmatory testing of BSL-3 agents (Figure 7-22). Sentinel laboratories provide routine diagnostic services and preliminary testing to determine if specimens need to be sent to a reference laboratory for further testing. The LRN provides these laboratories with:

- Standardized reagents and controls
- Agent-specific protocols
- Laboratory referral directory
- Secure communications
- Electronic laboratory reporting
- Training and technology transfer
- Proficiency testing
- Appropriate vaccinations for laboratory workers

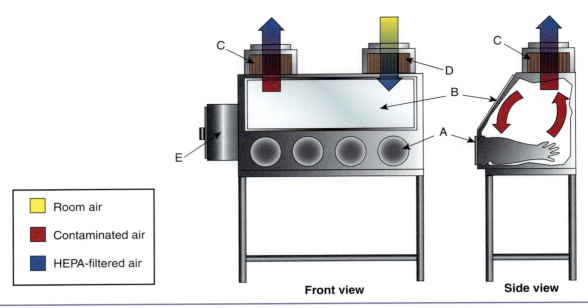

FIGURE 7-22 Diagram of air flow in a class III biological safety cabinet. The cabinet exhaust must be connected to the building exhaust system: (A) glove ports for attaching arm-length glove to cabinet; (B) sash; (C) HEPA exhaust filter; (D) HEPA supply filter; (E) pass-through box or autoclave

SUMMARY

Awareness of the threat of emerging infectious diseases is becoming a part of everyday life. Global changes in the environment, population movements, and travel have created environments favoring the emergence or re-emergence of diseases. It is the task of public health agencies to develop plans to contain and treat diseases when they surface, as well as to find ways to prevent disease occurrence.

REVIEW QUESTIONS

1. What is the difference between an emerging infectious disease and a re-emerging infectious disease?

2. What five factors can influence the emergence of a disease?

3. The most serious emerging infectious disease pathogens are currently not a problem in the United States. What conditions could cause the spread of these pathogens to the United States?

4. What characteristics do most emerging infectious diseases have in common?

5. Why is avian influenza, or bird flu, a problem for humans?

6. What must happen to an animal virus in order for it to cause a pandemic?

7. What are three viral hemorrhagic fevers? Why are they given this designation?

8. What methods must be used to prevent the spread of most emerging infectious diseases?

9. Why are insect control programs important in developing nations?

10. Why has tuberculosis resurfaced as a disease on the increase?

11. Explain the role of the LRN in responding to emerging diseases.

12. Explain how natural disasters can create a public health emergency.

13. Name five emerging diseases and explain transmission, symptoms, precautions for caregivers, and treatment.

14. Define avian influenza, biosafety level 4, bovine spongiform encephalopathy, Ebola virus, epidemic, epizootic, Laboratory Response Network, Marburg virus, *Mycobacterium tuberculosis*, pandemic, SARS, and zoonotic.

STUDENT ACTIVITIES

1. Complete the written examination for this lesson.

2. Find articles about emerging diseases in news magazines, newspapers, and other periodicals. Report on your findings.

WEB ACTIVITIES

1. Use the Internet to look up information on emerging infectious diseases on Web sites of the CDC, WHO, FDA, or USDA. Note how many diseases the CDC categorizes as emerging infectious diseases. Report on a disease that is not discussed in this lesson; include information about where it is found, how it is transmitted, as well as symptoms, treatment, and prevention.

2. Polio has not been a problem in the United States since the development of effective vaccines and institution of childhood vaccinations. Use the Internet to search for information on recent outbreaks of polio around the world. Report on the cause(s) of these outbreaks.

Public Health Threats: II. Biological Agents and Bioterrorism

LESSON OBJECTIVES:

After studying this lesson, the student will:

- List five pathogens that have potential use in bioterrorism or as biological weapons and explain how they are transmitted.
- Name six characteristics that make an agent useful as a biological weapon.
- Explain how the threat of bioterrorism affects the agricultural industry.
- Explain the role of laboratories and primary health care providers in recognizing and responding to potential bioterrorism agents.
- Define the glossary terms.

GLOSSARY

agroterrorism / acts of terrorism involving threats to agricultural products, including food animals and crops

botulinum intoxication / a condition where body tissues are affected by the botulinum toxin

botulinum toxin / a neurotoxin produced by *Clostridium botulinum*

Department of Homeland Security / a federal agency whose primary mission is to prevent, protect against, and respond to acts of terrorism on U.S. soil

intoxication / poisoning

virion / the infectious form of a virus

virulent / highly infectious

INTRODUCTION

For the past several decades, discussions about threats of biological weapons and bioterrorism have occasionally surfaced. However, since the September 11, 2001, attacks on the World Trade Center and the rise of terrorist activities around the world, serious attention is being given to these subjects. Investigations into the response to the 9/11 attacks showed that the United States was unprepared to handle a large-scale emergency.

In response to these concerns, the United States government created the **Department of Homeland Security** and charged it with the responsibility of planning for natural and manmade disasters as well as working to eliminate potential terror threats. Billions of dollars were distributed to city and state governments and emergency preparedness agencies to help them plan, equip, and train for preparedness. However, hurricanes Katrina and Rita, which ravaged the Louisiana, Mississippi, and Alabama coasts in 2005, demonstrated an alarming lack of disaster preparedness at all levels of government. Workable plans for evacuating, relocating, housing, and feeding large numbers of displaced persons were practically nonexistent. Backup communication systems failed. Systems to provide medical care were compromised. Although these disasters were located in one region, they brought the realization that disaster preparedness plans nationwide would likely have been deficient if faced with the same circumstances.

Federal, state, and local governments and public and private health care systems must be prepared to deal with the possibility that agents of terrorism might appear in civilian society. These terrorism threats could come in many forms, including chemical agents, radioactive agents, and biological agents. This lesson presents information about some biological agents that have the potential for use as weapons or bioterrorism agents, and outlines the role of the clinical laboratory in preparedness and reaction to a possible threat event.

BIOTERRORISM AGENTS

The Centers for Disease Control and Prevention (CDC) have identified pathogens that they consider to have high potential for use as a biological weapon. These have been placed on a high-priority list (class A list) that includes some organisms rarely seen in the United States and some that have been considered eradicated (Table 7-15). Characteristics that cause these organisms to be considered useful as biological weapons or terror agents include:

- Ease of person-to-person transmission
- Easily disseminated or dispersed
- Cause high mortality
- Outbreak would have potential for major public health impact
- Special measures would be required to reach a state of preparedness
- Might cause panic or disrupt society

Pathogens in the high-priority category that are discussed in this lesson include the bacteria and viruses that cause anthrax, smallpox, plague, atularemia, botulism, nd viral hemorrhagic fevers.

Anthrax

Anthrax is caused by infection with the spore-forming bacterium, *Bacillus anthracis* (Figure 7-23A). The disease occurs in domestic, wild, and exotic animals, including goats, sheep, cattle, hippos, elephants, lions, zebras, and camels. Humans usually become infected by contact with infected animals or contaminated articles and animal products, such as animal skins. Depending on the route of exposure, the victim can develop inhalation anthrax, gastrointestinal anthrax, or cutaneous anthrax. Because the spores of the anthrax organism persist in the environment, infection can occur when the spores deposited in the past become disturbed

AGENT	DISEASE
Bacillus anthracis	Anthrax
Variola virus	Smallpox
Francisella tularensis	Tularemia
Clostridium botulinum	Botulism
Yersinia pestis	Plague
Hemorrhagic viruses	Hemorrhagic fever

TABLE 7-15. Class A agents recognized by the Centers for Disease Control and Prevention (CDC) as having potential for use as biological weapons and the diseases they cause

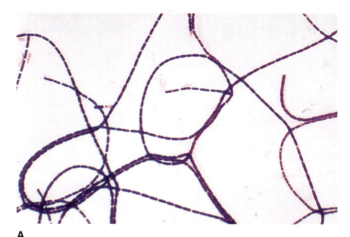

A

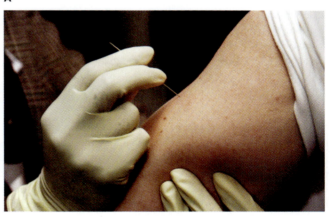

B

FIGURE 7-23 (A) Gram stain of *Bacillus anthracis*, the agent that causes anthrax; (B) demonstration of smallpox vaccination technique during a 2002 Centers for Disease Control and Prevention (CDC) workshop (*From CDC, Atlanta, GA*)

and aerosolized. Anthrax cases occur sporadically around the world in humans and livestock.

Anthrax has a long history. It is thought that the plagues described in Exodus were caused by anthrax in domestic animals and humans. In Europe, during the 1500s and the 1700s, anthrax was an important agricultural disease. Woolsorters in fifteenth century England were described as having inhalation anthrax, caused by inhaling anthrax-spore-containing aerosols generated during the processing of goat wool. Anthrax was also the first disease for which Louis Pasteur, in 1881, developed an effective live bacterial vaccine.

For decades, attention has been focused on the potential for anthrax to be used as a biological weapon. During World War I, attempts were made to use anthrax spores as a weapon against horses. Before and during World War II, the Japanese military developed the first relatively sophisticated anthrax biological weapons. Since World War II, many countries, including Russia, Great Britain, Canada, the United States, and Iraq, have shown an interest in the possible use of anthrax as a weapon.

Anthrax is uniquely suited for use as a weapon because:

- It is easy to produce large quantities. Using simple equipment, even individuals can produce gram quantities, as discovered when anthrax contaminated letters were sent to the Hart Senate building in 2001

- It has a long shelf life; dried spores remain viable for years

- It is dispersed easily and effectively

- It is environmentally stable. Areas can remain contaminated for months or years

- It has a high mortality rate, with systemic infection approaching 100% mortality within a few days after onset of symptoms

- Effective treatment for inhalation anthrax is lacking, especially once symptoms appear

In 1979, the accidental release of anthrax spores from a production facility in Sverdlosk, Russia, demonstrated on a small scale what the effects might be if anthrax were to be used as a weapon. Winds carried the organism 50 km from the facility, and at least 66 deaths due to inhalation anthrax were acknowledged, although some believe the number to be much higher.

Smallpox

Smallpox is a highly contagious, **virulent**, and often fatal disease caused by variola virus, a member of the family of pox viruses (Poxviridae). It is considered one of the most dangerous of the potential biological weapons. Smallpox also has a long history. It was endemic in India for over 2000 years and spread to other parts of Asia, including China and Japan, and also to Africa. In the twentieth century, the less virulent form of smallpox spread from Africa to the Americas and Europe.

A worldwide smallpox eradication program began in 1956 using vaccination with vaccinia virus, a related pox virus. Unvaccinated patients contracting the virulent form of the disease had a greater than 30% fatality rate. Smallpox was shown to have considerable potential as a biological weapon when outbreaks occurred in Europe in the 1970s and spread rapidly, despite a vaccinated population. Over 170 individuals were infected with smallpox during the epidemic in Yugoslavia in 1972. The outbreak began when a traveler infected with the deadly virus returned home to the Kosovo region of Yugoslavia.

In 1972, smallpox was considered eradicated in the United States and routine smallpox vaccinations were discontinued. From 1972 until 2001, the vaccine was provided to only a few hundred research scientists and medical professionals working with smallpox and similar viruses. After 9/11 and the anthrax scare of October 2001, the U.S. government developed a smallpox response plan. As part of this plan, enough vaccine has been stockpiled to vaccinate every person in the United States in the event of a smallpox emergency. In addition, a vaccination program that includes certain health care personnel and the military was initiated (Figure 7-23B).

At one time, supposedly only two high-security laboratories in the world had stores of the smallpox virus, the CDC in the United States and the Vector laboratory in the U.S.S.R (Russia). Although these stocks were supposed to be destroyed in 1999 (by resolution of the 1996 World Health Assembly), destruction was postponed and has not yet occurred. However, with the dissolution of the Soviet Union, it is believed that stocks of the virus may have been taken out of the country illegally. The U.S. government maintains a list of nations and groups suspected of having clandestine stocks of smallpox or of trying to obtain the virus. In 1999, this list was said to include Russia, China, India, Pakistan, Israel, North Korea, Iraq, Iran, Cuba, and Serbia, as well as possibly terrorist organizations such as al Qaeda.

Characteristics that make the smallpox virus of potential use as a terror agent include (1) infective dose is small, only 10 to 100 **virions**; (2) virions are stable in aerosols, which are a good way to deploy biological weapons; (3) the disease has a short incubation period and progresses rapidly; (4) the duration of the disease is long; (5) treatment requires complex transmission-based precautions and extensive medical support; and (6) there is a large susceptible civilian population because vaccinations of the general public ended in 1972 in the United States. However, smallpox virus is not as readily available and not as easily handled as some potential bacterial agents of bioterrorism such as anthrax (*Bacillus anthracis*) or plague (*Yersinia pestis*) organisms.

Plague

Plague is a zoonotic infection of rodents caused by the Gram-negative bacillus *Yersinia pestis*. The organism can be transmitted to humans by flea bites. Plague was the cause of the Black Death in mid-fourteenth century Europe, killing one-third of the European population (Figure 7-24A). Worldwide, cases of plague still have occurred. From 1970 to the present, in the United States, between 5 and 15 human cases occur each year, mostly in the southwestern states.

The disease normally occurs in three forms:

1. Bubonic plague, characterized by swollen lymph nodes (buboes), usually in the groin

2. Septicemic plague, blood infection

3. Pneumonic plague, development of secondary lung infection in patients with bubonic plague; the pneumonic form can be spread from person to person

Several times in human history there have been attempts to use the plague organism as a biological weapon. During the

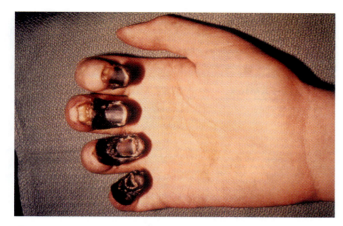

A

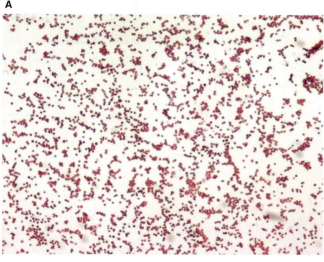

B

FIGURE 7-24 (A) Gangrenous fingertips of a plague patient, showing why this disease was called the "Black Death"; (B) Gram stain of *Francisella tularensis*, a tiny Gram-negative coccobacillus that causes tularemia (*From CDC, Atlanta, GA*)

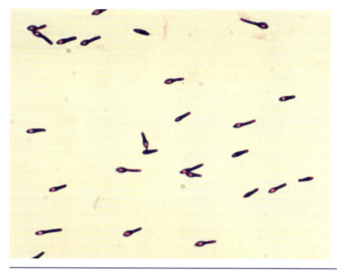

FIGURE 7-25 A photomicrograph of Gram-positive, spore-forming *Clostridium botulinum* (*From CDC, Atlanta, GA*)

Tularemia

Tularemia, also called rabbit fever, is caused by *Francisella tularensis*, a small, Gram-negative coccobacillus (Figure 7-24B). The organism occurs in wild and domestic animals in America, Europe, and Asia. Humans, such as rabbit hunters, become infected by contacting infected animals or animal products. Depending on the route of exposure, the organism can cause cutaneous infection, gastrointestinal symptoms (if ingested), or pneumonic disease (if inhaled). Tularemia has a short incubation period and causes symptoms that can be difficult to distinguish from anthrax or plague. Person-to-person transmission has not been documented.

F. tularensis has been considered a potential biological weapon for decades. It can be cultured easily, is stable in liquid and dry form, and causes infection at a low dose, less than 100 organisms. After World War II, weapons were developed by the United States with the capability of disseminating the organism. The Soviet Union was also developing weapons using tularemia from that period to the early 1990s. In both countries the work included modifying the organism's genetic makeup to create antibiotic-resistant strains or to enhance virulence.

A World Health Organization (WHO) committee estimated that dispersal of 50 kg of virulent *F. tularensis* in a city of 5 million inhabitants would result in approximately 19,000 deaths and cause long-lasting and/or relapsing illness in as many as a quarter million people. A study by the CDC estimated that the economic cost of an aerosol attack of *F. tularensis*, including treating the disease and decontaminating the area, would be $5.4 billion for every 100,000 persons exposed.

Botulism

Botulism is a life-threatening condition caused by **botulinum toxin**, a neurotoxin produced by the Gram-positive, spore-forming bacterium *Clostridium botulinum* (Figure 7-25). It is said that

years of the Black Death, Tartars, whose population was stricken with plague, catapulted corpses of their infected soldiers at the Genoese enemy. When plague broke out, the Genoese troops fled back to Italy. During World War II, the Japanese army secretly studied the plague organism for purposes of biological warfare, developing a way to use fleas to disseminate plague in a bomb or spray. Reports show that the Japanese used plague as a weapon in China at least three times during World War II. In the 1970s and 1980s, the Soviet Union also developed weapon forms of *Y. pestis*, using a dry, genetically engineered, antibiotic-resistant form of the bacterium. Other countries, including North Korea, Canada, and the United States, have had active plague research programs. Although plague has never been used as a weapon against U.S. forces, troops have been deployed in areas where plague is endemic, such as Hawaii and Vietnam. It was official policy during World War II to vaccinate U.S. troops with a killed plague vaccine.

these neurotoxins are the most potent toxins known and produce a muscular paralysis that can lead to respiratory failure. Botulism is not contagious and is not spread person to person. **Botulinum intoxication** is a public health emergency and must be immediately treated without waiting for laboratory confirmation. This includes notification of public health officials, administration of antitoxin, and hospitalization in a critical care unit with close monitoring for respiratory failure.

Natural cases of botulism occur as a result of ingestion of the toxin (foodborne), wound contamination, or intestinal proliferation of *Clostridium*. The toxin cannot penetrate intact skin. Nearly three-fourths of the more than 100 yearly botulism cases in the United States are infant botulism, caused by ingestion of *Clostridium* from sources such as contaminated honey. Infant botulism differs from foodborne botulism in that the bacteria survive and grow in the infant gut, producing toxins that are absorbed and gradually cause symptoms.

The remaining natural cases of botulism are acquired either through ingestion of food contaminated with the toxin, or by contamination of a wound by the *Clostridium* organism. Food botulism is usually associated with low-acid canned foods (beans, carrots, corn, etc.) that have not been heated properly, since heat inactivates the toxin. Botulinum toxin is also approved for some medical and cosmetic uses. Cases of botulinum intoxication have appeared caused by injections of improperly prepared botulinum toxin (Botox).

Another potential method of acquiring botulism is by inhalation of aerosolized toxin. State-sponsored biological weapons programs have produced botulinum toxins. Before the 1991 Gulf War, Iraq is said to have produced thousands of liters of botulinum toxin, with over half of its stock being incorporated into weapons designed to deliver aerosols of the toxin. This method of toxin dissemination has also been attempted by bioterrorists. Botulinum toxin can be produced using crude technology, so it is of potential use to bioterrorist groups.

In a bioterrorism attack, the routes of exposure to botulinum toxin would most likely be either oral or by inhalation. Since the toxins are rather unstable, the range of an aerosol attack would be limited. Cases might be clustered geographically at the time of exposure (building or work site). It is estimated that toxin in concentrations as low as 0.01 µg/kg of body weight is lethal to humans by inhalation, and 1.0 µg/kg is lethal by the oral route.

Hemorrhagic Fever Viruses

The viral hemorrhagic fevers (VHFs) are a group of viral diseases associated with significant bleeding. Many of these diseases are considered emerging infectious diseases. Viruses included in the VHF group include Ebola virus, Marburg virus, and the viruses causing Lassa Fever, Rift Valley fever, dengue, and yellow fever. (See the information on emerging infectious diseases in Lesson 7-3.) Naturally occurring outbreaks of these viral diseases, and subsequent person-to-person transmission in some cases, have shown that they could potentially be used as weapons (Table 7-16). In natural outbreaks of Ebola and Marburg, person-to-person spread has been prevented by use of contact and airborne precautions. Case fatality rates vary according to the virus, ranging from less than 5% to approximately 70% to 90% with the Ebola Zaire subtype.

TABLE 7-16. Four families of hemorrhagic viruses that have potential as biological weapons and the diseases caused

VIRUS FAMILY	DISEASES
Arenaviruses	Lassa fever
	New World hemorrhagic fevers
Filoviruses	Marburg VHF
	Ebola VHF
Bunyaviruses	Crimean-Congo hemorrhagic fever
	Rift Valley fever
Flaviviruses	dengue, yellow fever

Ebola and Marburg viruses, both members of the filovirus family, are considered to be the most dangerous and are categorized as category A bioweapon agents. Characteristics of these viruses include:

- High mortality and morbidity
- Person-to-person transmission
- Highly infectious at a low dose by the aerosol route
- Environmentally stable
- Large-scale production possible

State-sponsored programs have shown interest in hemorrhagic fever viruses as weapons. The Soviet Union produced large quantities of Marburg, Ebola, and Lassa viruses, as well as others. During the Kikwit Ebola outbreak in Zaire in the 1990s, the Aum Shinrikyo cult in Japan attempted to gain access to Ebola virus.

THREATS TO AGRICULTURE

While it is imperative to prepare for events that directly and immediately affect the health of citizens, it is also important to put measures in place to protect food sources from plant and animal diseases and from acts of terrorism on agriculture, or **agroterrorism**. Routine monitoring and surveillance programs of crops and livestock must be in place so that the presence of an exotic pathogen is detected rapidly and its source discovered. Enhanced security measures should also be adopted. In the United States, surveillance is primarily a function of the U.S. Department of Agriculture's (USDA) Animal and Plant Health Information Service (APHIS). This department has the tools to prevent the entry of foreign pests and to manage infestations, should they occur.

Plant and Animal Diseases

Several diseases affecting plants and animals can result in diminished food productivity. Animal diseases of concern include diseases such as BSE (bovine spongiform encephalopathy or mad cow disease), foot-and-mouth disease, and avian influenza. Insects also present a bioterrorism/agroterrorism risk, as most of the economically important insect pests in North America are not native but are introduced. Insects that can infect either livestock or crops are both of concern. If a new insect pest were discovered, it would be difficult to determine the source and whether or not it was introduced on purpose.

Whether a disease is deliberately brought in as an act of agroterrorism, or whether it is accidentally brought in, agricultural authorities must be prepared to respond promptly. Livestock illness and death can sometimes be noticed before authorities become aware of human health problems due to the same exposure. Farmers must be vigilant about security and report any abnormalities to veterinarians, law enforcement, or appropriate USDA authorities immediately to prevent problems from spreading. Introduction of harmful agents that would compromise farm products could be accomplished using low technology, but the impact and cost could be high. Losses from infectious agents would include animal suffering, injury, or death, as well as economic damage and public health danger from an unsafe food supply.

Foot-and-Mouth Disease

Foot-and-mouth disease (FMD) is a highly contagious viral disease of livestock and other hoofed animals. Concern has been expressed over the ease with which a disease such as FMD might be brought to America from countries where it is endemic, such as Afghanistan. About one-third of the al Qaeda September 11, 2001, hijackers had agricultural training; some had demonstrated an interest in aerial spraying of crops.

Threats to agriculture have also been used to try to influence or change government policies. For example, the agent causing foot-and-mouth disease has been used in extortion threats. In 2005, in New Zealand, a group demanding money and changes in governmental policy threatened to release the agent causing foot-and-mouth disease in a farming area, and claimed to have already released it on an island.

FOOD AND WATER SAFETY

Several pathogenic organisms have the potential to contaminate food or water supplies. These include the bacteria *Escherichia coli, Salmonella typhi, Shigella,* and *Vibrio cholerae.* The botulinum toxin is not stable in treated (chlorinated) water but is relatively stable in beverages. Heightened security measures and increased surveillance methods are needed to detect these organisms when they first occur.

LABORATORY ROLE IN BIOTERRORISM RESPONSE

The Laboratory Response Network (LRN), as described in Lesson 7-3, is a nationwide network of laboratories trained for rapid response to both biological and biochemical threats. Partners in the LRN include several governmental agencies and organizations including the CDC, Federal Bureau of Investigation (FBI), Defense Department, Agriculture Department, Environmental Protection Agency (EPA), Energy Department, Food and Drug Administration (FDA), Homeland Security, American Society of Microbiology (ASM), Association of Public Health Laboratories (APHL), and American Association of Veterinary Laboratory Diagnosticians (AAVDL). The LRN has played and will continue to play an important role in responding to biological threats.

Laboratory Response Network in Action

2001 Anthrax Attack

In October 2001, shortly after the World Trade Center attacks in New York City and the Pentagon attack in Washington, DC, letters containing anthrax spores were delivered to Florida, New York, and Washington. Twenty-two people subsequently became infected—11 with inhalation anthrax—and five died.

In Florida, a clinical specimen from one of the first victims revealed the anthrax bacillus. The identification was quickly confirmed by the Florida public health laboratory (an LRN member) and the CDC, setting in motion a large-scale investigation. Environmental and clinical samples were collected from the hospital, the victim's place of work, and places in North Carolina that he visited shortly before becoming ill. LRN laboratories performed tests on the samples and helped to determine that he had been exposed at work by a letter containing anthrax. As part of the investigation, testing was performed on samples from postal facilities, the U.S. Senate office buildings, and offices of news organizations.

By the time the investigation was completed in December 2001, 125,000 samples had been tested, which translates into more than 1 million separate tests. Before the recent cases of anthrax terrorism in 2001, only 15% of patients with inhalation anthrax would have been expected to survive. Because of rapid response and awareness, however, six of the 11 patients with inhalation anthrax survived that event.

SARS

The CDC and the LRN also played an important role in the investigation of the outbreak of SARS (Lesson 7-3). CDC laboratories sequenced the viral DNA of the coronavirus that causes SARS and laboratories of the LRN-developed tests and test materials that could be used by member laboratories to identify the virus.

BioWatch

The Department of Homeland Security has initiated an around-the-clock environmental surveillance program to sample air in certain densely populated cities. The samplers are maintained by the EPA and filters are removed daily and analyzed by LRN BioWatch laboratories. Using polymerase chain reaction (PCR) technology, biological agents can be rapidly identified. If a harmful agent were found, it would trigger a set of emergency response procedures.

Laboratory Preparedness

Members of the LRN have also developed materials to help smaller laboratories and sentinel laboratories reach a state of preparedness. Documents such as the Clinical Laboratory Bioterrorism (BT) Readiness plan, prepared by the ASM, provide a template for laboratories to follow to ensure that their readiness plan is comprehensive. Included in this material are detailed instructions for the handling and transport of the identified threat agents, as well as communication protocols, containment levels, detailed identification procedures, and training checklists.

SUMMARY

Several agents are currently recognized as having the potential to be used in biological weapons or as bioterrorism agents. Some of these are well-known pathogens that have been around a long time. Others cause diseases that have only been recognized in recent years. All have the potential to cause high rates of mortality as well as disrupt society. Many government agencies and scientific organizations have joined together to coordinate comprehensive readiness plans to respond rapidly to the emergence of a threat agent.

REVIEW QUESTIONS

1. Explain what is meant by agroterrorism and give examples of agents that might be used in this way.

2. For the following disease threats, list the causative agent and the reservoir of each: plague, tularemia, and smallpox.

3. What are six characteristics that make an agent useful as a threat agent?

4. Why is bioterrorism a hot topic?

5. What was the role of the LRN in the 2001 anthrax outbreak in the United States?

6. What is BioWatch?

7. What two threat agents have an ancient history of causing disease?

8. Define agroterrorism, botulinum intoxication, botulinum toxin, Department of Homeland Security, intoxication, virion, and virulent.

STUDENT ACTIVITIES

1. Complete the written examination for this lesson.

2. Ask your instructor to arrange a visit to a regional hospital, reference laboratory, or state public health laboratory. Find out what procedures they would follow if they suspected the presence of a threat agent. Ask if the laboratory is a sentinel or reference laboratory.

3. Look in newspapers, news magazines, or periodicals for information on recent natural outbreaks of agents such as the anthrax or plague bacterium. Find out what kind of disease was caused and what the mortality was.

WEB ACTIVITIES

1. Use the Internet to explore the Homeland Security Web site or another Web site with information about bioterrorism response. List six biological threat agents. Report which, if any, of these agents have caused animal or human illness in the last 5 years.

2. Use the Internet to search for outbreak information. Use reliable Web sources such as the CDC's *Morbidity and Mortality Weekly Reports* or Pro Med (Program for Monitoring Emerging Diseases) at www.promedmail.org.

7-5

Culture Techniques for Bacteria

LESSON OBJECTIVES

After studying this lesson, the student will:

- Explain the use of aseptic technique in bacteriology.
- Explain the differences between antiseptics and disinfectants and discuss how they are used.
- Describe the different types of biological safety cabinets.
- Explain the differences in primary, selective, and indicator media.
- Explain the use of transport media.
- Discuss safety precautions that must be observed when performing bacterial culture techniques.
- Explain the quality assessment procedures involved in culturing bacteria.
- Describe how to inoculate different forms of media.
- Demonstrate the methods for inoculating an agar plate and streaking for isolated colonies.
- Define the glossary terms.

GLOSSARY

agar / a seaweed derivative used to solidify microbiological media

antiseptic / a chemical used on living tissues to control the growth of infectious agents

aseptic technique / work practices used to prevent contamination when working with microorganisms

disinfectant / a chemical used on inanimate objects to kill or inactivate microbes

HEPA filter / high-efficiency particulate air filter used in biological safety cabinets

indicator medium / a bacteriological medium that detects certain chemical reactions of organisms growing on it; differential medium

inoculating loop / an instrument used to pick up and transfer bacteria

inoculation / the process of transferring a population of microorganisms to a growth medium

inoculum / a mass of bacteria being transferred from one medium to another

mycoplasma / the smallest free-living group of bacteria (class Mollicutes) that lack a cell wall and grow in the absence of oxygen; mollicutes

primary medium / a medium that provides nutritional requirements for an organism and is used to recover the organism from infectious material

quadrant / one-fourth of a circle; one-fourth of an agar plate

selective medium / a bacteriological medium that allows growth of some organisms while inhibiting growth of others

sterilization / the act of eliminating all living microorganisms from an article or area
transport medium / a medium that provides the proper environment for organisms during transport

INTRODUCTION

Certain basic techniques must be mastered to function effectively in the bacteriology laboratory. Personnel must be trained in the correct use of growth media, equipment, and reagents before beginning to work in bacteriology. Safe work practices must be followed when working with bacterial cultures to avoid exposure of the worker and the environment to the organism. Technicians must be proficient in aseptic techniques, use of inoculating loops, specimen preparation for reference laboratories, and proper culture techniques. Lesson 1-6 on biological safety should be reviewed before beginning this lesson.

ASEPTIC TECHNIQUE

   Aseptic technique is usually thought of as a set of procedures used to prevent spread of infection during surgical procedures. However, in the bacteriology laboratory, aseptic technique incorporates work practices used to prevent bacteria from infecting humans or contaminating surfaces, as well as to prevent contamination of the bacterial culture by unwanted organisms. Aseptic technique includes physical and chemical means of preventing contamination.

Physical Means of Preventing Contamination

Protective Clothing

There are several ways to incorporate aseptic technique into laboratory procedures. Wearing a fluid-resistant laboratory coat protects the technician from contamination, and the long sleeves protect the culture from contamination. The laboratory coat should be laundered at the hospital or laboratory and should never be worn home.

Safe Use of Equipment

Handling materials and equipment safely is important. The **inoculating loop**, used to transfer bacteria, must be sterilized and cooled before and after each use (Figure 7-26). It must be placed in the loop rack and never laid on the countertop.

Recent research has shown that the majority of laboratory-acquired infections occur by the respiratory route. Therefore, it is very important to avoid situations that create aerosols of infectious microorganisms. If sterile plastic disposable loops cannot be used, care should be taken to prevent aerosol formation when the inoculating loop is sterilized.

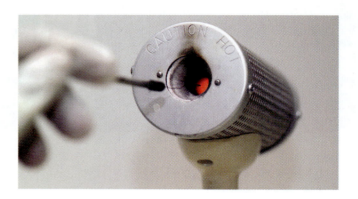

FIGURE 7-26 Sterilizing an inoculating loop using an electric incinerator

Microbiological Safety Cabinets

Microbiological safety cabinets are specially designed laminar flow cabinets that protect the worker from infectious agents. Most laboratories have a class I or class II safety cabinet. Class I cabinets protect the worker and the environment but do not protect the culture. Class II cabinets provide protection to the worker, the environment, and the culture (Figure 7-27). Although routine bacteriological work does not require the use of a safety cabinet, all work with fungi, *Mycobacterium*, and certain other infectious agents must be performed using a class II cabinet.

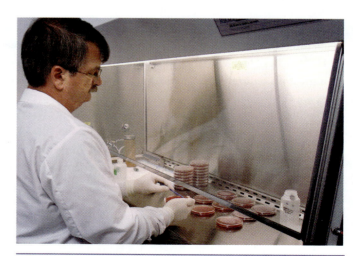

FIGURE 7-27 Using a biological safety cabinet in the microbiology laboratory (*From CDC, Atlanta, GA*)

TABLE 7-17. Disinfectants and antiseptics commonly used in microbiology

CHEMICAL NAME OR COMMON NAME	ORGANISMS EFFECTIVE AGAINST	USE
Alcohols, 70%–90% (isopropanol, ethanol)	Bacteria, *Mycobacterium*, and some viruses	Skin and surfaces
Iodine	Bacteria. fungi, viruses, protozoa	Skin
10% chlorine bleach	Especially good for viruses	Surfaces
Phenolics (Amphyl)	Most bacteria and viruses; *Mycobacterium*	Surfaces
Quaternary ammonium salts (QUATS)	Bacteria, some fungi	Surfaces

The class II cabinet operates by drawing air from the room, around the operator, into the front grille of the cabinet, and then into a special high-efficiency particulate air filter, called a **HEPA filter**. This filtered air then enters the work chamber from the top and is drawn downward, with the air flow splitting as it nears the work surface. Part of the air is drawn through the front grille and the rest through the back grille, providing a particulate-free environment inside the cabinet. The air then passes through the exhaust HEPA filter or the supply HEPA filter back into the hood. However, technicians must still use aseptic technique when working with cultures in a safety cabinet.

Chemical Means of Preventing Contamination

Disinfectants, chemicals used to kill or control the growth of microorganisms on inanimate objects, are used liberally and frequently in the bacteriology laboratory. Disinfectants are effective against most bacteria, as well as some viruses and fungi (Table 7-17). Disinfectants labeled bactericidal kill bacteria; those labeled bacteriostatic only slow the growth of bacteria. Disinfectants that kill microorganisms in their active, vegetative states (stages), may not be effective against the more resistant spore (resting) stages.

Because disinfection only reduces the number of microorganisms to a lower level, rather than killing all microorganisms present, disinfectants must be used liberally and often on work surfaces. Disinfectant should be applied to countertops before beginning a procedure and after the work is completed. In addition, work areas should be wiped with disinfectant any time a spill or splash occurs. The effectiveness of a disinfectant is influenced by its concentration, the number and type of microorganisms, and the pH, contact time, and temperature. The presence of interfering substances such as protein or other organic material can reduce the effectiveness of disinfectants (Table 7-18).

Antiseptics are chemicals used to control the growth of microorganisms on living tissue. Antiseptic soaps, gels, or foams are used to clean hands before donning gloves, after removing gloves, and any other time hands become contaminated. Labels on disinfectants and antiseptics provide information about the products' effectiveness against various microorganisms. Table 7-17 lists categories of disinfectants and antiseptics and the types of organisms for which they are effective.

Sterilization is a method that frees an article or area from all living organisms, including spores. Sterilization is most commonly performed by autoclaving. While sterilization by autoclave is preferable, items that cannot be heat-sterilized can be sterilized by exposure to chemicals such as aldehydes, peroxides, and either chlorine dioxide or ethylene oxide gas.

GROWTH MEDIA FOR CLINICAL BACTERIOLOGY

A bacteriological medium is a substance used to grow bacteria in the laboratory. The medium can be liquid, such as a broth, or solid, such as tubes or plates of media containing agar (Figure 7-28). **Agar** is a derivative of seaweed used to solidify liquid media.

In a clinical laboratory, the function of media is to help recover, grow, isolate, and identify microorganism(s). A good, all-purpose medium for bacteria must support the growth of a wide variety of microorganisms and be economical. One medium that fulfills these requirements is sheep's blood agar, commonly called blood agar (BA). Blood agar will support the growth of most microorganisms, from the tiny **mycoplasmas** to most of the yeasts.

TABLE 7-18. Factors affecting the action of disinfectants and antiseptics

Contact time

Temperature

pH

Concentration of chemical

Number of organisms present

Presence of organic matter, such as protein and blood

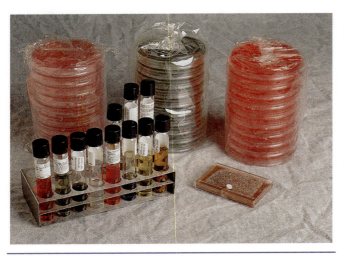

FIGURE 7-28 Various types of media used in bacteriology

Primary Media

The **primary medium** is the one on which the specimen collected from the patient is first inoculated. The choice of media is important and can determine the success of recovering the infection-causing agent. The primary medium is chosen based on the site of the infection; for example, the primary medium used for a wound culture would be different from that used for a urethral culture (Tables 7-19 and 7-20).

Selective Media

A **selective medium** contains ingredients that inhibit the growth of certain microorganisms while allowing the growth of others. Two examples of selective media are MacConkey's (MAC), shown in Figure 7-29, and EMB. Using a selective medium increases the chances of recovering a particular organism from a mixed bacterial population (Tables 7-19 and 7-20).

TABLE 7-19. Examples of common specimens, possible isolates, and media recommendations

SOURCE	POTENTIAL ORGANISMS	MEDIA	CO_2
Urine	E. coli	BA, EMB, or MAC	–
	Klebsiella		
	Proteus		
	Pseudomonas aeruginosa		
	Enterococcus		
Throat	Streptococcus pyogenes	BA	+
Sputum	Streptococcus pneumoniae	BA	+
Wounds	Staphylococcus sp.	BA, Choc, EMB or MAC, Thio	+
	Streptococcus sp.		
	Enterobactericae		
	Anaerobic bacteria		
Vaginal/urethral	Neisseria gonorrhoeae	BA, Choc, T-M	+
Stool	Salmonella	SS, HE, EMB or MAC, selenite	+
	Shigella		
	Pathogenic E. coli		
Cerebrospinal fluid	Neisseria meningitidis	BA, Choc, Thio	+
	Streptococcus pneumoniae		
	Haemophilus influenzae	H. isol. medium	+
Eye, ear	Neisseria gonorrhoeae	BA, Choc, T-M, EMB or MAC, Thio	+
	Haemophilus species		
	Staphylococcus aureus		
	Streptococcus pyogenes		
	Pseudomonas aeruginosa		
	Moraxella species		

BA = Blood agar; Choc = chocolate agar; MAC = MacConkey; SS = *Salmonella-Shigella*; HE = Hektoen enteric; T-M = Thayer Martin; Thio = Thioglycolate; H. isol. medium = *Hemophilus* isolation medium

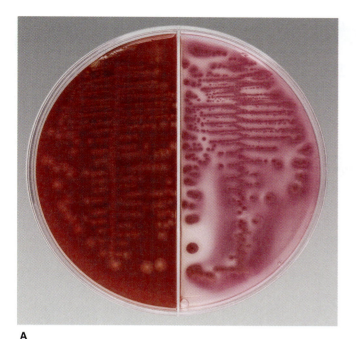

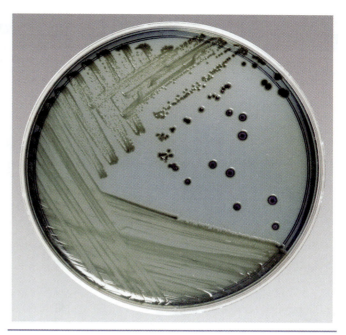

FIGURE 7-30 *Salmonella* growing on Hektoen enteric agar, an indicator medium. Note colonies with black centers. (*Courtesy Remel, Inc., Lenexa, KS*)

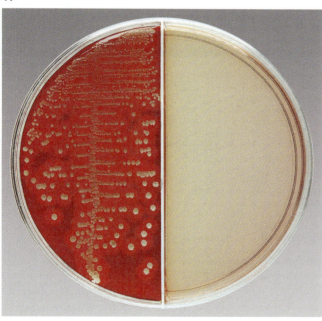

FIGURE 7-29 Bacterial growth on primary and selective media: (A) Gram-negative *Escherichia coli* and (B) Gram-positive *Staphylococcus aureus* inoculated to split plates of blood agar (left side of plates) and MAC (right side of plates). Blood agar supports growth of both organisms; MAC selects for Gram negatives. (*Courtesy Remel, Inc., Lenexa, KS*)

Indicator Media

An **indicator medium** (differential medium) detects metabolic activity of particular microorganisms. Indicator media can show chemical reactions of bacteria, such as fermentation of sugars, by a color change in the bacterial colony or in the medium. One example of an indicator medium is MAC, which produces a pink color when an organism ferments lactose (Figure 7-29A). Some media, such as EMB and MAC, contain ingredients that make them function as both indicator and selective media. The characteristics of growth on primary, selective, and indicator media can be valuable clues to a microorganism's identity (Figure 7-30). Table 7-20 gives examples of primary, selective, and indicator media, their principal ingredients, and reactions.

PERFORMING CULTURE TECHNIQUES

In the bacteriology laboratory, the technician often must transfer culture material from one type of medium to another. The process of transferring a population of microorganisms to a growth medium is called **inoculation**. The group of microorganisms being transferred is called the **inoculum**. The first transfer of inoculum is from the site of infection to the primary medium. For example, a throat swab would be inoculated to sheep's blood agar. Successful recovery and identification of the disease-causing agent depends on proper collection and transfer of the inoculum, and use of aseptic technique.

Safety Precautions

Technicians in the bacteriology laboratory must observe Standard Precautions, remembering that the specimens they handle can contain bacteria and other potentially infectious material (OPIM). Washing hands and wearing gloves are important when handling specimens. Other personal protective equipment (PPE) should be used as required. Aseptic technique, physical methods of preventing

TABLE 7-20. Common types of media for bacteriology

TYPE	USE	ACTIVE INGREDIENT(S)	PURPOSE
BA	Primary	Sheep or rabbit blood	Supports wide range of organisms
Choc, MTM	Primary	Heated blood	Provides hemoglobin and growth factors for fastidious organisms
EMB	Selective	Eosin y, methylene blue	Inhibits Gram-positive organisms
EMB	Indicator	Eosin-methylene blue complex	Indicates fermentation of lactose, sucrose
HE	Selective	Bile salts, acid fuchsin, bromthymol blue	Isolates and differentiates *Salmonella* and *Shigella*
SS	Selective	Bile salts, phenol red	
MAC	Selective	Bile salts, crystal violet	Inhibits Gram-positive organisms
MAC	Indicator	Neutral red	Indicates fermentation of lactose

BA = blood agar
Choc = chocolate agar
MTM = modified Thayer-Martin medium
EMB = eosin-methylene blue medium
MAC = MacConkey's medium
HE = Hektoen Enteric
SS = Salmonella-Shigella
These are just a few examples of the most common media used in small laboratories or physician office laboratories; there are many other types with specialized uses.

contamination, and chemical disinfection methods must be combined to ensure that the bacteriology laboratory is a safe working environment.

Work surfaces must be wiped with surface disinfectant before and after performing each procedure. Contaminated materials must never be included with general trash. Materials such as used culture media, disposable loops, specimen swabs, and any other supplies that have come in contact with live organisms must be packaged in special biohazard bags, decontaminated, and disposed of according to the facility's protocol. This might be done by autoclaving before disposal, by incineration, or by using a medical waste disposal service.

Quality Assessment

Quality assessment (QA) is an important aspect of bacteriology. A good quality program ensures that media are not contaminated, that they will support growth of organisms, and that indicator and selective media are reacting properly. A QA program will also help ensure that unknown isolates are correctly identified. The QA program can consist of internal and external components.

Internal Quality Assessment Program

The internal program includes specimen collection, media checks, reagent quality, equipment performance, and staff proficiency. Commercial control microorganism sets can be purchased

that meet CLSI requirements for testing commercially prepared media, antibiotic susceptibility testing, and help document a personnel assessment program. A QA program should also include monitoring and recording temperatures of all incubators and refrigerators.

External Quality Assessment Program

Laboratories must subscribe to one of several external QA or proficiency programs. These programs are a good way to ensure that staff is proficient in identifying organisms. Bacterial specimens are sent to the laboratory for identification at specified times during the year. Regulatory agencies responsible for laboratory inspection also offer microbiology proficiency programs.

Collecting and Transporting Specimens

It is important that bacterial specimens be collected correctly to ensure that culture results are valid. The type of swab used for collection must be chosen carefully. Most bacteriological procedures require the use of sterile swabs made of polyester (Dacron) or rayon because cotton contains ingredients that are toxic to many microorganisms. Once the specimen swab is delivered to the laboratory, the specimen should be placed on appropriate growth media as soon as possible.

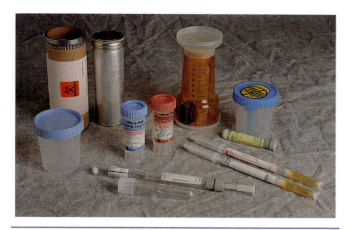

FIGURE 7-31 Transport media

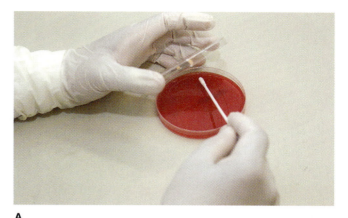

A

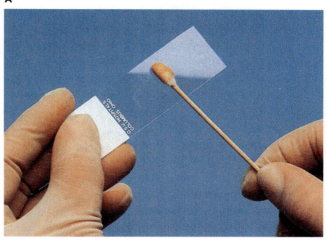

B

FIGURE 7-32 (A) Inoculating one quadrant of an agar plate using a swab; (B) preparing a bacterial smear using a swab

Smaller laboratories often send specimens to a reference laboratory for culture. These specimens are sent in a **transport medium**, one that provides the proper environment for microorganisms during transport (Figure 7-31). The transport supplies must be sterile and must include ingredients that will protect the microorganism from drying for several hours. Transport media are available to meet the growth requirements of different types of microorganisms, including aerobic and anaerobic. The reference laboratory should provide a procedure manual that includes the uses of the various media and a guide to media selection, usually based on the site of infection or source of the specimen. The reference laboratory also keeps the laboratory supplied with various types of transport media.

Inoculating Media

Aseptic conditions must be maintained during media inoculation. The lid of the petri dish should be raised just enough to allow streaking of the agar with the inoculating loop. Otherwise, the lid is always kept on the petri dish to prevent contaminating the medium and the culture. A reusable inoculating loop should be placed in its holder, not on the counter, after it is sterilized; a used, disposable loop should be discarded in the appropriate biohazard container. The risks of aerosol formation can be decreased by careful manipulation of the loop and use of sterile disposable loops that eliminate the need for heat-sterilization.

Agar Plate

The first step in inoculating an agar plate is labeling it with the patient's name and identification number. The petri dish is always labeled, on the *bottom*, not the lid, since the lid could be accidentally switched from one dish to another. Agar plates are always stored and incubated upside down to prevent the formation of condensate inside the lid.

Inoculating the Plate. The medium is inoculated by gently rolling the specimen swab onto one **quadrant** of the blood agar plate (Figure 7-32A). When only one swab is collected, a smear can be prepared from the same swab. After the swab has

been used to inoculate the plate, it is rolled across a glass microscope slide to produce a smear about 0.5 to 1 inch long (Figure 7-32B). The swab is then discarded in a biohazard waste container.

Streaking for Isolated Colonies. An inoculating loop is used to spread the inoculated material over the agar plate to produce isolated colonies. This is accomplished by transferring less culture material into each successive quadrant. Gentle pressure should be used to avoid tearing the agar's surface.

The loop is sterilized, cooled, and then used to spread the material from the first quadrant into the second quadrant (Figure 7-33). After the loop is sterilized again, it is used to spread material from the second quadrant into the third quadrant, and then from the third into the fourth. In the fourth quadrant, the procedure is done carefully to produce isolated colonies of the bacteria (Figure 7-33). Some workers choose to make the streaks in the fourth quadrant in the shape of a *tornado* to increase the distance between the developing colonies.

Agar Slant

Agar slant tubes can contain transport media, growth media, or reagents to test the biochemical reactions of bacteria. Agar slants are prepared by placing the tubes of media at an angle while the

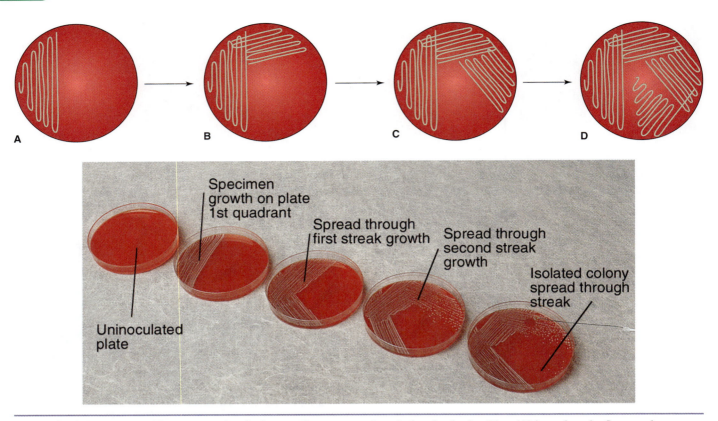

FIGURE 7-33 Streaking an agar plate in four quadrants to produce isolated colonies. Top: (A) inoculate the first quadrant; (B) turn the plate 90 degrees and use a sterile loop to streak into the second quadrant; (C) turn the plate another 90 degrees, sterilize the loop, and streak into the third quadrant; (D) turn the plate another 90 degrees, sterilize the loop, and make one streak in a "tornado" pattern into the fourth quadrant. Bottom: bacterial growth in each quadrant when streaked as shown in the top figure

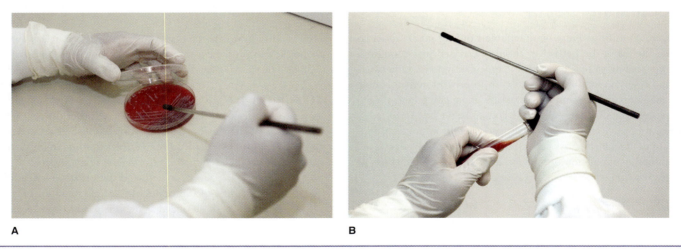

FIGURE 7-34 Transferring bacteria from an agar plate to an agar slant: (A) selecting a colony from an agar plate; (B) preparing to inoculate an agar slant

agar media solidifies. An agar slant tube should be labeled with date and patient information. Colonies are picked up from an agar plate with a sterile loop (Figure 7-34A). The slant tube is held in the other hand while the fourth and fifth fingers of the hand holding the loop are used to remove the tube's cap (Figure 7-34B).

The cap is not laid down but is held in this way until the tube is recapped after the procedure has been completed.

The loop is inserted into the tube and used to make a zig-zag pattern on the slant, starting on the slant's far end and ending at the top (Figure 7-35A). The loop is withdrawn, the tube is

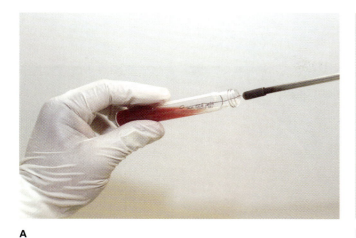

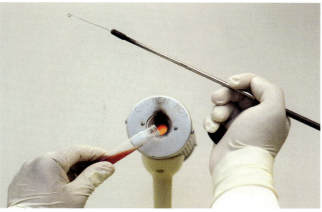

A   B

FIGURE 7-35 (A) Inoculating an agar slant and (B) sterilizing the mouth of the tube

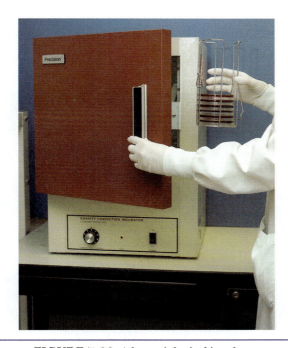

FIGURE 7-36 A bacteriological incubator

capped, and the loop is sterilized. If the loop or culture material touched the tube's rim the rim should be sterilized before recapping (Figure 7-35B). An agar slant can also be inoculated in a similar manner using a swab.

Indicator or Selective Medium

Additional types of media may be required to confirm an organism's identity. They are inoculated with the inoculating loop using the isolated colonies growing on the primary plate. The primary plate lid is raised just enough to insert the sterilized and cooled loop and pick up one or two isolated colonies. The loop is withdrawn, and the indicator/selective medium is inoculated and

streaked for isolated colonies. Split plates containing two kinds of media such as blood and EMB or MAC can be used. But the streaking method must be modified (Figure 7-29).

Observing the Culture after 24 Hours

Most human pathogens grow best at 35°C to 37°C. Inoculated plates are usually kept in a 35°C to 37°C incubator overnight (Figure 7-36); if growth is not evident or is insufficient, the plate is kept an additional 24 hours.

When the plate is removed from the incubator, bacterial growth can be observed through the lid. The plate should be inspected for the presence of isolated colonies (those colonies not touched by others) (Figure 7-37).

Hemolysis

Growth on blood agar should be observed for hemolysis. Some bacteria can completely lyse red blood cells, making the area around the bacterial growth almost transparent. This is called beta (β) hemolysis (Figure 7-37B). Other bacteria incompletely lyse the blood cells and produce green discoloration around the colonies. This is called alpha (α) hemolysis. Absence of hemolysis is called gamma (γ) hemolysis. Observation of hemolysis is especially important in diagnosing strep throat, since *Streptococcus pyogenes*, which causes strep throat, is beta hemolytic.

Colony Characteristics

Other bacterial colony characteristics that aid in identification are size, color, shape, and even odor. Bacterial colonies can be white, gray, yellow, or even red. Their size can range from almost too tiny to be seen to very large. Their shape is usually round and can be flattened or raised like a dome. Some organisms produce distinctive odors, such as one *Pseudomonas* species that smells like grapes and *Neisseria gonorrhoeae*, which smells to some like sweaty tennis shoes. *However, to avoid possible contact with bacteria, never place an open bacterial culture near your face.*

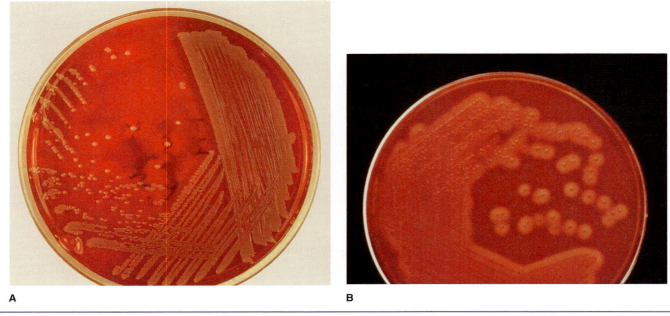

A

B

FIGURE 7-37 Growth of isolated bacterial colonies on blood agar: (A) *Staphylococcus aureus* and (B) beta-hemolytic *Streptococcus*

SAFETY Reminders

- Review safety section before beginning procedure.
- Observe Standard Precautions when handling specimens and cultures.
- Use a disposable inoculating loop when possible.
- Avoid formation of aerosols when sterilizing the inoculating loop.
- Sterilize reusable loops after use and return to holder.
- Wipe work surfaces frequently with surface disinfectant.
- Wear a fluid-resistant, buttoned laboratory coat to prevent clothing contamination.
- Do not wear or take the laboratory coat home.
- Do not place a bacterial culture near your face or try to smell it.

PROCEDURAL Reminders

- Review quality assessment section before beginning procedure.
- Sterilize the loop before and after each use.
- Keep agar slants or petri dishes open only long enough to transfer the culture.
- Use aseptic technique to prevent contaminating specimens or cultures.
- Perform quality checks on media and equipment.
- Transfer specimens to primary media as soon possible after collection.

SUMMARY

Good culture techniques are essential for accurate results in the bacteriology laboratory. Aseptic technique must be used to avoid contamination of the technician, the culture, and the environment. Sterile disposable loops should be used when possible to eliminate the risk of aerosol formation created by sterilizing the loop. Technicians must be able to successfully transfer organisms from the original specimen to primary, selective, and indicator media which can be in the form of agar plates or agar slants. The transfer must be accomplished without contamination of the specimen or loss of viability of the organism(s). Use of proper cul-

CRITICAL THINKING

Bill's work assignments in bacteriology included ensuring that countertops were wiped down appropriately and all contaminated materials disposed of properly. He used a surface disinfectant to wipe the counters every hour during the work day. Several times each shift he gathered all the used culture plates and other contaminated supplies into biohazard bags. After closing the bags securely, he placed them alongside the other trash to be picked up.

Should Bill be commended for ensuring the safety of everyone working in the laboratory? Explain your answer.

ture techniques ensures that the organism causing disease can be cultured and isolated successfully.

REVIEW QUESTIONS

1. Discuss aseptic technique in the bacteriology laboratory.
2. What are the differences between disinfectants and antiseptics?
3. Name two types of bacteriological safety cabinets and explain their uses.
4. What are the purposes of primary, selective, and indicator media?
5. Describe how to inoculate an agar plate using a swab.
6. Describe how to streak a plate for isolation.
7. Describe how to transfer an inoculum from an agar plate to an agar slant.
8. What are important colony characteristics that can be observed?
9. What hemolytic reactions of bacteria can be used to identify the organism?
10. Why are transport media used?
11. Discuss quality assessment in the bacteriology laboratory.
12. What safety techniques must be used in the bacteriology laboratory?
13. Define agar, antiseptic, aseptic technique, disinfectant, HEPA filter, indicator medium, inoculating loop, inoculation, inoculum, mycoplasma, primary medium, quadrant, selective medium, sterilization, and transport medium.

STUDENT ACTIVITIES

1. Complete the written examination for this lesson.
2. Inquire about the types of disinfectants used in local POLs.
3. Practice inoculating an agar plate using a swab and an inoculating loop, as outlined in the Student Performance Guide.

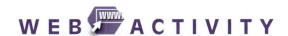

WEB ACTIVITY

Examine the labels of household disinfectants and compare their active ingredients with those of disinfectants used in health care settings. Use the Internet to find active ingredients of two disinfectant brands. Find out if the ingredients are bactericidal or bacteriostatic.

Student Performance Guide

LESSON 7-5 Culture Techniques for Bacteria: Inoculate and Streak an Agar Plate

Name _____ Date _____

INSTRUCTIONS

1. Practice inoculating and streaking an agar plate using a swab and an inoculating loop, following the step-by-step procedure.

2. Demonstrate the procedure satisfactorily for the instructor, using the Student Performance Guide. Your instructor will determine the level of competency you must achieve to obtain a satisfactory (S) grade.

NOTE: If sterile, disposable loops are used the manufacturer's instructions for use must be followed.

MATERIALS AND EQUIPMENT

- gloves
- antiseptic
- surface disinfectant
- Dacron or rayon sterile swabs, or, alternatively, the instructor may provide swabs with bacteria already applied, stored in capped culture tubes or transport tubes
- blood agar plates
- inoculating loops, sterile disposable preferred
- electric incinerator such as Bacti-Cinerator
- incubator set at 35°C to 37°C
- educational or nonpathogenic strains of *Escherichia coli* or *Staphylococcus aureus* growing on agar slants or in broth culture tubes
- waterproof marker for writing on plastic
- test tube rack
- loop holder
- biohazard container
- paper towels
- sharps container

PROCEDURE

Record in the comment section any problems encountered while practicing the procedure (or have a fellow student or the instructor evaluate your performance).

S = Satisfactory
U = Unsatisfactory

You must:	S	U	Comments
1. Assemble materials and equipment			
2. Turn on the electric incinerator (if using reusable wire loop)			
3. Wash hands and put on gloves			
4. Select an agar plate to be inoculated and label the bottom with the marker			
5. Select an inoculated swab or sterile swab and appropriate culture			

You must:	S	U	Comments
6. Place package of sterile disposable loops within reach; if using reusable wire loop, place it in loop holder within reach			
7. Remove the swab from package. If using a sterile swab, go to step 8. If using a pre-inoculated swab, go to step 11.			
8. Pick up tube of culture to be transferred in one hand; use fourth and fifth fingers of the hand holding the swab to remove the cap from the tube. (Hold cap with fingers for entire procedure; do not lay cap down)			
9. Insert tip of swab into culture and pick up a small amount			
10. Replace cap on culture tube and set tube in test tube rack. Be careful not to touch anything with the swab tip			
11. Lift the agar plate lid just enough to insert the swab and spread the inoculum over the surface of one quadrant of the agar plate			
12. Replace the lid on the petri dish			
13. Dispose of swab in biohazard container or as directed by instructor			
14. Streak the second quadrant of the plate: a. Use the sterile disposable loop following manufacturer's directions; alternatively, sterilize the wire inoculating loop using the electric incinerator and allow the wire to cool b. Lift the lid of the petri dish just enough to be able to insert the inoculating loop c. Touch the sterile loop in the first quadrant and streak all the way across the second quadrant d. Repeat step 14c six to eight times e. Follow manufacturer's instructions if disposable loop is used; or heat-sterilize the reusable loop and allow it to cool			
15. Streak the third quadrant of the plate using the disposable loop or the sterile wire loop: a. Lift the petri dish lid, touch the loop in the second quadrant, and streak all the way across the third quadrant b. Repeat step 15a six to eight times c. Follow manufacturer's instructions if disposable loop is used; or heat-sterilize the reusable loop and allow it to cool			

You must:	S	U	Comments

16. Streak the fourth quadrant of the plate to produce isolated colonies:
  a. Use the disposable loop or the sterile wire loop
  a. Lift the petri dish lid, touch the loop to the third quadrant, and spread the inoculum into the fourth quadrant. Use a continuous streak in a *tornado* pattern, decreasing the horizontal width of the streaks and increasing the vertical distance between the streaks			

17. Replace the lid on the petri dish			
18. Sterilize the loop and replace it in the holder or discard disposable loop into biohazard container			
19. Turn off the electric incinerator			
20. Place the agar plate upside down in the 35°C to 37°C incubator to incubate overnight (18 to 24 hours)			
21. Discard disposables in biohazard containers and clean work area with surface disinfectant			
22. Remove and discard gloves and wash hands with antiseptic			
23. The next day: Put on gloves and wipe work area with surface disinfectant. Remove the plate from the incubator and examine the growth (do not remove lid)			
24. Observe the colonies. Are they colored? What is the shape? Are they flat or raised? Record observations			
25. Look for hemolysis if blood agar was used. Record as no hemolysis, or alpha (α) or beta (β) hemolysis			
26. Dispose of used agar plate in biohazard container			
27. Wipe counter with surface disinfectant			
28. Remove gloves and wash hands with antiseptic			

Evaluator Comments:

Evaluator _____ Date _____

7-6

Preparing and Gram-Staining a Bacteriological Smear

LESSON OBJECTIVES

After studying this lesson, the student will:

- Prepare smears from a swab.
- Prepare smears from cultures growing on media.
- Heat-fix a bacteriological smear.
- Explain the principle of the Gram stain.
- Perform the Gram stain procedure.
- Identify Gram-positive organisms on a smear.
- Identify Gram-negative organisms on a smear.
- Demonstrate the use of aseptic techniques during bacteriological procedures.
- List the safety precautions to be observed when performing the Gram stain.
- Discuss quality assessment procedures that must be a part of preparing smears and performing Gram stains.
- Define the glossary terms.

GLOSSARY

bibulous paper / a special absorbent paper used to dry slides
counterstain / a dye that adds a contrasting color
mordant / a substance that fixes a dye or stain to an object

INTRODUCTION

The preparation and staining of a bacteriological smear is a relatively short and easy, but important, process. Smears can be prepared from cultures growing on media or directly from swabs collected from sites of infection. The smears are then stained to reveal the shape and structure of microorganisms present.

The most common bacterial stain is the Gram stain. By Gram-staining bacterial smears, bacteria can be separated into two broad groups, Gram positive and Gram negative, based on the structure of the bacterial cell wall. The Gram stain reaction and bacterial morphology provide clues to bacterial identity and serve as a guide to the tests that should be used for bacterial identification and determination of antibiotic susceptibility.

PREPARING THE BACTERIAL SMEAR

Safety Precautions

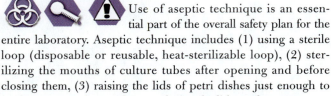 Use of aseptic technique is an essential part of the overall safety plan for the entire laboratory. Aseptic technique includes (1) using a sterile loop (disposable or reusable, heat-sterilizable loop), (2) sterilizing the mouths of culture tubes after opening and before closing them, (3) raising the lids of petri dishes just enough to perform a procedure and never placing the lids on the countertop, (4) discarding all contaminated materials in the proper biohazard containers, and (5) wiping the work area with surface disinfectant before beginning and after finishing a procedure (Lesson 7-5).

Additional rules include:

- Wearing gloves when transferring patient specimens to media or slides and when working with other potentially infectious material (OPIM)
- Wearing a fluid-resistant, buttoned laboratory coat to protect clothing and skin from contamination
- Keeping the work area free of clutter
- Wiping up all spills promptly with surface disinfectant
- Washing hands with antiseptic after every procedure and any other time they may have become contaminated
- Autoclaving all specimens and culture materials before disposal, being sure to follow all applicable local, state, and federal disposal regulations

Quality Assessment

Observing and interpreting bacterial morphology on a stained smear is an important part of bacteriology. The amount of culture material applied to the slide should be such that it is barely visible when dry. Heat-fixing must be performed carefully to prevent cracking the slide or damaging the organisms with extreme heat. Gram stain reagents should not be used after the expiration date. Control slides should be used to check the reliability of Gram stain reagents and technique of laboratory personnel. Each step in the Gram stain procedure should be timed, with special care taken to not allow decolorizer to remain on too long. Microscopes used to observe stained smears should be serviced on a regular basis. All lenses must be kept clean to allow accurate observations of the stained organisms.

Preparing a Smear from a Swab

Bacterial smears can be prepared from a specimen swab collected from a patient, such as a swab from a wound or lesion. It is preferable to obtain two swabs from a patient, one for culture and one for smear, but that is not always practical. If only one swab is collected, the swab must be used to inoculate the culture medium before the smear is made to prevent contamination of the swab from a non-sterile slide.

To prepare a smear of the specimen collected on a swab, a microscope slide is labeled with the patient's name and identification number. The swab is gently *rolled* across the surface of the slide (Figure 7-38). This action should leave just a thin film of material on the slide. When dry, the unstained smear should be barely visible on the slide. The swab should be replaced into its transport medium or discarded into a biohazard container.

Preparing a Smear from a Culture

A smear can be prepared from bacteria growing on tubed media, such as an agar slant, or on agar in a petri dish.

Using an Agar Slant

To prepare a smear from bacteria growing on a slant, a drop of sterile or filtered water is placed on a glass slide. The culture tube is held in one hand and the inoculating loop in the other. The fourth and fifth fingers of the hand holding the loop are used to unscrew the cap of the tube. The loop and the mouth of the tube are sterilized and allowed to cool briefly. Since several inches of the loop wire will enter the tube, the loop and about 2 to 2.5 inches of the wire above should be sterilized.

The loop is then used to pick up a very small amount of bacteria from the edge of the streak (Figure 7-39A). These bacteria are mixed with the drop of water on the slide and spread into a circle about the size of a nickel (Figure 7-39B). The mouth of the tube is sterilized again, the lid is replaced, and the tube is set in a test tube rack. The loop is then sterilized and replaced in its holder. The smear is allowed to air-dry.

Using a Petri Dish Culture

A drop of water is placed on a clean glass microscope slide. The petri dish lid should be raised just enough to insert the sterilized loop and touch it to an isolated colony. The bacteria are then mixed with the drop of water on the slide and spread into a circle about the size of a nickel. The smear is air-dried; the dry unstained smear should be just barely visible.

Heat-Fixing the Smear

When the smear is completely dry, it must be heat-fixed. Heat-fixing can be accomplished using an electric incinerator such as

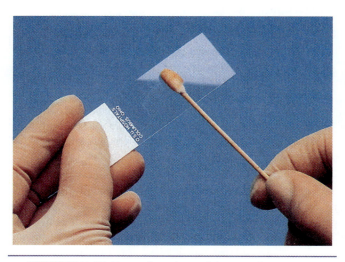

FIGURE 7-38 Preparing a bacterial smear from a swab

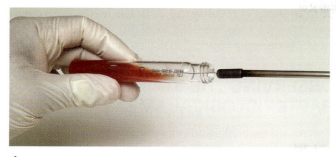

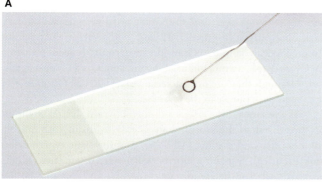

FIGURE 7-39 Prepare a smear from a culture: (A) touch sterile loop to bacterial growth; (B) mix bacteria with water on slide and spread to make a smear

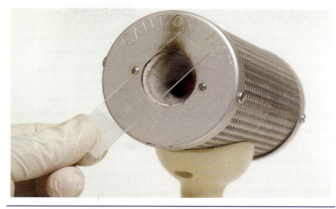

FIGURE 7-40 Heat-fixing a bacterial smear using an electric incinerator

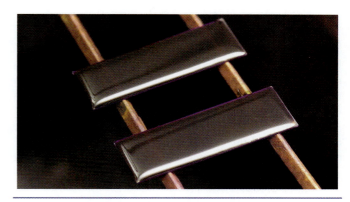

FIGURE 7-41 Slide staining rack

the Bacti-Cinerator (Figure 7-40), or an electric slide warmer. When a smear has been heat-fixed correctly, the slide should not feel hot if touched to the back of the hand.

Heat-fixing causes the organisms to adhere to the glass slide during the staining. Excessive heating will alter or destroy the microorganism's morphology and can break the slide. Under-heating will result in the organisms washing off the slide during staining, requiring that the specimen be recollected if the swab has already been discarded.

THE GRAM STAIN

The most frequently performed stain in the bacteriology laboratory is the Gram stain. Because most bacterial cells are so small and possess so little color, they are difficult to observe microscopically unless they are stained. The Gram stain is performed on a thin smear of bacteria that has been air-dried and heat-fixed.

The staining procedure consists of applying a sequence of primary stain, Gram's iodine, decolorizer, and **counterstain**. A counterstain is a dye that adds contrasting color to the object being stained.

Gram stain reactions are based on chemical differences in the structures of bacterial cell walls. The walls of Gram-negative cells are chemically more complex than the walls of Gram-positive cells. Both types of bacteria contain peptidoglycan in their cell walls, but the Gram-negative cell wall contains more lipid, polysaccharide, amino acids, and lipoprotein complexes than Gram-positive cell walls. Both types of cell walls take up the primary stain which is crystal violet. However, the components in

the cell walls of Gram-negative bacteria allow them to be decolorized (lose the crystal violet) and counterstained. The chemical composition of Gram-positive cell walls causes them to retain the crystal violet and resist decolorization.

Performing the Gram Stain

The air-dried and heat-fixed smear should be placed on a staining rack over a container to catch the staining reagents (Figure 7-41). This can be a beaker, pan, or a laboratory sink. Laboratories that have large volumes of work can use automated stainers.

Primary Stain

To begin the Gram stain procedure, the primary stain, a dye called crystal violet, is poured on the slide (Figures 7-41 and 7-42). The staining time is usually 1 minute, but the manufacturer's instructions must be followed. After 1 minute, the slide is rinsed by gently pouring tap water on it or by holding the slide with forceps under a gentle stream of tap water. The slide is then returned to the rack.

Gram's Iodine (Mordant)

Gram's iodine, a mordant, is then poured on the slide. A **mordant** is a substance that causes a dye or stain to adhere to the object being stained. After 1 minute, the slide is again rinsed with tap water.

Decolorizer

A decolorizer, such as alcohol or an alcohol-acetone mixture, is *briefly* added to the slide. This is best done while the slide is held with forceps and tilted downward at about a 30-degree angle. It is important that this not be done too long—3 to 5 seconds, or until no more purple runs off, is long enough. Immediately after decolorizing, the slide is rinsed with water to remove all decolorizer and stop the decolorization process (Figure 7-42).

The decolorization step is an important one. At this point in the staining process, the Gram-positive organisms will be dark purple-blue because their cell wall composition allows penetration and retention of the crystal violet. The Gram-negative organisms will appear rather colorless because their cell walls do not retain the crystal violet in the decolorization procedure. However, prolonged decolorization can eventually remove the primary stain from the Gram-positive organisms as well. This could cause incorrect identification of an organism.

Counterstain

In the last step, the slide is flooded with the counterstain, safranin. The safranin has no effect on the Gram-positive cells, which retained the crystal violet, but the colorless Gram-negative cells will be stained pink-red (Figure 7-42).

At the end of the counterstaining time, the slides are rinsed again and the excess water shaken off. The slides are then either placed in a rack to air-dry or dried by blotting between sheets of **bibulous paper** to remove the excess moisture. After the slides are completely dry, they are ready to be viewed microscopically.

OBSERVING THE STAINED BACTERIOLOGICAL SMEAR

The stained smear should be observed using the oil-immersion objective (100×) after the stained area has been located using the low-power (10×) objective. The Gram-negative organisms will appear pink-red, and the Gram-positive ones will appear dark blue-purple (Figures 7-42 and 7-43). Staphylococci and streptococci are common Gram-positive, round (coccus) bacteria. *Escherichia coli*, an inhabitant of the intestines, is a Gram-negative rod. Although they are not bacteria, yeasts such as *Candida albicans* stain dark purple in the Gram stain.

If the smear was prepared correctly, the bacteria should be spread out so the morphology is easy to distinguish and the color is crisp and distinct. All bacteria of the same type may not look identical, but the majority will be representative. Gram-negative rods can be slender and long, fat and long, or fat and short. Sometimes rods are so short that they appear round like the cocci and are called coccobacilli. The round bacteria can appear singly, in pairs, as grape-like clusters (staph), or in chains similar to strings of beads (strep). Figure 7-43 illustrates some of these variations in morphology.

STEP	TIME	PROCEDURE	RESULT
1	one minute	Primary stain: Apply crystal violet stain (purple) ↓ Rinse slide	All bacteria stain purple
2	one minute	Mordant: Apply Gram's iodine ↓ Rinse slide	All bacteria remain purple
3	three to five seconds	Decolorize: Apply alcohol ↓ Rinse slide	Purple stain is removed from Gram-negative cells
4	one minute	Counterstain: Apply safranin stain (red) ↓ Rinse slide	Gram-negative cells appear pink-red; Gram-positive cells appear purple

FIGURE 7-42 Steps in the Gram stain procedure

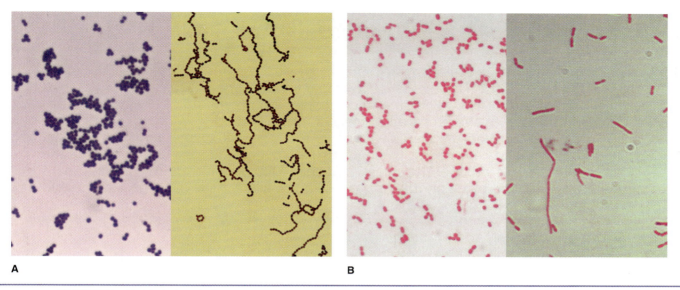

A   B

FIGURE 7-43 Variations in bacterial morphology: (A) cocci: left, grape-like clusters; right, bead-like chains; (B) rods: left, short and fat (coccobacilli); right, long and slender

SAFETY Reminders

- Review safety section before beginning procedure.
- Observe Standard Precautions when handling cultures and patient specimens.
- Wipe work surfaces with a surface disinfectant before and after procedures and anytime a spill occurs.
- Sterilize the loop before and after use and replace it in the holder. Use sterile disposable loops when possible.
- Avoid aerosol formation of bacterial cultures when preparing smears, heat-fixing slides, or sterilizing the loop.
- Use care to avoid burns or slide breakage while heat-fixing the slide or sterilizing the loop.
- Discard used slides in biohazard sharps container.
- Discard all contaminated materials in biohazard containers, as directed by the instructor.

PROCEDURAL Reminders

- Review quality assessment section before beginning procedure.
- Make smears thin enough to be just barely visible when unstained.
- Use gentle heat to fix the slide; too much heat will distort bacterial morphology or may cause the slide to break.
- Follow Gram stain instructions and timing carefully.
- Ensure that the microscope objectives and eyepieces are clean.

SUMMARY

Preparing and staining a smear for Gram stain is an important step in the process of identifying isolates from a specimen. The morphology and Gram stain reaction are valuable clues to the identity and eventually to the antibiotic susceptibility of the organism responsible for an infection. The staining process is relatively simple, but each step must be performed carefully. In the preparation of the smear, the procedures of the facility must be followed. Control slides should be used at prescribed intervals to

CRITICAL THINKING

Marion usually works in the chemistry section of the laboratory. Today, however, since she is cross-trained, she has been asked to help out in bacteriology because two of their employees are out. Marion did some microscope work, scanning Gram-stained slides for Christine, and then she prepared a smear from organisms growing on a blood agar plate. When she touched the sterilized loop to the bacterial colony, she noticed a sizzling sound. While Marion was at lunch, Christine stained the slide and looked at the smear under the microscope. The smear contained blobs of blue and red with no definite shapes. Christine made another smear from the same culture, stained it, and had no problem reading it.

1. Which is most likely the problem—Marion's smear technique or Christine's staining technique? Explain.
2. Which of the following could cause distorted, unrecognizable bacterial morphology in a Gram-stained bacteriological smear?
   a. Failing to heat-fix the smear
   b. Rubbing the swab across the slide
   c. Leaving decolorizer on too long
   d. Failing to sterilize the loop

check personnel technique and the performance of stain reagents. Because smears are made from the specimen or from a culture of the specimen, the swabs are potentially infectious and Standard Precautions must be observed.

REVIEW QUESTIONS

1. Discuss the use of Standard Precautions and aseptic technique in the bacteriology laboratory.
2. Why is it necessary to wear a laboratory coat when working with bacteria?
3. Why is it important to gently roll the swab across the slide when preparing a smear?
4. Why is the medium inoculated with the swab before the smear is made?
5. Explain the differences in the procedures for preparing smears from tube cultures and from petri dish cultures.
6. Why must the smear for Gram stain be heat-fixed before it is stained?
7. Explain how to perform a Gram stain.
8. Why are some bacteria Gram-positive and others Gram-negative?
9. What is the appearance of Gram-positive cocci? Of Gram-negative rods?
10. Why is it necessary to wipe countertops often with surface disinfectant?
11. What QA procedures must be followed when making and staining smears?
12. Define bibulous paper, counterstain, and mordant.

STUDENT ACTIVITIES

1. Complete the written examination for this lesson.
2. Obtain Gram-stained bacterial smears and practice recognizing bacterial morphology and Gram-stain reactions.
3. Practice preparing bacteriological smears, performing the Gram stain, and identifying Gram-negative and Gram-positive organisms as outlined in the Student Performance Guide.
4. Prepare duplicate smears from a culture of Gram-positive organisms. Gram stain the smears, decolorizing one smear for the normal time and the other for 30 seconds. Examine the smears microscopically, compare the staining results, and discuss your findings.

WEB 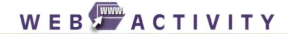 ACTIVITY

Use the Internet to find the morphology and Gram reactions of *Streptococcus pyogenes*, *Neisseria*, *Klebsiella*, *Pseudomonas*, *Clostridium*, and *Hemophilus*.

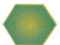 # Student Performance Guide

LESSON 7-6 Preparing and Gram-Staining a Bacteriological Smear

Name _____   Date _____

INSTRUCTIONS

1. Practice preparing and staining a bacteriological smear following the step-by-step procedure.
2. Demonstrate preparing and staining bacteriological smears satisfactorily for the instructor using the Student Performance Guide. Your instructor will determine the level of competency you must achieve to obtain a satisfactory (S) grade.

MATERIALS AND EQUIPMENT

- gloves
- timer
- antiseptic
- surface disinfectant
- nonpathogenic strains of *Escherichia coli* and *Staphylococcus aureus* growing on agar plates and/or slants
- microscope with 10×, 40×, and 100× (oil-immersion) objectives
- immersion oil
- electric incinerator
- glass microscope slides
- inoculating loop, disposable preferred
- holder for inoculating loops
- commercially prepared slides of Gram-negative and Gram-positive organisms
- diamond- or carbide-tip etching pencil or other slide-labeling pen
- sterile distilled H_2O or filtered H_2O
- test tube rack
- forceps or spring-type clothespins
- Gram stain kit or individual Gram stain reagents, including tap water for rinse
- staining rack and container or sink
- slide drying rack
- sterile Dacron swabs
- paper towels or laboratory tissue
- bibulous paper
- lens paper
- biohazard containers
- sharps containers

PROCEDURE

Record in the comment section any problems encountered while practicing the procedure (or have a fellow student or the instructor evaluate your performance).

S = Satisfactory
U = Unsatisfactory

You must:	S	U	Comments
1. Assemble equipment and materials			
2. Turn on the electric incinerator			
3. Wash hands and put on gloves			

4. Prepare one smear from each source listed below:
  a. Swab: prepare one smear from Gram-positive organism (*S. aureus*) and one from Gram-negative organism (*E. coli*), if available
    (1) Obtain a microscope slide and etch the I.D. (+) onto one end with etching pencil			

You must:	S	U	Comments
(2) Obtain a swab that has been inoculated with Gram-positive (+) organisms			
(3) Roll the swab gently across the surface of the slide to make a smear about the size of a nickel			
(4) Return the swab to its container or discard in biohazard container			
(5) Allow the smear to air-dry completely			
(6) Repeat steps a1 through a5, using a Gram-negative (–) organism; label slide with (–) sign			
(7) Hold the Gram-positive (+) slide by the edge using forceps or spring clothespin and place the slide flat against the opening of electric incinerator for a few seconds. Do not heat slide excessively			
(8) Heat fix the Gram-negative slide following step 4a7			
(9) Allow the slides to cool before staining			

b. Tubed media
  (1) Obtain a microscope slide and a culture of a Gram-positive organism and a Gram-negative organism growing on agar slants
  (2) Use sterile disposable loop or sterilize and cool the loop and transfer one drop of sterile water to the center of the microscope slide
  (3) Hold the tube of Gram-positive culture in one hand and the inoculating loop in the other
  (4) Use the fourth and fifth fingers of the hand holding the loop to twist the cap off the tube
  (5) Sterilize the loop and 2 to 2.5 inches of the wire above it and cool the loop
  (6) Sterilize the mouth of the culture tube and use the cooled loop to pick up a small amount of bacteria from the edge of the growth on the slant
  (7) Sterilize the mouth of the tube, replace the cap, and set the tube in a test tube rack
  (8) Mix the bacteria on the loop with the water on the slide and spread the mixture into a circle about the size of a nickel. Do not make the smear too thick
  (9) Repeat steps b1 to b8 using the Gram-negative culture
  (10) Allow smears through air-dry completely
  (11) Heat-fix the smears (as in 4a7)
  (12) Allow the slides to cool
c. Petri dish
  (1) Obtain microscope slides and a Gram-negative and a Gram-positive culture growing in petri dishes

You must:	S	U	Comments

(2) Sterilize and cool the inoculating loop and transfer one drop of sterile water to the microscope slides
    (3) Sterilize and cool the loop again
    (4) Lift the lid of the first petri dish just enough so the inoculating loop can fit into it
    (5) Touch the sterile loop to a bacterial colony and transfer a small amount to the drop of water on the slide
    (6) Replace the lid on the petri dish
    (7) Use the loop to mix the bacteria and water together and spread the mixture into a nickel-sized area
    (8) Repeat steps c1 through c7 using the second petri dish culture
    (9) Allow smears to air-dry completely
    (10) Heat-fix the smears (as in 4a7)
    (11) Allow the slides to cool			

5. Turn off the electric incinerator			
6. Assemble staining rack and reagents			
7. Place smears from all three sources on the staining rack, if space allows			
8. Flood the slides with crystal violet for the manufacturer's recommended time, usually 1 minute			
9. Rinse the stain off the slides with a gentle stream of water from a beaker, faucet, or plastic squeeze bottle and tilt the slides to remove excess water			
10. Flood the slides with Gram's iodine for the recommended time			
11. Rinse the slides as in step 9			

12. Decolorize and rinse smears one at a time:
  a. Hold slide using forceps or clothespin and add the decolorizer until no more purple color runs off the slide
  NOTE: Decolorize no longer than a few seconds to prevent over-decolorization
  b. Rinse the slide immediately to remove the decolorizer; tilt the slide to remove excess water and return slide to staining rack			

13. Repeat step 12 with the remaining slides			
14. Counterstain the smears by flooding the slides with safranin for the recommended time			
15. Rinse the slides, tilt to remove excess water; wipe the back of the slide with paper towel to remove stain; stand slides on end or blot between sheets of bibulous paper to dry			

You must:	S	U	Comments
16. Place the dry slide of the Gram-positive cocci on the microscope stage			
17. Use the low-power (10×) objective to locate the stained smear			
18. Observe the smear using the oil immersion objective			
19. Observe that the *Staphylococcus* organisms are Gram-positive cocci, with the majority being arranged in grape-like clusters			
20. Remove the slide and repeat the procedure, using the slide of Gram-negative rods			
21. Observe that the *E. coli* are Gram-negative rods			
22. Observe the third slide, observe the morphology and Gram stain reaction of the organisms present			
23. Rotate the low-power objective into place and remove the slide			
24. Clean the oil-immersion objective and the top of the microscope condenser with lens paper			
25. Return equipment to proper storage; wipe oil off slides gently and store slides, or discard in sharps container			
26. Return cultures to storage or discard in proper biohazard container to be autoclaved or picked up for disposal			
27. Clean work surfaces with disinfectant			
28. Remove and discard gloves in biohazard container and wash hands with antiseptic			

Evaluator Comments:

Evaluator _____ Date _____

Throat Culture and Rapid Tests for Group A *Streptococcus*

LESSON OBJECTIVES

After studying this lesson, the student will:

- Discuss the importance of identifying group A *Streptococcus*.
- Demonstrate the procedure for collecting a throat swab and performing a throat culture.
- Interpret the results of a throat culture.
- Use a bacitracin disk to identify group A *Streptococcus*.
- Discuss safety precautions that must be observed when performing throat cultures and rapid tests for group A *Streptococcus*.
- Discuss quality assessment procedures essential to the performance of throat cultures and rapid tests for group A *Streptococcus*.
- List two main types of technology used in rapid tests for group A *Streptococcus*.
- Perform a rapid test for group A *Streptococcus*.
- Define the glossary terms.

GLOSSARY

fossae / in the throat, shallow depressions where the tonsils were located before surgical removal

hemolysis / the rupture or destruction of red blood cells, resulting in the release of hemoglobin

pharyngeal / having to do with the back of the throat or pharynx

INTRODUCTION

The throat culture and rapid strep test are frequently performed microbiology laboratory tests, especially in children and young adults. The tests are performed when the patient's clinical symptoms suggest possible strep throat.

Strep tonsillitis is an infection by *Streptococcus pyogenes*, a Gram-positive coccus, which belongs to Lancefield group A. Therefore, it is often referred to as group A *Streptococcus*. Only 5% to 10% of patients with sore throats test positive for group

A strep. However, because the complications of untreated strep infection are serious, all patients who report symptoms should be tested. An untreated group A *Streptococcus* infection can result in scarlet fever, rheumatic fever, rheumatic endocarditis, or glomerulonephritis. These complications are most common in patients under the age of 25 years.

Group A *Streptococcus* (GAS) is just one of several Lancefield groups of streptococci that can cause tonsillitis and other infections in humans. Two other common groups are Lancefield group C and group G. These two groups can cause illness in some patients, while others are asymptomatic. *Streptococcus* grouping kits can be used to test for the other groups if a symptomatic patient tests negative for group A.

DETECTING GROUP A *STREPTOCOCCUS*

Confirmation of the preliminary diagnosis of Group A *Streptococcus* can be made either by identifying the organism in culture or by performing a rapid immunoassay test.

Safety Precautions

Personnel in smaller laboratories may be responsible for collecting the throat specimen and may also culture the organism or perform the rapid test for Group A *Streptococcus*. Appropriate personal protective equipment (PPE) must be worn; a buttoned, fluid-resistant laboratory coat will protect the technician's clothing from contamination. Gloves and protective eyewear should also be worn. A mask should be worn while collecting a throat culture if the patient is coughing excessively. Hands must be washed before gloving, after removing gloves, and after any time contamination is a possibility.

Technicians must not drink, apply cosmetics, or otherwise touch their eyes, nose, or mouth while working in the laboratory. Work surfaces must be wiped with a disinfectant before and after use. The area on which specimens are placed when brought to the laboratory should also be cleaned. Clutter should be removed to help prevent accidental spills. Electric incinerators must be used with caution. All waste must be placed in the appropriate biohazard containers and autoclaved before disposal.

Quality Assessment

The quality of results from bacteriology laboratory procedures is only as good as the quality of the work performed. Quality assessment programs must be in place to ensure reliability of media, stains, and test kits. Many commercial check systems are available for use with QA programs. (See Lesson 7-5 for a review.)

Each lot of blood agar media should be inoculated with a known culture of Group A *Streptococcus* to check for support of growth and demonstration of hemolysis. To ensure the quality of results from rapid tests for GAS, the manufacturer's instructions must be strictly followed. Reagents must not be used beyond the expiration dates and reagents from one kit cannot be used with another. Specified time limits for setting up the test and reporting results must be observed. Most test kits contain built-in (internal) controls. However, if a test system does not have an internal control, an external control must be run at recommended intervals. Results cannot be reported unless the controls give the expected reactions. New lots of swabs should be tested with stock cultures and latex kits to be sure the swabs support viability of organisms and do not interfere with the latex test, causing false reactions.

Performing the Throat Culture

Collecting the Specimen

The throat culture is performed using a sterile Dacron swab. If there will be a delay in getting the specimen to the laboratory, the swab must be placed in a transport medium suitable for streptococci. The throat culture is performed by swabbing the **pharyngeal** surfaces to pick up any organisms present. The swab should be gently passed across the surface of both tonsils or the **fossae** (if tonsils have been removed) and the back of the throat (Figure 7-44). The swab should not touch the tongue or the inside of the mouth; these surfaces are covered with normal flora of the mouth, which can grow on the medium and contaminate the culture.

Inoculating the Media

The throat swab is immediately used to inoculate one quadrant of a blood agar plate (Figure 7-45). A sterile loop is then used to streak for isolated colonies (Lesson 7-5). The loop can also be used to make two or three stabs into the blood agar. This is done by touching the inoculated area in the first quadrant with the

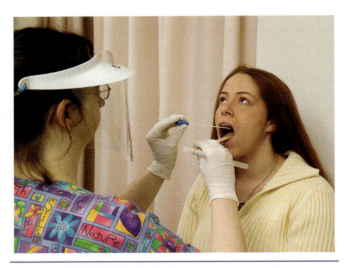

FIGURE 7-44 Performing a throat swab for culture or rapid strep test

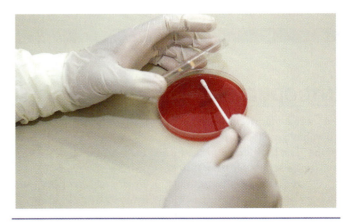

FIGURE 7-45 Inoculating an agar plate using a swab

sterile loop and then *stabbing* the loop into the agar two or three times in the fourth quadrant. A paper disk (the *A* disk) containing the antibiotic bacitracin can be placed on the concentrated streak in the first quadrant of the newly streaked plate before it is placed in the incubator.

Incubating the Culture

Growth of most streptococci is enhanced by incubation in an increased carbon dioxide (CO_2) environment. A CO_2 concentration of 10% increases the growth of hemolytic streptococci and inhibits the growth of other throat flora (Table 7-21). This can be accomplished with a special CO_2 incubator, or by using a candle jar (Figure 7-46). To use a candle jar, culture plates are placed inside a wide-mouth container, a short, lighted candle is placed on the top culture plate, and the lid is closed. The candle uses up most of the oxygen and extinguishes itself, leaving 5% to 10% CO_2 inside the jar. Commercial gas-generating systems are also available that accomplish this by chemical means.

TABLE 7-21. Characteristics of Group A *Streptococcus*

METHOD	CHARACTERISTIC/REACTION
Gram stain	Gram positive
Morphology	Coccus, grows in chains
Culture conditions	5% to 10% CO_2
Growth on blood agar	Beta (β) hemolysis
Antibiotic susceptibility	Bacitracin sensitive

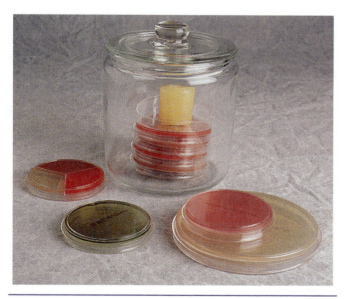

FIGURE 7-46 Candle jar: a lighted candle is set on the top agar plate to produce an atmosphere of 5% to 10% CO_2 after the jar lid is closed

Reading the Throat Culture Plate

After overnight incubation, the blood plate is examined for growth, which is noted as scant, moderate, or heavy. The agar is then examined for hemolysis and for growth around the bacitracin disk.

Hemolysis is indicated by clearing of the agar around colonies on the blood agar plate and in the stabs. Complete hemolysis is beta (β) hemolysis (giving a yellowish appearance to the agar); incomplete hemolysis, which produces a green coloration, is alpha (α) hemolysis. Absence of hemolysis is referred to as gamma (γ) hemolysis (Table 7-22). The stabs in the agar are closely examined because beta hemolysis will show up in the stabs even if it is difficult to see on the agar surface (Figure 7-47A).

The area around the bacitracin disk is also examined for bacterial growth. Bacitracin inhibits growth of Group A *Streptococcus*. The presence of beta-hemolytic colonies and a zone of inhibition (lack of bacterial growth) around the bacitracin disk indicates Group A *Streptococcus* (Table 7-21 and Figure 7-47B).

Some laboratories do not use a bacitracin disk on the original throat culture plate. If beta-hemolytic colonies are present after incubation of the culture, an isolated colony is streaked to another blood agar plate for confluent growth (produced by spreading the inoculum in close or overlapping streaks). A bacitracin disk is placed on the agar to be interpreted after overnight incubation.

If there is need to confirm group A, isolated beta-hemolytic colonies are tested with a panel of antibodies against the various groups of *Streptococcus*. These antibodies are available in kits.

Performing a Rapid Test for Group A *Streptococcus*

Although the throat culture is still performed, many rapid tests for Group A *Streptococcus* (GAS) are used by small and large laboratories to quickly identify the organism. Most of the kits produce test results in about 5 minutes. Two basic technologies used are lateral flow immunoassay and latex agglutination.

TABLE 7-22. Classification of hemolysis on blood agar

TYPE OF HEMOLYSIS	APPEARANCE
Beta (β)	Complete lysis of red blood cells around a colony, making agar almost transparent
Alpha (α)	Green discoloration of agar around a colony
Gamma (γ)	Absence of hemolysis

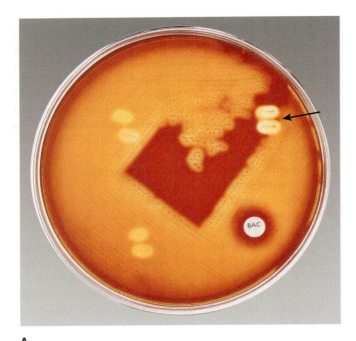

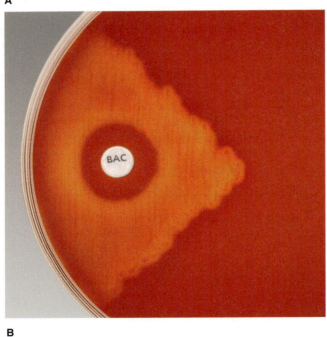

FIGURE 7-47 Beta-hemolytic *Streptococcus* growing on blood agar: (A) Beta hemolysis around stabs in agar (arrow); (B) closeup view of zone of inhibition by bacitracin disc (*Courtesy Remel Inc., Lenexa, KS*)

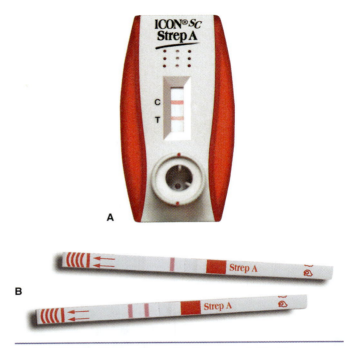

FIGURE 7-48 Rapid test kits for group A *Streptococcus:* (A) ICON SC Strep A test kit showing positive result; (B) ICON DS Strep A test strips; top strip shows negative result; bottom strip shows positive result (*Courtesy Beckman Coulter, Fullerton, CA*)

Immunoassays for Group A Streptococcus

The majority of rapid strep A tests are immunochromatographic assays that incorporate lateral flow technology. This test method is very sensitive and specific for the organism. These tests use an extract of the organisms from the throat swab. Some are two-step tests that include an acid extraction and the addition of the extract to the test system. Others have additional steps, such as adding a conjugate or a wash solution.

Results are displayed in different ways, based on the patterns the manufacturers used to apply the antibody to the test membrane. Some test systems produce a plus (+) sign for positive and a minus (−) sign for negative. If no group A antigen is present, the horizontal bar serves as a control to prove that the test is working. Any group A antigen present will bind and cause the vertical line to be visible, making a (+) sign. Other test kits use a colored dot or parallel colored lines on the test membrane to indicate results.

ICON Strep A Tests

The ICON SC Strep A and ICON DS strep A tests are CLIA-waived rapid immunoassays for detecting GAS antigen from throat swab specimens (Figure 7-48). They can aid in the diagnosis of Group A streptococcal infections. In the ICON SC strep A test, antibody specific to strep A antigen in the self-contained test device reacts with strep A antigen extracted from the patient throat swab. The antigen-antibody mixture travels through the membrane and generates a red line visible in the result window. The test device contains an internal control that will always turn red if the test has been performed correctly.

To perform the test, the patient's throat is swabbed using the special swab included in the test kit. Two different reagents are added to the swab chamber in the cassette. The swab is inserted

CURRENT TOPICS

INVASIVE GROUP A *STREPTOCOCCUS*

Nothing catches the attention of the public like headlines such as "Five victims of flesh-eating bacteria in local hospital" or "Girl loses lower arm to flesh-eating bacteria." News such as this is alarming, especially when readers are led to think that a brand-new organism is attacking humans and that scientists have no idea how to deal with it. Patients are afraid that their strep throat infection can change into this terrifying new form.

Actually, these bacteria have been around a long time. The condition in which the flesh is damaged is called *necrotizing fasciitis* (NF). The infection is caused by a subtype of Group A *Streptococcus pyogenes*, the group of bacteria that causes strep throat. Millions of people have strep throat every year and recover, while there are approximately only 10,000 to 15,000 who become infected with the invasive form of Group A *Streptococcus*.

The two subtypes of Group A *Streptococcus* that are invasive differ genetically from the noninvasive types. A method of genotyping called *emm* typing is used by researchers to detect these especially virulent types and track the epidemiology of outbreaks. In the United States, the rate of incidence of invasive strep A was stable between 2000 and 2005, while a peak in cases occurred in the time period of the 1980s to early 1990s.

Strep infections can be divided into noninvasive and invasive. Infection with noninvasive streptococci can cause strep throat, cellulitis, impetigo, glomerulonephritis, and rheumatic heart disease. The invasive types can cause NF, streptococcal toxic shock syndrome (STSS, not to be confused with toxic shock syndrome caused by staph), and rheumatic heart disease, to name a few. In cases of necrotizing fasciitis, destruction of muscle and other tissue occurs. Therefore, the news media has called it the *flesh-eating* organism.

Invasive strep A infections can begin as a sore or wound that shows redness, pain, drainage, or swelling. The wound rapidly changes to a painful purple or black patch, possibly within an hour. A health care provider must be consulted immediately if these symptoms occur. Other symptoms include fever, sweating, chills, nausea, dizziness, profound weakness, and finally shock. Treatment consists of administration of powerful, broad-spectrum intravenous antibiotics as soon as possible. Surgery is required to remove the damaged tissue and open and drain the infected areas. Amputation of an infected limb may be required to prevent spread of the infection. Although fatalities can occur, if infections are treated aggressively and early, patients can have a good prognosis.

Prevention consists of practicing good hygiene such as frequent handwashing, especially after coughing and sneezing. Any skin injuries should be immediately and thoroughly cleansed.

---

immediately, agitated 10 times around the chamber, and then is left undisturbed for 1 minute. After 1 minute has elapsed, the swab is rotated around the walls of the chamber 5 times while pressed up against the walls to express as much liquid sample from the swab as possible. The swab is then removed and discarded. The valve in the cassette is opened, allowing the mixture to flow into the membrane chamber, and a timer is set for 5 minutes. At the end of the 5 minutes, the result, visible on the front of the device, is read and interpreted. Two distinct red lines, one in the test (T) area and one in the control (C) area, indicate a positive result (Figure 7-48). A red line in the control area only indicates a negative result. If no line appears in the control region, the test is invalid and must be repeated after collecting a new specimen.

Latex Agglutination Tests

Latex agglutination kits use the antigen-antibody reaction to identify GAS. Microscopic latex beads coated with *antibodies* to GAS are reacted with an *antigen* preparation made from the throat specimen. Agglutination indicates presence of GAS. Absence of agglutination is a negative result.

Reliability of Rapid Tests for Group A *Streptococcus*

Rapid strep kits have high sensitivity and specificity when the number of bacteria in the throat is high. However, the results of these tests are not as accurate if the patient has a low number of bacteria in the throat or the swabbing is not thorough. The patient should not eat, drink, or gargle in the 30 minutes before the swab is taken. A false-negative result for Group A *Streptococcus* could cause a strep throat infection to be untreated, which could lead to serious complications in children and young adults. Any negative rapid strep test should be confirmed by a throat culture.

SAFETY Reminders

- Review safety section before beginning procedure.
- Follow Standard Precautions.
- Wear appropriate protective clothing.
- Treat all used swabs as if infectious.
- Wipe the work area frequently with surface disinfectant.
- Wear a mask and safety glasses when collecting the throat swab if the patient is coughing excessively.

PROCEDURAL Reminders

- Review quality assessment section before beginning procedure.
- Touch only the tonsils and back of the throat with the swab.
- Check the expiration date on media, disks, and kits.
- Follow the manufacturers' directions for the kit used.
- Incubate the culture in a 5% to 10% CO_2 atmosphere.
- Interpret any hemolysis carefully.

CRITICAL THINKING 1

Sue was working in the physician office laboratory when Jason came in to have a throat swab performed. His health care provider had ordered a rapid test for GAS because Jason had a fever and sore throat. The result from the rapid test was negative, so a throat culture for strep was ordered. Sue swabbed Jason's throat again and the health care provider gave Jason a prescription for an antibiotic. Sue inoculated the first quadrant of the plate using the specimen on the swab. She disposed of the swab in the appropriate biohazard container, sterilized the loop, and proceeded to begin to streak the inoculum into the other quadrants. A fellow worker interrupted her, and she had to lay the loop down momentarily. After overnight incubation of the plate at 35°C to 37°C in a CO_2 incubator, Tom, a coworker, examined the plate and observed atypical colonies that did not look like strep. He performed a Gram stain and saw some Gram-positive bacilli, similar in appearance to those commonly found on environmental surfaces.

1. What could cause the nonstrep bacteria to grow?
2. Were mistakes made in usual laboratory procedures? What were they?
3. Which laboratory technician needs a refresher course in culture techniques?
4. Was the throat culture needed?

CRITICAL THINKING 2

Maria worked the day shift in bacteriology. One of her first responsibilities each day was to examine cultures that had been incubating overnight. She saw that both throat and urine cultures had been set up on specimens from Shanda Mitchell. Maria pulled the plates to read the two cultures and found a blood agar plate for the throat culture, and blood agar and MAC plates that had been inoculated with urine, all in the 37°C aerobic incubator. The blood agar throat culture plate had scant growth.

Should the results be reported? Explain your answer.

SUMMARY

The rapid test for Group A *Streptococcus* and the throat culture are frequently performed. Both are performed from throat swabs and are important in the detection of strep infection. Most rapid strep A kits have a high specificity and high sensitivity. This means that they have the specificity to react only to strep A and are sensitive enough to detect small numbers of the organism. Manufacturer's instructions for performing rapid tests and interpreting results must be strictly followed. Test supplies must be used only with the kit for which they are intended. Blood agar plates should not be used after their expiration date. All materials used in the rapid test or culture must be discarded into appropriate biohazard containers in compliance with local regulations. It is important for the technician to wear appropriate PPE while performing the throat swab.

Because the complications from undiagnosed and untreated strep are very serious, the physician should order a throat culture if the rapid test is negative. Throat cultures are performed by inoculating throat swabs to blood agar. This medium supplies the required nutrients for growth of throat isolates and also demonstrates beta hemolysis, a characteristic of GAS.

REVIEW QUESTIONS

1. Why is early diagnosis of Group A *Streptococcus* infection important?

2. Explain why the tongue and mouth should not be touched when collecting a throat swab for strep.

3. Why is a throat culture inoculated to blood agar?

4. What is the purpose of the bacitracin disk?

5. What is the reason for making stabs in the agar?

6. Discuss the different types of hemolysis.

7. Discuss agglutination tests and rapid enzyme immunoassay tests for GAS.

8. Explain the possible consequence of a false-negative rapid strep test.

9. List four safety procedures that must be observed when collecting or processing throat culture swabs.

10. What quality assessment procedures are used in identifying GAS?

11. Define fossae, hemolysis, and pharyngeal.

STUDENT ACTIVITIES

1. Complete the written examination for this lesson.

2. Survey local POLs to find out which rapid tests for GAS are used and what procedure is followed when a rapid test is negative.

3. Practice performing a throat culture, as outlined in the Student Performance Guide.

4. Practice performing rapid tests for Group A *Streptococcus*, as outlined in the Student Performance Guide.

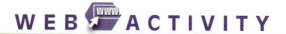

WEB ACTIVITY

Use the Internet to find two rapid strep tests that are not mentioned in this lesson. Report on your findings, including information such as test principle, test sensitivity and specificity, and CLIA complexity level.

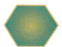

Student Performance Guide

LESSON 7-7 Throat Culture and Rapid Tests for Group A *Streptococcus*

Name _____ Date _____

INSTRUCTIONS

1. Practice performing a throat culture and rapid test for Group A *Streptococcus*, following the step-by-step procedure.

2. Demonstrate the procedures for throat culture and rapid tests for Group A *Streptococcus* satisfactorily for the instructor using the Student Performance Guide. Your instructor will determine the level of competency you must achieve to obtain a satisfactory (S) grade.

NOTE: The instructions given are for the ICON SC Strep A test (Beckman Coulter). Manufacturer's instructions must be followed for whichever test kit is used. Inclusion of this method does not constitute endorsement by the authors. If disposable loops are used, manufacturer's instructions for use must be followed.

MATERIALS AND EQUIPMENT

- face protection/face shield
- gloves
- timer
- sterile Dacron or rayon swabs
- blood agar plate
- inoculating loop, sterile disposable or sterilizable
- electric incinerator
- CO_2 incubator (35°C to 37°C) or incubator (35°C to 37°C) with candle jar
- bacitracin disks
- rapid test kit for Group A *Streptococcus*
- optional: stock culture of Group A *Streptococcus*
- biohazard container
- surface disinfectant
- antiseptic
- sharps container

PROCEDURE

Record in the comment section any problems encountered while practicing the procedure (or have a fellow student or the instructor evaluate your performance).

S = Satisfactory
U = Unsatisfactory

You must:	S	U	Comments
1. Assemble equipment and materials			
2. Wash hands, put on face shield, and put on gloves			
3. Collect throat specimen by swabbing the pharyngeal surfaces **NOTE:** Often the same swab can be used for the culture plate and the rapid test. However, some test kits recommend collecting two swabs			

You must:	S	U	Comments

4. Transfer the specimen to the properly labeled blood agar plate:
   a. Roll the swab gently on the surface of one quadrant of the blood agar plate. Save the swab for the rapid test or discard in biohazard container, if two swabs were collected
   b. Sterilize a loop for streaking the plate or use a sterile disposable plastic loop
   c. Streak the plate for isolated colonies as described in Lesson 7-5. Make two to three stabs in the fourth quadrant of agar. Place bacitracin disk on quadrant one (discard disposable loop in sharps container)
   d. Place the plate upside down in the 37°C CO_2 incubator overnight (or use candle jar in incubator)			

5. Perform ICON SC Strep A rapid test for Group A *Streptococcus* (Follow manufacturer's instructions on package insert)
   a. Allow test pack to come to room temperature (if not stored at room temperature)
   b. Remove test device from the foil pouch and begin the test immediately. Check to see that the marks on the chamber are in the position indicated on the package insert
   c. Hold reagent bottle A upright and add 5 full drops to the swab chamber
   d. Hold reagent bottle B upright and add 5 full drops to the swab chamber
   e. Perform the throat swab procedure and immediately add the swab to the chamber containing the reagents
   f. Hold the chamber base and vigorously agitate the swab in the chamber about 10 times
   g. Leave the swab in the chamber 1 minute. After 1 minute, hold the base of the chamber firmly with the thumb and index finger of one hand and remove the swab by bringing it halfway up the inside wall of the chamber and pressing it against the ribs on the inside of the wall. Rotate the swab 5 times while continuing to firmly press to expel as much liquid as possible
   h. Discard the swab in the appropriate biohazard container
   i. Open the valve into the device by turning the pink marks as shown on the package insert (If liquid does not appear in the window in 1 minute, discard the device and repeat the test with a new throat swab sample)
   j. Set the timer and read the results at 5 minutes. Note: Results are not reliable after 10 minutes			

You must:	S	U	Comments
k. Interpret the results: (1) Negative: A negative result will have a single red C line in the top of the window. This indicates that the procedure and reagents were correct but no Strep A was detected (2) Positive: A positive result will have two red lines, the C and T lines (3) Invalid: If no red lines are present or only the T line is red, the test is invalid			
6. Discard all contaminated materials into biohazard container			
7. Return all equipment to proper storage			
8. Wipe work area with surface disinfectant			
9. Remove and discard gloves in biohazard container			
10. Wash hands with antiseptic			
11. Observe the throat culture plate after overnight incubation a. Quantitate the growth: No growth, scant, moderate, or heavy growth. Record observation b. Observe for hemolysis and record the type: alpha, beta, or gamma (nonhemolytic). Be certain to examine the agar stabs c. Observe for zone of inhibition around the bacitracin disk if beta hemolysis is present. Record observation d. If hemolysis is observed, go to step 19. If not, go to step 12			
12. Wash hands and put on gloves			
13. Inoculate another blood agar plate using beta-hemolytic colonies from stock culture. Streak the whole plate for continuous growth. Place a bacitracin disk in the center of the plate. Incubate overnight at 35°C to 37°C in CO_2 incubator			
14. Clean equipment and return to storage			
15. Wipe work area with surface disinfectant			
16. Remove and discard gloves in biohazard container			
17. Wash hands with antiseptic			
18. Examine the plate from step 13 after overnight incubation. If beta-hemolytic colonies and a zone of inhibition (no growth) around the bacitracin disk are present, report as *beta-hemolytic streptococci present*			
19. Discard all contaminated materials into the biohazard container			

You must:	S	U	Comments
20. Wipe the counter with surface disinfectant			
21. Wash hands with antiseptic			

Evaluator Comments:

Evaluator _____ Date _____

Urine Culture and Colony Count

LESSON OBJECTIVES

After studying this lesson, the student will:

■ Select the correct primary medium and indicator medium for a urine culture.

■ Demonstrate the technique for streaking a urine culture for colony count.

■ Perform a colony count on a urine culture.

■ Discuss aspects of quality assessment that must be considered when performing urine culture and colony count.

■ Describe the safety precautions to observe when performing urine culture and colony count.

■ Define the glossary term.

GLOSSARY

colony count / an estimation of the number of organisms in urine made by counting the colonies on a urine culture plate

INTRODUCTION

The urine culture and colony count are frequently performed in the bacteriology laboratory. The physician orders a urine culture and colony count when a patient has UTI symptoms, such as frequent urination, pain and burning during urination, blood in the urine, and sometimes fever and backache (Table 7-23). The **colony count** gives an estimate of the number of organisms in the urine. The colony count is performed by counting the colonies that grow on the urine culture plate.

Urinary tract infection (UTI) occurs when bacteria migrate up the urethra into the bladder, or even further into the kidneys. Although females are prone to UTIs because of their anatomy, UTIs also occur in males. The microorganism most commonly respon-

sible is *Escherichia coli*, a Gram-negative rod that is part of the normal flora of the intestinal tract. Other Gram-negative rods, such as *Pseudomonas, Proteus*, and *Klebsiella*, can also cause UTI. A Gram-positive organism frequently found as the causative agent in urinary tract infections is *Staphylococcus saprophyticus* (Table 7-24).

PERFORMING THE URINE CULTURE

The urine culture is performed on a clean-catch specimen. The specimen is inoculated to a blood agar plate, which supports the growth of both Gram-negative and Gram-positive organisms; the blood agar plate is used for the colony count. The specimen is also inoculated to a selective medium such as EMB or MacConkey's (MAC).

TABLE 7-23. Symptoms associated with urinary tract infections
Frequent urination
Pain or burning sensation when urinating
Blood in urine
Fever
Backache

Safety Precautions

  The procedures performed in urine culture and colony count expose the technician to potentially infectious body fluids and to cultures of unidentified bacteria. Standard Precautions must be observed. Gloves must be worn when handling the urine and when handling the plates containing bacterial growth. The petri dish lid must be opened only as wide as required to pick up colonies for further testing. Disposable calibrated loops should be used when possible to eliminate the potential for aerosol formation. All contaminated materials must be discarded in biohazard waste containers, as directed by the instructor. All work surfaces must be wiped with a surface disinfectant. Hands must be washed with antiseptic after gloves have been removed.

Quality Assessment

Urine culture results are used to confirm a bacterial UTI. The specimen for culture must be collected before antibiotic therapy is begun. The patient must be instructed in the proper method of collecting a clean-catch urine specimen to avoid contamination of the urine. Since a bacterial UTI is usually caused by only one type of bacteria, the presence of three or more colony types on the primary culture plate suggests the urine was not clean-catch. If a routine urinalysis is also ordered on the specimen, the culture should be set up first, to prevent contamination of the specimen. Only calibrated inoculating loops should be used for the urine culture. The technician should verify the loop size and make sure the colony count is calculated correctly.

When each new shipment of media arrives, its contents should be visually inspected for contamination. To ensure that the media was not contaminated during manufacture, one plate or tube from each lot should be incubated overnight at 35°C to 37°C and then inspected for bacterial growth. In addition, the media can be inoculated with a known organism to ensure that the media contains all the ingredients required to support bacterial growth. Media must not be used beyond its expiration date.

Collecting the Specimen

The specimen must be collected by clean-catch, as described in Lesson 5-2. Females should be cautioned to avoid contaminating the specimen with vaginal material, which may contain microorganisms. If vaginal flora grow on the culture, they can interfere with the process of identifying the organism causing the infection.

The urine container should be labeled on the side (not on the lid) with the patient's name and identification number and the time of collection. The urine should be inoculated to culture media within 1 hour of collection. If the specimen is to be sent to a reference laboratory, the instructions and transport supplies of that laboratory must be used.

Streaking the Plates

Urine specimens are streaked onto two types of media:

- Primary medium, usually blood agar (BA), and
- Indicator/selective medium, such as EMB or MAC

Most urinary tract pathogens will grow on BA. Both EMB and MAC inhibit the growth of Gram-positive organisms and indicate fermentation reactions of Gram-negative organisms (Table 7-24).

A calibrated platinum or sterile plastic loop with a capacity of either 0.01 mL or 0.001 mL is used to inoculate the blood agar plate. The loop is sterilized and cooled and then dipped into a well-mixed urine sample. The loop is observed to be sure it is full of urine and then is used to make a vertical streak down the center of the BA plate. Fifteen to 20 horizontal cross streaks are then made all the way across the plate, crossing the vertical streak each time. In some laboratories, a third set of streaks is made at right angles to the second set (Figure 7-49). The EMB or MAC is inoculated in the same manner. The loop is sterilized after use and placed in its rack. If a sterile, disposable loop is used, it should be discarded into the sharps container. The culture plates are placed in the 35°C to 37°C incubator overnight.

Colony Count and Interpretation

After 18 to 24 hours or overnight incubation, the plates are removed from the incubator and observed for growth (Figure 7-50). Any distinguishing characteristics of the growth, such as colony color and morphology, and hemolysis on the BA plate, should be noted. Both Gram-positive and Gram-negative organisms can grow on the blood plate. Only Gram-negative organisms should grow on EMB or MAC.

The number of colonies on the BA plate is counted and reported as number of colonies per mL. If a 0.001-mL loop was used to inoculate the plate, the number of colonies counted is multiplied by 1000 to calculate the colony count per mL of urine. If a 0.01-mL loop was used, the number of colonies is multiplied by 100.

Urine cultures that have a significant colony count should be processed for bacterial identification and antibiotic susceptibility. A count of 100,000/mL or greater is evidence of UTI, whether or not the patient has symptoms. A colony of 30,000/mL or greater is considered significant in some facilities. In patients who have symptoms or have frequent UTIs, colony counts as low as 1000/mL can be significant. The technician must follow the standard operating procedures of the facility concerning when to perform identification and sensitivity procedures. These procedures are performed from colonies growing on the urine culture plates and are described in Lesson 7-9.

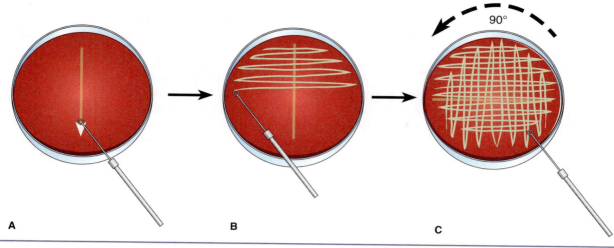

FIGURE 7-49 Streaking a urine culture plate: (A) make one streak down the center of the plate using a calibrated loop; (B) make several streaks at right angles to the initial streak, crossing over the original streak; and (C) make several streaks at right angles to the second set of streaks

TABLE 7-24. Organisms that commonly cause urinary tract infections

ORGANISM	MEDIA SUPPORTING GROWTH
E. coli	BA, EMB, MAC
Klebsiella	BA, EMB, MAC
Proteus	BA, EMB, MAC
Pseudomonas aeruginosa	BA, EMB, MAC
Enterococcus	BA, EMB, MAC
Staphylococcus saprophyticus	BA

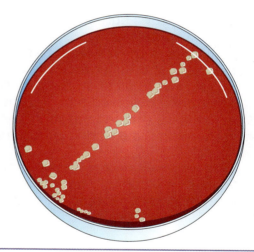

FIGURE 7-50 Examples of isolated colonies from a urine culture

SAFETY Reminders

- Review safety section before beginning procedure.
- Observe Standard Precautions.
- Wear a fluid-resistant, buttoned laboratory coat.
- Prevent aerosol formation.
- Wipe work surfaces with disinfectant before beginning work, when finished, and every time a spill occurs.

PROCEDURAL Reminders

- Review quality assessment section before beginning procedure.
- Instruct patient in proper method of clean-catch urine collection.
- Perform colony count from the blood agar plate.
- Consult facility's procedure manual if three or more colony types are present.
- Incubate the culture plates upside down.

CASE STUDY

Sharon is a technician in a small hospital laboratory. She rotates between the hematology, chemistry, and microbiology sections. On this morning, she was in microbiology examining culture plates which had been set up the previous day. She examined BA and MAC plates set up for a urine culture. Both plates had many colonies growing, and the colonies on each plate appeared to have the same morphology. Sharon counted 132 colonies on the MAC plate. From the requisition slip, she saw that the person who set the culture up had used a 0.001-mL loop. Sharon reported a colony count of 13,200/mL for the culture.

Discuss Sharon's performance in evaluating the urine culture. Does the patient have a urinary tract infection?

CRITICAL THINKING

Mrs. Miller went to her health care provider complaining of frequent, painful urination accompanied by a burning sensation, symptoms she had never had before. The provider ordered a routine urinalysis and a urine culture and colony count. In the laboratory, Mrs. Miller gave the lab order to Gina, who handed her a urine collection cup just as the phone rang. Mrs. Miller took the cup to the restroom and brought back a urine specimen, with her ID label on the cup. Gina performed a microscopic analysis of the urine sediment and observed 5 to 10 epithelial cells/LPF, mucus threads, and many bacteria. She then gave the urine to John, the other technician, to set up the urine culture. The next morning the BA urine culture plate had at least four different colony types growing on it.

1. Should the laboratory try to identify all four isolates?
2. What mistake(s) affected the routine urinalysis and culture?

SUMMARY

The urine culture and colony count are frequently ordered tests. Physicians use the results to determine whether or not the patient has a UTI. To ensure the quality of the results, the patient must be given specific instructions for collecting a clean-catch urine. A culture inoculated from a contaminated specimen can grow out many different organisms and prove confusing to those attempting to interpret the results. The facility's procedure manual must be followed in selecting the inoculating loop size, calculating the colony count and reporting the result. Standard Precautions must be observed and aseptic technique must be used. Disposable loops should be used if available. Facility rules for disposal of used agar plates and other contaminated supplies must be followed.

REVIEW QUESTIONS

1. Why must clean-catch urine be used for urine culture?
2. What types of media are used for urine culture?
3. Which culture plate is used to make the colony count?
4. Describe how to streak the BA plate for isolated colonies.
5. How does the loop used for streaking affect the colony count?
6. What measure(s) should be used in the urine culture procedure to increase safety?
7. Why is it important to perform quality assessment procedures on new shipments of media? How is this done?
8. Define colony count.

STUDENT ACTIVITIES

1. Complete the written examination for this lesson.

2. Practice performing the urine culture and colony count, as outlined in the Student Performance Guide.

WEB ACTIVITY

Use the Internet to find information on cystitis. Report on the complications that can occur if cystitis is untreated.

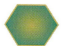

Student Performance Guide

LESSON 7-8 Urine Culture and Colony Count

Name _____ Date _____

INSTRUCTIONS

1. Practice performing the urine culture and colony count following the step-by-step procedure.

2. Demonstrate the procedure for urine culture and colony count satisfactorily for the instructor using the Student Performance Guide. Your instructor will determine the level of competency you must achieve to obtain a satisfactory (S) grade.

MATERIALS AND EQUIPMENT

- face protection and/or acrylic safety shield
- gloves
- clean-catch urine specimen
- blood agar plates
- EMB or MAC agar plates
- disposable or platinum calibrated loop (0.01 mL or 0.001 mL)
- electric incinerator
- wax pencil or marking pen
- surface disinfectant
- antiseptic
- sharps container
- biohazard container
- incubator set at 35°C to 37°C

PROCEDURE

Record in the comment section any problems encountered while practicing the procedure (or have a fellow student or the instructor evaluate your performance).

S = Satisfactory
U = Unsatisfactory

You must:	S	U	Comments
1. Assemble equipment and materials			
2. Turn on the electric incinerator			
3. Wash hands, put on face protection (or use acrylic safety shield), and put on gloves			
4. Obtain a clean-catch urine specimen			
5. Label the bottom of a blood agar plate and an EMB or MAC plate			
6. Mix the urine by swirling, and remove the lid from the urine container carefully, avoiding creating splashes or aerosols			
7. Select a sterile, disposable calibrated loop or sterilize and cool a platinum calibrated loop			

You must:	S	U	Comments
8. Insert the loop into the well-mixed urine sample. Remove the loop and check to see that the loop is filled with urine			
9. Transfer the loopful of urine to the surface of the blood agar plate by making a streak down the center of the plate			
10. Spread the urine over the plate by making 20 to 25 streaks at right angles to the center streak, crossing the center streak each time			
11. Turn the petri dish one-quarter turn (90 degrees) and streak 20 to 25 times at right angles to the first set, crossing all of them each time (follow facility policy for streaking)			
12. Replace the lid on the petri dish			
13. Repeat steps 7 through 12, using an EMB or MAC plate			
14. Discard disposable loop into sharps container or sterilize the platinum loop and return it to the holder			
15. Turn off electric incinerator			
16. Return equipment to proper storage			
17. Place agar plates upside down in 35°C to 37°C incubator for 18 to 24 hours (overnight)			
18. Discard contaminated materials into biohazard container			
19. Wipe counter with surface disinfectant			
20. Remove gloves and discard into biohazard container			
21. Wash hands with antiseptic			
22. The next day: Wash hands and put on gloves. Examine the plates			
23. Count the number of colonies on the blood agar plate			
24. Calculate the number of organisms by multiplying the number of colonies from step 23 by 1000 if the 0.001-mL loop was used, or by 100 if the 0.01-mL loop was used			
25. Record the results			
26. *Keep the plates to perform the antibiotic susceptibility test* (Lesson 7-9) or discard the plates in the biohazard container			
27. Wipe the counter with surface disinfectant			

You must:	S	U	Comments
28. Remove gloves and discard into biohazard container			
29. Wash hands with antiseptic			

Evaluator Comments:

Evaluator _____ Date _____

Bacterial Identification and Antibiotic Susceptibility Testing

LESSON OBJECTIVES

After studying this lesson, the student will:

- Select an isolated colony to perform a Gram stain.
- Use the microscope to identify Gram-positive and Gram-negative organisms.
- Explain how to perform the catalase and coagulase tests on Gram-positive organisms.
- Explain how to report the presumptive identification of Gram-positive and Gram-negative organisms.
- Discuss the use of manual and automated identification systems for bacteria.
- Perform the disk antibiotic susceptibility test.
- Interpret the results of the disk antibiotic susceptibility test.
- Discuss the safety precautions that must be observed when performing bacterial identification and antibiotic susceptibility tests.
- Discuss quality assessment procedures that must be followed when performing bacterial identification and antibiotic susceptibility tests.
- Define the glossary terms.

GLOSSARY

catalase test / a test to differentiate between *Streptococcus* and *Staphylococcus* sp.

coagulase test / a test to differentiate between *Staphylococcus aureus* and other *Staphylococcus* species

coliform / certain Gram-negative intestinal bacteria including *Escherichia coli*

minimum inhibitory concentration (MIC) / minimum concentration of an antibiotic required to inhibit the growth of a microorganism

pleomorphic / having varied shapes

INTRODUCTION

Identifying bacteria and determining their antibiotic susceptibility are important steps in the diagnosis and treatment of bacterial infections. For example when a urine culture yields a colony count considered clinically significant, it is usual to follow up with identification and susceptibility testing of the microorganism. The identification involves making a Gram stain of an isolated colony to determine if the predominant organism is Gram-positive or Gram-negative. Once the Gram reaction and morphology have been determined, biochemical tests are performed to further identify the microorganism. Although identity of the organism gives the physician guidance as to what antibiotic treatment would be best, antibiotic susceptibility tests should be performed to confirm that the antibiotic will be effective against the organism.

BACTERIAL IDENTIFICATION

Safety Precautions

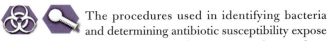 The procedures used in identifying bacteria and determining antibiotic susceptibility expose the technician to the organisms and reagents used to perform the tests. All safety policies, including Standard Precautions and aseptic techniques, must be followed to prevent contamination of the technician, the environment, and others working in the laboratory. Appropriate personal protective equipment (PPE) must be worn. The material safety data sheet (MSDS) accompanying reagents must be read by all personnel using the reagents.

Quality Assessment

Accurate bacterial identification and antibiotic susceptibility testing is essential in order for correct treatment to be administered. All quality assessment policies of the facility must be followed. Reagents, kits, or supplies must not be used beyond their expiration dates. Manufacturers' instructions for the use of bacterial identification systems and interpretation of antibiotic susceptibility must be followed. Control organisms must be tested at set intervals to ensure that antibiotic disks and reagents are reacting as expected.

Cultures of improperly collected urine can grow out three or more different organisms, making it difficult to determine which organism is causing infection. Many laboratories have a policy that, in these cases, the specimen will not be processed beyond the colony count. Each facility's standard operating procedure (SOP) manual must be followed.

Gram Stain and Selective Media Results

Observations of growth on the blood agar (BA) plate and the selective or indicator medium plate will give clues as to what type of organism is present. Gram-negative organisms will grow on BA as well as EMB and MacConkey's (MAC). Gram-positive organisms will grow only on the BA (Figure 7-51). Microscopic examination of a Gram stain performed on a colony will confirm the Gram reaction and will reveal or confirm the bacterial morphology—coccus or rod (bacillus). Growth characteristics can

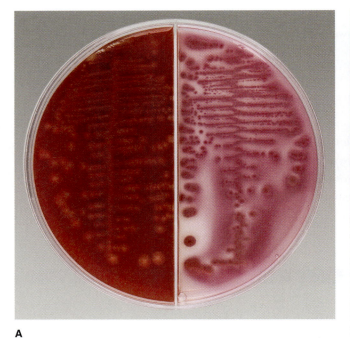

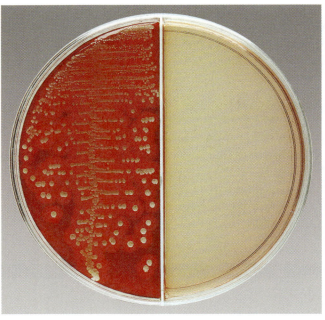

A   **B**

FIGURE 7-51 Bacterial growth on selective media: (A) *Escherichia coli* (Gram negative) and (B) *Staphylococcus aureus* (Gram positive) inoculated to split plates of blood agar (left side of plates) and MAC (right side of plates). Blood agar supports growth of both organisms; MAC selects for Gram negatives (*Courtesy Remel, Inc., Lenexa, KS*)

also be observed, such as whether the organism grows in clusters or chains or is **pleomorphic**, that is, has varied shapes.

Identification of Gram-Positive Bacteria

If an isolate is found to be a Gram-positive coccus, a **catalase test** must be run to determine if the organisms are *Staphylococcus* or *streptococcus* species. Staphylococci are catalase positive and streptococci are catalase negative. If the catalase test is positive and the organisms are Gram-positive cocci arranged in grape-like clusters, a **coagulase test** can help differentiate between *Staphylococcus aureus* and other *Staphylococcus* species. Latex agglutination tests can also be used to identify *S. aureus*.

Catalase Test

To perform the catalase test, a small portion of a colony is picked up with a sterile applicator stick and placed in a drop of 3% hydrogen peroxide on a clean microscope slide. The technician must be careful not to pick up blood agar since the hemoglobin in the blood will react with the catalase and cause a false positive reaction.

If bubbles appear within 10 seconds, the organism is catalase positive and can be presumptively identified as *Staphyloccus* species (Figure 7-52). Depending on the facility's microbiology reporting procedure, the report might read: "Gram-positive cocci morphologically resembling *Staphylococcus*, catalase positive." A positive catalase test should be followed by a coagulase test.

The absence of bubbles is a negative catalase test and is indicative of *Streptococcus* species. The result might be reported as "Gram-positive cocci, morphologically resembling *Streptococcus* species, catalase negative."

Coagulase Test

The coagulase test is used to differentiate between *S. aureus* and other staphylococci. Pathogenic staphylococci produce the enzyme coagulase that will cause fibrinogen in plasma to clot. The coagulase test can be performed by the slide or tube method, but the tube method is more reliable. Negative coagulase slide tests should be confirmed by a coagulase tube test.

A small amount of culture is mixed with a commercial *coagulase plasma* (rabbit plasma) on a slide or in a small test tube. The slide is examined for presence of clumping, which is a positive result. The inoculated tube is incubated at 37°C and checked each hour to see if the plasma has formed a fibrin clot, or solidified (Figure 7-53). It is important to check every hour because some *S. aureus* can also produce an enzyme that dissolves clots, causing a false-negative result.

A positive coagulase test could be reported as "Gram-positive cocci morphologically resembling *Staphylococcus*, coagulase positive." This is a presumptive identification of *S. aureus*.

A coagulase-negative organism would be reported as "Gram-positive cocci morphologically resembling *Staphylococcus* species, coagulase negative." This result indicates the organism is not *S. aureus* and could be *S. saprophyticus*, a common Gram-positive organism involved in urinary tract infections (UTIs).

Latex Agglutination Tests

Several latex agglutination tests are available to confirm the identification of *S. aureus*. Some examples of these are Staphyloslide by BD BBL, Sure-Vue Color Staph ID Latex Test Kit from Fisher Scientific, and Staphaurex test kit from Remel (Figure 7-54). These kits have colored latex particles coated with human fibrinogen and IgG specific for protein A found in *S. aureus*. A colony suspected of being *S. aureus* is mixed with the reagents on the special slide in the kit. If *S. aureus* is present, the coagulase will react with the fibrinogen and the IgG will react with the protein A to cause clumping. The latex particles are colored so that a positive reaction is easily visible.

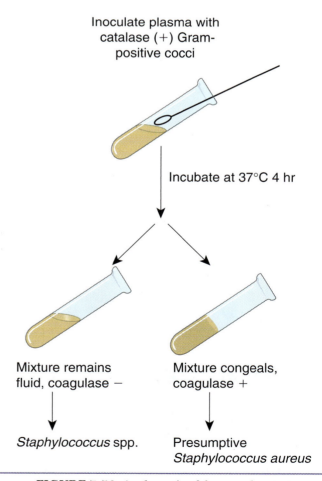

Inoculate plasma with catalase (+) Gram-positive cocci

Incubate at 37°C 4 hr

Mixture remains fluid, coagulase −

Mixture congeals, coagulase +

Staphylococcus spp.

Presumptive *Staphylococcus aureus*

FIGURE 7-53 A schematic of the coagulase test

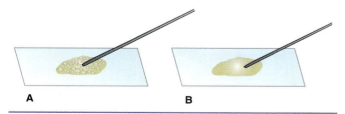

A   **B**

FIGURE 7-52 The catalase test: (A) bubbles indicate a positive test; (B) absence of bubbles indicates a negative test

CURRENT TOPICS

METHICILLIN-RESISTANT STAPHYLOCOCCUS AUREUS

In the nineteenth century, hospitals were increasingly used and extensive surgeries became more common because of the availability of anesthetics. There was an accompanying high mortality from hospital-acquired infections. The causative agent was most often *Streptococcus pyogenes*, but *S. aureus* also caused these infections. At the end of the century, when the antiseptic methods of Lister were implemented, mortality from infected wounds declined. This decline continued into the twentieth century, with *S. aureus* infections being the most common cause of mortality from surgery.

In the 1940s, penicillin, the miracle antibiotic, was introduced. However, by the 1950s penicillin-resistant strains of *S. aureus* developed and were responsible for additional problems in hospital-acquired infections. A particularly virulent strain was prevalent in neonatal units. For unknown reasons, this strain almost disappeared in the 1950s only to be replaced by other less-virulent penicillin-resistant strains. The ability of *S. aureus* strains to quickly adapt was demonstrated by their development of resistance to newly introduced antibiotics such as streptomycin, tetracycline, chloramphenicol, erythromycin, and others.

The medical community became disenchanted with antibiotic therapy until new forms of penicillin, such as methicillin and cloxicillin, were developed. Over the next few years, outbreaks of methicillin-resistant *S. aureus* (MRSA) were reported in Europe. The most severe infections were treated with vancomycin, a highly toxic drug. Then, in the 1970s, the number of serious infections caused by MRSA dropped dramatically along with the incidence of it in the hospitalized population. In 1970, the incidence of MRSA in the noses of patients was 8.0%, but by 1977 the incidence had dropped to 0.7%.

In the next few years, MRSA returned with a vengeance; in the 1980s a new epidemic strain emerged and spread around the world. The increase has continued into the twenty-first century. Some strains of MRSA have acquired a resistance to vancomycin. Although rare, this resistance is causing serious concern in the world medical community, since vancomycin is currently the last line of antibiotic defense against MRSA.

Methicillin resistance in *S. aureus* is due to the presence of cell wall proteins called Penicillin Binding Proteins (PBPs) which bind penicillin and prevent it from acting on the bacteria. Rapid tests to identify methicillin-resistant *S. aureus* are based on detection of these proteins (Figure 7-55).

The Centers for Disease Control and Prevention (CDC) has an active role in investigating, tracking, and characterizing strains of MRSA. It has been found that there is a growing incidence of MRSA infections in long-term care facilities. It also occurs in home-bound patients who develop bed sores. This makes it imperative that caretakers change gloves and observe careful handwashing between patients to avoid the rapid spread of the infection to the other debilitated patients.

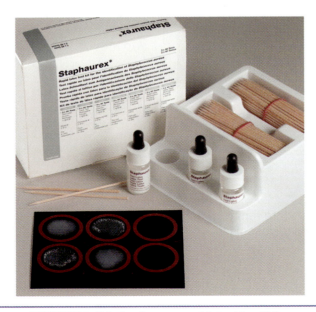

FIGURE 7-54 Staphaurex test kit for identifying *Staphylococcus aureus* (*Courtesy Remel, Inc., Lenexa, KS*)

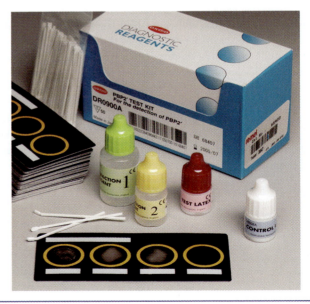

FIGURE 7-55 PBP2 test kit for identifying methicillin-resistant *Staphylococcus aureus* (MRSA) (*Courtesy Remel, Inc., Lenexa, KS*)

Identification of Gram-Negative Bacteria

Bacterial growth on EMB or MAC should be observed after overnight incubation to presumptively identify any Gram-negative rods that have grown. A Gram stain of bacteria growing on EMB or MAC should confirm that bacteria are Gram-negative, since both media inhibit growth of Gram-positive organisms.

Many Gram-negative microorganisms have a characteristic colony appearance on selective and indicator media. *Klebsiella* species has distinctive, bubblegum pink, mucoid colonies. *Escherichia coli* forms a green metallic sheen on EMB (Figure 7-56) and can be reported as "Gram-negative rods, **coliform** by EMB." Coliform refers to certain Gram-negative intestinal bacteria.

The physician can treat the patient on the basis of these preliminary reports and then check the results of antibiotic susceptibility tests to be sure that the prescribed antibiotic will be effective. However, the physician also may request a definitive identification of the isolated organism.

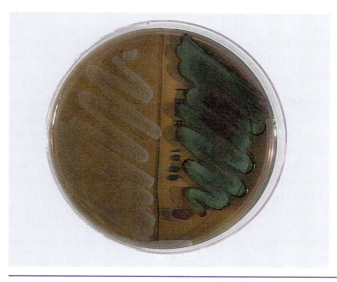

FIGURE 7-56 Metallic sheen produced by coliform bacteria (right half of plate) growing on EMB agar

Manual Bacterial Identification Systems

Both manual and automated systems are used to identify bacteria. Larger hospitals and reference laboratories use automated systems because of the high volume of cultures performed. Manual systems are used in smaller, low-volume laboratories or as backup to automated systems in larger laboratories. Manual systems contain several biochemical tests in a strip or tube (Figure 7-57). A single colony or a specific bacterial suspension of an organism is used to inoculate the test system.

API Microbial Identification Strips

The API systems consist of a flat tray with a series of wells containing reagents to test the organism for biochemical reactions such as fermentation of certain sugars. There are several types of API strips (Figure 7-57A). A few examples are API 20 E (Gram negatives), STAPH (staphylococci), and API 20 STREP (streptococci). A standardized suspension of the organism to be tested is added into the wells of the strip and the strip is then incubated for the prescribed time, usually 18 to 24 hours. The API 20 STREP can be read at 4 hours and again at 24 hours. The reactions are recorded and the organism is identified using an identification key. For quality control the company markets the API 20 E Reagent QC Test, which is used to check the reactivity of the reagents used in the strips.

Enterotube II

The Enterotube II (BD BBL) is used for rapid differential identification of Gram-negative bacteria (Figure 7-57B). It contains 15 tests, such as fermentation of certain sugars and other biochemical reactions. The inoculation is made with a single colony, the system is incubated for 18 to 24 hours at 37°C, and the results are read. The technician records the results of the biochemical reactions and uses an interpretation guide or key to make the identification.

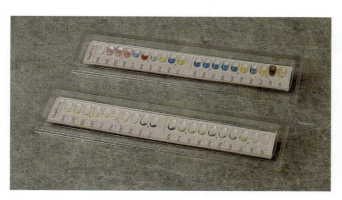

A

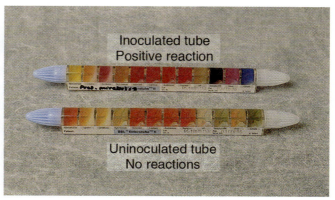

Inoculated tube
Positive reaction

Uninoculated tube
No reactions

B

FIGURE 7-57 Manual bacterial identification systems: (A) the API identification system; (B) Enterotube II

Automated Bacterial Identification Systems

Three automated systems are the MicroScan Walk-Away (Dade-Behring), the Phoenix (Becton Dickinson Diagnostic Systems), and the VITEK-2 (bioMérieux). These instruments use various methods to detect biochemical reactions and antibiotic susceptibility of organisms (Figure 7-58). Some measure turbidity to detect patterns of susceptibility or resistance to antimicrobials. Others use fluorometry and/or colorimetry to detect Gram-positive and Gram-negative bacteria.

ANTIBIOTIC SUSCEPTIBILITY TESTS

When a culture and antibiotic susceptibility test is requested, the susceptibility of the isolate(s) is assessed by exposing the organism to varying concentrations of antibiotics. Historically this has been accomplished manually using the method of Bauer and Kirby. Additional methods available are the semi-automated **minimum inhibitory concentration (MIC)** and fully automated MIC methods on instruments that also perform bacterial identification. The MIC is the minimum concentration of antibiotic required to inhibit growth of a particular microorganism.

Automated and Semi-Automated Methods

Larger laboratories with high volumes of cultures that require identification and susceptibility can use automated methods for determining both. Examples are the MicroScan Walk-Away (Dade-Behring), the Phoenix (Becton Dickinson Diagnostic Systems), and the VITEK-2 (bioMérieux). These instruments greatly increase the efficiency of the technicians working in hospital and reference laboratories.

Several instruments suitable for use in smaller laboratories are available that perform the MIC test. These instruments require that the technician make a standardized suspension of the organism and add it to wells in a microplate. Predetermined dilu-

tions of selected antibiotics are added to the inoculated wells. The plate is inserted into the instrument to incubate. At the end of the incubation time, the instrument reads the plates (Figure 7-59). Wells with no growth (susceptible to antibiotic) will be clear, and wells with bacterial growth (resistant to the particular antibiotic) will be turbid. The antibiotic susceptibility for each drug tested is reported as the MIC.

Manual Methods of Antibiotic Susceptibility

Manual methods of performing susceptibility tests involve streaking a Mueller-Hinton agar plate with a dilution of the culture to be tested. Disks or strips containing antibiotics are placed on the surface of the agar. After incubation the plate is checked to see which antibiotic inhibits growth of the particular organism.

Bauer-Kirby Susceptibility Test

The Bauer-Kirby test is a mainstay of smaller laboratories. It does not require the purchase of expensive equipment. The supplies for the test are readily available. Difficult or resistant organisms can be sent to a reference laboratory for further study.

Performing the Bauer-Kirby Test. To perform the Bauer-Kirby antibiotic susceptibility test, a standardized suspension is made of the organism in soy broth. The turbidity of the broth suspension is compared to a standard suspension, such as a McFarland's standard, available commercially in sets of varying concentrations. Alternatively, commercial kits such as the Prompt by BD-BBL can be used to standardize the procedure.

The suspension is thoroughly mixed just before use. A sterile swab is wet in the suspension, pressed against the inside of the tube to express any excess fluid, and then used to streak the surface of a Mueller-Hinton plate.

The entire plate is streaked by beginning at the top edge and making continuous streaks all the way across the agar to the bottom edge (Figure 7-60). The plate is then turned 90 degrees and streaked from the top edge all the way to the bottom edge,

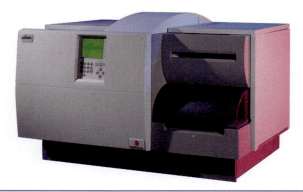

FIGURE 7-58 The VITEK-2 fully automated microbiology identification system (*Courtesy bioMérieux, Inc.*)

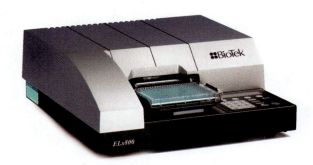

FIGURE 7-59 MIC plate reader system showing the welled plate (*Courtesy BioTek Instruments, Inc.*)

resulting in an almost continuous mat of growth after incubation. This is called a *lawn*.

The antibiotic disks, which are paper disks impregnated with antibiotics, are placed on the surface of the Mueller-Hinton agar while the surface of the plate is still wet from the inoculum. If only a small number of tests are being performed, sterile forceps are used to place the selected antibiotic disks. Disks should be evenly spaced in a circular pattern around the outer edge of the agar. Disk dispensers that dispense a set of 12 or more disks at a time are available from Difco and BBL (Figure 7-61). The disks must be well-tamped down onto the surface of the agar, so they will not fall off when the plate is turned upside down to incubate overnight.

Interpreting the Bauer-Kirby Test.
After overnight incubation at 35°C to 37°C, the plates are read for inhibition of growth around the antibiotic disks (Figure 7-62). The zones of inhibition can be measured using calipers, a ruler (Figure 7-63), or transparent templates with pre-printed zones for each antibiotic such as the Zone Interpretation Overlay Set by BBL.

Each antibiotic produces a specific zone size for each organism. The zone size is used to classify the organism as *sensitive (S)*, *resistant (R)*, or *intermediate (I)*, based on information in the package insert provided with each cartridge of antibiotic disks. The organism is said to be intermediate if the zone size is between sensitive and resistant.

AB Biodisk E

This method is similar to the traditional disk method in that a Mueller-Hinton plate is streaked with the organism to be tested. However, the antibiotics are contained on rectangular strips (Epsilometer) of plastic that are placed on the inoculated plate radiating out from the center. Each strip contains just one antibiotic. The strips contain a predefined continuous exponential gradient of antibiotic concentrations that correspond to MIC dilutions. Each strip has its own reading and interpretive scale.

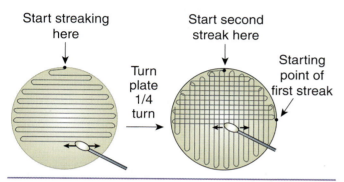

FIGURE 7-60 Streaking the Mueller-Hinton plate

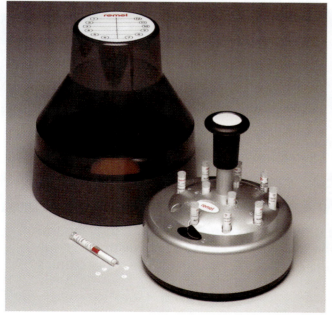

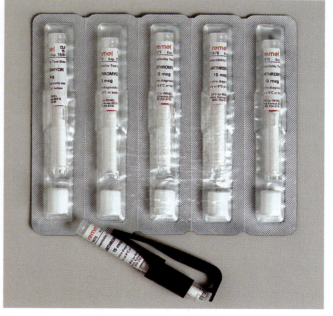

FIGURE 7-61 Antibiotic disk dispensers: (A) multi-disk dispenser; and (B) single antibiotic disk cartridge with ejector (*Courtesy Remel, Inc., Lenexa, KS*)

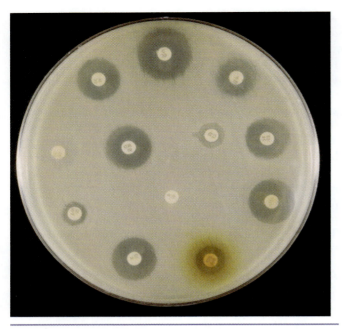

FIGURE 7-62 Antibiotic susceptibility plate showing zones of inhibition after 18 to 24 hour incubation

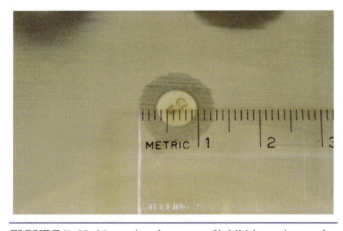

FIGURE 7-63 Measuring the zones of inhibition using a ruler

SAFETY Reminders

- Review safety section before beginning procedure.
- Observe Standard Precautions.
- Wear a fluid-resistant, buttoned laboratory coat.
- Consult MSDS for any reagents used.
- Avoid aerosol formation.
- Wipe work surfaces with disinfectant before beginning work, when finished, and every time a spill occurs.

PROCEDURAL Reminders

- Review quality assessment section before beginning procedure.
- Consult the facility's manual for the procedure to follow if three or more colony types are present in a urine culture.
- Incubate the culture plates upside down.
- Ensure that the Bauer-Kirby suspension is standardized when performing the antibiotic susceptibility test.

CASE STUDY

It was Natalie's day to read and interpret the urine cultures in the microbiology laboratory. When she examined Ms. Gonzalez's BA and EMB plates, she saw two distinct colony types on the BA plate and only one type on the EMB plate. Natalie counted 74 colonies total on the BA plate which had been streaked using a 0.001 mL loop.

1. What is the colony count on this patient's urine? Explain your answer.
2. What is the probable Gram-stain reaction of the colony(ies) growing on the EMB plate? Explain your answer.
3. Which colonies should be tested for the catalase reaction? Explain.

SUMMARY

The identification of a microorganism and determination of its antibiotic susceptibility can influence the treatment a patient receives for an infection. Bacterial identification can be as simple as observing a Gram-stained smear and performing catalase and coagulase tests, or as complex as processing the specimen in a semi-automated or automated system that can determine both the identity and the antibiotic susceptibility or MIC.

In many circumstances, the technician might be identifying and testing a bacterial culture isolated from urine of a patient suffering from recurrent UTI. The physician may only need to know the presumptive identity of the organism responsible and which antibiotic is effective against the bacterium. However, in cases where a patient is in serious condition from infection with an unknown microorganism, it is imperative that the most expedient methods be employed to confirm the bacterial identification and determine the MIC or antibiotic susceptibility.

All specimens and isolates must be treated as potentially infectious and Standard Precautions must be observed. The quality assessment procedures of the microbiology department must be followed to ensure that the identity and antibiotic susceptibility of the organism causing infection are correctly determined.

REVIEW QUESTIONS

1. What is indicated by the presence of three or more colony types on the BA plate in a urine culture?

2. Why is a correctly performed Gram stain important to the process of identifying bacteria?

3. How is the MIC determined?

4. In the Bauer-Kirby susceptibility test, what is indicated if there is a large area without bacterial growth around a disk?

5. Discuss how to presumptively identify bacteria.

6. Explain the catalase test.

7. Explain the coagulase test.

8. List two automated methods used to identify bacteria.

9. Give an example of a manual method of identifying bacteria by biochemical reactions.

10. Explain how to set up a disk antibiotic susceptibility test.

11. Describe how the zones of inhibition around the disks are measured.

12. Define catalase test, coagulase test, coliform, minimum inhibitory concentration, and pleomorphic.

STUDENT ACTIVITIES

1. Complete the written examination for this lesson.

2. Practice performing bacterial identification and antibiotic susceptibility tests as outlined in the Student Performance Guide.

WEB ACTIVITIES

1. Use the Internet to find recent information on microbial resistance to commonly prescribed antibiotics such as the z-pack, penicillin, or amoxicillin.

2. Use the Internet to go to a Web site such as WebMD; find the names of two antibiotics useful for treatment of urinary tract infections.

3. Use the Internet to find out which antibiotics are used to determine antibiotic susceptibility of both Gram-negative rods and Gram-positive cocci.

Student Performance Guide

LESSON 7-9 Bacterial Identification and Antibiotic Susceptibility Testing

Name _____ Date _____

INSTRUCTIONS

1. Practice performing the bacterial identification and antibiotic susceptibility tests following the step-by-step procedure.

2. Demonstrate the procedure for the antibiotic susceptibility test satisfactorily for the instructor, using the Student Performance Guide. Your instructor will determine the level of competency you must achieve to obtain a satisfactory (S) grade.

MATERIALS AND EQUIPMENT

- gloves
- Mueller-Hinton plates
- trypticase soy broth, 5 mL per tube, or a commercial kit such as Prompt by BBL
- McFarland's standard #2 or a commercial system for producing a standard suspension
- wax pencil or marking pen
- electric incinerator
- incubator set at 35°C to 37°C
- antibiotic disks (ampicillin, augmentin, norfloxacin, nitrofurantoin, trimethoprim, bactrim, and cephalothin are often used for urines)

- disk dispenser
- forceps
- calipers, ruler, or template to measure zones of inhibition
- sterile swabs
- culture plate from colony count, Lesson 7-8, or bacterial cultures growing on blood agar plates:
  — culture of *E. coli*, nonpathogenic strain
  — culture of Gram-positive coccus (*Streptococcus* or *Staphylococcus* sp.)
- materials for identification of Gram-positive bacteria
  — microscope slides
  — 3% hydrogen peroxide
  — sterile applicators
  — coagulase plasma and 13mm × 75mm test tubes (or use commercial kit)
- surface disinfectant
- antiseptic
- biohazard container
- sharps container

PROCEDURE

Record in the comment section any problems encountered while practicing the procedure (or have a fellow student or the instructor evaluate your performance).

S = Satisfactory
U = Unsatisfactory

You must:	S	U	Comments
1. Assemble materials and equipment			
2. Turn on the electric incinerator. Wash hands and put on gloves			

You must:	S	U	Comments
3. Write the identification on the bottom of Mueller-Hinton plate			

4. Prepare a bacterial suspension using broth and McFarland's standard #2 (or following the manufacturer's instructions if using a commercial system):
  a. Use sterile swab to pick up a few colonies from the culture plate
  b. Remove cap from broth and insert swab into broth, gently swishing the swab around to make a slightly turbid suspension of bacteria
  c. Compare with McFarland's #2 standard
  d. Press the swab against the side of the tube to express excess liquid. Replace cap on broth tube and set tube in rack			

5. Use the swab to streak the Mueller-Hinton agar: Starting at the top edge of the agar, make horizontal streaks the whole width of the plate, from top to bottom			
6. Turn the plate 90 degrees and streak from top to bottom, using the same swab; the agar surface should be almost completely covered with the broth inoculum (Figure 7-60)			
7. Discard swab into biohazard container			
8. Place antibiotic disks on the surface of the still-wet agar using either a disk dispenser or sterile forceps			
9. Sterilize the forceps (if used) and return them to storage. Turn off electric incinerator			
10. Replace the petri dish lid and incubate the plate upside down at 35°C to 37°C overnight (18 to 24 hours)			

11. Perform presumptive identification of Gram-positive colonies growing on the urine culture plate or use culture provided by instructor
  a. Perform Gram stain on a colony from the culture plate to confirm that the colony is Gram positive
  b. Perform the catalase test to distinguish *Streptococcus* from *Staphylococcus*:
    1) Place a small drop of 3% hydrogen peroxide on a microscope slide
    2) Pick up a tiny portion of the Gram-positive colony using a sterile applicator and mix the bacteria into the peroxide drop. Take care to avoid transferring any culture medium to the slide
    3) Observe for production of gas bubbles. After 10 seconds record as catalase positive (bubbles produced) or catalase negative (no bubbles produced). A positive reaction indicates a presumptive identification of *Staphylococcus* species; a negative reaction indicates a presumptive identification of *Streptococcus*			

You must:	S	U	Comments
c. Perform the coagulase test on a catalase-positive colony: 1) Remove the cap from the prepared rabbit plasma and mix a small amount of a catalase-positive colony into the plasma 2) Place the inoculated tube into a 37°C incubator for 4 hours 3) Check tube every hour to see if the plasma has clotted (solidified). If clotting occurs, report as "Gram-positive coccus morphologically resembling *Staphylococcus*, coagulase positive." This is a presumptive identification of *Staphylococcus aureus* 4) Report non-clotted tests as "Gram-positive coccus morphologically resembling *Staphylococcus* species, coagulase negative." This result indicates that the organism is a *Staphylococcus* species other than *Staphylococcus aureus*			
12. Remove gloves and wash hands with antiseptic			
13. The next day: Wash hands and put on gloves			
14. Remove Mueller-Hinton plate from incubator and observe for zones of inhibition through bottom of plate			
15. Measure zones, using a metric ruler, calipers, or a special transparent template			
16. Record the susceptibility of the organism to each antibiotic disk as sensitive (S), resistant (R), or intermediate (I), following the guidelines included on the package insert for each disk cartridge or the template markings			
17. Discard all contaminated materials into appropriate biohazard or sharps container			
18. Clean equipment and return to storage			
19. Wipe counter with surface disinfectant			
20. Remove gloves and discard in biohazard container			
21. Wash hands with antiseptic			

Evaluator Comments:

Evaluator _____ Date _____

7-10

Laboratory Detection of Sexually Transmitted Diseases

LESSON OBJECTIVES

After studying this lesson, the student will:

- Explain the importance of early detection of sexually transmitted diseases (STDs).
- Discuss the steady increase in the incidence of certain STDs.
- Explain why it is important for physician office laboratories and other small laboratories to be knowledgeable about STD testing.
- Discuss four basic types of tests used to detect STDs.
- List five STDs common in the United States.
- Name one method of detection for each of the five common STDs.
- Discuss the need for confirmatory tests for certain STDs.
- Explain the safety precautions that must be followed when performing tests for STDs.
- Discuss the quality assessment procedures involved in testing for STDs.
- Define the glossary terms.

GLOSSARY

Candida albicans / yeast that causes vaginitis and other infections, especially following antibiotic therapy

Chlamydia trachomatis / species of Gram-negative intracellular bacteria that is a cause of STDs

clue cells / vaginal epithelial cells covered with tiny, Gram-variable bacteria and seen in vaginal secretions of patients with bacterial vaginosis

gonorrhea / contagious infection spread by sexual contact and caused by *Neisseria gonorrhoeae*

herpes simplex virus, type 1 (HSV-1) / the virus causing oral herpes

herpes simplex virus, type 2 (HSV-2) / the virus causing genital herpes

human immunodeficiency virus (HIV) / the retrovirus that has been identified as the cause of AIDS

human papilloma virus (HPV) / a group of viruses, some of which are sexually transmitted

nongonococcal urethritis / gonorrhea-like STD caused by organisms other than gonococci

oxidase test / an enzyme test used to identify certain bacteria such as *Neisseria*

spirochetes / motile, helical or spiral bacteria of the family Spirochaeta

STD / sexually transmitted disease

syphilis / an infectious, chronic, sexually transmitted disease caused by a spirochete, *Treponema pallidum*

trichomoniasis / a sexually transmitted genitourinary tract infection caused by the parasitic protozoan, *Trichomonas vaginalis*

urethritis / infection or inflammation of the urethra

vaginitis / infection or inflammation of the vagina

venereal / having to do with, or transmitted by, sexual contact

INTRODUCTION

Sexually transmitted diseases (**STDs**) are transmitted primarily through sexual intercourse or other intimate contact. This lesson introduces basic laboratory methods used to detect STDs in males and females. STDs can be caused by bacteria, protozoa, fungi, or viruses. As sexual practices change, many microorganisms once limited to the genitourinary tract are found in other sites in the body. Tests for STDs should not be limited to specimens from the genitourinary tract. For example, in suspected cases of gonorrhea, urethral, rectal, and pharyngeal swabs can be collected.

Common STDs detected in the United States are Chlamydial infections, gonorrhea, herpes, hepatitis B, trichomoniasis, syphilis, HIV infection, human papilloma virus infection, and candidiasis (Table 7-25). In the United States, the incidence of STD cases rose dramatically until the appearance of AIDS in the 1980s. STDs then began to decline, and have continued to decline except for certain diseases, such as chlamydial infection, which continues to rise.

Formerly, most STD testing was performed in hospital or state public health laboratories because of the complexity of testing methods. A number of procedures are still performed in these larger laboratories, but several simple-to-use diagnostic kits that produce reliable results have been developed for detecting various STD agents. Many of these diagnostic methods are suitable for use in physician office laboratories (POLs).

Symptoms of Sexually Transmitted Diseases

Venereal disease, or STD, can have long-lasting effects in both males and females. In males, STDs usually produce symptoms such as a penile discharge or burning upon urination. However, evidence indicates that more males than previously thought can be positive for STDs, although asymptomatic. Any male whose sex partner is positive for an STD must be tested or treated. Females can be asymptomatic and go untreated for some STDs, a factor important in disease transmission and in infertility for many women.

DETECTION OF STDs IN FEMALES

Female patients may be tested for STDs because of findings during a routine examination and reporting of symptoms, or because a partner has tested positive for STDs. Many STDs cause **vaginitis**, an infection or inflammation of the vagina. Vaginitis can be caused by bacteria, fungi, or protozoa. Bacteria and yeast infections may occur because of changes in the vaginal pH or alteration in normal flora. Some of the most common organisms are *Gardnerella vaginalis* (formerly *Hemophilus vaginalis*), *Mobiluncus* species, *Streptococcus* group B, *Chlamydia trachomatis*, *Neisseria gonorrhoeae*, and *Candida albicans*.

Detection methods include Gram stain, culture, wet mounts, serum antibody tests, immunoassays, and DNA probes. Table 7-26 gives examples of STD detection methods.

The Three-Slide Test for Vaginitis

The three-slide test is an important part of discovering the cause of vaginitis. A relatively simple procedure, most of its results can be available in about 30 minutes, while the patient is still in the office. It is a Clinical Laboratory Improvement Amendments (CLIA)-waived physician-performed microscopy procedure (PPMP) test. Components of the three-slide test include:

- Saline wet mount preparation of vaginal secretions for *Trichomonas* and clue cells

TABLE 7-25. Common STDs detected in the United States and their causative agents

DISEASE	AGENT
Chlamydial infection	*Chlamydia trachomatis*
Genital warts	Human papilloma virus (HPV)
Gonorrhea	*Neisseria gonorrhoeae*
Herpes, type 1	Herpes simplex virus, type 1 (HSV-1)
Herpes, type 2	Herpes simplex virus, type 2 (HSV-2)
Hepatitis B	Hepatitis B virus (HBV)
HIV infection	Human immunodeficiency virus (HIV)
Trichomoniasis	*Trichomonas vaginalis*
Candidiasis	*Candida albicans*
Syphilis	*Treponema pallidum*

TABLE 7-26. STDs and examples of tests available for their detection

DISEASE	TEST METHODS
Chlamydial infection	EIA, ELISA, DNA probe, cell culture, FA
Gonorrhea	Culture, Gram stain, DNA probe, monoclonal antibody agglutination test
Herpes	Cell culture, EIA, serology for IgG and IgM
Candidiasis	KOH wet prep, culture, Gram stain, rapid chemical confirmation test
Trichomoniasis	Saline wet prep, antibody agglutination
Syphilis	
Screen	VDRL, RPR
Confirmatory	FTA-ABS, MHA-TP, direct smear
HIV infection	
Screen	EIA for anti-HIV-1
Confirmatory	Western blot, culture, p24 antigen
Hepatitis B	Anti-HBcAg (acute), anti-HBsAg (chronic), or hepatitis panel

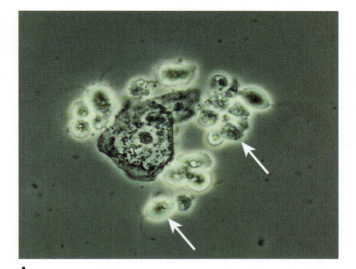

A

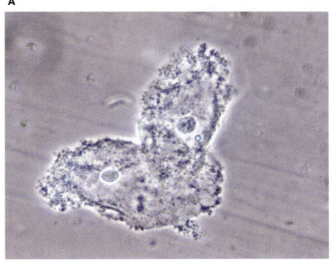

B

FIGURE 7-64 Saline wet mounts: (A) wet mount of vaginal discharge, showing *Trichomonas vaginalis* protozoa (arrows); (B) clue cells, vaginal epithelial cells covered with bacteria, indicating bacterial vaginosis (*From CDC, Atlanta, GA*)

- KOH (potassium hydroxide) preparation of vaginal secretions for yeasts and fungi

- Gram stain of endocervical secretions for bacteria and yeasts

Specimens for other tests can be collected at the same time, such as a swab for *N. gonorrhoeae* culture, or a swab for *C. trachomatis* or *N. gonorrhoeae* DNA probe tests. If suspected herpes lesions are present, a specimen can be collected from the lesions and sent to the reference laboratory in viral transport medium.

Saline Wet Preparation

The saline wet prep is prepared by mixing a drop of vaginal specimen with a drop of 0.85% saline on a microscope slide and adding a coverslip. A depression slide can also be used. The physician may examine the slide microscopically in the examination room or send it to the laboratory. It must be examined within 30 minutes of collection to detect *Trichomonas vaginalis*, a parasitic protozoan, which causes **trichomoniasis**. If *Gardnerella vaginalis* is present, **clue cells**, which are vaginal epithelial cells covered with the bacteria, may also be seen (Figure 7-64).

KOH Preparation

A drop of vaginal material is mixed with one to two drops of 10% KOH solution on a microscope slide or in a depression slide to look for fungi that can cause vaginitis, such as **Candida albicans**.

The KOH destroys structures such as epithelial cells and white blood cells; any fungi present will appear as tangled masses resembling hairs or threads (Figure 7-65).

Gram Stain

The swab used to inoculate the media for *Neisseria* culture can be used to prepare the smear for Gram stain. (The smear and staining procedures are described in Lesson 7-6.) The smear is Gram-stained and examined for the presence of bacteria and pus cells (white blood cells) using the oil-immersion objective of the microscope. Smears from uninfected females should have a moderate amount of *Lactobacillus* (Gram-positive rods), few or no white blood cells, and few epithelial cells (Figure 7-66A).

The smear is examined for the presence of *N. gonorrhoeae*, a Gram-negative, kidney bean–shaped diplococcus that causes gonorrhea. The organism can be found both inside neutrophilic leukocytes (intracellular) and also extracellular on smears from infected patients (Figure 7-67).

G. vaginalis is a Gram-variable microorganism, which means it may stain either Gram-negative or Gram-positive. If present on the smear, the tiny organisms will be scattered over the other constituents on the smear, especially the vaginal epithelial cells. If yeast cells are present, they will stain dark purple (Figure 7-66B).

Neisseria gonorrhoeae Culture

A sterile rayon or Dacron swab is used to collect the specimen for culture of *N. gonorrhoeae*, the organism that causes gonorrhea. The swab is used to streak the modified Thayer-Martin (MTM) agar in

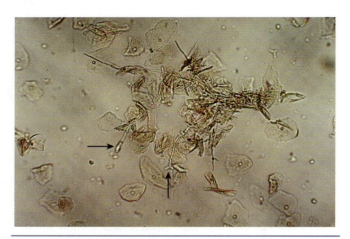

FIGURE 7-65 Vaginal smear showing fungal elements indicated by arrows (*From CDC, Atlanta, GA*)

the shape of a *Z* or a *W*. The culture must be transported to the laboratory where the plate is cross-streaked using a sterile loop (Figure 7-68). The culture plate is immediately placed in an increased carbon dioxide (CO_2) environment and incubated at 35°C to 37°C to prevent loss of viability of any organisms present.

Rapid Tests for Vaginitis and Vaginosis

Many rapid diagnostic tests are available for detection of organisms responsible for vaginosis and vaginitis. The tests are performed directly from the specimen swab. For example, the Genzyme OSOM BV BLUE kit for bacterial vaginosis/vaginitis (BV) can detect *Gardnerella vaginalis*, *Bacterioides* spp., *Prevotela*, and *Mobiluncus* spp. in less than 10 minutes. The Quidel Quick Vue ADVANCE is specific for *G. vaginalis*. Quidel also has a CLIA-waived kit for vaginal pH and presence of amines. One instrument, the BD Affirm VPIII, uses RNA probe technology to detect organisms causing BV. This method can detect *Candida* sp., *G. vaginalis*, and *T. vaginalis* from the same specimen swab.

DETECTION OF STDs IN MALES

Male STD patients usually have symptoms of **urethritis**, an inflammation of the urethra. The major symptoms are a burning sensation on urination or the presence of a penile discharge. Tests may include a urinalysis and culture, a Gram stain, a culture or DNA probe test for *N. gonorrhoeae*, immunoassay or DNA probe for *C. trachomatis*, and serology tests for herpes simplex virus (HSV), HIV, and syphilis.

Males also sometimes develop a *nonspecific* or **nongonococcal urethritis** in which the organisms causing the condition

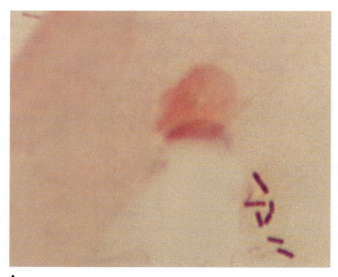

A

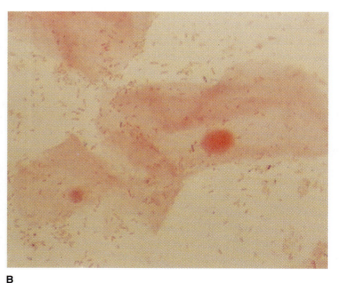

B

FIGURE 7-66 Gram-stained vaginal smears: (A) Gram positive lactobacilli (normal flora); (B) vaginal smear from patient with bacterial vaginosis (BV), showing clue cells with large numbers of small Gram-variable organisms, morphologically resembling *Gardnerella vaginalis*

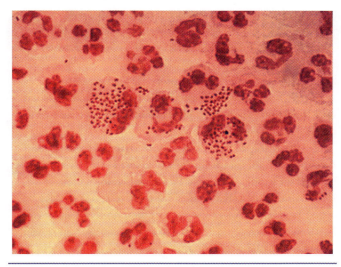

FIGURE 7-67 Gram-negative diplococci. Gram-stained vaginal smear showing white blood cells with intracellular Gram-negative diplococci, morphologically resembling *Neisseria gonorrhoeae*

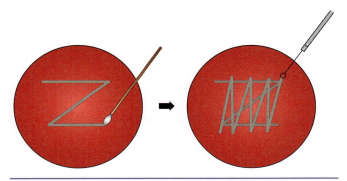

FIGURE 7-68 Cross-streaking the Thayer-Martin plate for vaginal culture

cannot be identified. In these cases, the patient is treated for the standard microorganisms usually implicated in urethritis.

Urinalysis and Urine Culture

If symptoms indicate possible STDs in a male patient, the specimens for those tests should be collected before the patient collects the urine sample.

The results of the urinalysis can help determine if the symptoms are due to urinary tract infection (UTI) or STD. If the midstream urine specimen contains red blood cells, bacteria, white blood cells, or protein, the patient may have a UTI instead of an STD. The results of urine culture can be used to confirm the urine microscopic findings. If the urine culture results are negative, the problems may be due to an STD.

Urethral Culture

The urethral discharge is collected on a urogenital swab and cultured for *N. gonorrhoeae*. It is inoculated onto an MTM plate

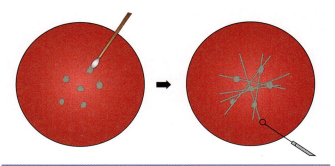

FIGURE 7-69 Cross-streaking a Thayer-Martin plate for urethral culture

by touching the urogenital swab to the plate five or six times. The plate is transported to the laboratory immediately, where it is cross-streaked using a sterile loop and placed into a 35°C to 37°C incubator in an increased CO_2 environment (Figure 7-69).

Urethral Gram Stain

A smear of the urethral discharge is made using the swab used for the culture. The smear is Gram-stained in the laboratory and examined microscopically. The entire smear is searched for evidence of bacteria, especially *N. gonorrhoeae*, other microorganisms, and white blood cells. The presence of many white blood cells is a strong indicator of bacterial infection.

IDENTIFICATION OF *NEISSERIA*

Appearance of Colonies

After overnight incubation, the Thayer-Martin plate is examined for bacterial growth. *N. gonorrhoeae* appear as tiny, shiny, grayish colonies growing along the streak pattern. If scant or no growth is present, the plate is incubated for an additional 24 hours. Other bacteria and yeasts can also grow on Thayer-Martin.

Confirmatory Tests from Culture

The **oxidase test** can be used to aid in identifying colonies of *N. gonorrhoeae*, an oxidase-positive organism. A purple-black color forms when oxidase-positive colonies are exposed to the oxidase reagent. If a suspected *Neisseria* colony gives a positive oxidase reaction, a smear and Gram stain should be performed on one of the oxidase-positive colonies. The presence of Gram-negative diplococci on the smear is presumptive for *N. gonorrhoeae* and a confirmatory test must be performed.

Several systems are available to confirm identification of *N. gonorrhoeae*. Examples are Dupont's Gonochek II that identifies *N. gonorrhoeae*, *N. lactima*, and *N. meningitidis*, and GonoGen (Becton Dickinson Microbiology Systems), a 15-minute agglutination test. DNA and RNA probe methods are also used to identify *Neisseria* species.

C U R R E N T   T O P I C S

HUMAN PAPILLOMA VIRUS

Human papilloma virus (HPV) infects the genital skin and mucus membranes of men and women. More than 30 of approximately 100 types of the virus are sexually transmitted. Most infected individuals have no symptoms, are unaware that they are infected, and unknowingly pass it on to their sexual partners. Most people clear the infection on their own within 2 years. However, some of these viruses are classified as high-risk types and can cause malignant tumors, leading to cancer of the cervix, vulva, vagina, anus, or penis. These high-risk types can also cause women to have abnormal Papanicolaou (Pap) smears that are indicative of the infection. According to the American Cancer Society, about 10,500 women develop cervical cancer each year and 3,900 die from it. Low-risk HPV types cause mild Pap smear abnormalities or genital warts, single or multiple growths or bumps in the genital area that are sometimes cauliflower shaped.

Approximately 20 million people in the United States are currently infected with HPV. At least 50% of sexually active men and women will acquire HPV at some point. By age 50 at least 80% of women will have acquired a genital HPV infection. About 6.2 million Americans get a new genital HPV infection each year.

According to the Centers for Disease Control and Prevention (CDC), a specific test to detect HPV DNA should be used for women with mild Pap smear abnormalities. Also, it is recommended that women 30 years of age and older be tested for HPV DNA at the time of their annual Pap smear. In 2006, a vaccine to prevent HPV infection was approved for use in preadolescent girls.

Traditional methods for culturing viruses cannot be used for HPV. Examination of tissue biopsies has been one method of detection, but it is not very specific or sensitive. In 2004 the Food and Drug Administration (FDA) approved a DNA HPV detection method, the HC 2 from Digene. In this test, the HPV DNA is hybridized to RNA probes. These hybrids are detected by a chemiluminescent system. The sensitivity is similar to PCR assays.

Nucleic Acid Methods for Detection of *Neisseria gonorrhoeae*

Several manufacturers have test methods for detecting organisms using RNA or DNA probes or PCR (polymerase chain reaction). PCR is more specific and sensitive but technically more difficult. The BD ProbeTec ET System is a DNA amplification assay. It reduces the time required for sample handling and amplification and produces rapid results in the detection of *N. gonorrhoeae*.

TESTS FOR OTHER STDs

Many types of tests are available for detecting other STDs such as herpes, hepatitis, syphilis, and HIV and chlamydial infections. Methods include negative staining, electron microscopy, fluorescent antibody techniques, enzyme immunoassays (EIAs), serological tests, monoclonal antibody agglutination, and nucleic acid (DNA and RNA) probes (Table 7-26). The physician may order tests for one or more of these other diseases, depending on the patient's symptoms and/or sexual history.

An increasing number of easy-to-use test systems are becoming available, so that more testing can be performed in the smaller laboratory and the physician office laboratory (POL). However, tests for some organisms are more time-consuming, technically advanced, or infrequently performed; specimens for these tests must be sent to a reference laboratory for testing.

Tests for Herpes Infection

Two herpes viruses commonly cause disease in humans. **Herpes simplex virus, type 1 (HSV-1)** causes oral herpes and **herpes simplex virus, type 2 (HSV-2)** causes genital herpes. HSV infections have chronic, painful, recurring episodes.

Two methods of testing for herpes infection are cell culture and detection of serum antibody levels of anti-HSV. If herpes lesions are present, a vesicle can be broken with a sterile swab or needle and the vesicle fluid collected using another sterile swab. The swab is then inserted into viral transport medium and sent to a reference laboratory for culture. Cell culture results are available in 24 to 48 hours.

A sample of the patient's blood can also be sent to a reference laboratory for measurement of serum titers of IgG and IgM to HSV-1 or HSV-2. The titers indicate whether the patient has active herpes or has ever had herpes type 1 or type 2 in the past. Rapid diagnostic tests are available to test for antibodies to HSV-2. The Fisher Sure-Vue test uses a few drops of the patient's blood. The result can be read on the test cassette in 7 to 10 minutes.

Tests for *Chlamydia* Infection

Chlamydia trachomatis infection can be detected by EIA, cell culture, fluorescent antibody (FA), and DNA probes. In the female patient, *C. trachomatis* infection may cause the cervix to bleed easily just from the touch of a swab during examination. The cervix is said to be *friable*.

C. trachomatis infection is a common cause of urethritis in males, especially in young adults. Since urination temporarily flushes out any microorganisms inhabiting the urethra, for best chances of detection, the patient should not have urinated in the 1 to 2 hours before the specimen collection.

There are several tests for *C. trachomatis*. In some DNA probe tests, the same patient swab can be used to test for both *Chlamydia* and *N. gonorrhoeae*. DNA probe tests have high sensitivity and specificity. A piece of DNA with a specific sequence of nucleic acids, called the *probe DNA*, is added to a mixture containing the DNA from any organisms in the patient specimen. If the patient specimen contains the specific organism being tested, the DNA probe will combine with the DNA of the organisms and produce a color or luminescence. This signal will be measured by the instrumentation.

Immunoassay tests are also available for *C. trachomatis*. Two of these are the Premier *Chlamydia* by Meridian and CLEARVIEW *Chlamydia* from Wampole Laboratories. These tests have built-in positive and negative controls. The tests can be used to screen urines for *Chlamydia* in male patients, but their lower urine test sensitivity means negative results should be confirmed by another method. The PathoDX *Chlamydia trachomatis* FA direct test is a fluorescent antibody technique from Remel. This test has the advantage of detecting the organism directly from urethral and endocervical swab specimens.

Each of the various tests has its own instructions and supplies. For example, procedures and supplies will be different for each manufacturer's DNA probe test. The technologist and the clinician must be sure to follow instructions for the method being used.

Tests for Syphilis

Syphilis is the venereal disease caused by *Treponema pallidum*, a **spirochete** or spiral bacterium. Early (primary) syphilis is characterized by skin lesions. Organ or tissue damage occurs in the secondary stage. Late-stage (tertiary) syphilis can affect the cardiovascular and central nervous systems.

Because of the difficulty in growing *Treponema* in culture, the screening method of choice has been detection of serum antibody. The *Venereal Disease Research Laboratory (VDRL)* test and the *rapid plasma reagin (RPR)* test are screening tests for syphilis. The VDRL test can only be performed by laboratories certified in its use. The RPR is a simpler procedure.

The Venereal Disease Research Laboratory Test

Patients infected with *T. pallidum* produce a nonspecific, antibody-like substance called reagin. When the VDRL antigen mixture, made of cardiolipin, cholesterol, and lecithin, is reacted with serum containing reagin, a visible reaction—flocculation—occurs. The test is *reactive* in 70% to 99% of primary and secondary syphilis cases, but is usually nonreactive in tertiary cases.

The Rapid Plasma Reagin Test

The RPR test has a carbon-containing cardiolipin antigen that reacts with the antibody-like substance (reagin) produced in response to syphilis and some other conditions. The RPR is also a flocculation test, with the carbon causing black clumps on a white background in a reactive test. Test results are reported as *reactive* or *nonreactive*. A reactive result is not diagnostic for syphilis, but only indicates the presence of these nonspecific antibodies.

Confirmation of a Reactive Syphilis Screening Test

A *reactive* result in a serum VDRL or RPR screening test must be confirmed by a more specific test method, since *biologic false positives* (BFPs) can occur. Several nonsyphilitic conditions can cause BFPs, including tuberculosis, hepatitis, pneumonia, pregnancy, and rheumatoid arthritis.

The fluorescent treponemal antibody-absorption (FTA-ABS) test is a specific test that uses *Treponema* antigen to detect patient serum *Treponema* antibodies. The *T. pallidum* microhemagglutination assay (MHA-TP) also detects serum antibodies to the syphilis organism. Both the FTA-ABS and the MHA-TP are specific treponemal antigen tests that are used to confirm a reactive RPR or VDRL test. Newer test methods use enzyme-linked immunosorbent assays (ELISAs).

Tests for HIV

Human immunodeficiency virus (HIV) is transmitted sexually and by contact with infectious body fluids. The main approach to HIV testing is to assay for anti-HIV in the patient's serum. Since this antibody usually does not appear until several months to a year after exposure, a negative test must be followed by another test in about 6 months. These tests are usually performed in reference laboratories and state public health laboratories.

Since saliva and urine from HIV-infected patients contain HIV antibodies, tests have been developed to detect HIV antibodies in saliva, urine, and blood. One rapid blood test for antibodies to HIV-1 is the Trinity Biotech Uni-Gold Recombigen HIV test. The test can be performed on whole blood, plasma, or serum. The sample is added to the sample well in the test cassette, and a wash solution is added. Ten minutes later, the result is shown in the result window. The test is CLIA-waived when whole blood is used.

As HIV infections progress, the virus multiplies and can be cultured and isolated. Some tests detect viral components such as the p24 antigen. The p24 antigen can be detected very early after HIV infection, then disappears, and cannot be detected again until the late stages of the disease.

Tests for Hepatitis B Infections

The hepatitis B virus (HBV) can cause serious illness and even be fatal because of its effects on the liver. A patient can remain chronically infected with HBV even when asymptomatic. The chronic infection can lead to liver cancer (hepatocarcinoma).

HBV is highly infectious and can be transmitted through sexual contact, exposure to infectious blood or other body fluids, or exposure to contaminated food. An HBV vaccine is available that provides lifelong immunity for immunocompetent individuals who complete the entire three-shot series. At-risk health care workers must be immunized or must sign a refusal statement waiving employer liability.

A wide range of tests are available for detecting HBV antigens and antibodies. Test methods include radioimmunoassays, EIA, and ELISA. The most common screening test is the test for HBV surface antigen (HBsAg). A positive result indicates the patient has, or recently has had, an acute HBV infection. The finding of HBsAg several months after infection indicates the person is a chronic HBV carrier. The anti-HBsAg titer is used to check for immunity after receiving the HBV vaccine. Detecting antibody to the HBV core antigen (anti-HBcAg) is another test for HBV infection.

SUMMARY

This lesson has introduced basic laboratory methods used to detect STDs. Agents that cause STDs include bacteria, protozoa, fungi, and viruses. Screening tests for STDs and confirmation of positive results were formerly performed only in large hospitals or state or reference laboratories. However, many STD test kits are now available for use in POLs and other smaller laboratories. Rapid tests are available for detection of BV, HSV-2, and antibodies to HIV-1. Use of these rapid tests makes it possible to screen for STDs on-site. Reference or state laboratories are used primarily for confirmation of STD screening tests.

REVIEW QUESTIONS

1. Explain the importance of early detection of STDs.
2. Discuss the correlation between STD incidence and the number of HIV infections.

3. Why should personnel in POLs and other small laboratories be knowledgeable about STDs and the methods used to detect them?
4. List five STDs common in the United States.
5. Name one method of detection for each of five STDs.
6. What does the presence of HBsAg indicate about a patient?
7. What is the danger of chronic HBV infection?
8. Why should patients be tested for both HSV-1 and HSV-2?
9. Define *Candida albicans; Chlamydia trachomatis;* clue cells; gonorrhea; herpes simplex virus, type 1; herpes simplex virus, type 2; human immunodeficiency virus; human papilloma virus; nongonococcal urethritis; oxidase test; spirochetes; STD; syphilis; trichomoniasis; urethritis; vaginitis; and venereal.

STUDENT ACTIVITIES

1. Complete the written examination for this lesson.
2. Survey POLs in your community to find out the extent of STD testing performed.
3. Determine how a nearby reference laboratory confirms positive HIV tests and reactive RPR tests.
4. Tour your state's public health laboratory. Ask for copies of their epidemiology reports on STD incidence in your state.

WEB ACTIVITIES

1. Use the Internet to search for the *Morbidity and Mortality Weekly Reports* (MMWR). Find statistics for the incidence of *Chlamydia* cases for the last 10 years.
2. Use the internet to find information about PCR or DNA and RNA probe technology. Report on the use of one of these technologies in detecting an STD.

Fecal Occult Blood Test

LESSON OBJECTIVES

After studying this lesson, the student will:

- Discuss the purpose of the fecal occult blood test.
- Explain the principle of the guaiac reaction.
- List two causes of false-positive guaiac reactions.
- List one cause of a false-negative guaiac reaction.
- Explain how the immunochemical test (ICT) for occult blood differs from guaiac tests.
- Instruct a patient on how to collect a specimen for the fecal occult blood test.
- Perform a test for fecal occult blood.
- List safety precautions to be observed in performing the fecal occult blood test.
- Discuss the quality assessment procedures and policies that must be followed when performing the fecal occult blood test.
- Define the glossary terms.

GLOSSARY

guaiac / a chemical derived from the resin of the *Guaiacum* tree
malignant / cancerous; not benign
occult / concealed or hidden

INTRODUCTION

The fecal occult blood test is a simple, inexpensive screening test that detects bleeding in the gastrointestinal tract. Although the test is not specific for any disease, it is widely used as a screening test for colon cancer, a leading cause of death in the United States. The fecal occult blood test is CLIA-waived.

As **malignant** or cancerous cells grow, they cause microscopic bleeding in the intestine that might not be detected by the naked eye. The fecal occult blood test detects this hidden, or **occult**, bleeding in the colon through a chemical test for blood on a small portion of stool specimen. Early detection of intestinal bleeding aids the physician in discovering colon and other intestinal cancers, and other diseases of the gastrointestinal tract.

PRINCIPLES OF FECAL OCCULT BLOOD TESTS

The fecal occult blood test is a good screening procedure, since it can detect amounts of blood too small to be visible. Several manufacturers offer test kits for fecal occult blood. Beckman Coulter markets the Hemoccult family of test kits (Figure 7-70). Coloscreen is distributed by Helena Laboratories. Two types of fecal occult blood tests are in use—the guaiac test and the immunochemical test.

Guaiac Test

The test for fecal occult blood that has been used for years is also called the guaiac test. It is performed using a slide that contains paper squares coated with **guaiac**, a chemical derived from tree resin. A small portion of stool (fecal) specimen is applied to the paper in the slide. A developer solution containing hydrogen peroxide (H_2O_2) is added to the paper. If blood is present in the specimen, the iron (Fe) in the hemoglobin catalyses the reaction between the guaiac in the paper and the (H_2O_2). The completed reaction forms a blue color. A simplified reaction equation is:

$$\text{Alpha guaiaconic acid} + H_2O_2 \xrightarrow{\text{hemoglobin (Fe)}} \text{Blue quinone compound}$$

The guaiac reaction is not specific for blood. Certain foods and drugs can interfere with the test causing a false result (Table 7-27). The peroxidase enzyme, found in horseradish and turnips, will produce a false-positive result; in addition, the iron in red meat will react positively. Cimetidine, a medication for ulcers, contains a blue pigment that can interfere with interpretation of the test result. Excess dietary vitamin C can inhibit the reaction and cause a false-negative result.

Immunochemical Test for Fecal Occult Blood

A method of testing for fecal occult blood has been developed based on the immunochemical detection of hemoglobin in fecal specimens. An example is the Hemoccult ICT (Figure 7-71), by Beckman Coulter, which also makes the Hemoccult guaiac-based test kits.

The immunochemical test (ICT) for fecal occult blood uses an antibody to the globin chain in hemoglobin to detect blood. The ICT has some advantages over the guaiac test:

- The hemoglobin is stable in a dried specimen and testing can be delayed for several days without loss of reactivity

TABLE 7-27. Dietary factors causing false-negative and false-positive guaiac tests	
FALSE POSITIVES	**FALSE NEGATIVES**
Turnips	Excess vitamin C
Horseradish	
Excess red meat (in diet)	
Any food containing peroxidase enzyme	
The ulcer medication cimetidine contains a blue pigment that can interfere with test interpretation	

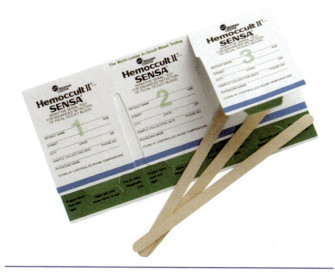

FIGURE 7-70 Hemoccult II Sensa slides (*Courtesy Beckman Coulter, Fullerton, CA*)

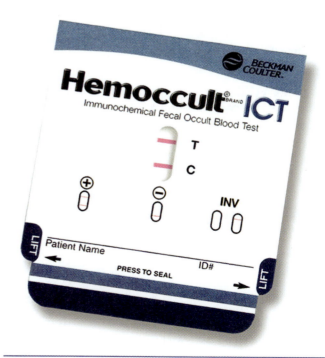

FIGURE 7-71 Hemoccult ICT test showing a positive result (*Courtesy Beckman Coulter, Fullerton, CA*)

- Dietary restrictions are not necessary since the test is specific for hemoglobin
- The test has high sensitivity (that is, will detect low levels of blood)
- The test gives a clear endpoint, a colored line

A disadvantage of the ICT is that it detects mainly colon bleeding, while the guaiac test can detect bleeding in the stomach, small intestine, and large intestine.

PERFORMING THE GUAIAC FECAL OCCULT BLOOD TEST

Safety Precautions

 Standard Precautions must be observed when handling fecal specimens or slides that have had fecal specimens applied to them. Slides mailed to the laboratory for testing must be shipped in a safety pouch or container approved by the carrier and labeled as containing a biological specimen.

Quality Assessment

 Manufacturer's instructions for the fecal occult test being used must be followed exactly. Patients must be instructed in the proper diet and drug restrictions to follow before collecting the fecal specimens because dietary substances, as well as some drugs, can interfere with the guaiac reaction, causing false results. Most procedures require that patients be instructed to eliminate large doses of vitamin C and red meat from their diet for at least 3 days before obtaining the fecal specimen. Table 7-27 lists other factors that can cause false-negative and false-positive guaiac reactions.

If the slides are prepared by the patient, generally they should be delivered to the laboratory and tested within 3 days, since further delay has been shown to cause a false-negative result. This time can vary depending on the test method and brand of slide used. Because the end point of the test is a visible color reaction, technicians must pass a color blindness test before being allowed to report the results.

Slides and developer should be stored at room temperature protected from light, heat, and volatile chemicals. Developer should not be used with slides from another kit. Slides for the guaiac test contain built-in positive and negative control areas (performance monitors) that should only be developed after the patient specimen is developed and interpreted, to avoid any crossover from the control area to the specimen area. The test must be considered invalid if the performance monitor areas fail to react properly.

Specimen Collection

The fecal sample can be collected by the physician during a rectal examination or sigmoidoscopy. Alternatively, the patient can collect specimens at home, apply the samples to the test slides, and bring or send the slides to the laboratory to be tested.

Patient Instructions

The patient should be given a list of instructions including dietary and drug restrictions. Detailed instructions can be found in the manufacturers' product inserts. Collection containers such as urine cups can be provided to the patient for home use. Patients should be instructed not to allow the specimen to be contaminated with water, urine, or blood from bleeding hemorrhoids or menstrual periods.

Application of Specimen to Slide

After the specimen has been obtained, the patient should use an applicator stick provided in the kits to spread a thin layer of stool to one of the specimen areas (boxes). The applicator should be reused to obtain a second sample from another area of the specimen and apply it to the remaining box. To increase the likelihood of detecting occult blood, specimens should be collected from bowel movements on three successive days and applied to three different test slides.

Developing the Guaiac Test

If the slide preparation was done at home, the patient information on the front side of the slides should be confirmed when the slides arrive in the laboratory. The flap on the back of the slide is opened, and two drops of developer are applied to each sample area. Any blue color developing around the fecal smears within 60 seconds is a positive test (Figure 7-72). Color photos of positive and negative smears are included with every test kit for comparison.

Using the Performance Monitors

Controls or performance monitors are built into each card. The monitor(s) should be developed only after the patient sample has been tested and interpreted. One negative and one positive control spot are included near the test areas. One drop of developer is applied between the positive and negative spots. If the slide and developer are functioning properly, within 10 seconds, a blue color will appear in the positive control (monitor) area; the negative control (monitor) area will have no blue color (Figure 7-72).

Test Interpretation

The fecal occult blood test is only a screening test and is not specific for any one disease. It has been shown to be very effective in detecting bleeding associated with colon cancer, but detection is not 100%. Positive tests should be followed with more definitive tests such as colonoscopy or X-ray studies.

Some occult blood tests have a higher sensitivity than others, a factor that should be considered when interpreting the test results. Some minor bowel lesions can bleed intermittently, so a test can be negative even in the presence of disease. For this reason, specimens are usually tested on three different days, and samples from different parts of the fecal specimen are applied to the two test squares. Patients who continue to have intestinal symptoms and negative occult blood tests should be tested further using more specific methods.

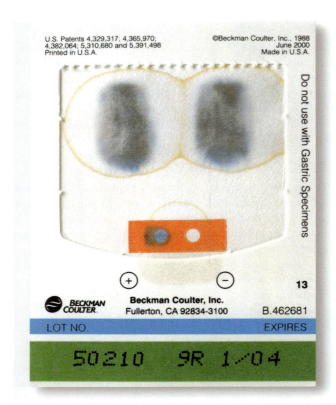

FIGURE 7-72 Positive Hemoccult guaiac test. Any trace of blue at the edge of the fecal smear is a positive test. Performance monitor area (orange rectangle) shows positive and negative control reactions. (*Courtesy Beckman Coulter, Fullerton, CA*)

SAFETY Reminders

- Review safety section before beginning procedure.
- Observe Standard Precautions.
- Treat patient specimens and all materials that come in contact with them as potentially infectious.
- Avoid contacting eyes and skin with developer.

PROCEDURAL Reminders

- Review quality assessment section before beginning procedure.
- Be sure slides are tested within the specified time.
- Protect the slides from heat and light.
- Interpret test results before applying developer to the performance monitors.
- Wait 3 to 5 minutes after applying the fecal sample to the paper before adding developer.
- Do not use slides after expiration date.

CASE STUDY

At his yearly checkup, Mr. Simpson was given three guaiac test slides. He was instructed to take them home, obtain three different specimens, prepare the slides and return them to the laboratory for developing. He was also given a card listing dietary restrictions. A month later, Mr. Simpson returned to the laboratory with the prepared slides. He apologized for taking so long, but said that the slides had been in his car for a week and he had forgotten to drop them off at the laboratory. The technician developed the slides. All three were negative in the patient test areas. On two of the slides both performance monitors were negative; one slide had a positive and a negative performance monitor result.

1. The best interpretation for these results is:
   a. The results were correct and should be reported as negative and charted
   b. The H_2O_2 developer reagent was defective and should be replaced
   c. The tests are invalid, likely because of exposure to extreme temperatures
   d. The expiration date on the slides had passed
2. What is the best next step?

SUMMARY

Colon cancer is a leading cause of death in the United States. However, it has been shown that a program of regular screening can detect cases early that are treatable and often curable. The fecal occult blood test is a simple, inexpensive screening tool to detect intestinal bleeding, often a symptom of serious intestinal disease. Several kits are available, and these can be taken home by patients to apply the fecal specimen then returned to the laboratory for developing and interpretation of results. Although the tests are simple to perform, there are interferences and patient compliance in restricting their diet prior to testing is important. Positive fecal occult blood tests should be followed by more definitive diagnostic techniques to determine the exact cause of the bleeding.

REVIEW QUESTIONS

1. What is the purpose of the fecal occult blood test?
2. What is the principle of the guaiac reaction?
3. List two causes of false-positive guaiac tests and tell why they occur.
4. List one cause of a false-negative guaiac test result.
5. Explain how to instruct a patient in collecting the fecal specimen and preparing the slides.
6. Why should patient samples be regarded as potentially infectious?
7. Why is colon cancer a leading cause of death?
8. Why should the fecal occult blood test be performed in a series of three?
9. How does the ICT differ from the guaiac test?
10. Define guaiac, malignant, and occult.

STUDENT ACTIVITIES

1. Complete the written examination for this lesson.
2. Practice instructing a patient in collecting the specimen and applying it to the slides.
3. Practice performing a test for fecal occult blood as outlined in the Student Performance Guide.

WEB ACTIVITIES

1. Use the Internet to search for package inserts for fecal occult blood tests. Find inserts from two different manufacturers. Compare the procedures and sensitivities of the two tests.
2. Use the information from one manufacturer's instructions to prepare a patient instruction card, listing the dietary restrictions and instructions to the patient on how to collect the specimen(s) and prepare the slides.
3. Use the Internet to find information about using the fecal occult blood test as a screening test for colon cancer and other gastrointestinal diseases. Visit Web sites such as the American Cancer Society site. Report on the use of the fecal occult blood test as a screening test for colon cancer.

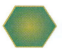

Student Performance Guide

Lesson 7-11 Fecal Occult Blood Test

Name _____ Date _____

INSTRUCTIONS

1. Practice performing a test for fecal occult blood following the step-by-step procedure.

2. Demonstrate the test for fecal occult blood satisfactorily for the instructor, using the Student Performance Guide. Your instructor will determine the level of competency you must achieve to earn a satisfactory (S) grade.

NOTE: Procedure given is general. Package insert for test kit used should be consulted for specific instructions before performing the test.

MATERIALS AND EQUIPMENT

- gloves
- antiseptic
- surface disinfectant
- timer
- test kits for fecal occult blood
- applicator sticks
- cups for collecting fecal specimens
- fecal specimens
- biohazard container
- laboratory tissues and paper towels
- aerosol air deodorizer
- fume hood or biosafety cabinet
- sharps container

PROCEDURE

Record in the comment section any problems encountered while practicing the procedure (or have a fellow student or the instructor evaluate your performance).

S = Satisfactory
U = Unsatisfactory

You must:	S	U	Comments
1. Wash hands and put on gloves			
2. Assemble materials and equipment			
3. If the specimen has already been applied to the slide, proceed to step 5. If slides are to be taken home, practice instructing a patient in collecting the specimen and preparing and labeling the slides. Show the patient the instructions on the slide cover and ask if there are any questions			
4. If the specimen is available, but not applied to the slide, proceed as follows: a. Fill out the patient information on the front of the slide package			

You must:	S	U	Comments
b. Working in a fume hood or biosafety cabinet, open the flap on the front to expose the two paper guaiac squares. Follow the directions and obtain a small portion of the stool sample on the applicator stick. Apply a thin smear to box A c. Reuse the applicator stick to obtain a second sample from a different part of the specimen. Apply a thin smear to box B d. Close the cover and discard applicator into biohazard container e. Wait 3 to 5 minutes for the smears to dry			
5. Turn the slide over and open the perforated flap to expose the backs of boxes A and B, and the performance monitor (control) area			
6. Apply two drops of the developer onto each smear (boxes A and B) and start the timer			
7. Read the results after the appropriate time interval			
8. Compare the colors on the slide to the color guide in the package insert. Any blue color at the edge of the smear is a positive test			
9. Apply *one* drop of developer between the positive (+) and the negative (–) performance monitor areas. Read the results after the appropriate time interval. The positive monitor should have a blue color; the negative monitor should have no blue color. If the performance monitors do not react properly, repeat the test, using a new slide			
10. Record the results			
11. Discard all contaminated materials in the appropriate biohazard or sharps container			
12. Wipe the counter with surface disinfectant			
13. Return supplies to proper storage			
14. Remove gloves and discard into biohazard container			
15. Wash hands with antiseptic			

Evaluator Comments:

Evaluator _____ Date _____

UNIT 8

Basic Parasitology

UNIT OBJECTIVES

After studying this unit, the student will:

- Discuss the functions of the parasitology section of the clinical laboratory.
- Discuss mechanisms of parasitic infection.
- Describe parasite control methods.
- Describe diagnostic techniques for blood, tissue, and intestinal parasites.
- Explain the procedures for the proper collection and processing of specimens for parasite examination.
- Perform a test for pinworms.
- Prepare fecal specimens for microscopic parasite examination.
- Prepare blood smears for parasite examination.

UNIT OVERVIEW

Parasitology is usually a part of the microbiology department. Only in large reference or research laboratories is parasitology a stand-alone department. Because of the variety of parasites and the infrequency with which they are found, most laboratory workers do not gain much experience in parasite identification. Therefore, many laboratories routinely send specimens for parasite examination to a reference or state health laboratory.

The stool, or fecal, specimen is the specimen most frequently examined for parasites. However, parasites can be present in and on all parts of the body, so the proper specimen varies with the patient's symptoms. Since the malarial parasite infects red blood cells, the hematology technician is usually the first to detect that organism. *Trichomonas*, a flagellated parasite, can inhabit the genitourinary tract and can be detected during the microscopic part of a routine urinalysis. Organisms such as lice can infest body hair. Tapeworms, round-worms, amoebae, *Giardia*, and *Cryptosporidium* infect the intestinal tract. Organisms such as *Toxoplasma* are found in tissue and can be detected by immunological methods.

Many types of parasitic organisms cause human disease. Most parasitic diseases in the United States have been brought under control with education, improved sanitation techniques, and insect control measures. However, worldwide, millions of people are infected with parasites, and in many parts of the world parasites remain a major cause of disease and death.

As world travel has become common-place, parasitic infections are detected more frequently in U.S. clinical laboratories. Additionally, organisms such as *Toxoplasma* and *Cryptosporidium* are becoming an increasing problem because they can cause severe disease in immunocompromised AIDS, transplant, and chemotherapy patients.

Unit 8 provides information about basic parasitology concepts and laboratory procedures. Lesson 8-1 is a brief introduction to the field of parasitology. Groups of the more common human parasites, modes of transmission, life cycles, and diagnostic methods are outlined. Lesson 8-2 describes specimen collection and processing for parasite examination and describes the procedure for the pinworm test. Methods of preparing fecal specimens for microscopic examination for parasites are presented in Lesson 8-3. Lesson 8-4 describes the procedure for preparing, staining, and examining blood smears for parasites.

This unit represents only an introduction to the field of clinical parasitology. Becoming expert in parasite identification requires much practice and study. Specimens must be collected and processed correctly to increase the likelihood of detecting any parasite(s) present. Personnel should also have a solid knowledge of parasites and be able to recognize parasitic forms. Technicians in laboratories that do not perform frequent parasitology procedures may not be able to identify all parasites, but they must be alert enough and sufficiently trained to recognize that something unusual in the specimen requires expert evaluation.

READINGS, REFERENCES, AND RESOURCES

Ash, L. R. & Orihel, T. C. (1997). *Atlas of human parasitology* (4th ed.). Chicago: ASCP Press.

Bogitsh, B., et al. (2005). *Human parasitology* (3rd ed.). San Diego: Academic Press.

Forbes, B. A., et al. (2002). *Bailey & Scott's diagnostic microbiology* (10th ed.). St. Louis: C. V. Mosby.

Garcia, L. S. (2001). *Diagnostic medical parasitology* (4th ed.). Washington, DC: American Society for Microbiology.

Heelan, J. S. & Ingersoll, F. W. (2001). *Essentials of human parasitology*. Clifton Park, NY: Thomson Delmar Learning.

Henry, J. B. (Ed.) (2006). *Clinical diagnosis and management by laboratory methods* (21st ed.). Philadelphia: W. B. Saunders.

Leventhal, R. & Cheadle, R. F. (2002). *Medical parasitology: a self-instructional text* (5th ed.). Philadelphia: F. A. Davis Company.

Roberts, L. S. & Janovy, J. (2004). *Foundations of parasitology* (7th ed.). St. Louis: McGraw-Hill.

Zeibig, E. A. (1997). *Clinical parasitology: a practical approach*. Philadelphia: W. B. Saunders.

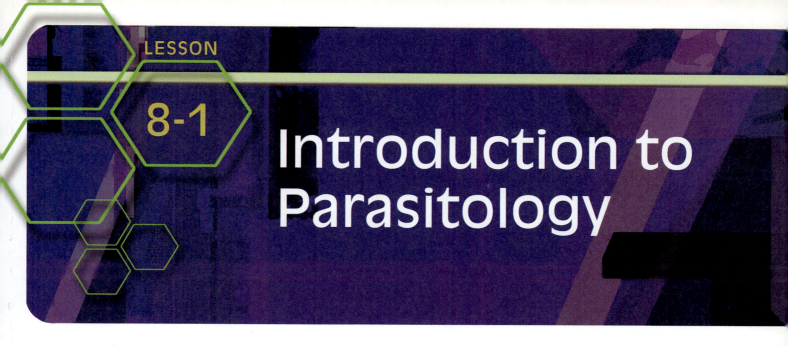

Introduction to Parasitology

LESSON OBJECTIVES

After studying this lesson, the student will:

- Name the three major morphological parasite groups.
- List three ways in which parasite infections are transmitted.
- List four ways to control or prevent parasitic infections.
- List three methods used to diagnose parasitic infections.
- List four specimens that are examined for parasites.
- Name three blood parasites.
- Name three intestinal protozoan parasites.
- Name three types of parasitic helminths.
- Explain how immunological tests are useful in the parasitology laboratory.
- Explain how eradication of guinea worm is a successful model for eradication of parasitic disease.
- Define the glossary terms.

GLOSSARY

arthropod / a member of the phylum Arthropoda, which includes crustaceans, insects, and arachnids

atrial / of or relating to a body cavity

cestode / tapeworm; member of the class Cestoda

commensal / an organism that lives with, on, or in another, without injury to either

congenital / acquired during fetal development, and present at the time of birth, but not inherited

cyst / the dormant stage of an organism surrounded by a resistant covering; the nonmotile, nonfeeding stage of a protozoan parasite

definitive host / the host in which the sexual or adult form of the parasite is found

ectoparasite / a parasite that lives on the outer surface of a host

endemic / recurring in a specific location or population

helminth / a worm, especially a parasitic worm; in parasitology, the group comprising the roundworms and flatworms

host / the organism from which a parasite obtains nutrients and in which some or part of the parasite's life cycle is completed

immunocompromised / having reduced ability or inability to produce a normal immune response

intermediate host / the host in which the asexual, immature, or larval form of the parasite is found

larva / immature stage of an invertebrate

nematode / roundworm; any unsegmented worm of the class Nematoda

opportunistic parasite / an organism that causes disease only in immunocompromised hosts

ova / eggs

parasite / an organism that lives in or on another species and at the expense of that species

pathogenic / capable of causing damage or injury to the host

proglottid (pl. proglottids) / the tapeworm body segment that contains the male and female reproductive organs

protozoa / unicellular eukaryotic organisms, both free-living and parasitic

reservoir host / the host, other than the usual host, in which the parasite lives and is infectious

trematode / fluke; any parasitic flatworm of the class Trematoda

vector / an agent that transports a pathogen from an infected host to a noninfected host

INTRODUCTION

Parasites are organisms that live in or on another organism, the **host**, and live at the expense of the host organism. In other words, the parasite depends on the host for nutrients, which causes injury to the host. Clinical parasitology is the study of parasites and parasitic diseases, including methods of diagnosing, treating, and controlling parasitic diseases.

Some parasites cause little obvious harm to the host, for example head lice. Others, such as the malarial parasite, can cause severe disease and even death if left untreated. These are called **pathogenic** parasites. **Opportunistic parasites** are those organisms that cause few or no symptoms in healthy hosts but can cause severe disease in **immunocompromised** hosts.

Parasites can be classified in several ways. They can be grouped according to the site in which they normally are found; for example, intestinal parasites, blood parasites, or **ectoparasites** (parasites on the exterior of the host). Or they can be grouped according to morphological characteristics; for example, worms (tapeworms, roundworms, and flukes), protozoa, and arthropods (insects and arachnids).

Parasitic infections are usually diagnosed by finding and identifying the parasite, either macroscopically or microscopically, or by immunological tests. This lesson presents an overview of the field of clinical parasitology as it relates to clinical laboratory procedures. Clinical parasitology textbooks and atlases should be consulted for more comprehensive information.

CHARACTERISTICS OF PARASITES

Several characteristics are considered when identifying parasites. These include morphology, host specificity, geographical distribution, life cycle, and vectors.

Morphological Classification

Parasites, like other living organisms, can be grouped according to international rules of zoological classification based on morphology and other characteristics. Although organisms are often called by various common names, such as hookworm or beef tapeworm, they have two-part latinized scientific names that are recognized internationally. The scientific name of an organism is always italicized, with the genus name also capitalized. For example, the scientific name for one species of malarial parasite is *Plasmodium ovale*.

Types of Hosts

To complete their life cycles, most parasites have specific requirements. Although essentially all animal species have parasites, these parasites are often very host-specific. However, if conditions are right, parasites normally found in one host can survive or even thrive in an unnatural host. An example of this is the dog heartworm, *Dirofilaria immitis*. This parasite is considered to be host-specific, with dogs being the natural host. However, the dog heartworm can infect other animals, such as cats. These infections are not usually as serious as infections in dogs.

The **definitive host**, or main host, is the organism in which the sexually mature (adult) form of a parasite is found. Some parasites require two or more different host species to complete their life cycle.

The **intermediate host** is an organism required to complete a parasite's life cycle in addition to the definitive host. The intermediate host usually harbors an asexual or **larval** (immature) form of the parasite. For example, *Plasmodium*, which causes malaria, lives in both humans and mosquitoes. In humans, *Plasmodium*'s intermediate host, the parasite reproduces asexually. Sexual reproduction of *Plasmodium* occurs in the mosquito, the definitive host.

A **reservoir host** is an organism other than the main host that can harbor a parasite and serve as a source of infection. A **vector** is a living carrier that transmits the parasite to an uninfected host. A *biologic vector* is a host essential to the life cycle, for example the biologic vector for *Plasmodium* is the mosquito. *Mechanical vectors* transmit the parasite mechanically. For example, flies that land on infected feces and then land on food can carry infective parasite stages from one site to another.

Geographic Distribution

Parasites are only found where the appropriate hosts, vectors, or animal reservoirs are available to allow the organism's life cycle to develop and be perpetuated. Environmental factors, such as humidity and temperature, are important to the survival of most parasites, especially those that require arthropod vectors. Temperature extremes and dry conditions are often detrimental to parasitic forms. Therefore, the majority of parasites are found in temperate to tropical climates.

Life Cycles

A parasitic life cycle is the complete process of a parasite infecting (or infesting) a host, growing, developing, reproducing, and being transmitted to a new host (Figure 8-1). Parasite life cycles can be simple or complex. Some parasites spend their entire life in one host. Others require different types of hosts during different parts of their life cycles. Still others are only parasitic for a portion of their life and are free-living at other times. Knowledge of the specific life-cycle requirements of each type of parasite is valuable in preventing parasitic infections and in determining the appropriate specimen to examine when parasitic infection is suspected.

Infective Stage Versus Diagnostic Stage

The *infective stage* of the parasite is the stage of the life cycle during which the parasite is capable of infecting a host. The *diagnostic stage* is the life cycle stage that can be detected in a specimen and helps in diagnosis. Knowledge of the infective stage is required to understand how to prevent transmission. Knowledge of the diagnostic stage is required to select the proper diagnostic method. Sometimes the diagnostic stage and infective stage are the same, particularly for the intestinal parasites. For example, in the life cycle diagram of *Giardia* shown in Figure 8-1, the **cyst** is the infective stage as well as a diagnostic stage.

Infection Versus Infestation

Parasites, such as lice, that live on external body surfaces cause *infestations*. Parasites that live within the host cause *infections*. Parasites can infect (or infest) external body surfaces, external body cavities, the intestinal tract, blood, and organs such as the liver, bone marrow, and other tissues. Many parasites have specific tissue requirements and will migrate through the body to locate in a specific organ. The site infected by a parasite is determined by how the parasite enters the body, the parasite's tissue specificity, and the host's immunity.

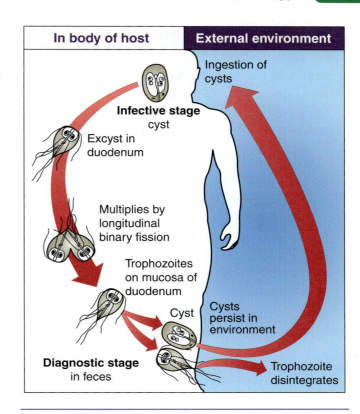

FIGURE 8-1 Example of parasite life cycle diagram. Shown is life cycle of *Giardia intestinalis*

Transmitting Parasitic Infections

Most parasitic infections are acquired through contact with an infected person, ingestion of an infective form in food or water, or insect bites. A few organisms can be acquired through **congenital** infection and some organisms, such as hookworm, can penetrate intact skin. Table 8-1 lists some parasitic diseases, their usual routes of transmission, and their infective stages.

HOW PARASITES CAUSE DISEASE

Parasitic disease occurs when the damage caused to the host by the parasite becomes severe enough to cause pathologic changes in the host. Parasitic infections can be asymptomatic (without symptoms), cause to mild to moderate symptoms, or even cause death.

Many factors determine the effect a parasitic infection will have on the host, including the parasite's number, size, location, and toxicity. The host's condition is also a factor. Damage can be mechanical, such as obstruction of an organ or vessel; irritative or toxic, caused by substances produced or released by the parasite; or damage can be caused by an allergic reaction. Some infections are self-limiting. Common problems seen with parasitic infections include anemia, jaundice, secondary bacterial infections, organ dysfunction, and interference with normal physiological processes.

TABLE 8-1. Examples of parasitic diseases, their transmission routes, and their infective stages

DISEASE	CAUSATIVE ORGANISM	TRANSMISSION ROUTE	INFECTIVE STAGE
Amebiasis	*Entamoeba histolytica*	Ingestion	Cyst
Giardiasis	*Giardia intestinalis*	Ingestion	Cyst
Malaria	*Plasmodium*	Mosquito bite	Sporozoite
Toxoplasmosis	*Toxoplasma gondii*	Ingestion or congenital	Oocysts or zoite
Trichomoniasis	*Trichomonas vaginalis*	Sexual contact	Trophozoite
Babesiosis	*Babesia*	Tick bite	Sporozoite
Cryptosporidiosis	*Cryptosporidium*	Ingestion	Oocyst
Trichinosis	*Trichinella spiralis*	Ingestion	Larva
Enterobiasis	*Enterobius vermicularis*	Ingestion	Ova
Hookworm	*Necator, Ancylostoma*	Skin penetration	Larva
Ascariasis	*Ascaris lumbricoides*	Ingestion	Ova
Chagas disease	*Trypanosoma cruzi*	Ingestion, mucous membrane, blood	Trypomastigote
Dracunculiasis	*Dracunculus medinensis*	Ingestion	Larvae

Immunity to Parasites

Absolute immunity to parasites is rare unless the individual (species) is an unsuitable host. In general, resistance to parasitic infection increases with age. Hosts with good nutrition and health are less likely to develop severe symptoms than hosts from impoverished socioeconomic conditions.

Parasites stimulate immune responses much like those stimulated by viruses or bacteria. This means antibodies can develop against the infecting parasite and the cell-mediated immune response can be stimulated. Immunological tests can be used to aid in diagnosing some parasitic infections. These are especially useful when it is difficult to obtain a specimen for examination, such as in tissue or organ infections. For example, toxoplasmosis is a parasitic disease that can be diagnosed by measuring serum antibody to *Toxoplasma*.

Treating Parasitic Infections

Several drugs are effective against parasites, but most have some level of toxicity. The degree of treatment success depends on the infecting parasite, the magnitude of the infection, the host's health, and the infection site. In some cases, surgery is required to remove the parasite.

Parasite Infections in Immunocompromised Patients

Immunocompromised patients, such as AIDS, organ transplant, chemotherapy, or radiation patients, are especially vulnerable to parasitic infection. Infections with organisms such as *Toxoplasma* and *Cryptosporidium* can be life-threatening to these patients and must be treated with vigorous drug therapy. Immunodiagnosis in immunocompromised patients can be difficult because blood antibody levels are often below detection limits.

DIAGNOSIS OF PARASITIC INFECTIONS

Most parasitic diseases have generalized symptoms such as fever, pain, chills, diarrhea, or fatigue and loss of vitality, symptoms that could be caused by a variety of conditions or diseases. A definitive diagnosis of parasitic infections usually depends upon finding and identifying the parasite's diagnostic stage.

Specimens that are examined for evidence of parasites include feces, urine, sputum, aspirations, and blood and other tissues. For some parasites, immunological tests are available. Patient history is also very important in the diagnosis of parasitic infections, particularly if the patient has any history of travel to **endemic** areas, areas where the organism occurs naturally.

PREVENTING PARASITIC INFECTIONS

The key to preventing parasitic infections is to understand the transmission methods and the location of the parasite's infective stages. Parasite-control methods include:
- Blocking transmission of the infective form
- Providing health education
- Improving sanitation
- Identifying and treating infected individuals to prevent the spread of infection
- Developing vaccines (in research stage)

Blocking Transmission

One of the most important ways of preventing parasite infections is to block transmission of the parasite's infective stage by breaking a link in the organism's life cycle. For this reason, it is important to understand the life history of the parasite, where it is found, the host required for its reproduction, and how transmission occurs.

CURRENT TOPICS

OUTBREAKS OF PARASITIC INFECTIONS

Although the incidence of parasitic infections is not high in the United States, a small lapse in sanitation or other preventive techniques can allow parasite infections to emerge and cause disease and sometimes death. Most U.S. outbreaks can be traced to failures in infrastructure, such as water or sewage treatment, or to unsafe food processing and preparation procedures. Another potential source of outbreaks is natural disasters, such as major flooding and hurricanes. These increase the risk of water becoming contaminated with untreated sewage or animal wastes, creating potential for parasitic infections. Examples of recent food- and water-borne parasitic outbreaks in the United States include:

- In the 1990s, a water treatment plant failure in Milwaukee, Wisconsin, caused more than 400,000 people to become infected with *Cryptosporidium*, an intestinal parasite. *Cryptosporidium* causes severe diarrhea of 1- to 2-week duration in healthy, immunocompetent individuals, but can cause life-threatening illness in immunocompromised individuals. Several fatalities occurred as a result of the Milwaukee cryptosporidiosis outbreak.
- Between 1999 and 2003, all 50 states reported cryptosporidiosis cases, averaging over 3,000 cases annually.

- In the last decade, several outbreaks of cyclosporiasis have been reported in the United States and Canada. Cyclosporiasis is caused by infection with *Cyclospora*, a coccidian parasite causing symptoms similar to those caused by *Cryptosporidium*. Most of these outbreaks were traced to ingestion of contaminated raw produce, primarily raspberries. Improved sanitation techniques in food harvesting and processing could have prevented most of these outbreaks.
- In California in 2006, lung infections with *Paragonimus*, the lung fluke, were diagnosed in patients who had eaten raw or undercooked imported freshwater crabs.
- Outbreaks of giardiasis, caused by the intestinal flagellate *Giardia intestinalis*, are reported fairly frequently in the United States. Examples include:
  - Waterborne outbreaks in New York State (1975, 1995, 1997), New Hampshire and Montana (1980), Colorado, (1981), Nevada (1982), Oregon (1997), Florida (1998), and Ohio (2004)
  - Foodborne outbreaks (1990s) caused by contaminated salad bars and taco ingredients
  - Outbreaks after playing in recreational waters such as swimming pools, lakes, or public spraying fountains (Florida, 2006)
  - Outbreaks in institutions such as nursing homes and day care centers

When the infective stage of the parasite is known, it is possible to plan effective control and prevention methods. For example, in the 1800s in North America, malaria was found as far north as southern Canada. When it was discovered that the malarial parasite was transmitted to man through the bite of infected mosquitoes, mosquito control measures were implemented in the United States. The use of DDT and other pesticides rapidly and drastically reduced the malaria infection rate, so that by the 1950s, the United States was not considered endemic for malaria. However, because of the banning of effective (but toxic) pesticides such as DDT and increases in worldwide travel, occasional new cases of malaria have been seen in the United States since 2000. Some of these have occurred in individuals who have no history of travel to endemic areas.

Health Education and Improved Sanitation

Health education about proper personal hygiene and food handling has contributed to a drop in parasitic diseases. Improved sanitation techniques and standards in water quality, sewage treatment, and waste disposal reduce the incidence of infection with waterborne parasites.

ORGANISMS PARASITIC FOR HUMANS

The parasites that infect humans can be grouped into three large groups: **protozoa**, **helminths**, and **arthropods** (Figure 8-2).

Protozoa

Protozoa are single-celled eukaryotic organisms that are larger than most bacteria. Parasitic protozoa include amoebae, flagellates, ciliates, and apicomplexans (formerly sporozoa; see Table 8-2). All four of these groups contain organisms parasitic to man and other animals. Protozoa can infect most body sites, including blood, tissues, the intestinal and genitourinary tracts, and the oral cavity.

Helminths

Helminth is the common name used for parasitic worms. These include **trematodes** (flukes), **cestodes** (tapeworms), and **nematodes** (roundworms; see Table 8-3). Most helminth infections occur in the intestinal tract. However, other tissues are sometimes infected by certain helminths.

CURRENT TOPICS

ERADICATING PARASITIC DISEASES: GUINEA WORM DISEASE—A SUCCESS STORY

Parasitic diseases such as malaria cause millions of deaths worldwide each year. Parasites also cause painful, debilitating disease and loss of productivity for millions worldwide. However, efforts by various organizations such as the Centers for Disease Control and Prevention (CDC), World Health Organization (WHO), UNICEF, Bill and Melinda Gates Foundation, and The Carter Center, to name a few, are succeeding in controlling, reducing, and in some cases eradicating some parasitic diseases. Partnering with these organizations are industry, drug companies, and governments of many countries around the world. Three parasitic diseases that are currently targeted for eradication by worldwide cooperation are *dracunculiasis* caused by the guinea worm, lymphatic *filariasis*, and *onchocerciasis*, also called river blindness.

Guinea Worm Disease

Guinea worm disease is an ancient disease, known to have been around for thousands of years. The worm has been found in ancient Egyptian mummies. Before eradication efforts began, Guinea worm was found in Africa, Asia

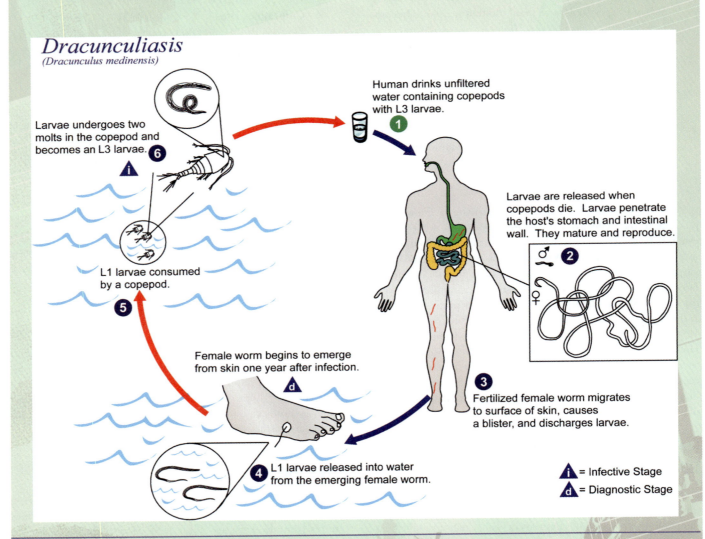

Dracunculiasis
(Dracunculus medinensis)

Larvae undergoes two molts in the copepod and becomes an L3 larvae. **6** **i**

L1 larvae consumed by a copepod. **5**

Female worm begins to emerge from skin one year after infection. **d**

4 L1 larvae released into water from the emerging female worm.

Human drinks unfiltered water containing copepods with L3 larvae. **1**

Larvae are released when copepods die. Larvae penetrate the host's stomach and intestinal wall. They mature and reproduce.

♂ **2**
♀

3 Fertilized female worm migrates to surface of skin, causes a blister, and discharges larvae.

i = Infective Stage
d = Diagnostic Stage

Guinea worm life cycle (*From CDC, Atlanta, GA*)

CURRENT TOPICS (continued)

(including India and Pakistan), and some parts of South America. Rather than being a rapid *killer* disease, Guinea worm disease causes painful crippling, resulting in children who cannot attend school and adults who cannot work. This spells economic disaster for agricultural communities.

Life Cycle

Guinea worm disease (dracunculiasis) is caused by the roundworm *Dracunculus medinensis*. It is contracted by ingesting water contaminated with microscopic water fleas (copepods) carrying infective larvae, as shown in the life cycle diagram. Once ingested, the larvae migrate to the small intestine, penetrate the wall of the intestine, and pass into the body cavity. There, over a period of about a year, the female Guinea worm matures to an adult (approximately 2 to 3 feet long and the diameter of a cooked spaghetti noodle). She then migrates to a subcutaneous site, usually on the lower leg, where she emerges through a painful, burning skin blister, creating a lesion where secondary infections often occur.

The Guinea worm life cycle is perpetuated when victims immerse their affected limbs in water to relieve pain caused by the emerging worm, or when they wade into water to collect drinking water. When an emerging Guinea worm senses water, the worm releases millions of immature larvae into the water, thus contaminating the water supply. The worm is capable of doing this for several days after emerging from the ulcer when it comes in contact with water. The larvae are ingested by microscopic copepods, where they develop into the infective stage in about 2 weeks. The transmission cycle continues when people drink water containing copepods harboring the infective Guinea worm larvae.

Once an individual is infected with Guinea worm, there is no effective drug treatment. Instead, once the adult worm begins emerging from the blister, it is removed by wrapping the end of the worm around a small stick and extracting it gradually over a period of weeks, a slow and painful process.

Disease Control and Eradication

Guinea worm disease is expected to be the first infectious disease eradicated from the world without a vaccine or treatment. Efforts to control Guinea worm disease have focused on education about disease transmission and use of low technology methods. Since infection only occurs by drinking contaminated water, education of communities about measures to create safe drinking water can eliminate disease. These include:

- Preventing people with open Guinea worm ulcers from entering waters used for drinking
- Obtaining drinking water from deep, uncontaminated wells
- Filtering drinking water to remove copepods
- Treating unsafe drinking waters with larvicides

Because of eradication efforts beginning in 1986, Guinea worm disease has been reduced worldwide by more than 99.5%. In 1986, there were an estimated 3.5 million cases annually; in 2005 reported cases numbered less than 11,000. By 2006, more than 170 countries had been declared free of Guinea worm disease, and only a handful of African countries—including Sudan, Ghana, and Mali—accounted for the remaining fraction of 1% of the disease. Through continued cooperative efforts, this debilitating disease can be completely eradicated.

TABLE 8-2. Examples of medically important protozoa

PROTOZOAN GROUP	EXAMPLES
Amoebae	*Entamoeba*
Flagellates	*Trichomonas, Giardia*
Ciliates	*Balantidium*
Apicomplexa	*Plasmodium, Toxoplasma*

TABLE 8-3. Examples of medically important helminths

HELMINTH GROUP	EXAMPLES
Trematodes (flukes)	Liver fluke, lung fluke
Cestodes (tapeworms)	Beef tapeworm, pork tapeworm
Nematodes (roundworms)	Pinworm, hookworm, whipworm

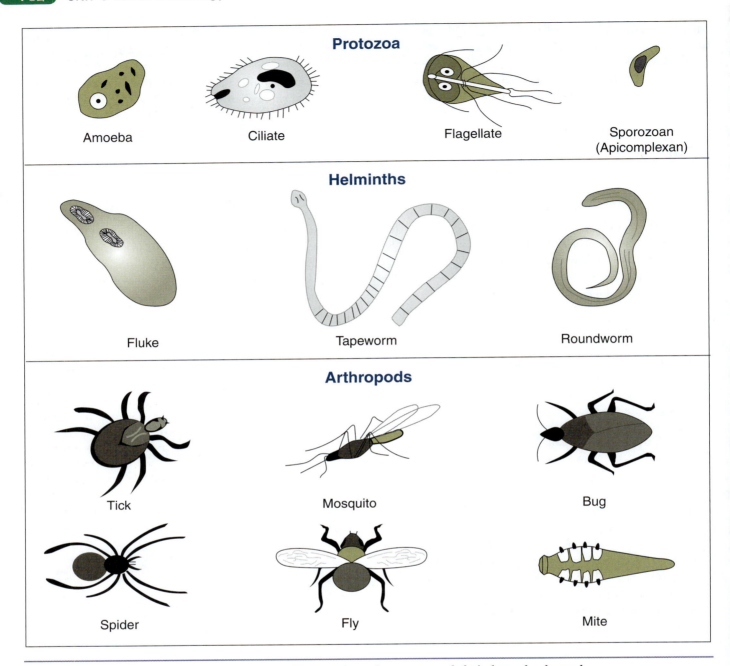

FIGURE 8-2 Three major groups of parasites: protozoa, helminths, and arthropods

Arthropods

Arthropods include arachnids, such as spiders, ticks, and mites, and insects, such as lice, bugs, fleas, flies, and mosquitoes (Table 8-4). Some arthropods, such as lice, fleas, and mosquitos, are parasitic to humans, while others, such as flies, are important in transmitting the infective stage of parasites to humans.

TABLE 8-4. Medically important arthropods

ARTHROPOD GROUP	EXAMPLES
Arachnids	Spiders, ticks, mites
Insects	Lice, bugs, fleas, flies, mosquitoes

LABORATORY IDENTIFICATION OF PARASITES

A useful parasite classification for the clinical laboratory is based on the organ system in which the parasites are found. The ecto-parasites are usually easily seen and identified. However, endo-parasites present more of a problem and require special specimen preparation. Two broad categories of endoparasites are:

- Intestinal and atrial parasites
- Blood and tissue parasites

Intestinal and Atrial Parasites

Of the several types of organisms that can infect the intestinal tract (Table 8-5), some are pathogenic, whereas others are **commensal**, that is, not harmful.

Atrial Protozoa

Atrial parasites infect body cavities. *Entamoeba gingivalis* is an amoeba that can be present in the mouth but is usually consid-ered commensal. *Trichomonas vaginalis* is a flagellate that can infect the urogenital tract.

Intestinal Protozoa

Pathogenic intestinal protozoa include *Entamoeba his-tolytica, Giardia intestinalis, Cyclospora, Isospora belli*, and *Cryptosporidium. Giardia* is the most common intestinal pro-tozoan pathogen in the United States and is a frequent cause of diarrhea in children in day care centers.

Nonpathogenic protozoa common to the intestinal tract include other *Entamoeba* sp., *Endolimax, Chilomastix*, and *Iodamoeba*.

Intestinal Helminths

The most common helminths are nematodes. These include *Enterobius vermicularis* (pinworm), *Trichuris trichiura* (whip-worm), *Ascaris lumbricoides* (large roundworm), and hookworms (*Necator* and *Ancylostoma*). Trematodes found in the intestinal tract include *Fasciolopsis, Fasciola, Heterophyes, Metagonimus*, and *Clonorchis*.

The most common tapeworm infection in the U.S. is caused by the dwarf tapeworm, *Hymenolepis nana*. Other tapeworms that can infect humans include the beef tapeworm (*Taenia sagi-nata*), the pork tapeworm (*Taenia solium*), the fish tapeworm (*Diphyllobothrium latum*), and the dog tapeworm (*Dipylidium caninum*; see Table 8-5).

Laboratory Detection of Intestinal and Atrial Parasites

Intestinal and atrial parasites are usually identified by the mor-phology seen during microscopic examination of fecal or oral specimens. Atlases of parasite morphology are indispensable in the parasitology laboratory. Intestinal protozoa are identified by the morphology of cysts, trophozoites, or oocysts in fecal speci-mens. Because protozoa are so small, identification of genus and

TABLE 8-5. Examples of intestinal parasites

PROTOZOA	
Amoebae	*Entamoeba*
Ciliates	*Balantidium*
Flagellates	*Giardia*
Apicomplexans	*Cryptosporidium, Isospora, Cyclospora*
HELMINTHS	
Trematodes	*Fasciolopsis*
Cestodes	*Taenia, Dipylidium, Hymenolepis*
Nematodes	*Enterobius, Ascaris*

species can be difficult. However, it is very important to distin-guish pathogens from commensals.

Roundworm infections are diagnosed by identifying **ova** (eggs), larvae, or adults in fecal or perianal specimens. Trematode infections can also be diagnosed by identifying ova in fecal speci-mens. *Paragonimus* and *Schistosoma* worms inhabit the lungs and blood vessels, respectively, but their eggs are often found in feces or urine (*Schistosoma*). Tapeworms are identified by finding ova or **proglottids** (tapeworm segments) in feces.

Immunological tests have been developed to detect a few intestinal protozoa. These tests are coming into wider use because they have some advantages over traditional microscopic methods. The technician does not need to have morphological expertise to be able to interpret the results of immunoassays. The assays often have high sensitivity, that is, they can detect low levels of antigen, levels that might require microscopic examination of several specimens before the parasite could be detected.

Antigen capture immunoassays (modified enzyme immuno-assays) are available for detecting some parasite antigens in fecal specimens. An example is the Triage Parasite Panel by Biosite Diagnostics (Figure 8-3). *Entamoeba histolytica, Giardia*, and *Cryptosporidium* antigens can be detected in less than 20 minutes using a single self-contained test cassette that also includes con-trols for the three organisms.

Other immunological tests available include kits that detect serum antibody to *E. histolytica* and fluorescent antibody kits to detect *Giardia* and *Cryptosporidium* in fecal specimens as well as in water supplies.

Blood and Tissue Parasites

Worldwide, the blood and tissue parasites are a diverse group (Table 8-6). However, only a few blood and tissue parasites are endemic in the United States.

Blood Parasites

The most common blood parasite is the malarial parasite (*Plasmodium* sp.). Other blood parasites include the trypano-somes, *Babesia*, and the filarial worms.

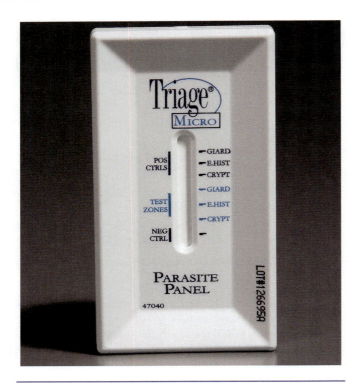

FIGURE 8-3 Biosite triage panel
(*Photo courtesy Biosite, Inc., San Diego, CA*)

TABLE 8-6. Examples of blood and tissue parasites

PARASITES FOUND IN BLOOD	PARASITES FOUND IN TISSUE
Plasmodium	*Toxoplasma*
Babesia	*Trichinella*
Trypanosoma	*Leishmania*
Filarial worms	*Trypanosoma*
	Amoebae
	Schistosoma
	Filarial worms

Tissue Parasites

Tissue parasites include *Toxoplasma*, free-living and parasitic amoebae (*Naegleria* and *Acanthamoeba*), *Leishmania, Schistosoma*, some filarial worms, microsporidia, trypanosomes, and *Trichinella*.

Laboratory Detection of Blood and Tissue Parasites

The specimen required for detecting blood and tissue parasites is determined by the location or site of infection and the organism suspected. Blood parasites are identified by microscopic examination of stained blood smears, described in Lesson 8-4.

Tissue parasites can be identified by microscopic examination of stained biopsy material, aspirates, sputum, skin snips, or by immunological tests, such as tests of serum for antibody to *Toxoplasma*.

Pneumocystis carinii is an opportunistic pathogen found in the lungs. It causes pneumonia in immunocompromised individuals and has been responsible for many AIDS deaths. In the past, *Pneumocystis* was grouped with protozoa because it can be identified with stains typically used for protozoan parasites. Although it is accepted that *Pneumocystis* should be grouped with the fungi, many parasitology laboratories continue to provide diagnostic testing for *Pneumocystis*.

SUMMARY

Organisms capable of parasitizing humans are quite diverse, and belong to three major groups—protozoa, helminths, and arthropods. Knowledge of parasite life cycles, geographic distribution, infective stages, and diagnostic stages are all key to understanding, diagnosing, and preventing parasitic infections. In the laboratory, most parasitic infections are diagnosed by finding a parasitic form in a clinical specimen. However, in recent years immunochemical tests have been developed for some intestinal and tissue parasites.

In the United States, parasites are not frequently observed in clinical specimens. Because of this, many laboratory personnel do not have much experience in parasite identification and specimens for parasite examination are often sent to reference or state public health laboratories.

Clinical laboratory personnel should be familiar with characteristics of common parasitic infections so the appropriate specimens are collected and correctly processed for examination. This greatly increases the chances of discovering parasites in the laboratory examination. Lesson 8-2 gives the procedures for processing specimens to examine for parasites.

REVIEW QUESTIONS

1. How are parasitic infections usually diagnosed?
2. What are the three major groups of organisms that contain human parasites?
3. How does geography or climate affect the incidence of parasites?
4. What body sites can be infected by parasites?
5. Name three factors that affect the severity of parasitic infections.
6. Name three ways parasitic diseases can be transmitted.
7. Name four methods used to prevent or control parasite infections.
8. Name four groups of protozoan parasites.
9. Name three groups of parasitic helminths.
10. How are intestinal parasitic infections usually diagnosed?
11. How are infections with blood or tissue parasites usually diagnosed?

12. What is Guinea worm disease? What measures have been used to eradicate the disease?

13. Define arthropod, atrial, cestode, commensal, congenital, cyst, definitive host, ectoparasite, endemic, helminth, host, immunocompromised, intermediate host, larva, nematode, opportunistic parasite, ova, parasite, pathogenic, proglottid, protozoa, reservoir host, trematode, and vector.

STUDENT ACTIVITIES

1. Complete the written examination for this lesson.

2. Research a parasitic disease. Report on the life cycle, transmission, symptoms, diagnostic methods, and recommended course of treatment.

WEB ACTIVITIES

1. Use the Internet to look at the CDC or National Institutes of Health (NIH) Web sites and find the sections on parasitic diseases. Report on a protozoan intestinal parasite. Include life cycle, diagnostic stage, and infective stage information. Find photographs of the organism.

2. Use the Internet to find the section on the CDC Web site that archives the *Morbidity and Mortality Weekly Report*. Find out what parasitic diseases are considered reportable.

3. Use the Internet to find information about the incidence of leishmaniasis in the United States. Explain why recent increased findings of parasites in U.S. clinical laboratories might correlate with deployment of military personnel to the Middle East.

Collecting and Processing Specimens for Parasite Examination

LESSON OBJECTIVES

After studying this lesson, the student will:

■ Explain the procedure for collecting fecal specimens for parasite examination.

■ Name two preservatives commonly used for fecal specimens.

■ Describe safety precautions to observe when handling fecal specimens.

■ Describe the proper transport procedure for fecal specimens.

■ Demonstrate the preparation of a cellophane tape swab.

■ Name two nonfecal specimens that can be examined for parasites.

■ Discuss transmission and detection of enterobiasis.

■ Explain how toxoplasmosis is transmitted and how it can be prevented.

■ Explain how quality assessment policies are important in specimen collection and processing.

■ Define the glossary terms.

GLOSSARY

pinworm / *Enterobius vermicularis*, a small parasitic nematode; also called seatworm

proglottid / the tapeworm body segment that contains the male and female reproductive organs

PVA / polyvinyl alcohol, a preservative used for fecal specimens

trophozoite / the motile, feeding stage of protozoan parasites

INTRODUCTION

Although small laboratories do not usually perform the microscopic examination for parasites, laboratory personnel must provide patient instructions for specimen collection when appropriate, and must process specimens before they are sent to a reference laboratory. A basic understanding of parasite life cycles is required to be sure the most appropriate specimen is obtained, and thus increase the chances that any parasites present will be discovered. The two most common parasitology laboratory tests requested are for fecal examination for ova and parasites (O & P) and blood examination for malarial parasites. The O & P test requires a fecal specimen, and the malarial smear requires a fresh blood specimen.

This lesson describes routine specimen collection and processing to detect intestinal parasites and the procedure for detecting pinworms. Lesson 8-3 describes the procedures for preparing fecal wet mounts and fecal smears for staining, as well as fecal-concentration techniques. The procedure for preparing and staining blood smears for detection of blood parasites is described in Lesson 8-4.

TYPES OF SPECIMENS FOR PARASITE EXAMINATION

Fecal (Stool) Specimens

The fecal specimen is examined when infection with intestinal parasites is suspected. Helminths, amoebae, and other intestinal protozoa can be identified during microscopic examination of unstained, stained, and concentrated fecal specimens. Fecal specimens are also used for immunological tests that detect *Giardia*, *Cryptosporidium*, and *Entamoeba histolytica* antigens.

Blood Specimens

Blood is examined when infection with blood parasites such as the malarial parasite, filiarial worms, or certain trypanosomes is suspected. Specially prepared and stained blood smears or wet mounts of blood are prepared. Blood to be tested for malaria must be collected at timed intervals. The collection of blood and preparation of blood smears for examination for parasites is described fully in Lesson 8-4.

Specimens for Immunological Tests

Although immunological tests are being developed for many parasites, only a few have widespread use. Kits to detect and differentiate parasitic diarrheal diseases caused by *Cryptosporidium*, *Giardia*, or *Entamoeba histolytica* are used by many laboratories. Fresh specimens are centrifuged and filtered for use in the kits. Parasite antigens in the filtered specimen, if present, are detected using a rapid colorimetric enzyme immunoassay that contains antibodies against specific parasite antigens.

Immunological tests can also be used to detect the presence of anti-parasite antibody in patient serum, as in the test for *Toxoplasma*. In the case of suspected acute infection, paired serum samples (samples collected 2 to 3 weeks apart) are tested for the presence of IgM and IgG, or for a rising antibody titer. Toxoplasmosis is discussed further in Current Topics in this lesson.

Other Specimens

Specimens other than blood or stool can be tested or examined for parasites. The type of specimen required depends on the organism(s) suspected based on the patient's symptoms and medical history. For example:

- Sputum specimens are examined for *Paragonimus*
- Vaginal secretions are examined for *Trichomonas*
- Tissue specimens, usually processed and stained by the histology laboratory, are examined when *Trichinella*, *Toxoplasma*, or other tissue parasites are suspected

Examples of organisms that can be found in nonfecal specimens are listed in Table 8-7.

COLLECTING AND PROCESSING FECAL SPECIMENS

Safety Precautions

 Several potential hazards are present when collecting and processing specimens for parasite examination. These include possible exposure to infective parasite cysts, oocysts, eggs, or larvae in stool specimens as well as to nonparasitic pathogens that can be present in stool and biological fluids. Workers must use Standard Precautions, as well as standard microbiology safety practices. Standard Precautions must be used even with preserved (fixed) specimens, because some parasite forms can remain viable for weeks after fixation.

TABLE 8-7. Examples of organisms found in nonfecal specimens	
TYPE OF SPECIMEN	**POSSIBLE ORGANISMS**
Sputum	*Paragonimus, Ascaris*
Blood	*Plasmodium, Babesia, Trypanosoma*
CSF	Amoebae, *Toxoplasma, Trypanosoma*
Liver	Amoebae, *Leishmania, Schistosoma*
Urine	*Trichomonas, Schistosoma*
Muscle	*Trichinella*
Duodenal aspirates	*Giardia, Isospora*
Vaginal secretions	*Trichomonas*

CURRENT TOPICS

TOXOPLASMOSIS

One of the most common human infections worldwide is toxoplasmosis, caused by the single-celled protozoa *Toxoplasma gondii*. In the United States, over 20% of the population (more than 60 million people) test positive for *Toxoplasma* antibodies. The two infective forms of *Toxoplasma* are *oocysts* and *tissue cysts*.

Life Cycle and Epidemiology

The definitive hosts of *Toxoplasma gondii* are domestic and wild cats. Humans and many other animal species are intermediate hosts. Cats become infected by ingesting *T. gondii* tissue cysts present in meat/animals or by ingesting oocysts. After ingestion, parasites released from the tissue cysts or oocysts invade the epithelial cells of the cat's small intestine, replicate, and form oocysts, which are excreted in the feces. One to 5 days after excretion, the oocysts sporulate (develop to the infective stage). These oocysts, which are resistant to disinfectants, freezing, and drying, can remain viable for months in the environment, but are destroyed by heating to 70°C for 10 minutes.

Humans and other animals become infected by ingesting viable oocysts or tissue cysts. This can occur by:

- Accidentally ingesting viable oocysts from hands or food contaminated with cat feces (such as by touching hand to mouth after cleaning a litter box, gardening, or touching anything that has contacted cat feces)
- Touching hands to mouth after handling or eating contaminated raw or undercooked meat, especially pork, lamb, or venison. This transmission method is estimated by the U.S. Department of Agriculture to account for 50% of U.S. cases, and is also estimated to be an important cause of death due to a foodborne organism
- Ingesting water contaminated with *Toxoplasma*
- Transplacental transmission
- Organ transplant or blood transfusion from infected donor (rare occurrence)

Once the infective form is ingested by an intermediate host, the parasites released (called tachyzoites) invade tissue and form tissue cysts—usually in skeletal muscle, heart muscle, or brain—that can remain for the host's lifetime. In the dormant tissue cysts, the parasites are called bradyzoites. In the healthy individual, tissue cysts are usually few in number and are kept dormant by the immune system. This photomicrograph shows a *Toxoplasma* tissue cyst stained with fluorescent antibody technique.

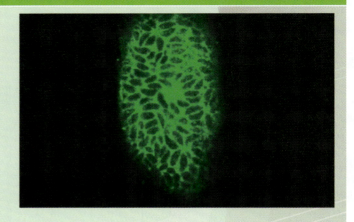

Toxoplasma cyst stained with immunofluorescent stain and showing numerous banana-shaped parasites in the cyst (*Photo courtesy C. A. Sundermann, Auburn University, AL*)

Clinical Symptoms and Complications

Symptoms of toxoplasmosis vary depending on the health and immune competency of the individual. For the healthy population, toxoplasmosis is rather benign. Most people have very few symptoms, and some may not even be aware they have an infection. Others experience mild flulike symptoms, with muscle aches and swollen lymph nodes.

For immunocompromised individuals and pregnant women, *Toxoplasma* infection can cause serious complications. In HIV/AIDS, chemotherapy, or transplant patients, toxoplasmosis can cause brain, eye, and organ damage. Reactivation of previous infection can occur when the immune system becomes unable to keep the infection dormant and tissue cysts rupture, releasing parasites. Complications develop such as disseminated disease or toxoplasmic encephalitis, the most frequent severe neurologic infection among persons with AIDS in the United States.

Congenital toxoplasmosis can occur in infants born to women who become infected during (or just before) pregnancy. Many infants with congenital toxoplasmosis are born with serious eye or brain damage, including hydrocephaly. The severity of the complications can be reduced by prompt diagnosis and treatment of the mother. Infants can also be born with subclinical infection and remain asymptomatic until their teens or twenties, when ocular toxoplasmosis develops causing a condition called *retinochoroiditis*.

CURRENT TOPICS (continued)

Laboratory Diagnosis of Toxoplasmosis

Since *Toxoplasma gondii* antibodies appear early in infection and remain detectable for life, the primary method of detecting *T. gondii* infection in immunocompetent individuals is serological testing. Patient serum is tested for IgG and/or IgM *T. gondii*-specific antibodies using immunofluorescent assay (IFA) methods available in various commercial kits. In adults, a rising IgG titer, or presence of IgM in acute serum and IgG in convalescent serum indicates recent or active infection.

In immunocompromised patients, serology results are not always reliable because antibody levels are often low even when infection is present. In these patients, the parasites can be observed in blood, body fluids, bronchoalveolar lavage fluids, and lymph node or other biopsy tissue. If congenital toxoplasmosis is suspected, the newborn should be tested for IgA as well as IgM, since the test for IgA is more sensitive in infants. Molecular methods such as polymerase chain reaction (PCR) can be used for detecting congenital infections *in utero*. Because kit sensitivity and specificity varies, and tests are complex and not always easily interpreted, tests for *T. gondii* antibodies should be performed by laboratories where the tests are frequently performed.

Prevention

Females, before becoming pregnant, and individuals with weakened immune systems should be tested for *Toxoplasma*-specific IgG antibodies. For immunocompetent females, a positive IgG test means that they have been infected sometime previously, have immunity, and generally do not need to worry about passing the infection to the fetus, should they become pregnant. For immunocompromised individuals who test positive, drug therapy may be indicated to prevent reactivation of infection. A negative test for either of these patient populations indicates that they have not been infected, are most likely susceptible to infection, and should take precautions to avoid exposure to the parasite. These precautions include:

- Wearing gloves when gardening or handling soil
- Washing hands well with soap and water after outdoor activities
- Having someone else change the cat's litter box daily, before oocysts have time to become infectious
- Washing hands well after handling raw meat and before eating or preparing other foods
- Thoroughly washing cutting boards, knives, and all utensils used to prepare raw meat
- Cooking all meat to an internal temperature of 160° F until it is no longer pink or the juices become colorless.

Good safety practices include, but are not limited to, wearing fluid-resistant protective clothing and gloves, using biological safety cabinets, decontaminating work surfaces frequently, washing hands before donning gloves and after removing gloves, and disposing of all sharp objects in a sharps container for biohazards.

Specimens should be processed in a fume hood to avoid inhaling preservative fumes and to minimize unpleasant odors. All specimens and processing materials should be disposed of in the same manner as bacterial or biohazardous specimens.

Quality Assessment

Specimens must be collected and processed according to established laboratory procedures. The timing of specimen collection is critical for some tests, such as blood smears for malaria and the pinworm test.

- Specimens must be collected from patients before anti-parasite drugs are administered.
- Fecal specimens should not be collected within 7 days after administration of antacids, mineral oil, barium, bismuth, or certain antidiarrheal medications or within 3 weeks after certain antimicrobial agents and dyes.

- Specimens must be processed as quickly as possible after collection to ensure that parasite morphology is maintained.
- Microscopic examination of unfixed specimens must be performed within 30 minutes to 1 hour of collection to increase the chance of finding motile forms.

Specimen Collection

Fecal samples should be collected in a clean, dry, wide-mouth, leakproof container that has a tight-fitting lid. Specimens can be collected in a bedpan and transferred to the container, but the sample *must not* be contaminated with urine or water. Patients should wait 1 week after ingesting antidiarrheal medication, radiopaque compounds (barium), or oily laxatives before fecal specimens for parasite examination are collected.

The specimen container must be labeled with the patient's name and the date and time of collection. It is recommended that at least three separate specimens be collected over a period of 3 to 5 days. Specimens should be delivered to the laboratory as soon as possible (within 2 hours of collection). If specimen transport must be delayed, kits containing vials with preservatives and containers for mailing are available (Figures 8-4 and 8-5).

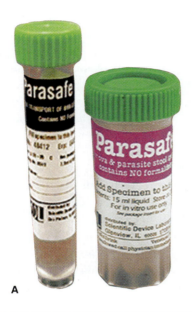

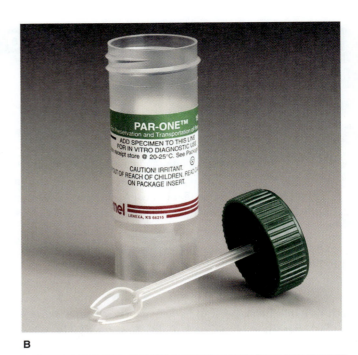

A

B

FIGURE 8-4 Fixative vials for preserving fecal specimens (*Photo* **A** *courtesy Scientific Device Lab, Inc., Des Plaines, IL*; *Photo* **B** *courtesy Remel, Inc., Lenexa, KS*)

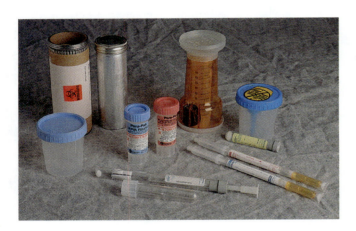

FIGURE 8-5 Containers for transporting or mailing biological specimens

Specimen Processing

Specimens should be processed and examined as soon as possible after arrival at the laboratory. It is especially important to process watery specimens within 30 minutes to 1 hour, because forms such as protozoan **trophozoites** deteriorate rapidly.

Specimen consistency should be observed and recorded (watery, loose, soft, or formed). In helminth infections, adult worms or tapeworm **proglottids** can sometimes be seen and should be reported. If blood or mucus is present in the fecal sample, portions of these areas should be selected for examination. In protozoan infections, trophozoite forms are more likely to be found in the more fluid specimens and cyst forms in the more formed specimens.

Preservation

Portions of the specimen should be preserved for future examination and for staining. In the past, it was necessary to use two separate preservatives, formalin and **PVA** (polyvinyl alcohol), because a single preservative was not available that could preserve parasite morphology, and also provide satisfactory results with the trichrome parasite stain and immunochemical tests. However, formalin and PVA had the disadvantages of producing toxic fumes (formalin) and containing mercury (PVA). To meet Occupational Safety and Health Administration (OSHA) requirements for safety and disposal, environmentally-safe zinc and copper-based PVA preservatives are now used that are formalin- and mercury-free (Figure 8-4). These new preservatives, such as Para-Pak EcoFix (Meridian Diagnostics), Parasafe (Scientific Device Laboratory), and Par-One (Remel), provide satisfactory morphology, staining, and immunochemical results with the use of just one preservative.

Specimen Transport

Fecal specimens to be mailed or otherwise transported should be placed in a fixative vial and appropriately labeled. The vial should be enclosed in a leakproof container or bag and placed in a labeled mailing/transport carton (Figure 8-5). Transport containers must be approved for biological materials by the United States Postal Service or other carrier.

PROCEDURE: DETECTION OF PINWORM (ENTEROBIUS) INFECTION

Enterobiasis

The most common roundworm infection in the United States is enterobiasis, caused by infection with *Enterobius vermicularis*, the human **pinworm** or seatworm. This parasite is frequently found in young children in day care centers and elementary schools. It is estimated that, in the United States, approximately 40 million people are infected at any one time.

Life Cycle, Transmission, and Clinical Symptoms

Pinworm infections are acquired by ingesting pinworm ova. The ova hatch in the small intestine, releasing larvae that mature into tiny adult worms within about 30 days. The adult female pinworm lives in the colon and migrates out of the anus during the night to deposit microscopic-size ova in the perianal folds. This leads to the characteristic symptom, anal itching, and contributes to reinfection when children scratch and their hands become contaminated. Pinworm infections are also easily spread when ova from contaminated clothing and bedding become airborne and are inhaled and then ingested.

Specimen Collection

Pinworm infections are rarely detected by examining fecal specimens. Rather, the specimen for pinworm is a perianal specimen. A simple collection technique is to provide a perianal *paddle* swab for the patient or parent to take home. A typical commercial pinworm collection device consists of a flat plastic paddle or spatula with one sticky surface in a sterile sealed container (Figure 8-6). The perianal specimen is obtained by gently spreading the buttocks apart and pressing the paddle swab several times around the anal opening between 9 PM and midnight or in the early morning before bathing. It may be necessary to collect several specimens over a period of days because the female worm does not migrate

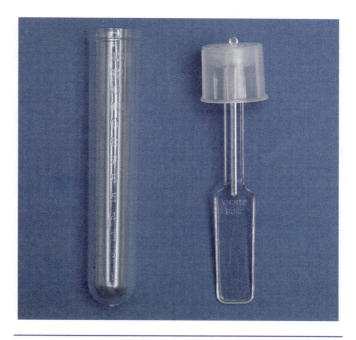

FIGURE 8-6 Commercial perianal "paddle" swab. Pinworm ova adhere to surface of paddle

every night. The specimen should be delivered to the laboratory the morning of collection.

If a commercial collection device is not available, a perianal swab can be prepared from clear cellophane tape, a microscope slide, and a wooden tongue depressor. A piece of cellophane tape 4 to 5 inches long is attached to the back of a microscope slide, wrapped around the end of the slide, and smoothed into place on the top of the slide. A paper tab is attached to the free end of the tape for labeling (Figure 8-7). These slides can be stored in a cool place for weeks until used.

To collect the perianal specimen using the cellophane tape slide, the slide is placed against a tongue depressor, and the tape is lifted and looped over the end of the depressor, sticky

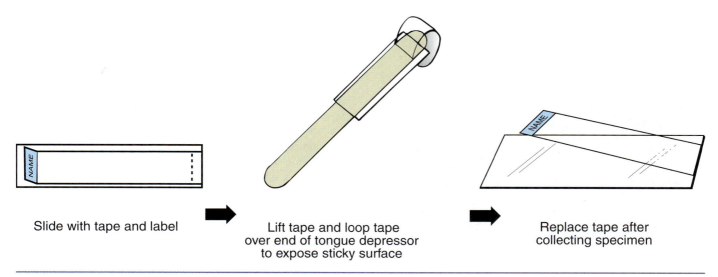

Slide with tape and label

Lift tape and loop tape over end of tongue depressor to expose sticky surface

Replace tape after collecting specimen

FIGURE 8-7 Technique for preparing a cellophane tape swab

side out (Figure 8-7). The sticky surface of the tape is gently pressed against the perianal region several times. The tape is then smoothed back onto the slide, sticky side down, and the slide is delivered to the laboratory for examination.

Microscopic Identification

Because the location and appearance of *Enterobius* ova are so characteristic, identification of pinworm ova is a parasitology procedure that can be performed in most laboratories and usually does not require the services of a reference laboratory. Diagnosis is confirmed by finding *Enterobius* ova in the perianal swab specimen. The paddle (or slide) is microscopically examined for ova using the 10× objective. When examining a cellophane tape preparation, a nontoxic clearing agent (xylene substitute) can be placed under the tape to dissolve the adhesive and allow for easier ova identification.

Enterobius ova have a characteristic appearance (Figure 8-8). They are 20 to 32 μm × 50 to 60 μm in size, colorless, flattened on one side, have a thick-walled shell, and contain a developing larva.

Special Precautions

Pinworm ova remain viable for weeks as do other helminth ova. Infection is easily transmitted when airborne ova are accidentally ingested or when the mouth is touched with contaminated fingers. Therefore, special care must be taken when collecting the specimen, handling the swab, and examining the swab for ova. The microscope must be decontaminated after examining the preparation. The used collection device or slide should be discarded into a biohazard sharps container.

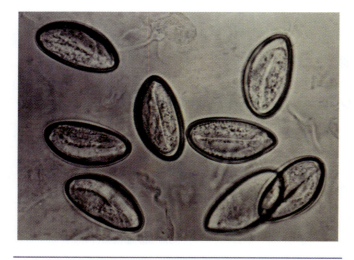

FIGURE 8-8 Microscopic appearance of *Enterobius* ova from cellophane tape prep (*From CDC, Atlanta, GA*)

SAFETY Reminders

- Review safety precautions section before performing procedure.
- Observe Standard Precautions when handling specimens.
- Wear appropriate PPE when handling specimens.
- Avoid skin contact with preservatives and inhalation of fumes.
- Handle preserved specimens as if infectious.
- Dispose of specimens properly.

PROCEDURAL Reminders

- Review quality assessment section before performing procedure.
- Collect specimens according to established procedures.
- Collect specimens at proper time intervals.
- Process specimens promptly.

SUMMARY

Examinations of blood, stool, tissues, and other biological specimens are essential to the diagnosis of parasitic infections. Successful detection of parasites depends on having properly collected and prepared specimens. Although parasite examination is often performed in a reference laboratory, the local laboratory must process the specimens and prepare them for transport. Established procedures for collection and processing must be carefully followed to ensure that specimens meet acceptable testing criteria. Standard Precautions must be used when handling all specimens in case infective parasite forms are present.

Some tests for parasites can be easily performed in local laboratories. The pinworm test is one such test because the distinguishing characteristics of pinworm ova and the symptoms of pinworm infection make it easily identified and diagnosed. Tests to detect antigens of intestinal protozoa that cause diarrheal disease (*Cryptosporidium, Giardia,* and *Entamoeba histolytica*) are available as rapid enzyme immunoassay kits. Tests for *Toxoplasma* based on detection of anti-toxoplasma antibodies in patient serum are, in general, more complex to interpret and should be performed by personnel experienced in testing for toxoplasmosis.

REVIEW QUESTIONS

1. Explain the proper method for collecting fecal specimens.

2. Which type of fecal specimen must be processed quickly? Why?

3. What terms are used to describe the consistency of fecal specimens?

4. What safety precautions must be observed when handling and processing fecal specimens? Why?

5. What characteristics are required of a preservative that is to be used with fecal specimens?

6. What parasite is best detected from a perianal swab?

7. How are commercially available sticky paddles used to collect perianal specimens?

8. Explain how to prepare and use a cellophane tape swab.

9. What specimens other than feces are examined for parasites?

10. Name three parasites found in nonfecal specimens.

11. Explain why the timing of specimen collection and rapid processing of the specimen can be important to recovery of the parasite.

12. How are pinworm infections transmitted? How are they diagnosed?

13. What is the scientific name of the pinworm? To what parasite category does it belong?

14. How is toxoplasmosis transmitted to humans? How is it prevented?

15. Define pinworm, proglottid, PVA, and trophozoite.

STUDENT ACTIVITIES

1. Complete the written examination for this lesson.

2. Practice instructing a patient to properly collect a fecal specimen for parasite examination as outlined in the Student Performance Guide.

3. Practice preparing a perianal swab (cellophane tape swab) as outlined in the Student Performance Guide. Practice instructing a patient to collect a perianal specimen using a paddle or slide preparation as outlined in the Student Performance Guide.

4. Practice processing fecal specimens for parasite examination as outlined in the Student Performance guide.

WEB ACTIVITIES

1. Use the Internet to find distributors of parasitology supplies. What preservatives are used in the collection vials?

2. Use the Internet to find information about the preferred treatments for enterobiasis and toxoplasmosis.

Student Performance Guide

Lesson 8-2 Collecting and Processing Specimens for Parasite Examination

Name _____ Date _____

INSTRUCTIONS

1. Practice the procedures, or practice giving instructions, for collecting and preserving fecal specimens for parasite examination, following the step-by-step procedure.

2. Practice instructing a patient to collect a perianal specimen using a pinworm paddle or cellophane tape slide following the step-by-step procedure.

3. Demonstrate these procedures satisfactorily for the instructor, using the Student Performance Guide. Your instructor will determine the level of competency you must achieve to receive a satisfactory (S) grade.

MATERIALS AND EQUIPMENT

- gloves
- face shield and/or acrylic safety shield
- antiseptic
- surface disinfectant
- biohazard container
- sharps container
- fume hood or biological safety cabinet (optional)
- microscope
- disposable applicator sticks
- fecal collection containers with lids
- fecal preservative vials (environmentally safe brand)
- leakproof transport containers
- fecal specimens (students can bring pet specimens for practice)
- commercial perianal paddle swabs
- materials for preparing cellophane tape swabs
  - microscope slides with beveled edges
  - clear (not frosted) cellophane tape
  - wooden or plastic tongue depressors
- visuals and prepared microscope slides of *Enterobius* ova
- atlas of parasite morphology containing illustrations of *Enterobius* ova

PROCEDURE

Record in the comment section any problems encountered while practicing the procedure (or have a fellow student or the instructor evaluate your performance).

S = Satisfactory
U = Unsatisfactory

You must:	S	U	Comments

1. Instruct a patient in the proper procedure for collecting a fecal specimen (steps 1a and 1b):
  a. Give patient a lidded fecal specimen container, label, and transport container
  b. Explain the fecal collection procedure to the patient, emphasizing the following precautions:
    (1) Specimen must not be contaminated with urine or water			

You must:	S	U	Comments
(2) Outer surface of specimen container must not be contaminated (3) Container must be labeled with the patient's name, date, and the time of collection (4) Unpreserved specimens must be transported to a laboratory immediately following collection (within 2 hours) (5) Specimens should not be collected until at least 7 days after ingesting interfering substances such as oily laxatives, barium or radiopaque contrast media, or antidiarrheal medications (6) Labeled specimen container must be placed in outer transport container			

2. Preserve a fecal specimen, or instruct patient in the proper way to preserve the specimen (steps 2a through 2n)
  a. Wash hands and put on gloves. Put on face protection or place acrylic safety shield on work surface (Optional: work in a biological safety cabinet or fume hood)
  b. Obtain a fecal specimen, preservative vial, and transport container. Check label to be sure required patient information is present (name, date, time of collection)
  c. Open container and observe consistency of specimen. Record as watery, loose, soft, or formed
  d. Use applicator in cap of preservative vial or disposable applicator to obtain a portion of specimen
  e. Add specimen to the *fill* line on the preservative vial, or add amount of specimen equal to approximately one-third the volume of the preservative in vial
  f. Mix specimen with preservative thoroughly using applicator
  g. Replace cap on vial and tighten
  h. Discard used applicator (if applicable) into biohazard container
  i. Label vial with patient information
  j. Insert labeled vial into transport container, seal container, and label
  k. Discard specimen into biohazard container
  l. Disinfect work area with surface disinfectant
  m. Remove gloves and discard into biohazard container
  n. Wash hands with antiseptic			

You must:	S	U	Comments
3. Prepare a cellophane tape slide following steps 3a through 3e. (If materials are not available, skip to step 4.) a. Obtain clear cellophane tape, clean microscope slide, and paper tab b. Attach a 4- to 5-inch section of tape to one end of the back of the slide c. Bring the tape over the end of the slide and smooth the tape down over top surface of the slide, leaving a small portion of tape free at the end (see Figure 8-7) d. Attach a small paper tab to the free end of the tape for use as a label and lifting tab e. Store the slide in a cool, dust-free location			
4. Explain the proper collection of a pinworm specimen using a commercial pinworm paddle following steps 4a through 4e. (If commercial paddle is not available, skip to step 5.) Instruct patient (or parent) to: a. Wash hands and put on gloves b. Remove paddle from sterile container c. Obtain specimen by gently touching the sticky surface of the swab/paddle to the perianal region several times d. Return the swab to its container being careful to avoid touching the sticky swab, and seal the container e. Label container with name, date, and time and transport to the laboratory			
5. Explain the proper collection of a pinworm specimen using a cellophane tape slide following steps 5a through 5i. (If cellophane tape slide is not available, skip to step 6.) Instruct patient (or parent) to: a. Wash hands and put on gloves b. Obtain cellophane tape slide, tongue depressor, and transport container c. Label tab on slide with patient information d. Place slide against tongue depressor near the end, tape side up e. Lift the cellophane tape and form a loop around the end of the tongue depressor, sticky side of tape to the outside (see Figure 8-7) f. Obtain specimen by gently touching the sticky surface of the tape to the perianal region several times g. Lift the tape from the tongue depressor carefully and smooth the sticky side back down onto the microscope slide, being careful not to touch the sticky surface h. Place slide in transport container and seal. Remove and discard gloves and wash hands i. Label transport container with name, date, and time and arrange for transport to the laboratory			

You must:	S	U	Comments
6. Optional: If available, practice identifying *Enterobius* ova by examining prepared microscope slides using the 10× objective. Make several drawings of the ova seen. If an ocular micrometer is available, measure length and width of five ova			
7. Optional: Practice the procedure for microscopic examination of the pinworm swab/slide a. Wash hands and put on gloves b. Place the pinworm paddle on the microscope stage, sticky side up and scan the paddle area using the 10× objective c. Place the cellophane tape slide on the microscope stage and demonstrate how to observe for ova using the low-power (10×) objective d. Discard used slide or swab into appropriate biohazard container and disinfect microscope stage			
8. Return supplies to storage			
9. Disinfect work area with surface disinfectant			
10. Remove gloves and discard into biohazard container			
11. Wash hands with antiseptic			

Evaluator Comments:

Evaluator _____   Date _____

Microscopic Methods of Detecting Intestinal Parasites

LESSON OBJECTIVES

After studying this lesson, the student will:

- Name three types of preparations used for the microscopic examination of fecal specimens.
- Explain how to prepare saline and iodine wet mounts for microscopic examination.
- Explain the use of flotation and sedimentation procedures to concentrate fecal specimens.
- Prepare fecal smears from fresh or fixed fecal specimens.
- Discuss giardiasis, including modes of transmission and methods of diagnosis.
- List safety precautions to be observed when preparing fecal specimens for microscopic examinations.
- Discuss why adherence to quality assessment procedures is important when preparing fecal specimens for microscopic examination.
- Define the glossary terms.

GLOSSARY

micrometer / a ruled device for measuring small objects

ocular micrometer / a micrometer that fits in the microscope eyepiece and that is used to measure microscopic objects

trichrome stain / a stain commonly used to identify parasites in fecal smears

INTRODUCTION

The majority of parasitic infections are diagnosed by the microscopic identification of the parasite in blood, tissue, or fecal specimens. Much experience is required to become expert in parasite identification.

This lesson describes the methods of preparing fecal specimens for microscopic parasite examination. The procedures for examining blood for parasites are described in Lesson 8-4. The preparation of tissues for parasite examination is usually performed in the histology laboratory, where tissues are fixed, sectioned, and stained with special stains for parasite detection.

MICROSCOPIC EXAMINATION OF FECAL SPECIMENS

The routine fecal specimen examination for parasites includes microscopic examination of:

- Wet mounts from fresh or fixed specimens
- Wet mounts of concentrated specimens
- Stained fecal smears

A schematic illustrating how to prepare fecal specimens for microscopic examination is shown in Figure 8-9.

Safety Precautions

 Preparing fecal specimens for microscopy exposes the technician to biological and chemical hazards. Standard Precautions must be followed when handling fecal specimens. Even after fixative is added, specimens are still potentially infectious, since some parasites (particularly helminth eggs and protozoan cysts) are not immediately killed by fixatives.

Procedures that use fixatives and volatile chemicals should be performed in a fume hood to eliminate the possibility of inhaling fumes. Appropriate personal protective equipment (PPE), including chemical-resistant gloves, must be worn to prevent exposing skin to the fixatives.

Quality Assessment

 The laboratory procedure manual and manufacturer's instructions must be carefully followed when preparing fecal specimens for examination. Specimens must be processed promptly to prevent deterioration of any viable organisms in the specimen. Reagents should not be interchanged between fecal concentration kits or diagnostic kits. Reagent containers must remain tightly capped when not in use to prevent evaporation or changes in specific gravity. Centrifuge speed should be checked and recorded at designated intervals using a tachometer. Timing requirements of concentration techniques must be followed.

Wet Mounts

Wet mounts are prepared from fresh or preserved fecal specimens. Motile trophozoites (trophs) can be observed in wet mounts of *fresh* specimens. Observing motility is helpful, because preserved trophozoites are very small, lack many distinguishing characteristics, and can be easily overlooked by the microscopist. Wet mounts from fixed specimens are used to detect cysts, ova, and larva.

Preparing Wet Mounts

Wet mounts are prepared by mixing a small amount of fresh or fixed specimen with a drop of saline on one end of a microscope slide (Figure 8-10). A similar portion of specimen is mixed with a

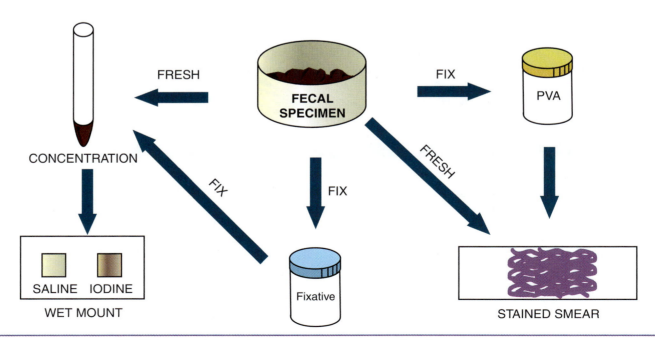

FIGURE 8-9 Schematic for preparing fecal specimens for microscopic examination

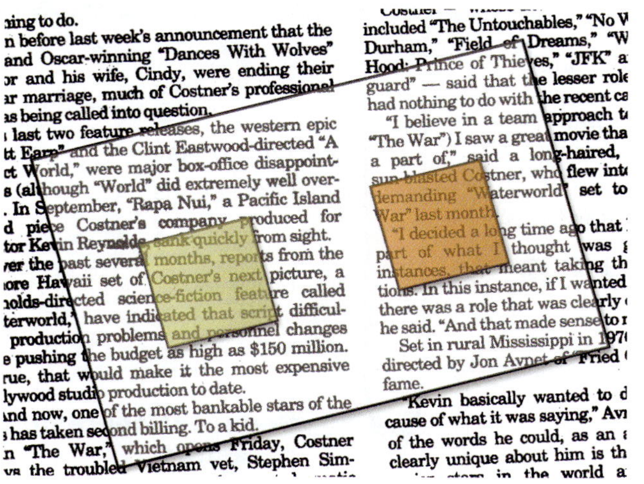

FIGURE 8-10 Wet mounts of fecal material for microscopic examination; density of saline and iodine wet mounts is checked by placing over newsprint

drop of iodine solution on the other end of the slide and a coverglass is placed over each mixture. If desired, the coverglass edges can be sealed with petroleum jelly to retard drying. The preparations should be thin enough to read newsprint through the specimen when the slide is placed on newspaper (Figure 8-10).

Examining Wet Mounts

The entire wet mount preparation should be examined using the 10× or 20× objective. Most ova and larvae can be seen at this magnification. The 40× (high-power) objective should be used to examine the preparation for protozoa. Helminth eggs retain better morphology in the saline mount: iodine provides good morphology of protozoan cysts. An **ocular micrometer** should be used to measure any organisms seen.

Concentration Techniques for Fecal Specimens

Concentration techniques increase the likelihood of detecting the parasite. Fresh or preserved specimens can be concentrated by *sedimentation* or *flotation* techniques.

Sedimentation Techniques

Sedimentation techniques use solutions of lower specific gravity (sp. gr.) than the sp. gr. of the parasites, causing the parasites to collect in the sediment when the specimen is centrifuged. Parasites such as helminth ova and larvae and protozoan oocysts can be detected. In the sedimentation technique, the specimen is filtered, washed by centrifugation, and ethyl acetate is added to the specimen and mixed. The specimen is centrifuged, the top layers of supernatant are removed, and the sediment in the bottom of the tube is used to prepare saline and iodine wet mounts for microscopic examination (Figure 8-11). The formalin-ethyl acetate sedimentation method has been modified for use in several fecal concentrator kits.

Flotation Techniques

Flotation techniques use solutions of high specific gravity to cause the less dense parasitic forms to float to the solution's top while fecal debris settles to the bottom (Figure 8-11). Most organisms and ova can be recovered with these methods. Two solutions used for flotation are zinc sulfate ($ZnSO_4$) and Sheather's, particularly useful for protozoa such as *Cryptosporidium* oocysts and *Giardia* cysts. In flotation techniques, the specimen is filtered, washed by centrifugation, and mixed with a solution such as zinc sulfate (sp. gr. 1.190 to 1.200) or Sheather's solution (sp. gr. 1.18). During centrifugation, parasite forms rise to the top of the solution. The fluid surface is collected using a loop or coverslip, and wet mounts are prepared for microscopic examination.

Commercial systems for fecal concentration are available, such as Para-Pak CON-trate and Macro-CON by Meridian Diagnostics, Fecal Concentrator II by Remel, and Parasep by Diasys Corporation. These disposable kits filter and concentrate fecal specimens, using modified sedimentation techniques. Some kits are designed as completely closed systems, in which the concentrator tube fits onto the preservative vial and all steps take place within the closed system. This minimizes exposure of the technician to the specimen.

Fecal Smears

Smears should be prepared from all fecal specimens. The smears can be made from fresh or fixed specimens.

Preparing Fecal Smears

Smears from modified polyvinyl alcohol (PVA)-fixed specimens are prepared by removing a portion of well-mixed specimen and spreading over a large area extending from the top edge to the bottom edge of the slide (Figure 8-12). The smear should dry for at least 4 hours (or overnight) at 35°C before staining.

Smears from fresh specimens are prepared similarly. A portion of the specimen is spread over a large area of the slide. Smears of fresh specimens must be placed in modified-PVA fixative *before* they are allowed to dry. Smears can remain in fixative several days. After fixation, the smears can be stained.

Staining Fecal Smears

Stained smears are particularly important for positive identification of protozoan parasites. Several stains are useful for parasite identification. Most laboratories use a modification of the **trichrome stain**, which seems to be the easiest to perform and gives the most consistent results. Trichrome-stained protozoa are blue-green to purple with red nuclei; helminths are purple. Immunofluorescent stains or modified acid-fast stains are used to identify *Cryptosporidium*.

Staining techniques for fecal specimens are complex and time-consuming. Most laboratories prepare the smears when processing the specimens and save the smears to stain in a batch. For this reason, final laboratory ova and parasites (O & P) reports are often not available until several days after the specimen is received.

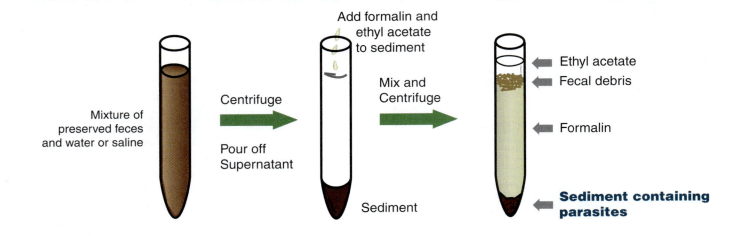

SEDIMENTATION

Mixture of preserved feces and water or saline

Centrifuge

Pour off Supernatant

Add formalin and ethyl acetate to sediment

Mix and Centrifuge

Sediment

Ethyl acetate
Fecal debris

Formalin

Sediment containing parasites

FLOTATION

Mixture of preserved feces and water or saline

Centrifuge

Pour off Supernatant

Add ZnSO$_4$ to sediment

Sediment

Mix

Coverglass
Parasites

ZnSO$_4$

Fecal debris

FIGURE 8-11 Sedimentation (top) and flotation (bottom) techniques

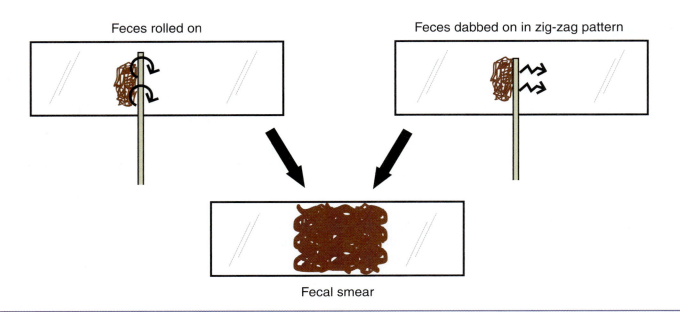

Feces rolled on

Feces dabbed on in zig-zag pattern

Fecal smear

FIGURE 8-12 Two methods of preparing fecal smears

Organisms Seen in Fecal Specimens

Intestinal protozoa are identified by the morphology of cysts, trophozoites, or oocysts in fecal specimens. Pathogenic intestinal protozoa include *Entamoeba histolytica, Dientamoeba fragilis, Giardia intestinalis, Balantidium coli, Isospora belli, Cryptosporidium, Cyclospora,* and possibly *Blastocystis hominis.* Nonpathogenic intestinal protozoa include other *Entamoeba* sp., *Endolimax, Chilomastix,* and *Iodamoeba.*

Helminths are identified by ova, larvae, or adults in fecal specimens. Any helminth found in a fecal specimen is considered of clinical importance.

Figures 8-13, 8-14, and 8-15 contain diagrams of amoebic, flagellate, ciliate, apicomplexan, and helminth forms of the more common human parasites. More information on these parasites can be found in Lesson 8-1 and textbooks of clinical parasitology.

CURRENT TOPICS

GIARDIASIS

Giardiasis is caused by infection with the single-celled flagellated protozoan *Giardia intestinalis* (also called *Giardia lamblia*). *Giardia*, a cause of diarrheal disease worldwide, and a common cause of diarrhea in travelers, is found in every region in the United States. It is one of the most common causes of waterborne enteric disease in the United States. In 2002, giardiasis was added to the Centers for Disease Control and Prevention (CDC) list of nationally notifiable diseases. The Food and Drug Administration (FDA) estimates that approximately 2% of the U.S. population is infected with *Giardia*.

Transmission

Giardia infections are transmitted by the fecal-oral route, most commonly by eating or drinking contaminated food or water. *Giardia* parasites live in the small intestine of infected humans and animals in a motile form called a *trophozoite*. As trophozoites move through the intestine, they form protective, resistant cysts (shown in the micrographs) that are eliminated in the feces into the environment. Infection occurs when the cysts are ingested by:

■ Swallowing recreational water (swimming pools, hot tubs, fountains, lakes, springs, etc.) contaminated with animal or human feces or sewage containing *Giardia*

■ Eating uncooked food contaminated with *Giardia*

■ Accidentally swallowing *Giardia* picked up from surfaces (such as bathroom fixtures, changing tables, diaper pails, or toys) contaminated with feces from an infected person

Clinical Symptoms and Laboratory Diagnosis

Symptoms of giardiasis begin a week or two after infection and include diarrhea, nausea, flatulence, abdominal cramps, and fatty stools that tend to float. In healthy individuals the symptoms can last from a couple of weeks to several weeks, and the infection can become chronic. In immunocompro-mised individuals, the disease can be long-lasting and debilitating, requiring supportive therapy as well as drug treatment.

Giardiasis is diagnosed by microscopic examination of fecal specimens for the presence of *Giardia* cysts. Examination of wet mounts (iodine-stained or unstained) using the high-power objective is sometimes all that is required to find *Giardia* cysts. If wet mounts are negative, the specimen can be concentrated and re-examined, providing a higher probability of finding the organism in light infections. The figure shows an iodine-stained *Giardia* cyst (top) and a trichrome-stained cyst (bottom).

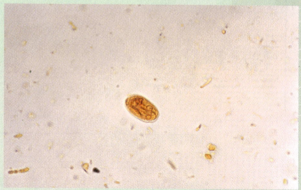

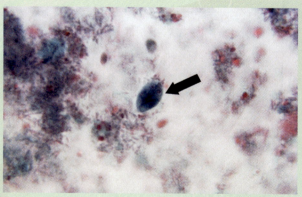

Giardia intestinalis: (top) iodine-stained cyst in fecal wet mount; (bottom) cyst (arrow) in a fecal smear stained with trichrome stain (*From CDC, Atlanta, GA and Dr. Mae Melvin*)

AMEBAE					
Entamoeba histolytica	*Entamoeba hartmanni*	*Entamoeba coli*	*Endolimax nana*	*Iodamoeba butschlii*	*Dientamoeba fragilis*

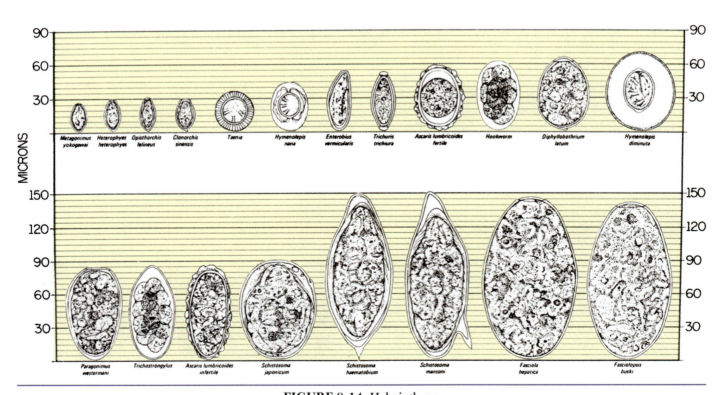

FIGURE 8-13 Intestinal amoebae (*Dientamoeba* is a flagellate)
(*From Centers for Disease Control Publication No. 84-8116, U.S. Department of Health and Human Services*)

FIGURE 8-14 Helminth ova
(*From Centers for Disease Control Publication No. 84-8116, U.S. Department of Health and Human Services*)

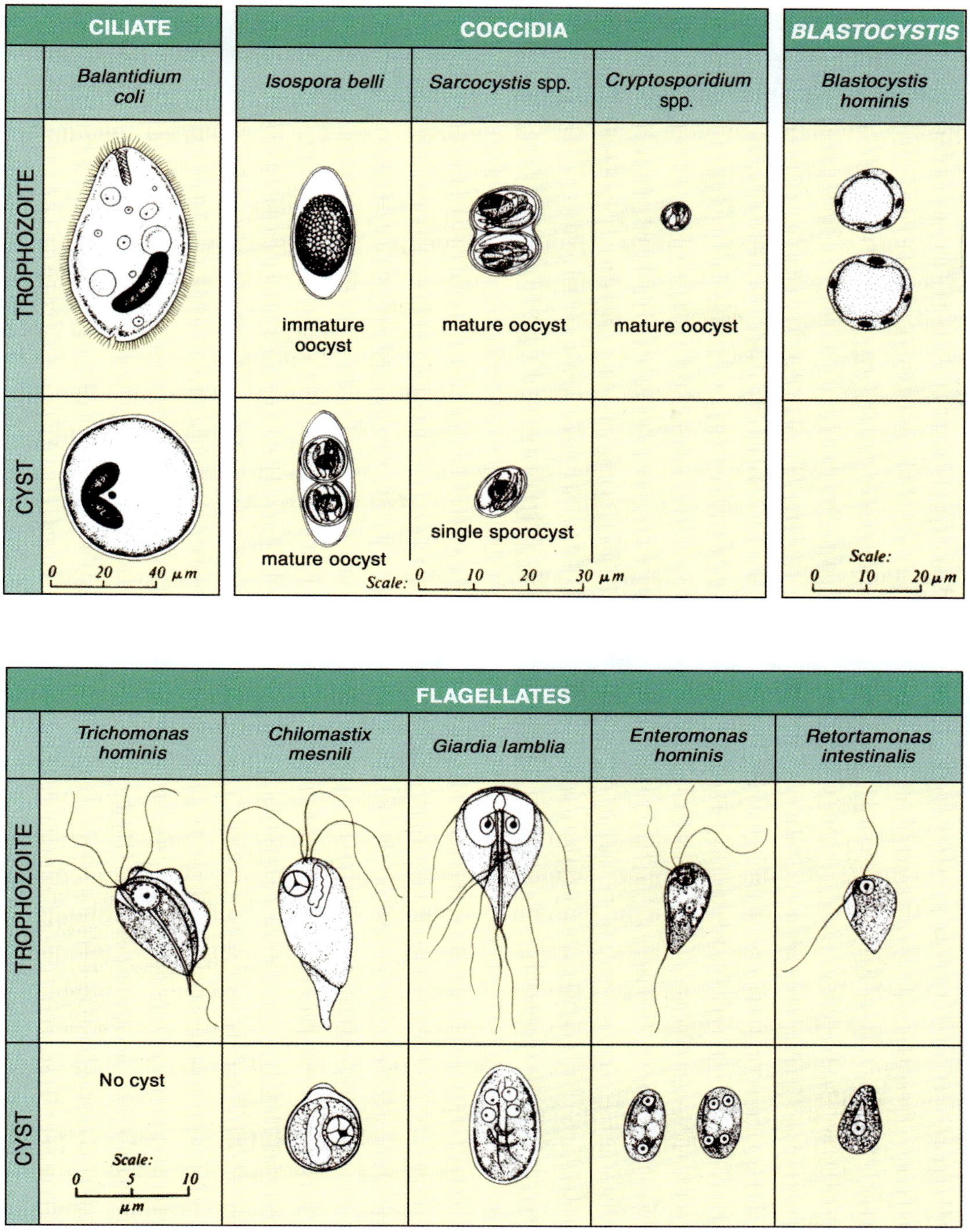

FIGURE 8-15 Intestinal ciliates, coccidia, and flagellates
(*From Centers for Disease Control Publication No. 84-8116, U.S. Department of Health and Human Services*)

SAFETY Reminders

- Review safety section before beginning procedure.
- Use Standard Precautions when handling fresh and preserved fecal specimens.
- Balance load before turning on centrifuge.
- Do not open centrifuge lid until rotor has completely stopped.
- Avoid exposure to fixatives and other chemicals by working in a fume hood and wearing protective clothing and gloves.
- Dispose of specimens in biohazard containers.

PROCEDURAL Reminders

- Review quality assessment section before beginning procedure.
- Follow laboratory procedure manual for concentration technique(s).
- Observe proper centrifugation times and speeds.
- Check specific gravity of solutions regularly.
- Do not use reagents after expiration dates.
- Allow fecal smears from fixed specimens to dry several hours or overnight before staining.
- Place smears from fresh specimens in fixative before the smears dry.

SUMMARY

Intestinal parasites are discovered and identified by microscopic examination of direct wet mounts, wet mounts prepared from concentrated fecal specimens, and trichrome-stained fecal smears. Large laboratories generally perform these procedures in house, while many smaller laboratories process specimens and send them to a reference laboratory for analysis. Whichever protocol is followed, Standard Precautions must always be observed when handling all fecal specimens, even preserved ones, because some parasite forms remain infective even in preservative. Use of a sedimentation or flotation concentration method increases the likelihood of finding parasites in light infections. Kits for fecal concentration, which use closed systems, provide technicians increased protection from exposure to the specimen.

One intestinal parasite that is common worldwide, including in the United States, is *Giardia intestinalis*. Infection with *Giardia* occurs through ingestion of infectious cysts present in contaminated food or water. *Giardia* cysts have a characteristic appearance and are easily identified in fecal specimens.

REVIEW QUESTIONS

1. What three types of preparations are used for microscopic examination for intestinal parasites?
2. What specimens are used for wet mounts?
3. What diluents are used for wet mounts?
4. Name two methods of concentrating fecal specimens. Where are the concentrated parasites found in each method?
5. How are fecal smears prepared for staining?
6. What stain is used for fecal specimens?
7. What are symptoms of giardiasis? How is it acquired?
8. Why must Standard Precautions be used when handling preserved fecal specimens?
9. Define micrometer, ocular micrometer, and trichrome stain.

STUDENT ACTIVITIES

1. Complete the written examination for this lesson.
2. Practice preparing fecal specimens for microscopic examination as outlined in the Student Performance Guide.

WEB ACTIVITIES

1. Use the Internet to search the CDC Web site. Find out how many *Giardia* outbreaks have been reported in the United States in the last 10 years.
2. Use the Internet to find the drug of choice (trade name and generic name) for treating *Giardia* infections. For what other conditions is the drug used?

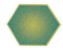

Student Performance Guide

Lesson 8-3 Microscopic Methods of Detecting Intestinal Parasites

Name _____ Date _____

INSTRUCTIONS

1. Practice preparing fecal specimens for microscopic examination for intestinal parasites, following the step-by-step procedure.

2. Demonstrate the procedure for preparing fecal specimens for microscopic examination satisfactorily for the instructor, using the Student Performance Guide. Your instructor will determine the level of competency you must achieve to obtain a satisfactory (S) grade.

MATERIALS AND EQUIPMENT

- gloves
- face shield and/or acrylic safety shield
- antiseptic
- surface disinfectant
- absorbent lab paper
- sharps container
- biohazard containers
- applicator sticks
- preserved fecal specimens
- fume hood or biological safety cabinet

Materials for Wet Mounts:

- coverglasses, 22 mm^2
- glass microscope slides, 2 × 3 inch preferable
- saline (0.85% NaCl)
- iodine solution for fecal wet mounts (Lugol's, Dobell and O'Connors, or D'Antoni's)

  D'Antoni's iodine:
  - add 1.0 gram potassium iodide (KI) and 1.5 gram iodine crystals to 100 mL distilled water in a dark bottle. Shake well and filter daily before use.
- disposable transfer pipets

Materials for Preparing Fecal Smears for Staining:

- 35°C incubator or laboratory oven
- microscope slides, 1 × 3 inch
- applicator sticks

Materials for Fecal Concentration:

- fecal concentrator kit(s) and package insert
- clinical centrifuge capable of spinning conical tubes at 500g
- applicator sticks

OPTIONAL: Preserved fecal specimens containing parasites, atlases, diagrams, stained microscope slides, photographs, or videos of intestinal parasites

PROCEDURE

Record in the comment section any problems encountered while practicing the procedure (or have a fellow student or the instructor evaluate your performance).

S = Satisfactory
U = Unsatisfactory

You must:	S	U	Comments
1. Assemble equipment and materials			
2. Prepare a work area by placing absorbent lab paper on counter or in fume hood			
3. Put on face protection or position acrylic safety shield on work surface			
4. Wash hands and put on gloves			

5. Demonstrate the procedure for preparing a fecal smear for staining, following steps 5a through 5d
  a. Obtain preserved fecal specimen and two 1 × 3 inch microscope slides
  b. Use applicator stick to mix specimen and remove a small portion
  c. Spread specimen evenly on slide by rolling applicator stick across slide or smearing in a zig-zag fashion (as in Figure 8-12). Smear should cover one-third to one-half the length of the slide and should extend from the slide's top edge to bottom edge. Prepare a second slide from the same specimen
  d. Label slides and place them in 35°C incubator to dry for at least 4 hours, preferably overnight			

6. Demonstrate the procedure for preparing saline and iodine wet mounts from a preserved fecal specimen, following steps 6a through 6i
  a. Obtain a preserved specimen
  b. Place a glass slide on work area
  c. Place one drop of saline on left half of slide and one drop of iodine solution on right half of slide
  d. Use applicator stick to mix specimen
  e. Remove a small portion of specimen with applicator stick and mix with saline drop. Place a coverglass over the drop
  f. Remove another small portion of fecal specimen and mix with iodine drop. Place a coverglass over the drop. Discard applicator in biohazard container
  g. Place slide over newsprint and check thickness of wet mounts (letters should be readable through the specimen)
  h. *Optional:* Place slide on microscope stage and scan specimens with the low-power and high-power objectives. Use visual aids such as atlases, diagrams, or photographs to help recognize parasitic forms
  i. Discard slide in biohazard sharps container			

You must:	S	U	Comments

7. Perform a fecal concentration procedure, following steps 7a through 7k. (If not available, skip to step 8)
  a. Obtain a preserved fecal specimen and a fecal concentrator kit
  b. Follow the manufacturer's specific directions (general directions are given below)
  c. Add surfactant to the preservative vial that contains the specimen
  d. Attach the filtration unit with conical tube to the vial securely
  e. Invert unit and tap to force specimen into the tube
  f. Remove filtration unit and vial and discard appropriately
  g. Add appropriate volumes of ethyl acetate, or other solutions indicated, to the tube
  h. Cap tube tightly and shake the tube
  i. Centrifuge the tube at the proper speed and for the proper time
  j. Decant supernatant as directed
  k. Resuspend pellet, prepare wet mounts (as in step 6), and examine microscopically			

8. Discard all contaminated materials in appropriate biohazard containers			
9. Discard or store preserved specimens, as directed by instructor			
10. If available, use the microscope to examine prepared slides containing fecal parasites. Using atlases and figures in this lesson, try to identify parasite forms			
11. Disinfect work area with surface disinfectant. Remove face protection			
12. Remove and discard gloves in biohazard container and wash your hands with antiseptic			

Evaluator Comments:

Evaluator _____ Date _____

LESSON

8-4

Preparing and Staining Smears for Blood Parasites

LESSON OBJECTIVES

After studying this lesson, the student will:

- Describe how to properly collect a blood specimen for parasite examination.
- Diagram the *Plasmodium* life cycle.
- Describe the symptoms of malaria.
- Discuss the epidemiology and symptoms of Chagas disease.
- Explain the purpose of preparing thin and thick blood smears for detecting blood parasites.
- Prepare and stain thin and thick blood smears.
- List safety precautions to be observed when preparing and staining blood smears for parasites.
- Discuss quality assessment procedures to follow when preparing blood smears for parasite examination.
- Define the glossary terms.

GLOSSARY

Anopheles / the genus of mosquito that is the definitive host for the human malaria parasites (genus *Plasmodium*) and that is capable of transmitting the organism to humans

Giemsa stain / a polychromatic stain used for staining blood cells and blood parasites

malaria / in humans, a disease caused by infection with protozoan parasites of the genus *Plasmodium*

microfilaria (pl. microfilariae) / immature form of a filarial worm

parasitemia / parasites in the blood

paroxysm(s) / the cycle(s) of chills and fever associated with malaria and that occur 36 to 72 hours apart, depending on the *Plasmodium* species

Plasmodium / the protozoan genus that includes the organisms causing human malaria

741

INTRODUCTION

Several parasites have forms or stages that are present in the blood of infected individuals during part of the parasite's life cycle. Examples of these are the parasites that cause malaria, sleeping sickness (African trypanosomiasis), Chagas disease (American trypanosomiasis), babesiosis, and dog heartworm disease.

The best method for detecting blood parasites is microscopic blood examination. This lesson explains the proper techniques of preparing and staining blood smears for detecting and identifying blood parasites. Much experience is required to recognize and identify the various species of blood parasites. Identifying specific blood parasites is beyond the scope of this lesson.

BLOOD PARASITES

Parasites found in blood during some part of their life cycle include *Plasmodium*, *Babesia*, *Trypanosoma*, and *Leishmania*. Table 8-8 gives information about blood parasites, including modes of transmission.

Human Malaria

Human **malaria** is caused by any one of four species of parasitic protozoa of the genus *Plasmodium* (Table 8-9). The parasites are transmitted to humans through the bite of *Anopheles* mosquitoes (the definitive host) or, rarely, through transfusion of infected blood. Mosquitoes become infected when they ingest blood from an infected person. Figure 8-16 shows a malarial parasite's life cycle.

Malaria is the most widely known parasitic disease of the blood and has high morbidity and mortality. Forty-one percent of the world's population lives in malaria endemic areas, which include parts of Africa, Asia, the Middle East, Central and South America, Hispaniola, and Oceania. It is estimated that between 700,000 and 2.7 million persons die of malaria each year, a majority of them children. The recent increase in insecticide-resistant mosquitoes and drug-resistant *Plasmodium* strains has made malaria prevention and treatment more difficult. Despite over 50 years of research, an effective malarial vaccine approved for human use has yet to be developed, although some are in trials.

Malaria has been considered eradicated in the United States since the early 1950s, but an average of over 1,000 cases are still reported annually. Most of these cases are imported, acquired by travelers to malaria-endemic countries. However, a few locally transmitted outbreaks of mosquito-borne malaria still occur. These are caused when local mosquitoes become infected after taking a blood meal from an infected individual who acquired the parasite in an endemic area. If these mosquitoes bite other individuals, the organisms can be transmitted to local residents.

TABLE 8-9. *Plasmodium* species that cause human malaria

SPECIES	DISEASE CAUSED	PAROXYSMS
P. vivax	Benign tertian malaria	Every 48 hours
P. ovale	Ovale malaria	Every 48 hours
P. malariae	Quartan malaria	Every 72 hours
P. falciparum	Malignant malaria	Every 36 to 38 hours

TABLE 8-8. Examples of parasites found in blood, their modes of transmission, and the diseases they cause

ORGANISM	TRANSMISSION	DISEASE CAUSED
Plasmodium spp.	Mosquito bite	Malaria
Babesia	Tick bite	Babesiosis
Trypanosoma brucei	Tsetse fly bite	African sleeping sickness, trypanosomiasis
Trypanosoma cruzi	Reduviid bug bite contaminated with bug's infected feces	Chagas disease, American trypanosomiasis
Wuchereria bancrofti	Mosquito bite	Filariasis, elephantiasis
Brugia spp.	Mosquito bite	Filariasis, elephantiasis
Leishmania donovani	Sand fly bite	Visceral leishmaniasis, Kala azar, dumdum fever
Toxoplasma gondii	Ingestion of oocysts, eating under-cooked infected meat, congenital	Toxoplasmosis

Malaria
(Plasmodium spp.)

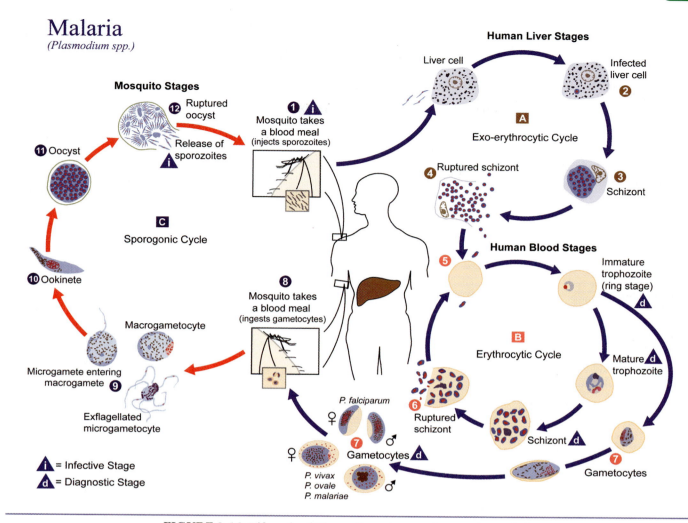

FIGURE 8-16 Life cycle of *Plasmodium*, the organism causing malaria
(*From CDC, Atlanta, GA*)

Because the two species of *Anopheles* mosquito that can transmit malaria are still widely found in the United States, there is a risk that malaria could be reestablished. Since the early 1960s over 90 cases of transfusion-transmitted malaria have been reported in the United States, cases that could have been prevented if blood donor guidelines had been followed.

Other Blood Parasites

Among the several other blood parasites are the protozoa *Babesia* and *Trypanosoma* and the filarial worms (Table 8-8). Although these organisms are not seen frequently in the United States, their incidence is increasing owing to increased worldwide travel and, in the case of *Trypanosoma cruzi*, expansion of the endemic area from Mexico into the southwestern United States. One filarial animal parasite transmitted by mosquitoes and common in the United States is the dog heartworm, *Dirofilaria immitis*. Heartworm infection is diagnosed by examination of dog blood for **microfilariae**, immature forms of the heartworm (Figure 8-17).

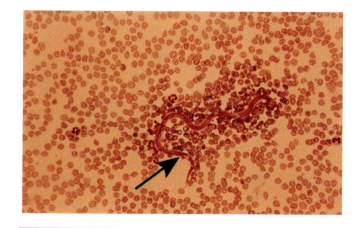

FIGURE 8-17 Canine heartworm microfilariae
in stained blood smear

CURRENT TOPICS

CLINICAL SYMPTOMS AND LABORATORY DIAGNOSIS OF MALARIA

Human malaria is usually associated with distinct, recognizable symptoms. Diagnosis can be confirmed by identification of the malarial parasite in a blood smear.

Symptoms

Plasmodium infection causes anemia, enlarged spleen, and cycles of chills, fever, and sweats called **paroxysms**. The parasites infect liver cells and red blood cells. As the parasites develop in red blood cells, they eventually cause the infected cells to rupture, releasing toxins and parasites and initiating the cycle of paroxysms. Malaria should be considered a possible cause of unexplained fever even for patients in malaria-free countries, and these patients should be questioned about their recent travel history.

Laboratory Identification

Malarias can range from mild to fatal, depending on the species of *Plasmodium* causing the infection. *Plasmodium falciparum* is the most deadly species. Rapid species identification is important since treatment may vary according to the species. *Plasmodium* species can be identified by careful microscopic examination of stained thick and thin blood smears by experienced personnel. The stained smears are examined extensively using the oil-immersion objective and the back-and-forth serpentine motion to scan adjacent fields as for the differential count. Thin smears are examined for 30 minutes, looking for parasitic red blood cell inclusions; 100 to 200 microscopic fields are examined in the thick film, looking for the presence of parasitic forms (see figures). Species identification is beyond the scope of this lesson. However, the photos shown here depict blood stages of *Plasmodium falciparum* and *P. vivax* as they appear in thin and thick smears.

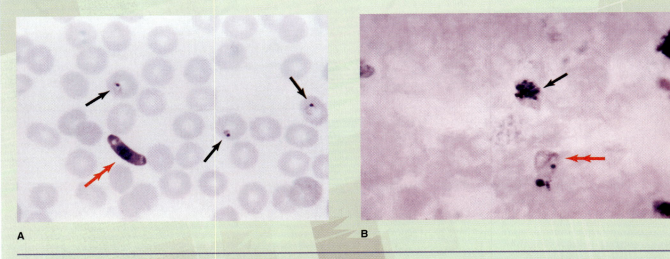

A

B

Malarial parasites in blood smears: (A) micrograph of Giemsa-stained thin smear showing a *Plasmodium falciparum* gametocyte (bottom, double arrow) and several ring forms within erythrocytes (arrows). *Photo from CDC, Atlanta, GA and Steven Glenn.* (B) thick film micrograph showing a mature *Plasmodium vivax* schizont (top arrow) and a growing trophozoite (bottom double arrow) *Photo from CDC, Atlanta, GA and Dr. Mae Melvin.*

CURRENT TOPICS

AMERICAN TRYPANOSOMIASIS— CHAGAS DISEASE

American trypanosomiasis, also called Chagas disease, is caused by the protozoan parasite *Trypanosoma cruzi*. The disease is found in the Americas from the southern United States through Central and South America to southern Argentina. Chagas disease is a major health problem in many Latin American countries, affecting an estimated 16 to 18 million people and causing approximately 50,000 deaths per year. As immigration from Latin and South America has increased, the potential of transmission of Chagas disease by blood transfusion has become more substantial in the United States, with some transfusion-related cases already being reported in North America. In addition, in recent years, the infection has been transmitted to organ transplant recipients through infected donated organs.

Epidemiology

T. cruzi can be transmitted to both humans and animals by a bug called the reduviid, triatomine, or kissing bug (shown in figure A), which lives primarily in cracks and holes of substandard housing in the tropics and subtropics of the Americas. The bug becomes infected by taking a blood meal from an infected individual. The infective stage then develops in the bug and is passed in its feces. People can become infected by:

- Touching their eyes, mouth, or open cuts after hands have come in contact with infective bug feces
- Bugs directly depositing infected feces in their eyes
- Congenital infection acquired from mother during pregnancy or at birth
- Receiving transfused blood or transplanted organ containing the parasite

Clinical Symptoms and Laboratory Diagnosis

Chagas disease is a serious disease that develops over many years. Infection often begins in childhood, and victims may not experience severe symptoms in the early stages. If symptoms are present during the acute phase, they can include fever, enlarged spleen and lymph nodes, and fatigue. Diagnosis is made by microscopic examination of a fresh blood specimen to look for motile forms, examination of a stained blood smear (shown in figure B), or by blood culture. Drug treatment is usually successful in the early acute phase.

About one-third of infected persons develop chronic disease 10 to 30 years after initial infection. Enlarged heart, heart failure, and cardiac arrest can occur, all caused by growth of the parasite in the heart tissue. In chronic disease, parasite numbers in the blood are usually too low to be detectable in smears, so culture, immunological, or molecular testing methods are used for diagnosis. Drug treatment is usually not successful in the chronic phase.

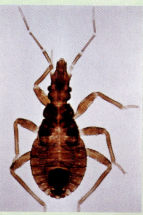

A

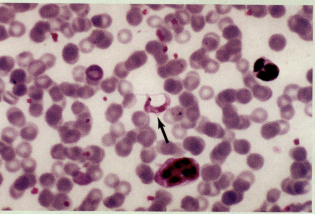

B

Chagas disease: (A) the kissing bug, *Triatoma infestans*, a vector for Chagas disease (*Photo from CDC, Atlanta, GA and WHO*); (B) micrograph of Giemsa-stained *Trypanosoma cruzi* (arrow) in a blood smear (*From CDC, Atlanta, GA and Dr. Mae Melvin*)

LABORATORY DETECTION OF BLOOD PARASITES

Safety Precautions

 Standard Precautions must be followed to protect health care workers and patients. Appropriate personal protective equipment (PPE) must be worn when collecting blood specimens and handling any biological specimens. Hands should be washed before donning and after removing gloves. Safety needles and lancets must used. These should be discarded in sharps container. Skin contact with chemicals and inhalation of chemical fumes should be avoided.

Quality Assessment

The procedure for preparing and staining blood smears for parasite examination will be explained in each laboratory's procedure manual and must be followed to ensure a quality specimen. Only qualified personnel shown to be competent in parasite identification should interpret and report results from blood smears for parasites. Considerations unique to preparing and staining these smears include:

- Timing of blood collection—Because some **parasitemias**, such as malaria, exhibit periodicity (the number of parasites in the blood fluctuates with time), the timing of collection is critical. Blood should be collected between paroxysms. Collection at several intervals over a period of 2 to 3 days may be required to ensure obtaining a specimen containing the parasites.

- Blood specimens should be collected before any drug treatment is initiated.

- Capillary blood is the preferred specimen, especially for malaria, because anticoagulants can alter parasite morphology and staining characteristics.

- Smears should be prepared at least in duplicate, with only one set being stained initially.

- Blood smears should be stained and examined as soon as possible after collection; parasite morphology deteriorates with time.

- Positive control smears should be stained with each fresh dilution of Giemsa stain.

Specimen Collection

Blood for parasite examination can be obtained by capillary puncture or venipuncture. However, blood to be examined for parasites should *not* be anticoagulated. Anticoagulants distort parasite morphology and interfere with staining of parasitic stages.

Timing of blood collection in suspected malaria cases is important. Blood should be collected between paroxysms, which can occur from 36 to 72 hours apart depending on the infecting species (Table 8-9).

Preparing the Blood Smears

Thick and thin blood smears are prepared. The thick smear is used for screening; it contains 10 to 30 times as much blood per microscopic field as a thin smear. Therefore, examining thick smears increases the chance of detecting parasites in a *light infection* because of the greater volume of blood screened. The thin film or smear is used to identify the parasite because the morphology is better in thin than in thick smears. Thick and thin smears can be prepared on separate slides (Figures 8-18 and 8-19) or on the same slide (Figure 8-20).

Preparing a Thin Smear

A thin smear is prepared from freshly collected *anticoagulant-free* blood in the manner described in Lesson 2-7.

- A drop of blood is spread on a clean glass slide in the same way as for a differential count (Figure 8-18).

- The smear is allowed to air-dry in a slide rack.

- The smear is then immersed in absolute methanol for 30 to 60 seconds to fix the smear and is again allowed to air-dry.

- A minimum of two thin smears should be prepared from each blood collection.

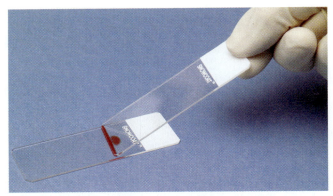

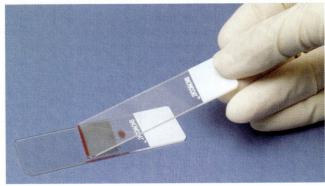

FIGURE 8-18 Preparing a thin blood smear

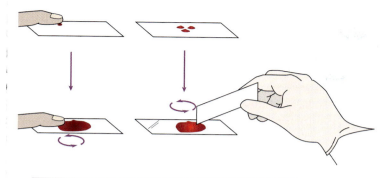

FIGURE 8-19 Two methods of preparing thick blood smears: (Left) make smear directly from finger puncture; (Right) use slide to spread a few drops of blood to form a thick smear

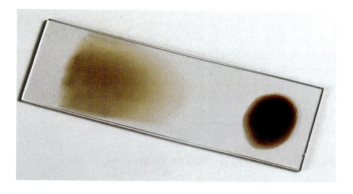

FIGURE 8-20 Thin (left) and thick (right) smears prepared on the same slide and stained with Giemsa stain (*Photo from CDC, Atlanta, GA and Steven Glenn*)

Preparing a Thick Smear

Two methods of preparing thick blood smears are shown in Figure 8-19. A few small drops of blood can be placed on a slide and spread into a dime-sized (approximately 2 cm) circle with the corner of another glass slide; or a large drop of capillary blood can be touched from a fingerstick to a slide and spread in a circular motion using slight pressure against the finger.

■ A *minimum* of two thick smears should be prepared from each blood collection.

■ Thick smears should be allowed to dry flat at room temperature several hours or overnight before staining.

■ A properly prepared thick film should be thin enough to read through when the slide is laid on a newspaper; smears that are too thick can peel off the slide during staining.

■ Thick smears are *not* fixed before staining.

■ Thick smears should be stained within 24 hours of preparation.

Staining the Blood Smears

The preferred stain for identifying parasites in blood is **Giemsa stain**. This polychromatic stain is similar to Wright's but does not have fixative incorporated into it. Wright's stain, which is routinely used for hematological studies, can be used for thin smears if rapid results are needed. However, parasites do not stain as well with Wright's as with Giemsa stain and results from Wright's-stained smears should be confirmed by examination of a Giemsa-stained smear.

Giemsa stain can be purchased as a stock solution to be diluted before use. Optimal dilutions and staining times should be determined for the brand and stain lot used. Staining times range from 20 minutes to 2 hours, depending on the stain dilution. Quick Giemsa stains are available that do not require the long staining times, but staining results are usually not as good as with traditional Giemsa stain.

Preparing the Stain

A fresh dilution of Giemsa stain should be made daily. The stock Giemsa solution should be diluted with phosphate-buffered water, pH 7.0 to 7.2. Commonly used dilutions are 1:20, 1:50, or 1:100, with 1:50 being the most common (Table 8-10).

Staining the Smears

Only one set of smears should be stained initially. This leaves a backup set in case a problem occurs during staining or smears must be sent to a reference laboratory.

Thin Smears. A thin smear previously fixed in absolute methanol should be immersed in freshly diluted Giemsa stain for the appropriate time (see Table 8-10). After staining, the slide should be rinsed briefly in phosphate-buffered water and air-dried in a slide rack. Stained slides should be stored in covered slide boxes protected from light.

TABLE 8-10. Dilutions and staining times for blood smears using commercial Giemsa stain

DILUTION	STAINING TIME	DIRECTIONS FOR MAKING DILUTION
1:20	20 minutes	2 mL Giemsa* + 38 mL bH₂O**
1:50	50 minutes	1 mL Giemsa + 49 mL bH₂O
1:100	2 hours	1 mL Giemsa + 99 mL bH₂O

* stock Giemsa stain, available commercially
** phosphate-buffered water, pH 7.0 to 7.2

SAFETY Reminders

- Review safety section before beginning procedure.
- Follow Standard Precautions when collecting and handling blood.
- Use caution in handling methanol; do not inhale fumes or allow it to contact skin.

PROCEDURAL Reminders

- Review quality assessment section before beginning procedure.
- Use only fresh anticoagulant-free blood to make the smears.
- Do not make thick smears too thick.
- Make fresh dilutions of Giemsa stain daily.
- Blood smears should always be screened and interpreted by qualified workers experienced in parasite identification.
- Include positive control slides each time a new batch of stain is used.

Thick Smears. The dry smear should be immersed in Giemsa stain diluted 1:50 for 50 minutes (for other staining options see Table 8-10). The smear is then rinsed for 3 to 5 minutes in buffered water and allowed to air-dry in a slide rack. The dry, stained smears should be stored in slide boxes.

Since thick films are not fixed, during staining the red blood cells will be lysed (destroyed) and only white blood cells, platelets, and parasites (if present) will remain intact. This makes it possible to microscopically scan the thick areas without the red blood cells obscuring the field of view.

SUMMARY

Several parasites are identified by microscopic examination of specially prepared and stained blood smears. Human blood parasites include *Plasmodium* species, the organisms causing malaria; the trypanosomes, which cause African sleeping sickness and American trypanosomiasis or Chagas disease; and *Babesia*, which causes babesiosis. Animal blood parasites, such as the dog heartworm, are also diagnosed by microscopic examination of blood.

In diseases such as malaria, patients' clinical symptoms, such as the interval between paroxysms, must be considered when choosing blood collection times. The procedures for collecting the blood specimen and preparing and staining these smears must be carefully followed to ensure the best chance of finding and identifying parasites. Examination of both thin and thick smears increases the chances of finding parasites in light infections. All safety precautions must be observed, and quality assessment policies must be followed for reliable results. Smear results must be reviewed, interpreted, and reported only by qualified personnel trained in parasite identification.

CASE STUDY

Tommy Rogers, a regular patient at a small internal medicine clinic, came in complaining of episodes of chills, fever, and sweats. Upon questioning, he revealed that he had returned from India 3 weeks previous. Tommy's physician ordered blood smears to be prepared and stained so that she could examine them for malarial parasites. Adrian, the laboratory assistant, prepared thin and thick smears. Not finding Giemsa stain in the laboratory, he stained both smears using Wright's stain. Before the physician even looked at the smears microscopically, after a glance at the stained smears, she immediately said that the smears and stain needed to be redone.

1. Was there anything wrong with the types of smears prepared? If so, what?
2. Was there anything wrong with the stain procedure? If so, what?
3. What did the physician see by glancing at the thick smear that caused her to request that the smears be redone?

REVIEW QUESTIONS

1. What blood specimen is used to make smears for parasite examination?

2. Why are both thin and thick smears prepared?

3. Explain the procedure for making the thin blood smear.

4. Explain the procedure for making the thick blood smear.

5. What is the preferred stain for blood smears for parasite examination?

6. What safety precautions must be observed when preparing malarial smears?

7. Why is the blood-collection time important when malaria is suspected?

8. Diagram the life cycle of malaria. Indicate points where the life cycle could be interrupted to stop transmission of the parasite.

9. What organism causes Chagas disease and how is it transmitted? Where is Chagas disease endemic?

10. Give reasons why cases of malaria and Chagas disease might increase in the United States.

11. Define *Anopheles*, Giemsa stain, malaria, microfilaria, parasitemia, paroxysm, and *Plasmodium*.

STUDENT ACTIVITIES

1. Complete the written examination for this lesson.

2. Practice the procedure for preparing and staining smears for blood parasites as outlined in the Student Performance Guide.

3. Optional: Heartworm infection is diagnosed by examining dog blood for microfilariae, which are immature forms (larvae) of the heartworm. To examine blood for heartworm, obtain freshly collected canine blood (less than 1 day old) from a local veterinary practice. Prepare and stain thin and thick smears from the blood. If the dog is infected with heartworm (*Dirofilaria* sp.), the stained microfilariae can be seen with the low-power objective. (Microfilariae will stain even in anticoagulated blood.) Stained microfilariae will appear as long, purple worm-like organisms. Wet preps can also be performed: Place a small drop of blood on a glass slide and place a coverslip over it. Observe the specimen using the low-power objective. If the blood specimen is fresh and contains microfilariae, they will be seen moving under the coverslip.

W E B www A C T I V I T I E S

1. Search the Internet to find recommendations for malaria prevention for U.S. citizens traveling to foreign countries. Find out where malaria is endemic. Report on prophylactic drugs that are prescribed for travelers and list countries that have a risk of malaria transmission.

2. Report on a blood parasite other than *Plasmodium* or *Trypanosoma cruzi* (Table 8-8 lists some examples). Search the Internet for information about the parasite, including geographical distribution, life cycle, symptoms of infection, diagnosis, and treatment.

Student Performance Guide

Lesson 8-4 Preparing and Staining Smears for Blood Parasites

Name _____ Date _____

INSTRUCTIONS

1. Practice preparing and staining smears for blood parasites, following the step-by-step procedure.

2. Demonstrate the procedure for preparing and staining smears for blood parasites satisfactorily for the instructor, using the Student Performance Guide. Your instructor will determine the level of competency you must achieve to receive a satisfactory (S) grade.

MATERIALS AND EQUIPMENT

- gloves
- antiseptic
- surface disinfectant
- biohazard container
- sharps container
- face protection or acrylic safety shield
- timer
- slide drying rack
- materials for capillary puncture
- microscope slides
- staining jars (Coplin jars)
- absolute methanol
- stock Giemsa stain
- phosphate-buffered water, pH 7.2 Recipe for Giemsa buffer (phosphate-buffered water):
  - 39 mL 0.067 M NaH_2PO_4
  - 61 mL 0.067 M Na_2HPO_4
  - 900 mL distilled water
  - check pH; should be 7.0 to 7.2
- microscope
- immersion oil
- lens paper
- slide box

OPTIONAL VISUAL AIDS: commercially prepared stained slides of *Plasmodium, Trypanosoma,* and *Babesia*; commercially prepared stained slides of filarial worms, such as dog heartworm (*Dirofilaria* sp.); charts, Kodachrome slides, and figures showing morphology of blood parasites

NOTE: Consult manufacturer's instructions accompanying Giemsa stain for recommended optimal dilution and staining time.

PROCEDURE

Record in the comment section any problems encountered while practicing the procedure (or have a fellow student or the instructor evaluate your performance).

S = Satisfactory
U = Unsatisfactory

You must:	S	U	Comments
1. Assemble equipment and materials for capillary puncture. Put on face protection or set up acrylic safety shield			
2. Wash hands and put on gloves			

You must:	S	U	Comments
3. Perform a capillary puncture			
4. Wipe away the first drop of blood			

5. Prepare thick smears:
  a. Allow one or two large drops of blood from the capillary puncture to fall onto the center of a microscope slide
  b. Spread the blood evenly into a dime-sized circle using *slight* pressure against the fingertip (or use the corner of a clean glass slide to spread the blood)
  c. Make a second thick smear
  d. Check the thickness of the smears by placing slides on printed material. The print should be readable through the blood film
  e. Place the slides on a flat surface in a dust-free place and allow them to completely air-dry at room temperature. DO NOT FIX			

6. Prepare thin smears:
  a. Apply a small drop of blood to a glass slide and use a clean spreader slide to form a thin blood film
  b. Make a second thin smear and set both smears aside to air-dry
  c. Immerse dried thin smears in absolute methanol for 30 to 60 seconds and air-dry			

7. Apply pressure to puncture site with sterile gauze when satisfactory smears have been obtained. (If staining is to be done another day, clean work area, remove gloves, and wash hands. Reglove before handling smears for staining procedure)			

8. Stain smears:
  a. Immerse slides in a freshly prepared 1:50 dilution of Giemsa stain for 50 minutes. (Be sure thin smear has been fixed and thick smear has dried for several hours)
  b. Rinse stained smears in buffered water: rinse thin smear 1 to 2 minutes; rinse thick smear 3 to 5 minutes
  c. Place rinsed slides in slide rack and allow to air-dry			

9. Place thin smear on microscope stage and observe cells using oil-immersion objective. Observe quality of stain: red blood cells should be pinkish. White blood cell nuclei should be blue-purple. Examine red blood cell for stained intracellular parasitic inclusions. (Refer to charts, figures, or commercially prepared slides, if available)			

You must:	S	U	Comments
10. Remove thin smear from microscope stage and place thick smear in position. Examine thick smear using oil-immersion objective. White blood cells and platelets should be visible, but red blood cells should have been destroyed in the staining process. If parasites were present in the blood specimen, they will be stained. (Refer to charts, figures, or commercially prepared slides, if available.)			
11. If available, examine commercially prepared malaria smears. Use an atlas to aid in identifying parasite forms			
12. Remove slide from microscope stage and clean oil from microscope objective with lens paper			
13. Place slides in covered slide box			
14. Discard capillary puncture materials in appropriate biohazard and sharps containers			
15. Clean equipment and return to proper storage			
16. Clean work area with surface disinfectant			
17. Remove and discard gloves in biohazard container			
18. Wash hands with antiseptic			

Evaluator Comments:

Evaluator _____ Date _____

Glossary

AABB / see American Association of Blood Banks

AAMA / see American Association of Medical Assistants

abbreviation / the shortening of a word, often by removing letters from the end of the word

absorbance (A) / a logarithmic expression of the amount of light absorbed by a substance containing colored molecules; optical density (O.D.)

accessioning / the process by which specimens are logged in, labeled, and assigned a specimen identification code

accreditation / a voluntary process in which a private, independent agency grants recognition to institutions or programs that meet or exceed established standards of quality

accuracy / a measure of how close a determined value is to the true value

acidosis / an abnormal condition in which blood pH falls below 7.35

acquired immunodeficiency syndrome (AIDS) / a form of severe immunodeficiency caused by infection with the human immunodeficiency virus (HIV)

acronym / combination of the first letters or syllables of a group of words to form a new group of letters that can be pronounced as a word

acute phase proteins / proteins that increase rapidly in serum during acute infection, inflammation, or following tissue injury

adhesion / the act of two parts or surfaces sticking together

aerobic / requiring oxygen

aerosol / liquid in the form of a very fine mist

agar / a seaweed derivative used to solidify microbiological media

agglutination / the clumping or aggregation of particulate antigens due to reaction with a specific antibody

agglutination inhibition / interference with, or prevention of, agglutination

aggregate / the total substances making up a mass; a cluster or clump of particles

aggregation / the collecting of separate objects into one mass

agroterrorism / acts of terrorism involving threats to agricultural products, including food animals and crops

Airborne Precautions / a CDC isolation category designed to prevent the transmission of infectious diseases, such as measles, that are spread by the airborne route

alanine aminotransferase (ALT) / an enzyme present in high concentration in liver tissue and that is measured to assess liver function; also called SGPT

albumin / the most abundant protein in normal plasma; a homogeneous group of plasma proteins that are made in the liver and that help maintain osmotic balance

alimentary tract / the digestive tube from the mouth to the anus

alkaline phosphatase (ALP or AP) / an enzyme widely distributed in the body, especially in the liver and bone

alkalosis / an abnormal condition in which blood pH rises above 7.45

allele / one of two or more alternate forms of a gene responsible for hereditary variation

allergy / a condition resulting from an exaggerated immune response; hypersensitivity

American Association of Blood Banks (AABB) / international association that sets blood bank standards, accredits blood banks, and promotes high standards of performance in the practice of transfusion medicine

American Association of Medical Assistants (AAMA) / professional society and credentialing agency for medical assistants

American Medical Technologists (AMT) / professional society and credentialing agency for clinical laboratory personnel

American Society for Clinical Laboratory Science (ASCLS) / professional society and credentialing agency for clinical laboratory personnel

American Society for Clinical Pathology (ASCP) / professional society and credentialing agency for clinical laboratory personnel and allied health personnel

American Society of Phlebotomy Technicians (ASPT) / professional society and credentialing agency for phlebotomists

amperometry / the technology that uses electrodes and electrode potential to measure electron generation

amorphous / without definite shape

AMT / see American Medical Technologists

anaerobic / growing in the absence of oxygen

analyte / a chemical substance that is the subject of chemical analysis

anamnestic response / rapid increase in blood immunoglobulins following a second exposure to an antigen; booster response or secondary response

anemia / a condition in which the red blood cell count or hemoglobin level is below normal; a condition resulting in decreased oxygen-carrying capacity of the blood

angioplasty / surgical repair of a vessel

anion / a negatively charged ion

anisocytosis / marked variation in the sizes of erythrocytes when observed on a peripheral blood smear

Anopheles / the genus of mosquito that is the definitive host for the human malaria parasites (genus *Plasmodium*) and is capable of transmitting the organism to humans

antibiotic susceptibility testing / determining the susceptibility of bacteria to specific antibiotics

antibody (Ab) / serum protein that is induced by, and reacts specifically with, a foreign substance (antigen); immunoglobulin

anticoagulant / a chemical that prevents blood coagulation

antigen (Ag) / foreign substance that induces an immune response by causing production of antibodies and/or sensitized lymphocytes that react specifically with that substance; immunogen

antihuman globulin test / a sensitive test using a commercial antihuman globulin reagent to detect human globulin coated on red blood cells; antiglobulin test; Coombs' test

antiseptic / a chemical used on living tissues to control the growth of infectious agents

antiserum / serum that contains antibodies

anuria / absence of urine production; failure of kidney function and suppression of urine production

aperture / an opening

apheresis / the process of removing a specific component, such as platelets, from donor blood, and returning the blood to donor circulation

arteriosclerosis / abnormal thickening and hardening of the arterial walls, causing loss of elasticity and impaired blood circulation

artery / a blood vessel that carries oxygenated blood from the heart to the tissues

arthritis / inflammation of the joints

arthropod / a member of the phylum Arthropoda, which includes crustaceans, insects, and arachnids

ASCLS / see American Society for Clinical Laboratory Science

ASCP / see American Society for Clinical Pathology

aseptic technique / work practices used to prevent contamination when working with microorganisms

aspartate aminotransferase (AST) / an enzyme present in many tissues, including cardiac, muscle, and liver, and that is measured to assess liver function; also called SGOT

ASPT / see American Society of Phlebotomy Technicians

atherosclerosis / a form of arteriosclerosis in which lipids, calcium, cholesterol, and other substances deposit on the inner walls of the arteries

atrial / of or relating to a body cavity

atypical lymphocyte / lymphocyte that occurs in response to viral infections and that is common in infectious mononucleosis; reactive lymphocyte

autoantibody / an antibody directed against the self (one's own tissues)

autoclave / an instrument that uses pressurized steam for sterilization

autoimmune disease / disease caused when the immune response is directed at one's own tissues (self-antigens)

average / the sum of a set of values divided by the number of values; the mean

avian influenza / an infection of birds with one of the influenza A viruses; bird flu

B

B lymphocyte (B cell) / the type of lymphocyte primarily responsible for the humoral immune response

bacillus / a rod-shaped bacterium

bacteriology / the study of bacteria

band cell / an immature granulocyte with a nonsegmented nucleus; a "stab cell"

basilic vein / large vein on inner side ("pinky" side) of arm

basophil / a leukocyte containing basophilic-staining granules in the cytoplasm

basophilia / abnormal increase in the number of basophils in the blood

basophilic / blue in color; having affinity for the basic stain

basophilic stippling / remnants of RNA and other nuclear material remaining inside the erythrocyte after the nucleus is lost from the cell and which appear as small purple granules in red blood cells stained with Wright's stain

beaker / a wide-mouthed, straight-sided container with a pouring spout formed from the rim and used to make estimated measurements

Beer's Law / a mathematical relationship that demonstrates the linear relationship of concentration to absorbance and that forms the basis for spectrophotometric analysis

bibulous paper / a special absorbent paper used to dry slides

bilirubin / a product formed in the liver from the breakdown of hemoglobin

binocular / having two oculars or eyepieces

biohazard / risk or hazard to health or the environment from biological agents

biological safety cabinet / a special work cabinet that provides protection while working with infectious microorganisms

biosafety level 4 (BSL-4) / a designation requiring the use of a combination of work practices, equipment, and facilities to prevent exposure of individuals or the environment to pathogens that can be transmitted by aerosol and that pose a high risk of life-threatening disease for which treatment or vaccine is not generally available

blast cell / an immature blood cell normally found only in the bone marrow

blind sample / an assayed sample that is sent as an unknown to laboratories participating in proficiency testing programs

blood bank / clinical laboratory department where blood components are tested and stored until needed for transfusion; immunohematology department; transfusion services; also the refrigerated unit used for storing blood components

blood group antibody / a serum protein (immunoglobulin) that reacts specifically with a blood group antigen

blood group antigen / a substance or structure on the red blood cell membrane that stimulates antibody formation and reacts with that antibody

bloodborne pathogens (BBP) / pathogens that can be present in human blood (and blood-contaminated body fluids) and that cause disease

Bloodborne Pathogens (BBP) Standard / OSHA guidelines for preventing occupational exposure to pathogens present in human blood and body fluids, including, but not limited to, human immunodeficiency virus (HIV) and hepatitis B virus (HBV); final OSHA standard of December 6, 1991, effective March 6, 1992

borosilicate glass / non-reactive glass with high thermal resistance and commonly used to make high quality laboratory glassware

botulinum intoxication / condition where body tissues are affected by the botulinum toxin

botulinum toxin / a neurotoxin produced by *Clostridium botulinum*

bovine spongiform encephalopathy (BSE) / a fatal, neurological disease of cattle caused by an unconventional transmissible agent called a prion; commonly called mad cow disease

Bowman's capsule / the portion of the nephron that receives the glomerular filtrate

buffer / a substance that lessens change in pH of a solution when acid or base (alkali) is added

buffy coat / a light-colored layer of leukocytes and platelets that forms on top of the RBC layer when a sample of blood is centrifuged or allowed to stand undisturbed

BUN / blood urea nitrogen; a test measuring urea in blood

C

CAAHEP / see Commission on Accreditation of Allied Health Education Programs (formerly CAHEA)

calibration / the process of checking, standardizing, or adjusting a method or instrument so that it yields accurate results

Candida albicans / a yeast that causes vaginitis and other infections, especially following antibiotic therapy

CAP / see College of American Pathologists

capillary / a minute blood vessel that connects the smallest arteries to the smallest veins, and that serves as an oxygen exchange vessel

capillary action / the action by which a fluid enters a tube because of the attraction between the fluid and the tube

capillary tube / a slender glass or plastic tube used for laboratory procedures

carcinogen / a substance with the potential to produce cancer in humans or animals

cardiopulmonary circulation / the system of blood vessels that circulates blood from the heart to the lungs and back to the heart

carrier / a person who harbors an organism, has no symptoms or signs of disease, but is capable of spreading the organism to others

cast / in urinalysis, a protein matrix formed in the kidney tubules and washed out into the urine

catalase test / a test to differentiate between *Streptococcus* and *Staphylococcus* sp.

cation / a positively charged ion

caustic / a chemical substance having the ability to burn or destroy tissue

CBC / see complete blood count; a commonly performed group of hematological tests

CDC / Centers for Disease Control and Prevention

cell diluting fluid / a solution used to dilute blood for cell counts

cell-mediated immunity / immunity provided by T lymphocytes and cytokines

Celsius (C) scale / temperature scale having the freezing point of water at zero (0°) and the boiling point at 100°

Centers for Disease Control and Prevention (CDC) / central laboratory for the national public health system

Centers for Medicare and Medicaid Services (CMS) / the agency within DHHS responsible for implementing CLIA '88

centi / prefix used to indicate one-hundredth (10^{-2}) of a unit

centrifuge / an instrument with a rotor that rotates at high speeds, in a closed chamber

cephalic vein / a superficial vein of the arm (thumb side) commonly used for venipuncture

cerebrospinal fluid (CSF) / fluid surrounding the spinal cord and bathing ventricles of the brain

cestode / tapeworm; member of the class Cestoda

chemical hygiene plan / comprehensive written safety plan detailing the proper use and storage of hazardous chemicals in the workplace

Chlamydia trachomatis / a species of gram-negative intracellular bacteria that is a cause of STDs

chromogen / a substance that becomes colored when it undergoes a chemical change

chronic fatigue syndrome (CFS) / a syndrome characterized by prolonged fatigue and other non-specific symptoms and for which the cause remains unknown

clean-catch urine / a midstream urine sample collected after the urethral opening and surrounding tissues have been cleansed

CLIA '88 / see Clinical Laboratory Improvement Amendments of 1988

clinical chemistry / the laboratory section that uses chemical principles to analyze blood and other body fluids

Clinical Laboratory Improvement Amendments of 1988 (CLIA '88) / a federal act that specifies minimum performance standards for clinical laboratories

clinical laboratory science / the health profession concerned with performing laboratory analyses used in diagnosing and treating disease as well as in maintaining good health; medical technology

clinical laboratory scientist (CLS) / a professional who has a baccalaureate degree from an accredited college or university, has completed clinical training in an accredited clinical laboratory science (medical technology) program, and has passed a national certifying examination; medical technologist

Clinical and Laboratory Standards Institute (CLSI) / an international, nonprofit organization that establishes standards of best current practice for clinical laboratories; formerly National Committee for Clinical Laboratory Standards (NCCLS)

clinical laboratory technician (CLT) / a professional who has completed a minimum of two years of specific training in an accredited clinical laboratory technician (medical laboratory technician) program and has passed a national certifying examination; medical laboratory technician

CLSI / see Clinical and Laboratory Standards Institute

clue cells / vaginal epithelial cells covered with tiny, Gram-variable bacteria and seen in vaginal secretions of patients with bacterial vaginosis

CMS / see Centers for Medicare and Medicaid Services

coagulase test / a test to differentiate between *Staphylococcus aureus* and other *Staphylococcus* species

coagulation / the process of forming a fibrin clot; the laboratory department that performs tests of hemostasis

coagulation factors / a group of plasma proteins (and the mineral calcium) involved in blood clotting

coarse adjustment / control that adjusts position of microscope objective and is used to initially bring objects into focus

coccus / a spherical bacterium

codocyte / target cell

codominant / in genetics, a gene that is expressed in the heterozygous state, that is, in the presence of a different allelic gene

coefficient of variation / a calculated value that compares the relative variability between different sets of data

COLA / see Commission on Office Laboratory Accreditation

coliform / certain gram-negative intestinal bacteria, including *Escherichia coli*

collagen / a protein connective tissue found in skin, bone, ligaments, and cartilage

College of American Pathologists (CAP) / agency that offers accreditation to clinical laboratories and certification to clinical laboratory personnel

colony / a defined mass of bacteria assumed to have grown from a single organism

colony count / an estimation of the number of organisms in urine by counting the colonies on a urine culture plate

commensal / an organism that lives with, on, or in another, without injury to either

Commission on Accreditation of Allied Health Education Programs (CAAHEP) / agency that accredits educational programs for clinical laboratory personnel; formerly CAHEA

Commission on Office Laboratory Accreditation (COLA) / agency that offers accreditation to physician office laboratories

communicable / able to be transmitted directly or indirectly from one individual to another

complement / a group of plasma proteins that can be activated in immune reactions, can cause cell lysis, and can help initiate the inflammatory response

condenser / apparatus located below the microscope stage that directs light into the objective

congenital / acquired during fetal development, and present at the time of birth, but not inherited

Contact Precautions / CDC isolation category designed to prevent transmission of diseases spread by close or direct contact

controls / solutions usually made from human serum and with a known concentration of the same constituents as those being measured in the patient sample

cortex / the outer layer or portion of an organ

Coumadin / an anticoagulant derived from coumarin that is administered orally to prevent or slow clotting

counterstain / a dye that adds a contrasting color

creatine kinase (CK) / an enzyme present in large amounts in brain tissue and in heart and skeletal muscle and that is measured to aid in diagnosing heart attack

creatinine / a breakdown product of creatine that is normally excreted in the urine

crenated cell / a shrunken red blood cell with scalloped or toothed margins

critical measurements / measurements made when the accuracy of a solution's concentration is important; measurements made using glassware manufactured to strict standards

culture / growth of microorganisms in a special medium; the process of growing microorganisms in the laboratory

cyanmethemoglobin / a stable colored compound formed when hemoglobin is reacted with Drabkin's reagent; hemiglobincyanide (HiCN)

cyst / dormant stage of an organism surrounded by a resistant covering; the nonmotile, nonfeeding stage of a protozoan parasite

cystitis / inflammation of the urinary bladder

cytokine / any of various nonantibody proteins secreted by cells of the immune system and that help regulate the immune response; lymphokine

cytoplasm / the fluid portion of the cell surrounding the nucleus

D

D-dimer / one of the products formed from the breakdown of fibrin by plasmin

deci / prefix used to indicate one-tenth of a unit

deep vein thrombosis (DVT) / occurrence of a thrombus within a deep vein, usually of the leg or pelvis

definitive host / the host in which the sexual or adult form of the parasite is found

deionized water / water that has had most of the mineral ions removed

dendritic cells / cells in lymphoid tissues that form a network to trap foreign antigens

deoxyhemoglobin / the hemoglobin formed when oxyhemoglobin releases oxygen to tissues

Department of Health and Human Services (DHHS) / the governmental agency that oversees public health care matters; commonly called HHS

Department of Homeland Security / a federal agency whose primary mission is to prevent, protect against, and respond to acts of terrorism on United States soil

DHHS / see Department of Health and Human Services

diabetes mellitus / a disorder of carbohydrate metabolism characterized by a state of hyperglycemia due to insulin deficiency

dialysate / in kidney dialysis, a solution used to draw waste products and excess fluid from the body

differential count / a determination of the relative numbers of each type of leukocyte; white blood cell differential count; leukocyte differential count

diluent / a liquid added to a solution to make it less concentrated

dilution / a solution made less concentrated by adding a diluent; the act of making a dilute solution; the degree to which a solution is made less concentrated

dilution factor / reciprocal of the dilution

disinfectant / a chemical used on inanimate objects to kill or inactivate microbes

disseminated intravascular coagulation (DIC) / a bleeding disorder characterized by widespread thrombotic and secondary fibrinolytic reactions

distal convoluted tubule / the portion of a renal tubule that empties into the collecting tubule

distilled water / the condensate collected from steam after water has been boiled

diurnal / having a daily cycle

DNA / the nucleic acid that carries genetic information and that is found primarily in the nucleus of all living cells; deoxyribonucleic acid

Drabkin's reagent / a hemoglobin diluting reagent that contains iron, potassium, cyanide, and sodium bicarbonate

drepanocyte / sickle cell

Droplet Precautions / a CDC isolation category designed to prevent the transmission of diseases spread through the air over short distances

dysfunction / impaired or abnormal function

E

Ebola virus / a highly infectious filovirus that causes a hemorrhagic fever

ectoparasite / a parasite that lives on the outer surface of a host

ectopic pregnancy / development of fetus outside the uterus; extrauterine pregnancy

EDTA / ethylenediaminetetraacetic acid; an anticoagulant commonly used in hematology

EIA / see enzyme immunoassay

electrolyte solution / a solution that conducts an electrical current

electrolytes / the cations and anions important in maintaining fluid and acid-base balance

electron microscope / a microscope that uses an electron beam to create images from a specimen and that is capable of much greater magnification and resolving power than a light microscope

elliptocyte / elongated, cigar-shaped red blood cell

embolus (pl. emboli) / a mass (clot) of blood or foreign matter carried in the circulation

endemic / recurring in a specific location or population

endogenous / produced within; growing from within

endothelium / the layer of epithelial cells that lines blood vessels and the serous cavities of the body

engineering control / use of available technology and equipment to protect the worker from hazards

English system of measurement / system of measurement in common use in the United States for nonscientific measurements; sometimes called U. S. customary system

enzyme / a protein that causes or accelerates changes in other substances without being changed itself

enzyme immunoassay (EIA) / an assay that uses an enzyme-labeled antibody as a reactant

eosin / a red-orange stain or dye

eosinophil / a leukocyte containing eosinophilic granules in the cytoplasm

eosinophilia / abnormal increase in the number of eosinophils in the blood

epidemic / disease affecting many persons at the same time, spread from person-to-person, and occurring in an area where the disease is not prevalent

epidemiology / the study of the factors that cause disease and determine disease frequency and distribution

epitope / the portion of an antigen that reacts specifically with an antibody; antigenic determinant

epizootic / an outbreak of disease in an animal population

Epstein-Barr virus (EBV) / a virus that infects lymphocytes and is the cause of infectious mononucleosis

erythrocyte / see red blood cell

erythrocyte indices / see red blood cell indices

erythrocytosis / an excess of RBCs in the peripheral blood; sometimes called polycythemia

ethics / a system of conduct or behavior; rules of professional conduct

exogenous / originating from the outside

exposure control plan / a plan identifying employees at risk of exposure to bloodborne pathogens and providing training in methods to prevent exposure

exposure incident / an accident, such as a needlestick, in which an individual is exposed to possible infection through contact with body substances from another individual

eyepiece / ocular

F

Fahrenheit (F) scale / temperature scale having the freezing point of water at 32° and the boiling point at 212°

fastidious bacteria / bacteria that require special nutritional factors to survive

FDA / see Food and Drug Administration

femtoliter (fL) / a unit of volume; 10^{-15}L

fibrin / a protein formed from fibrinogen by the action of thrombin

fibrin degradation products (FDP) / degradation products formed when plasmin cleaves fibrin or fibrinogen; formerly fibrin split products

fibrin split products / see fibrin degradation products

fibrinogen / a plasma protein produced in the liver and converted to fibrin through the action of thrombin

fibrinolysis / enzymatic breakdown of a fibrin clot

field diaphragm / adjustable aperture attached to microscope base

fine adjustment / control that adjusts position of microscope objectives and is used to sharpen focus

fission / reproductive process in which the parent cell divides into two identical independent cells

fixative / preservative; a chemical that prevents deterioration of cells or tissues

flagellum (pl., flagella) / slender, lash-like appendage that serves as organ of locomotion for sperm cells and some protozoa

flask / a container with an enlarged body and a narrow neck

flint glass / inexpensive glass with low resistance to heat and chemicals

fluorescent / having the property of emitting light of one wavelength when exposed to light of another wavelength

folic acid / a member of the B vitamin complex

fomites / inanimate objects, such as bed rails, linens, or eating utensils, that may be contaminated with infectious organisms and serve as a means of their transmission

Food and Drug Administration (FDA) / the division of DHHS responsible for protecting the public health by assuring the safety and efficacy of foods, drugs, biological products, medical devices, and cosmetics

formula weight (F.W.) / weight of the entity represented by a chemical formula; molecular weight

forward grouping / the use of known antisera (antibodies) to identify unknown antigens on a patient's cells; forward typing; direct grouping

fossae / in the throat, shallow depressions where the tonsils were located before surgical removal

fume hood / a device that draws contaminated air out of an area and either cleanses and recirculates it, or discharges it to the outside

G

gamma glutamyl transferase (GGT) / an enzyme present in liver, kidney, pancreas, and prostate, and that is measured to assess liver function

gauge / a measure of the diameter of a needle

Gaussian curve / a graph plotting the distribution of values around the mean; normal frequency curve

genes / segments of DNA that code for specific proteins or enzymes and that are the structural units of heredity

genotype / the allelic genes that are responsible for a trait

Giemsa stain / a polychromatic stain used for staining blood cells and blood parasites

globin / the protein portion of the hemoglobin molecule

globulins / a heterogeneous group of serum proteins with varied functions

glomerular filtrate / the fluid that passes from the blood into the nephron and from which urine is formed

glomerulonephritis / inflammation of the glomeruli

glomerulus (pl. glomeruli) / a small bundle of capillaries that is the filtering portion of the nephron

glucagon / a pancreatic hormone that increases blood glucose concentration by promoting the conversion of glycogen to glucose

glucose dehydrogenase / enzyme that converts glucose to gluconolactone and is used in glucose analytical methods

glucose oxidase / an enzyme that converts glucose to gluconic acid and that is used in glucose analytical methods

glycated hemoglobin (GHb) / see Hemoglobin A1c

glycogen / the storage form of glucose found in high concentration in the liver

glycolysis / energy production as a result of the metabolic breakdown of glucose

glycosuria / glucose in the urine; glucosuria

gonorrhea / a contagious infection spread by sexual contact and caused by *Neisseria gonorrhoeae*

gout / a painful condition in which blood uric acid is elevated and urates precipitate in joints

graduated cylinder / an upright, straight-sided container with a flared base and a volume scale

gram (g) / basic metric unit of weight or mass

gram-formula weight / the weight in grams of the entity represented by a chemical formula

Gram negative / designation for bacteria that lose the crystal violet (purple stain) and retain the safranin (red stain) in the Gram stain procedure

Gram positive / designation for bacteria that retain the crystal violet (purple stain) in the Gram stain procedure

Gram stain / a differential stain used to classify bacteria

granulocyte / a leukocyte containing granules in the cytoplasm; any of the neutrophilic, eosinophilic, or basophilic leukocytes

guaiac / a chemical derived from the resin of the *Guaiacum* tree

H

hCG / human chorionic gonadotropin, the hormone of pregnancy produced by the placenta; uterine chorionic gonadotropin (uCG)

HDL cholesterol / high-density lipoprotein fraction of blood cholesterol; "good" cholesterol

Health Care Financing Administration (HCFA) / see Centers for Medicare and Medicaid Services (CMS)

Health Insurance Portability and Accountability Act (HIPAA) / 1996 Act of Congress, a part of which guarantees protection of privacy of an individual's health information

helminth / a worm, especially a parasitic worm; in parasitology, the group comprising the roundworms and flatworms

hemacytometer / a heavy glass slide made to precise specifications and used to count cells microscopically; a counting chamber

hemacytometer coverglass / a special coverglass of uniform thickness used with a hemacytometer

hematocrit / the volume of erythrocytes packed by centrifugation in a given volume of blood and expressed as a percentage; abbreviated "crit" or Hct

hematology / the study of blood and the blood-forming tissues

hematoma / the swelling of tissue around a vessel due to leakage of blood into the tissue

hematopoietic stem cell / see hemopoietic stem cell

hematuria / the presence of blood in the urine

heme / the iron-containing portion of the hemoglobin molecule

hemiglobincyanide (HiCN) / cyanmethemoglobin

hemoconcentration / increase in the concentration of cellular elements in the blood

hemoglobin (Hb, Hgb) / the major functional component of red blood cells that is the oxygen-carrying protein

hemoglobin A1c (HbA1c) / hemoglobin modified by the binding of glucose to the beta globin chains of hemoglobin; also called glycated or glycosylated hemoglobin

hemolysis / rupture or destruction of red blood cells resulting in the release of hemoglobin

hemolytic disease of the newborn (HDN) / a condition in which maternal antibody targets fetal red blood cells for destruction

hemophilia / a bleeding disorder resulting from a hereditary coagulation factor deficiency or dysfunction

hemopoiesis / the process of blood cell formation and development; hematopoiesis

hemopoietic stem cell / an undifferentiated bone marrow cell that gives rise to blood cells

hemorrhage / uncontrolled bleeding

hemostasis / the process of stopping bleeding, which includes clot formation and clot dissolution

HEPA filter / high-efficiency particulate air filter used in biological safety cabinets

heparin / an anticoagulant used in certain laboratory procedures and in treatment of thrombosis

hepatitis B virus (HBV) / the virus that causes hepatitis B infection and is transmitted by contact with infected blood or other body fluids

hepatitis C virus (HCV) / the virus that causes hepatitis C infection and is transmitted by contact with infected blood or other body fluids

hepatosplenamegaly / enlargement of the liver and spleen

herpes simplex virus, type 1 (HSV-1) / the virus causing oral herpes

herpes simplex virus, type 2 (HSV-2) / the virus causing genital herpes

heterophile antibodies / antibodies that are increased in infectious mononucleosis

hexokinase / an enzyme that converts glucose to glucose-6-phosphate and that is used in glucose analytical methods

HIPAA / see Health Insurance Portability and Accountability Act of 1996

histocompatibility testing / performance of assays to determine if donor and recipient tissue are compatible

histogram / a graph that illustrates the size and frequency of occurrence of articles being studied

HIV / human immunodeficiency virus, a retrovirus that has been identified as the cause of acquired immunodeficiency syndrome (AIDS)

homeostasis / the tendency toward steady state or equilibrium of body processes

host / the organism from which a parasite obtains nutrients and in which some or part of the parasite's life cycle is completed

Howell-Jolly body / nuclear remnant remaining in red blood cells after the nucleus is lost, commonly seen in pernicious anemia and hemolytic anemias

human chorionic gonadotropin (hCG) / the hormone of pregnancy, produced by the placenta; also called uterine chorionic gonadotropin, uCG

human immunodeficiency virus (HIV) / the retrovirus that has been identified as the cause of AIDS

human leukocyte antigen (HLA) / any of several antigens present on leukocytes and other body cells that are important in transplant rejection

human papilloma virus (HPV) / a group of viruses, some of which are sexually transmitted

humoral immunity / immunity provided by B lymphocytes and antibodies

hyaline / transparent, pale

hypercalcemia / blood calcium levels above normal

hyperglycemia / blood glucose concentration above normal

hyperkalemia / blood potassium levels above normal

hyperlipidemia / excessive amount of fat in blood

hypernatremia / blood sodium levels above normal

hyperthyroidism / excessive functional activity of the thyroid gland; excessive secretion of thyroid hormones

hyphae / filaments of a mold that make up the mycelium

hypoalbuminemia / marked decrease in serum albumin concentration

hypocalcemia / blood calcium levels below normal

hypochromic / having reduced color or hemoglobin content

hypodermic needle / a hollow needle used for injections or for obtaining fluid specimens

hypoglycemia / blood glucose concentration below normal

hypokalemia / blood potassium levels below normal

hyponatremia / blood sodium levels below normal

hypothyroidism / thyroid function deficiency

I

immunity / resistance to disease or infection

immunization / the process of producing immunity to an antigen

immunoassay / a diagnostic method using antigen-antibody reactions

immunocompetent / capable of producing a normal immune response

immunocompromised / having reduced ability or inability to produce a normal immune response

immunoglobulins (Ig) / antibodies; serum proteins that are induced by and react specifically with antigens (immunogens)

immunohematology / the study of the human blood groups; in the clinical laboratory, often called blood banking or transfusion services

immunology / the branch of medicine encompassing the study of the immune processes and immunity

immunosuppression / suppression of the immune response by physical, chemical, or biological means

impedance / resistance in an electrical circuit

implantation / attachment of the early embryo to the uterus

incubation period / the time elapsed between exposure to an infectious agent and the appearance of symptoms

index of refraction / the ratio of the velocity of light in one medium, such as air, to its velocity in another material

indicator medium / a bacteriological medium that detects certain chemical reactions of organisms growing on it; differential medium

infection / a pathological condition caused by growth of microorganisms in the host

infectious mononucleosis / a contagious viral disease caused by Epstein-Barr virus

inflammation / a nonspecific protective response to tissue injury brought about primarily by release of chemicals such as histamine and serotonin and action of phagocytic cells

inoculating loop / an instrument used to pick up and transfer bacteria

inoculation / process of transferring a population of microorganisms to a growth medium

inoculum / mass of bacteria being transferred from one medium to another

insulin / the pancreatic hormone essential for proper metabolism of blood glucose and maintenance of blood glucose levels

intermediate host / the host in which the asexual, immature, or larval form of the parasite is found

international normalized ratio (INR) / a way of reporting a prothrombin time that takes into consideration the sensitivity of the thromboplastin used and the mean of the normal prothrombin time in the facility's population

international sensitivity index (ISI) / a value assigned to each lot of thromboplastin to compensate for variations in sensitivities of thromboplastin from different sources

intoxication / poisoning

intravascular / within the blood vessels

ionized calcium / in the body, a mineral that plays an important role in hemostasis

ion-selective electrode / an electrode manufactured to respond to the concentration of a specific ion

iris diaphragm / device that regulates the amount of light striking the specimen being viewed through the microscope

isolation / the practice of limiting the movement and social contact of a patient who is potentially infectious or who must be protected from exposure to infectious agents; quarantine

isotonic solution / a solution that has the same concentration of dissolved particles as the solution or cell with which it is compared

J

JC / see Joint Commission

Joint Commission (JC) / an independent agency that accredits hospitals and large health care facilities

K

keratocyte / a red blood cell deformed by mechanical trauma

ketones / a group of chemical substances produced during increased fat metabolism; ketone bodies

ketonuria / ketones in the urine

kidney / the organ in which urine is formed

kilo / prefix used to indicate one thousand (10^3) units

Köhler illumination / alignment of illuminating light for microscopy; double diaphragm illumination

L

Laboratory Response Network (LRN) / a nationwide network of laboratories coordinated by the CDC with the ability for rapid response to threats to public health

labware / article(s) or container(s) intended for laboratory use

lactate dehydrogenase (LD or LDH) / an enzyme widely distributed in the body that is measured to assess liver function

lancet / a sterile, sharp-pointed blade used to perform a capillary puncture

larva / immature stage of an invertebrate

laser / a narrow intense beam of light of only one wavelength going in only one direction

latent / dormant; in an inactive or hidden phase

lateral / toward the side

LDL cholesterol / low-density lipoprotein fraction of blood cholesterol; "bad" cholesterol

lens / a curved transparent material that spreads or focuses light

lens paper / a special nonabrasive material used to clean optical lenses

leukemia / a chronic or acute disease involving unrestrained growth of leukocytes

leukocyte / see white blood cell

leukocytosis / increase above normal in the number of leukocytes (white blood cells) in the blood

leukopenia / decrease below normal in the number of leukocytes (white blood cells) in the blood; leukocytopenia

Levey-Jennings chart / a quality control chart used to record daily quality control values

lipemic / having a cloudy appearance due to excess lipid content

lipids / any one of a group of fats or fat-like substances

liter (L) / basic metric unit of volume

loop of Henle / the U-shaped portion of a renal tubule between its proximal and distal portions

lumen / the open space within a tubular organ or tissue

lymphadenopathy / a condition in which the lymph glands are enlarged or swollen

lymphocyte / a small basophilic-staining leukocyte having a round or oval nucleus and playing a vital role in the immune process

lymphocytosis / an increase above the normal number of lymphocytes in the blood

lymphokines / nonantibody proteins produced by lymphocytes in response to antigen stimulation and that play a role in regulating the immune response; cytokines

lyophilize / remove water from a frozen solution under vacuum; freeze-dry

M

macrocytic / having a larger-than-normal cell size

macrophages / long-lived phagocytic tissue cells derived from blood monocytes and that function in destruction of foreign antigens and serve as antigen-presenting cells

major histocompatibility complex (MHC) / the group of genes responsible for producing antigens, such as HLA, that contribute to the failure of organ and tissue transplants

malaria / in humans, a disease caused by infection with protozoan parasites of the genus *Plasmodium*

malignant / cancerous; not benign

Marburg virus / a filovirus that causes a hemorrhagic fever

material safety data sheet (MSDS) / written safety information that must be supplied by manufacturers of chemicals and hazardous materials

mean / the sum of a set of values divided by the number of values; the average

mean cell hemoglobin (MCH) / mean corpuscular hemoglobin; average red blood cell hemoglobin expressed in picograms (pg)

mean cell hemoglobin concentration (MCHC) / mean corpuscular hemoglobin concentration; comparison of the weight of hemoglobin in a red blood cell to the size of the cell expressed in percentage or g/dL

mean cell volume (MCV) / mean corpuscular volume; average red blood cell volume; in a blood sample, expressed in femtoliters (fL) or cubic microns (μ^3)

median cubital vein / a superficial vein located in the bend of the elbow (cubital fossa) that connects the cephalic vein to the basilic vein

medical laboratory technician (MLT) / clinical laboratory technician

medical technologist (MT) / clinical laboratory scientist

medical technology / clinical laboratory science

medium / a substance used to provide nutrients for growing microorganisms

medulla / the inner or central portion of an organ

megakaryocyte / a large bone marrow cell from which platelets are derived

melanin / a dark pigment of skin, hair, and certain tumors

meniscus / the curved upper surface of a liquid in a container

meter (M) / basic metric unit of length or distance

methylene blue / a blue stain or dye

metric system / the decimal system of measurement used internationally for scientific work

MIC / see minimum inhibitory concentration

micro / prefix used to indicate one-millionth (10^{-6}) of a unit

microalbumin / small amount of albumin in urine, not detectable by routine reagent strip

microalbuminuria / condition in which small amounts of albumin are present in the urine

microbiology / the branch of biology dealing with microbes

microcytic / having a smaller-than-normal cell size

microfilaria (pl. microfilariae) / immature form of a filarial worm

microfuge / a centrifuge that spins microcentrifuge tubes at high rates of speed; microcentrifuge

microhematocrit / a hematocrit performed in capillary tubes using a small quantity of blood; packed cell volume (PCV)

microhematocrit centrifuge / an instrument that spins capillary tubes at a high speed to rapidly separate cellular components of the blood from the liquid portion of the blood

micrometer / a ruled device for measuring small objects

microorganism / a single-celled microscopic organism

micropipet / a pipet that measures or holds one mL or less

micropipetter / a mechanical pipetter that can measure or deliver very small volumes, usually less than 1.0 mL

microscope arm / the portion of the microscope that connects the lenses to the base

microscope base / the portion of the microscope that rests on the table and supports the microscope

midstream urine / a urine sample collected from the mid-portion of a urine stream

milli / prefix used to indicate one-thousandth (10^{-3}) of a unit

minimum inhibitory concentration (MIC) / the minimum concentration of an antibiotic required to inhibit the growth of a microorganism

molar solution (M) / solution containing one mole of solute per liter of solution

mole / formula weight of a substance expressed in grams

molecular weight (M.W.) / sum of atomic weights of the formula unit; formula weight

monochromator / a device that isolates a narrow portion of the light spectrum

monoclonal antibody / antibody derived from a single cell line or clone

monocular / having one ocular or eyepiece

monocyte / a large leukocyte usually having a convoluted or horseshoe-shaped nucleus

mordant / a substance that fixes a dye or stain to an object

morphology / the form and structure of cells, tissues, and organs

mutagen / a substance with the potential to make a stable change in a gene that then can be passed on to offspring

mycelium / a mass of hyphae that makes up the vegetative body of molds

Mycobacterium tuberculosis / an acid-fast bacillus that causes tuberculosis

mycology / the study of fungi

mycoplasma / the smallest free-living group of bacteria (Class Mollicutes) that lack a cell wall and grow in the absence of oxygen; mollicutes

mycosis / infection caused by fungi

myocardial infarction (MI) / heart attack caused by obstruction of the blood supply to or within the heart

myoglobin / a pigmented, oxygen-carrying protein found in muscle tissue

N

NAACLS / see National Accrediting Agency for Clinical Laboratory Sciences

nano / prefix used to indicate one-billionth (10^{-9}) of a unit

National Accrediting Agency for Clinical Laboratory Sciences (NAACLS) / agency that accredits educational programs for clinical laboratory personnel

National Committee for Clinical Laboratory Standards (NCCLS) / see Clinical and Laboratory Standards Institute (CLSI)

National Credentialing Agency for Laboratory Personnel (NCA) / credentialing agency for clinical laboratory personnel

National Institute for Occupational Safety and Health (NIOSH) / federal agency responsible for workplace safety research and that makes recommendations for preventing work-related illness and injury

National Institute of Standards and Technology (NIST) / a federal agency that promotes international standardization of measurements; formerly the National Bureau of Standards

National Phlebotomy Association (NPA) / professional society and credentialing agency for phlebotomists

NCA / see National Credentialing Agency for Laboratory Personnel

NCCLS / see Clinical and Laboratory Standards Institute

nematode / roundworm; any unsegmented worm of the class Nematoda

nephron / the structural and functional unit of the kidney composed of a glomerulus and its associated renal tubule

nephrotoxic / toxic or destructive to kidney cells

neutrophil / a neutral-staining leukocyte, usually the first line of defense against infection

neutrophilia / abnormal increase in the number of neutrophils in the blood

nocturia / excessive urination at night

noncritical measurements / estimated measurements; measurements made in containers that estimate volume (such as beakers)

nongonococcal urethritis / a gonorrhea-like STD caused by organisms other than gonococci

nonpathogenic / not normally causing disease in a healthy individual

normal flora / microorganisms that are normally present at a specific site

normochromic / having normal color

normocytic / having a normal cell size

nosepiece / revolving unit to which microscope objectives are attached

nosocomial / hospital-acquired; acquired as a result of being hospitalized or institutionalized

nosocomial infection / an infection acquired in a hospital or health care facility

nucleated red blood cell / a red blood cell that has not yet lost its nucleus; NRBC

nucleus (pl. nuclei) / the central structure of a cell that contains DNA and controls cell growth and function

O

objective / magnifying lens closest to the object being viewed with a microscope

occult / concealed or hidden

Occupational Safety and Health Act (OSH Act) / Congressional act of 1970 created to help reduce on-the-job illnesses, injuries, and deaths, and requiring employers to provide safe working conditions

Occupational Safety and Health Administration (OSHA) / the federal agency that creates workplace safety regulations and that enforces the Occupational Safety and Health Act of 1970

ocular / eyepiece of the microscope that contains a magnifying lens

ocular micrometer / micrometer that fits in microscope eyepiece and that is used to measure microscopic objects

oliguria / decreased production of urine

opalescent / having a milky iridescence

opportunistic parasite / an organism that causes disease only in immunocompromised hosts

opportunistic pathogen / a microorganism that causes disease in the host only when normal defense mechanisms are impaired or absent

oral glucose tolerance test (OGTT) / analysis of blood glucose at timed intervals following ingestion of a standard glucose dose

OSHA / Occupational Safety and Health Administration; the federal agency that monitors the Occupational Safety and Health Act of 1971

other potentially infectious materials (OPIM) / any and all body fluids, tissues, organs, or other specimens from a human source

ova / eggs

oxidase test / an enzyme test used to identify certain bacteria, such as *Neisseria*

oxyhemoglobin / the form of hemoglobin that binds and transports oxygen

P

packed cell column / the layers of blood cells that form when a tube of whole blood is centrifuged

palpate / to examine by touch

pandemic / widespread disease transmitted person-to-person and occurring over an entire country, continent, or even worldwide

parasite / an organism that lives in or on another species and at the expense of that species

parasitemia / parasites in the blood

parasitology / the study of parasites

parenteral / any route other than by alimentary canal; intravenous, subcutaneous, intramuscular, or mucosal

parfocal / having objectives that can be interchanged without varying the instrument's focus

paroxysm(s) / the cycles of chills and fever associated with malaria and that occur from 36 to 72 hours apart, depending on the *Plasmodium* species

partial thromboplastin / the lipid portion of thromboplastin, available as a commercial preparation; formerly cephaloplastin

pathogen / an organism or agent capable of causing disease in a host

pathogenic / capable of causing damage or injury to the host

pathologist / a physician specially trained in the nature and cause of disease

percent solution / a solution made by adding units of solute needed per 100 units of solution

percent transmittance (%T) / the percentage of light that passes through a solution

pericardial fluid / fluid within the pericardial cavity

peritoneum / a membrane lining the abdominal cavity and containing a fluid which keeps abdominal organs from adhering to abdominal wall; parietal peritoneum

peroxidase / the enzyme that converts hydrogen peroxide to water and oxygen

personal protective equipment (PPE) / specialized clothing or equipment used by workers to protect from direct exposure to blood or other potentially infectious or hazardous materials; includes, but is not limited to, gloves, laboratory apparel, eye protection, and breathing apparatus

petechiae / small, purplish hemorrhagic spots on the skin

petri dish / a shallow, covered dish made of plastic or glass

pH / a measurement of the hydrogen ion concentration expressing the degree of acidity or alkalinity of a solution

phagocytosis / the ingestion of a foreign particle or cell by another cell

pharyngeal / having to do with the back of the throat or pharynx

phenotype / in blood banking, the blood type determined by blood typing tests

phlebotomist / a health care worker trained in blood collection; venipuncturist

phlebotomy / venipuncture; entry of a vein with a needle

Physician Office Laboratory (POL) / small medical laboratory located within a physician office, group practice, or clinic

physiological saline / 0.85% (0.15M) sodium chloride solution

pico / prefix used to indicate 10^{-12}

picogram (pg) / micromicrogram; 1×10^{-12} gram

pinworm / *Enterobius vermicularis,* a small parasitic nematode; also called seatworm

pipet / a slender tube used in the laboratory for measuring and transferring liquids

plasma / the liquid portion of blood in which blood cells are suspended; the straw-colored liquid remaining after blood cells are removed from anticoagulated blood

plasma cell / a differentiated B lymphocyte that produces antibodies

plasmin / an enzyme that binds to fibrin and initiates breakdown of the fibrin clot (fibrinolysis)

plasminogen / the inactive precursor of plasmin

Plasmodium / the protozoan genus that includes the organisms causing human malaria

platelet / a formed element in circulating blood that plays an important role in blood coagulation; a small disk-shaped fragment of cytoplasm derived from a megakaryocyte; a thrombocyte

pleomorphic / having varied shapes

pleural fluid / the fluid in the space between the pleural membrane of the lung and the inner chest wall

POCT / see point-of-care test(ing)

poikilocytosis / significant variation in the shape of erythrocytes

point-of-care testing (POCT) / testing outside the traditional laboratory setting; also called bedside testing, off-site testing, or alternate-site testing

POL / see physician office laboratory

polychromatic / having many colors

polyclonal antibodies / antibodies derived from more than one cell line

polycythemia / an excess of red blood cells in the peripheral blood

polyethylene / plastic polymer of ethylene used for containers

polypropylene / lightweight plastic polymer of propylene that resists moisture and solvents and is heat-sterilizable

polystyrene / clear, colorless polymer of styrene used for labware

polyuria / excessive production of urine

population / the entire group of items or individuals from which the samples under consideration are presumed to have come

porphyrins / a group of light-sensitive, pigmented, ringed chemical structures that are required for the synthesis of hemoglobin

postprandial / after eating

precipitation / formation of an insoluble antigen-antibody complex

precision / reproducibility of results; the closeness of obtained values to each other

prefix / modifying word or syllable(s) placed at the beginning of a word

primary lymphoid organs / organs in which B and T lymphocytes acquire their special characteristics; in humans, the bone marrow and thymus

primary medium / a medium that provides nutritional requirements for an organism and is used to recover the organism from infectious material

proficiency testing (PT) / a program in which a laboratory's accuracy in performing analyses is evaluated at regular intervals and compared to the performance of similar laboratories

progeny / offspring or descendants

proglottid (pl. proglottids) / the tapeworm body segment that contains the male and female reproductive organs

proportion / relationship in number or amount of one portion compared to another portion or to the whole; ratio

protective isolation / an isolation category designed to protect highly susceptible patients from exposure to infectious agents; reverse isolation

proteinuria / protein in the urine, usually albumin

prothrombin / the precursor of thrombin; factor II

prothrombin time (PT) / a coagulation screening test used to monitor oral anticoagulant therapy

protozoa / unicellular eukaryotic organisms, both free-living and parasitic

Provider Performed Microscopy Procedures (PPMP) / a Certificate category under CLIA '88

proximal convoluted tubule / the portion of a renal tubule that collects the filtrate from Bowman's capsule

pulmonary embolism / occlusion of a pulmonary artery or one of its branches, usually produced by an embolus that originated in a deep vein of the leg or pelvis

PVA / polyvinyl alcohol, a preservative used for fecal specimens

pyelitis / inflammation of the renal pelvis

pyelonephritis / inflammation of the kidney and the renal pelvis

Q

quadrant / one-fourth of a circle; one-fourth of an agar plate

quality assessment (QA) / in the laboratory, a program that monitors the total testing process with the aim of providing the highest quality patient care; a synonym for "quality assurance"

quality assurance (QA) / see quality assessment

quality control (QC) / a system that verifies the reliability of analytical test results through the use of standards, controls, and statistical analysis

quality systems (QS) / in an institution, a comprehensive program in which all areas of operation are monitored to ensure quality with the aim of providing the highest quality patient care

quartz glass / expensive glass with excellent light transmission; glass used for cuvettes; silica glass

R

radioimmunoassay (RIA) / an assay using a test component labeled with a radioisotope

radioisotope / an unstable form of an element that emits radiation and can be incorporated into diagnostic tests, medical therapies, and biomedical research; radioactive isotope

random error / error whose source cannot be definitely identified

random urine specimen / a urine specimen collected at any time, without regard to diet or time of day

ratio / relationship in number or degree between two things

reactive lymphocyte / see atypical lymphocyte

reagent / substance or solution used in laboratory analyses; substance involved in a chemical reaction

reciprocal / inverse; one of a pair of numbers (as 2/3 and 3/2) that has a product of one

red blood cell (RBC) / blood cell that transports oxygen (O_2) to the tissues and carbon dioxide (CO_2) to the lungs; erythrocyte

red blood cell indices / calculated values that compare the size and hemoglobin content of RBCs in a blood sample to reference values; erythrocyte indices

reference laboratory / an independent regional laboratory that offers routine and specialized testing services to hospitals and physicians

reflectance photometer / an instrument that measures the light reflected from a colored reaction product

refractometer / an instrument for measuring the refractive index of a substance

renal hilus / the concavity in the kidneys where nerves and vessels enter or exit

renal pelvis / the funnel-shaped expansion of the upper portion of the ureter that receives urine from the renal tubules

renal threshold / the blood concentration above which a substance not normally excreted by the kidneys appears in the urine

renal tubule / a small tube of the nephron that collects and concentrates urine

reservoir host / the host, other than the usual host, in which the parasite lives and is infectious

resolving power / the ability of a microscope to produce a separate image of two closely-spaced objects; resolution

reticulocyte / an immature erythrocyte that has retained RNA in the cytoplasm

reticulocytopenia / a decrease below the normal number of reticulocytes in the circulating blood

reticulocytosis / an increase above the normal number of reticulocytes in the circulating blood

reticulum / a network

reverse grouping / the use of known cells (antigens) to identify unknown antibodies in the patient's serum or plasma

reverse osmosis / purification of water by forcing water through a semi-permeable membrane

Rh (D) immune globulin (RhIG) / a concentrated, purified solution of human anti-D antibody used for injection; RhoGam

rheumatoid arthritis (RA) / an autoimmune disease characterized by pain, inflammation, and deformity of the joints

rheumatoid factors (RF) / autoantibodies that are directed against human IgG and are often present in the serum of rheumatoid arthritis patients

RNA / the nucleic acid that is important in protein synthesis and that is found in all living cells; ribonucleic acid

rotor / the part of a centrifuge that holds the tubes and rotates during the operation of the centrifuge

rouleau(x) / group(s) of red blood cells arranged like a roll of coins

S

sample / in statistics, a subgroup of a population

SARS / the acronym for severe acute respiratory syndrome, a condition caused by a coronavirus

schizocyte / a fragmented red blood cell; formerly schistocyte

secondary lymphoid tissue / tissues in which lymphocytes are concentrated, such as the spleen, lymph nodes, and tonsils

sediment / solids that settle to the bottom of a liquid

sedimentation / the process of solid particles settling to the bottom of a liquid

selective medium / a bacteriological medium that allows growth of some organisms while inhibiting the growth of others

seroconversion / the appearance of antibody in the serum of an individual following exposure to an antigen

serological centrifuge / a centrifuge that spins small tubes such as those used in blood banking; serofuge

serology / the study of antigens and antibodies in serum using immunological methods; laboratory testing based on the immunological properties of serum

serum / the liquid obtained from blood that has been allowed to clot

shift / an abrupt change from the established mean indicated by the occurrence of all control values on one side of the mean

shift to the left / the appearance of an increased number of immature neutrophil forms in the peripheral blood

SI units / standardized units of measure; international units

sickle cell / crescent- or sickle-shaped red cell; drepanocyte

sickle cell anemia / inherited blood disorder in which RBCs can form a sickle shape due to the presence of Hemoglobin S

solid-phase chemistry / an analytical method in which the sample is added to a strip or slide containing, in dried form, all the reagents for the procedure

solute / the substance dissolved in a given solution

solution / a homogeneous mixture of two or more substances

solvent / a dissolving agent, usually a liquid

specific gravity / the ratio of the weight of a solution to the weight of an equal volume of distilled water; a measurement of density

spectrophotometer / an instrument that measures intensities of light in different parts of the light spectrum

spiral bacteria / motile bacteria having a helical or spiral shape

spirochetes / motile, helical or spiral bacteria of the family Spirochaeta

stage / platform that holds the object to be viewed microscopically

standard / a chemical solution of a known concentration that can be used as a reference or calibration substance

standard deviation / a measure of the spread of a population of values around the mean

Standard Precautions / a set of comprehensive safety guidelines designed to protect patients and healthcare workers by requiring that all patients and all body fluids, body substances, organs, and unfixed tissues be regarded as potentially infectious

statistics / the branch of mathematics that deals with the collection, classification, analysis, and interpretation of numerical data; a collection of quantitative data

STD / sexually transmitted disease

stem / main part of a word; root word; the part of a word remaining after removing the prefix or suffix

stem cell / an undifferentiated cell

sterilization / the act of eliminating all living microorganisms from an article or area

stomatocyte / red blood cell with an elongated, mouth-shaped central area of pallor

suffix / modifying word or syllable(s) placed at the end of a word

supernatant / the clear liquid remaining at the top of a solution after centrifugation or settling out of solid substances; the liquid lying above a sediment

supravital stain / a dye that stains living cells or tissues

synovial / of or relating to the lubricating fluid of the joints

synovial fluid / viscous fluid secreted by membranes lining the joints

syphilis / an infectious, chronic, sexually transmitted disease caused by a spirochete, *Treponema pallidum*

syringe / a hollow, tube-like container with a plunger, used for injecting or withdrawing fluids

systematic error / a variation that can influence results to be consistently higher or lower than the real value

systemic circulation / the system of blood vessels that carries blood from the heart to the tissues and back to the heart

T

T lymphocyte (T cell) / the type of lymphocyte responsible for the cell-mediated immune response

target cell / abnormal red blood cell with "target" appearance; codocyte

TC / on pipets, a mark indicating to contain

TD / on pipets, a mark indicating to deliver

teratogenic / relating to a substance capable of causing birth defects or interfering with normal fetal development

terminology / terms used in any specialized field

thalassemia / an inherited condition in which abnormal hemoglobin is produced, resulting in anemia

thrombin / a protein formed from prothrombin by the action of thromboplastin and other factors in the presence of calcium ions; factor II$_a$

thrombocyte / a blood platelet

thrombocytopenia / abnormal decrease in the number of platelets in the blood

thrombocytosis / abnormal increase in the number of platelets in the blood

thromboplastin / a lipoprotein found in endothelium and other tissue; coagulation factor III, also called tissue factor

thrombus (pl. thrombi) / a blood clot that obstructs a blood vessel

thymus / a gland, located near the thyroid, that is a primary lymphoid tissue

thyroid stimulating hormone (TSH) / a hormone synthesized by the anterior pituitary gland and that regulates the activity of the thyroid gland; thyrotropin

thyroxine / a thyroid hormone, commonly called T$_4$

titer / in serology, the reciprocal of the highest dilution that gives the desired reaction; the concentration of a substance determined by titration

tourniquet / a band used to constrict blood flow

Transmission Based Precautions / specific safety practices used in addition to Standard Precautions when treating patients known to be or suspected of being infected with pathogens that can be spread by air, droplet, or contact

transplant / living tissue placed into the body; the placing of living tissue into the body

transport medium / a medium that provides the proper environment for organisms during transport

trematode / fluke; any parasitic flatworm of the class Trematoda

trend / an indication of error in the analysis, detected by increasing or decreasing values in the control sample

trichomoniasis / a sexually transmitted genitourinary infection caused by the parasitic protozoan, *Trichomonas vaginalis*

trichrome stain / a stain commonly used to identify parasites in fecal smears

triglycerides / the major storage form of lipids; lipid molecules formed from glycerol and fatty acids

triiodothyronine / one of the thyroid hormones, commonly called T$_3$

trophoblastic / relating to embryonic nutritive tissue

trophozoite / the motile, feeding stage of protozoan parasites

tubular necrosis / death of the tissue comprising the renal tubules

turbid / having a cloudy appearance

U

Universal Precautions / a method of infection control in which all human blood and other body fluids containing visible blood are treated as if infectious

ureter / the tube carrying urine from the kidney to the urinary bladder

urethra / the canal through which urine is discharged from the urinary bladder

urethritis / infection or inflammation of the urethra

uric acid / breakdown product of nucleic acids

urinary bladder / an organ for the temporary storage of urine

urine / excretory fluid produced by the kidneys

urinometer / a float with a calibrated stem used for measuring specific gravity of urine; hydrometer

urobilinogen / a breakdown product of bilirubin formed by the action of intestinal bacteria

urochrome / the yellow pigment that gives urine its color

UTI / urinary tract infection

V

vacuole / a membrane-bound compartment in cell cytoplasm

vaginitis / infection or inflammation of the vagina

variance / the square of the standard deviation; mean square deviation

vasoconstriction / a narrowing of the diameter of a blood vessel

vector / an agent that transports a pathogen from an infected host to a noninfected host

vein / a blood vessel that carries deoxygenated blood from the tissues to the heart

venereal / having to do with, or transmitted by, sexual contact

venipuncture / entry of a vein with a needle; a phlebotomy

virion / the infectious form of a virus

virology / the study of viruses

virulent / highly infectious

vitamin B$_{12}$ / a vitamin essential to the proper maturation of blood cells and other cells in the body

vitamin K / a vitamin essential for production of coagulation factors II, VII, IX, and X

VLDL cholesterol / very low density lipoprotein fraction of blood cholesterol

W

Westergren tube / a slender pipet marked from 0-200 mm used in the Westergren erythrocyte sedimentation rate method

Westgard's rules / a set of rules used to determine when a method is out of control

white blood cells (WBC) / blood cells that function in immunity; leukocytes

Wintrobe tube / a slender thick-walled tube, used in the Wintrobe erythrocyte sedimentation rate

work practice controls / methods of performing tasks that reduce the worker's exposure to blood and other potentially hazardous materials

working distance / distance between the microscope objective and the microscope slide when the object is in sharp focus

Wright's stain / a combination of eosin and methylene blue in methanol; a polychromatic stain

X

XDP / fibrin-degradation products that contain the D-dimer cross-linked region

Y

yeast / a small single-celled eukaryotic fungus that reproduces by fission or budding

Z

zone of inhibition / in the antibiotic susceptibility test, the area around an antibiotic disk that contains no bacterial growth

zoonotic / infection or disease that can be transmitted from vertebrate animals to humans

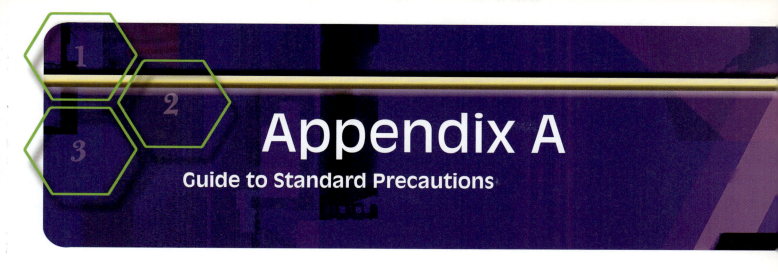

Appendix A
Guide to Standard Precautions

Wash Hands. Wash hands **before putting on gloves** and **immediately after removing them,** using antiseptic soap, foam, or gel. Follow the manufacturer's instructions for the amount of antiseptic to use and the length of time the product should remain on the skin to be effective against infectious agents. Hands must be washed after patient contact, before going to another patient. In addition, hands must be washed anytime there is inadvertent contact with blood or OPIM.

Wear Gloves. Wear gloves anytime there is potential exposure to blood or OPIM. Change gloves between tasks and between patients to avoid the possible transfer of infectious agents. Wash hands with antiseptic before putting on gloves and immediately after removing them. Immediately remove torn or punctured gloves, wash hands with antiseptic, and put on a clean pair.

Wear Mask and Eye Protection or Face Shield. Protect mucous membranes of the eyes, nose, and mouth during laboratory procedures and patient-contact activities that are likely to generate **splashes** or **sprays of blood, body fluids, secretions,** or **excretions.**

Wear Fluid-Resistant Laboratory Coat. Protect skin and clothing from chemicals, stains, and biocontamination by wearing a fluid-resistant laboratory coat when performing laboratory procedures. Never wear or take a laboratory coat home or wear it outside of the healthcare facility.

Wear Gown. Wear gown in appropriate transmission-based precautions conditions to protect skin and prevent contamination of clothing during patient procedures that are likely to generate **splashes** or **sprays of blood, body fluids, secretions,** or **excretions.** Remove soiled gown promptly, discard appropriately, and wash hands with antiseptic. Do not wear gown out of immediate work area.

Bloodborne Pathogens. Prevent needlestick injuries by using safety needles and needle safety devices. Discard all such devices in a sharps container immediately after use. Lancets must be discarded into a sharps container. Sharps containers should be located as near to the point of use as possible.

Never Recap Used Needles Do not remove used needles from disposable syringes, and do not bend, break, or otherwise manipulate used needles. Place used disposable syringes and needles, scalpel blades, and other sharp items in sharps containers immediately after use.

Use Resuscitation Devices as an alternative to mouth-to-mouth resuscitation.

Patient-Care Equipment. Handle used patient-care equipment soiled with **blood, body fluids, secretions,** or **excretions** in a manner that prevents skin and mucous membrane exposures, contamination of clothing, and transfer of infectious agents to other patients or the environment. Be sure that single-use items are used for only one patient and then properly discarded. Ensure that reusable equipment is not used for the care of another patent until it has been appropriately decontaminated and reprocessed.

Environmental Control. Follow hospital procedures for routine care, cleaning, and disinfection of environmental surfaces, beds, bedrails, bedside equipment and other frequently-touched surfaces.

Linen. Handle, transport, and process used linen soiled with **blood, body fluids, secretions,** or **excretions** in a manner that prevents exposure and contamination of clothing, and avoids transfer of infectious agents to patients and environments.

Patient Rooms. Always read and follow all infection control or transmission-based precautions posted outside a patient's room. Ask at the nearest nurses' station if the instructions are unclear or if you have questions concerning appropriate personal protective equipment or work practices.

Appendix B
Laboratory Reference Values

HEMATOLOGY AND COAGULATION

TEST	REFERENCE RANGE	SI
Hemoglobin:		
Newborn	16–23 g/dL	160–230 g/L
Children	10–14 g/dL	100–140 g/L
Adult males	13–17 g/dL	130–170 g/L
Adult females	12–15 g/dL	120–150 g/L
Microhematocrit:		
Newborn	51–61%	.51–.61
One year	32–38%	.32–.38
Six years	34–42%	.34–.42
Adult males	42–52%	.42–.52
Adult females	36–48%	.36–.48
Reticulocyte Percentages:		
Newborn	2.5–6.5%	
Adult	0.5–1.5%	
Erythrocyte Sedimentation Rate (ESR)		
Wintrobe method (one-hour)		
Adult males	0–9 mm	
Adult females	0–20 mm	
One hour Sediplast ESR		
Males	< 50 years	0–15 mm
	> 50 years	0–20 mm
Females	< 50 years	0–20 mm
	> 50 years	0–30 mm
ZSR (all ages)		
Normal	40–51%	
Borderline	51–54%	
Elevated	≥55%	

TEST	REFERENCE RANGE
ACT (Hemochron Jr.)	89–153 sec
Prothrombin Time	10–13 sec
Activated Partial Thromboplastin Time	31–39 sec
Bleeding Time:	
Ivy method	2–9 min
Duke method	1–3 min
White Blood Cell Counts:	
Newborn	$9.0–30.0 \times 10^9$/L
One year	$6.0–14.0 \times 10^9$/L
Six years	$4.5–12.0 \times 10^9$/L
Adult	$4.5–11.0 \times 10^9$/L
Red Blood Cell Counts:	
Adult males	$4.5–6.0 \times 10^{12}$/L
Adult females	$4.0–5.5 \times 10^{12}$/L
Red Blood Cell Indices:	
Mean Corpuscular Volume (MCV)	86–98 fL
Mean Corpuscular Hemoglobin (MCH)	27–32 pg
Mean Corpuscular Hemoglobin Concentration (MCHC)	32–37%
Platelet Count	$1.5–4.0 \times 10^{11}$/L

White Cell Differential Count:

Leukocyte	one month	six-year-old	twelve-year-old	adult	Absolute Counts (cells/μL) adult
Neutrophil (seg)	15–35%	45–50%	45–50%	50–65%	2250–7150
Neutrophil (band)	7–13%	0–7%	6–8%	0–7%	0–770
Eosinophil	1–3%	1–3%	1–3%	1–3%	45–330
Basophil	0–1%	0–1%	0–1%	0–1%	0–110
Monocyte	5–8%	4–8%	3–8%	3–9%	135–990
Lymphocyte	40–70%	40–45%	35–40%	25–40%	1125–4400
Platelets	An average of 7–20 platelets per oil immersion field is considered normal				

URINE REFERENCE VALUES

Urine Volume

AGE	REFERENCE RANGE (mL/24 HOURS)
Newborn	20–350
One year	300–600
Ten years	750–1500
Adult	750–2000

Components of Urine Sediment

	REFERENCE VALUES
RBC/HPF	0–4
WBC/HPF	0–4
Epith/HPF	occasional (may be higher in females)
Casts/LPF	occasional hyaline
Bacteria	negative
Mucus	negative to 2+
Crystals	only crystals such as cystine, leucine, tyrosine, and cholesterol are considered clinically significant

Physical and Chemical Characteristics of Urine

	REFERENCE VALUES
Color	pale yellow to amber
Transparency	clear
Specific gravity	1.005–1.030
pH	4.5–8.0
Protein	negative to trace
Glucose	negative
Ketone	negative
Bilirubin	negative
Blood	negative
Urobilinogen	0.1–1.0 mg/dL
Bacteria (nitrite)	negative
Leukocyte esterase	negative

CLINICAL CHEMISTRY REFERENCE VALUES

SUBSTANCE MEASURED	REFERENCE RANGES	
	CONVENTIONAL UNITS	SI UNITS
Alanine aminotransferase (ALT)	3–30 U/L	3–30 U/L
Albumin	3.8–5.0 g/dL	38–50 g/L
Alkaline phosphatase (AP)	20–130 U/L	20–130 U/L
Aspartate aminotransferase (AST)	10–37 U/L	10–37 U/L
Bicarbonate (HCO_3^-)	22–28 mEq/L	22–28 mmol/L
Bilirubin (Total)	0.1–1.2 mg/dL	2–21 μmol/L
Bilirubin, Direct	0–0.3 mg/dL	0–6 μmol/L
BUN	8–18 mg/dL	2.9–6.4 mmol/L
Calcium	8.7–10.5 mg/dL	2.18–2.63 mmol/L
Chloride	98–108 mEq/L	98–108 mmol/L
Cholesterol, Total	140–250 mg/dL (desirable level <200 mg/dL)	3.64–6.50 mmol/L
Creatine kinase (CK)	30–170 U/L	30–170 U/L
Creatinine	0.7–1.4 mg/dL	62–125 μmol/L
Gamma glutamyl transferase (GGT)	3–40 U/L	3–40 U/L
Glucose	70–110 mg/dL	3.9–6.2 mmol/L
Iron	65–165 μg/dL	11.6–29.5 μmol/L
Lactate dehydrogenase (LD)	110–230 U/L	110–230 U/L
Phosphorus	3.0–4.5 mg/dL	0.96–1.44 mmol/L
Potassium	3.5–5.4 mEq/L	3.5–5.4 mmol/L
Sodium	135–148 mEq/L	135–148 mmol/L
TSH	0.35–5.0 μIU/mL	0.35–5.0 mIU/L
Total Protein	6.0–8.0 g/dL	60–80 g/L
Triglycerides	10–190 mg/dL	0.11–2.15 mmol/L
Uric Acid	3.5–7.5 mg/dL	0.21–0.44 mmol/L

Appendix C
Abbreviations and Acronyms Commonly Used in Medical Laboratories

A	absorbance
Ab	antibody
ACT	activated clotting time
AFB	acid-fast bacillus
Ag	antigen
AHG	anti-human globulin
AIDS	acquired immunodeficiency syndrome
ALL	acute lymphocytic leukemia
ALP, AP	alkaline phosphatase
ALT	alanine aminotransferase (formerly SGPT)
AML	acute myelogenous leukemia
ANA	anti-nuclear antibody
APTT	activated partial thromboplastin time
ARC	AIDS-related complex
AST	aspartate aminotransferase (formerly SGOT)
BA	blood agar
bacti	bacteriology
BBP	bloodborne pathogen
BP	blood pressure
BSI	body substance isolation
BT	bleeding time
BUN	blood urea nitrogen
C	Celsius, centigrade
CBC	complete blood count
cc, ccm	cubic centimeter
CCU	coronary care unit
CDC	Centers for Disease Control and Prevention
CFU	colony forming unit
CGL	chronic granulocytic leukemia
chol	cholesterol
CK	creatine kinase
Cl	chloride
CLA	clinical laboratory assistant
CLL	chronic lymphocytic leukemia
CLS	clinical laboratory scientist

CLT	clinical laboratory technician
cm	centimeter
CNS	central nervous system
CO	carbon monoxide
CO_2	carbon dioxide
CPD	citrate-phosphate-dextrose
CPK	creatine phosphokinase
crit	hematocrit
C & S	culture and sensitivity
CSF	cerebrospinal fluid, colony stimulating factor
cu mm	cubic millimeter, mm^3
DAT	direct antiglobulin test
DIC	disseminated intravascular coagulation
diff	leukocyte (white blood cell) differential
EBV	Epstein-Barr virus
EDTA	ethylenediaminetetraacetic acid
EIA	enzyme immunoassay
EMB	eosin-methylene blue
ESR	erythrocyte sedimentation rate
EU	Ehrlich units
F	Fahrenheit
FBS	fasting blood sugar
FDP	fibrinogen degradation products
FUO	fever of unknown origin
g, gm	gram
GGT	gamma glutamyl transferase
GI	gastrointestinal
GTT	glucose tolerance test
GU	genitourinary
HAV	hepatitis A virus
Hb, Hgb	hemoglobin
HBV	hepatitis B virus
hCG	human chorionic gonadotropin
HCl	hydrochloric acid
HCO_3^-	bicarbonate

Hct	hematocrit	nm	nanometer
HCV	hepatitis C virus	O.D.	optical density
HDL chol	high density lipoprotein cholesterol	OGTT	oral glucose tolerance test
HDN	hemolytic disease of newborn	O & P	ova and parasites
H & H	hemoglobin and hematocrit	OPIM	other potentially infectious material
HIV	human immunodeficiency virus	OSHA	Occupational Safety and Health Administration
HLA	human leukocyte antigen		
H_2O	water	PCV	packed cell volume
HPF	high power field	pH	hydrogen ion concentration
HSV	herpes simplex virus	PMN	polymorphonuclear neutrophil
ICU	intensive care unit	POCT	point-of-care testing
Ig	immunoglobulin	POL	physician office laboratory
IgG	immunoglobulin G	PP	postprandial
IgM	immunoglobulin M	PPE	personal protective equipment
IM	infectious mononucleosis	ppm	parts per million
i.m.	intramuscular	PRC	packed red cells
ITP	idiopathic thrombocytopenic purpura	PSA	prostate specific antigen
IU	international unit	PT	prothrombin time, pro-time
IV, i.v.	intravenous	QA	quality assessment
K	potassium	QC	quality control
kg	kilogram	qns	quantity not sufficient
L	liter	qs	quantity sufficient
LD, LDH	lactate dehydrogenase	RA	rheumatoid arthritis
LDL chol	low density lipoprotein cholesterol	RBC	red blood cell
LPF	low power field	RF	rheumatoid factors
m	meter	RhIG	Rh immune globulin
M	molar	RIA	radioimmunoassay
MCH	mean cell hemoglobin	RNA	ribonucleic acid
MCHC	mean cell hemoglobin concentration	RPR	rapid plasma reagin
MCV	mean cell volume	sed rate	erythrocyte sedimentation rate
μg	microgram	SEM	scanning electron microscope
μL, μl	microliter	SGOT	serum glutamic oxaloacetic transaminase
μmol	micromole	SGPT	serum glutamic-pyruvic transaminase
mEq	milliequivalent	SI	international units (Le Systéme International d'Unités)
mg	milligram		
MI	myocardial infarction	SICU	surgical intensive care unit
mIU	Milli International Unit	SP	Standard Precautions
mL, ml	milliliter	sp.gr.	specific gravity
MLT	medical laboratory technician	staph	*Staphylococcus*
mm	millimeter	stat	immediately
mmol	millimole	STD	sexually transmitted disease
mol	mole	STI	sexually transmitted infection
MRI	magnetic resonance imaging	strep	*Streptococcus*
MRSA	methicillin-resistant *Staphylcoccus aureus*	STS	serological tests for syphilis
MSDS	material safety data sheet	TEM	transmission electron microscope
MT	medical technologist	TIA	transient ischemic attack
N	normal, normality	TIBC	total iron binding capacity
Na	sodium	UA	urinalysis, uric acid
NaCl	sodium chloride	UP	Universal Precautions

URI	upper respiratory infection
UTI	urinary tract infection
UV	ultraviolet
VD	venereal disease
VDRL	Venereal Disease Research Laboratory

VLDL	very low density lipoproteins
vWF	von Willebrand factor
WBC	white blood cell
XDP	fibrin degradation products

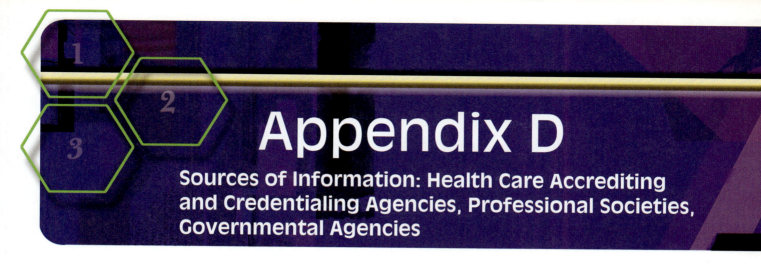

Appendix D

Sources of Information: Health Care Accrediting and Credentialing Agencies, Professional Societies, Governmental Agencies

Accrediting Agencies

American Association of Blood Banks (AABB)
8101 Glenbrook Road
Bethesda, MD 20814-2749
301.907.6977
www.aabb.org

College of American Pathologists, Laboratory Accreditation Program
325 Waukegan Road
Northfield, IL 60093-2750
800.323.4040
www.cap.org

Commission on Accreditation of Allied Health Education Programs (CAAHEP)
35 E. Wacker Dr., Suite 1970
Chicago, IL 60606-2208
312.553.9355
e-mail: caahep@caahep.org
www.caahep.org

Commission on Office Laboratory Accreditation (COLA)
9881 Broken Land Pkwy., Suite 200
Columbia, MD 21046–1158
410.381.6581
800.981.9883
e-mail: info@COLA.org
www.cola.org

Council for Higher Education Accreditation
One Dupont Circle NW, Suite 510
Washington, DC 20036-1135
202.955.6126
e-mail: chea@chea.org
www.chea.org

Joint Commission (formerly known as the Joint Commission on Accreditation of Healthcare Organizations [JCAHO])
One Renaissance Blvd.
Oakbrook Terrace, IL 60181
630.792.5000
www.jcaho.org

National Accrediting Agency for Clinical Laboratory Sciences (NAACLS)
8410 W. Bryn Mawr Ave., Suite 670
Chicago, IL 60631-3415
773.714.8880
e-mail: naaclsinfo@naacls.org
www.naacls.org

Credentialing Agencies, Professional Societies and Other Sources of Information

Advance for Medical Laboratory Professionals
2900 Horizon Drive, Box 61556
King of Prussia, PA 19406-0956
800.355.1088
www.advanceweb.com

American Association for Clinical Chemistry
2101 L. Street NW, Suite 202
Washington, DC 20037
800.892.1400 or 202.857.0717
www.aacc.org
Journal/Publications: *Clinical Laboratory News, Clinical Chemistry*

American Association of Bioanalysts (AAB)
Associate Member Section (formerly ISCLT)
917 Locust Street, Suite 1100
St. Louis, MO 63101-1413
314.241.1445
www.aab.org

American Association of Blood Banks (AABB)
8101 Glenbrook Road
Bethesda, MD 20814-2749
301.907.6977
www.aabb.org

American Association of Medical Assistants (AAMT)
20 N. Wacker Dr., Suite 1575
Chicago, IL 60606-2903
312.899.1500
www.aama-ntl.org
Journal: *PMA-The AAMA Journal*

American Medical Association
515 North State Street
Chicago, IL 60610
312.464.5000
www.ama-assn.org

American Medical Technologists (AMT)
710 Higgins Road
Park Ridge, IL 60058-5765
847.823.5169
www.amt1.com

American Society for Clinical Laboratory Science (ASCLS)
7910 Woodmont Avenue, Suite 530
Bethesda, MD 20814
301.657.2768
e-mail: ascls@ascls.org
www.ascls.org

Board of Registry, American Society for Clinical Pathology (ASCP)
P.O. Box 12277
Chicago, IL 60612-0277
312.738.1336
e-mail: info@ascp.org
www.ascp.org

American Society for Microbiology (ASM)
1325 Massachusetts Ave. NW
Washington, DC 20005-4171
202.942.9319
www.asmusa.org
Journals: *Journal of Clinical Microbiology, Clinical Microbiology Reviews, Clinical and Diagnostic Laboratory Immunology, Journal of Virology*

American Society of Hematology
1200 19th St. NW, #300
Washington, DC 20036
202.857.1118
www.hematology.org
Journal: *Blood*

American Society of Phlebotomy Technicians (ASPT)
1109 2nd Ave. S.W.
P.O. Box 1831
Hickory, NC 28602
704.322.1334
www.aspt.org

Association for Professionals in Infection Control and Epidemiology (APIC)
1275 K Street NW, Suite 1000
Washington, DC 20005-4006
202.789.1890
e-mail: APICinfo@apic.org
www.apic.org
Journal: *American Journal of Infection Control*

Association of Schools of Allied Health Professions
1730 M Street, Suite 500
Washington, DC 20036
202.293.4848
e-mail: asahp1@asahp.org
Journal: *Journal of Allied Health*

Centers for Disease Control and Prevention
1600 Clifton Road
Atlanta, GA 30333
404.639.3534
404.639.3311
800.311.3435
www.cdc.gov

Centers for Medicare and Medicaid Services (CMS)
7500 Security Blvd.
Baltimore, MD 21244
410.786.3000
www.cms.hhs.gov

Clinical Laboratory Management Association
989 Old Eagle Road, Suite 815
Wayne, PA 19087-1704
610.995.9580
www.clma.org
Journals: *Clinical Laboratory Management Review, Vantage Point*

Clinical and Laboratory Standards Institute (CLSI)
940 West Valley Road, Suite 1400
Wayne, PA 19087-1898
610.688.0100
www.clsi.org

Food and Drug Administration (FDA)
5600 Fishers Lane
Rockville, MD 20857
888.INFO.FDA
www.fda.gov

National Credentialing Agency for Laboratory Personnel (NCA)
P.O. Box 15945-289
Lenexa, KS 66285
913.438.5110
www.applmeapro.com/nca/

National Institute for Occupational Safety and Health (NIOSH)
200 Independence Ave. S.W., Room 715H
Washington, DC 20201
800.35NIOSH
www.cdc.gov/niosh

National Institutes of Health (NIH)
Bethesda, MD 20892
e-mail: NIHInfo@OD.NIH.GOV
www.nih.gov

National Technical Information Service (NTIS)
U.S. Dept. of Commerce
Springfield, VA 22161
703.605.6000
800.553.6847
www.ntis.gov

Occupational Safety and Health Administration (OSHA)
U. S. Dept. of Labor
Public Affairs Office, Room 3647
200 Constitution Ave. NW
Washington, DC 20210
202.693.1999
www.osha.gov

Superintendent of Documents
U. S. Government Printing Office
Washington, DC 20402
202.512.1800
FAX 202.512.2250
www.access.gpo.gov

Proficiency Testing

Several agencies as well as some state public health laboratories have DHHS approved proficiency testing programs. Contact individual state agencies or CMS for additional information. A listing of approved proficiency testing programs may be obtained through the CDC's Public Health Practice Program Office, Division of Laboratory Systems, www.phppo.cdc.gov/dls/

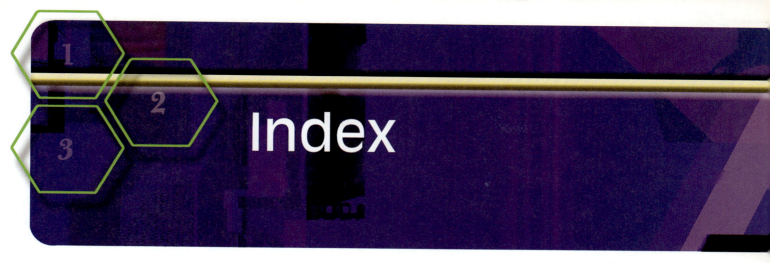

Index